Men's Health

Men's Health

Third Edition

Edited by

Roger S Kirby MA MD FRCS(Urol) FEBU
Director
The Prostate Centre
London
UK

Culley C Carson III MD
Division of Urology
University of North Carolina at Chapel Hill
Chapel Hill, NC
USA

Alan White PhD RN
Centre for Men's Health
Faculty of Health
Leeds Metropolitan University
Leeds
UK

and

Michael G Kirby
Visiting Professor
University of Hertfordshire and the Prostate Centre
London
UK

informa
healthcare

Informa Healthcare USA, Inc.
52 Vanderbilt Avenue
New York, NY 10017

© 2009 by Informa Healthcare USA, Inc.
Informa Healthcare is an Informa business

No claim to original U.S. Government works
Printed and bound in India by Replika Press Pvt. Ltd.
10 9 8 7 6 5 4 3 2 1

Library of Congress Cataloging-in-Publication Data
Men's health / edited by Roger S. Kirby ... [et al.]. – 3rd ed.
  p. ; cm.
  Includes bibliographical references and index.
  ISBN 978-0-415-44733-1 (hb : alk. paper)   1.   Men–Health and hygiene.   2.   Men–Medical
care.   3.   Men–Diseases.   I. Kirby, R. S. (Roger S.)
  [DNLM: 1. Men's Health.   WA 306 M548 2009]
  RC48.5.M462 2009
  613'.04234–dc22   2008047504

For Corporate Sales and Reprint Permissions call 212-520-2700 or write to: Sales Department, 52 Vanderbilt Avenue, 16th floor, New York, NY 10017.

Visit the Informa Web site at
www.informa.com

and the Informa Healthcare Web site at
www.informahealthcare.com

Composition by Exeter Premedia Services Pvt Ltd, Chennai, India

Dedicated to Professor Ken Kirby FRS

Contents

Contents

Contents

List of contributors

Richard A Anderson MD PhD FRCOG
Division of Reproductive and Developmental
Science
University of Edinburgh
Edinburgh, Scotland
UK

William R Anderson MB FRCS(Ed) FRCS(Glas)
Urology Research Fellow
Department of Urology
St Mary's Hospital
Portsmouth
UK

Ian Banks
Professor of Men's Health
Leeds Metropolitan University
Leeds
and President
European Men's Health Forum
London
UK

John A Bartlett
Kilimanjaro Christian Medical Centre
Moshi
Tanzania
and Division of Infectious Diseases
Department of Medicine
Duke University Medical Center
Durham, NC
USA

Simon E Barton BSc MD FRCP(Ed) FRCP
Consultant Physician GUM/HIV
Chelsea & Westminster NHS Foundation Trust
London
UK

D John Betteridge MD PhD
University College London
London
UK

Steven Boorman MBBS MRCGP FFOM FRCP
Director Corporate Responsibility
Chief Medical Adviser
Royal Mail Group
London
UK

Frances Bunn
Faculty of Health and Human Sciences
University of Hertfordshire
Hertfordshire
UK

Culley C Carson III MD
Division of Urology
University of North Carolina at Chapel Hill
Chapel Hill, NC
USA

Andrew L Clark
University of Hull
Castle Hill Hospital
Kingston-upon-Hull
UK

John GF Cleland
University of Hull
Castle Hill Hospital
Kingston-upon-Hull
UK

Alison P Coletta
Medical Writer
European Journal of Heart Failure
University of Hull
Castle Hill Hospital
Kingston-upon-Hull
UK

Katherine M Coyne BA MRCP
Specialist Registrar GUM/HIV
Chelsea & Westminster NHS Foundation Trust
London
UK

Keliegh S Culpepper MD
Harvard Dermatopathology Fellow
Department of Pathology
Brigham and Women's Hospital
Harvard Medical School
Boston, MA
USA

Melanie E Cunningham
Faculty of Health and Human Sciences
University of Hertfordshire
Hertfordshire
UK

Joseph Dall'Era MD
Division of Urology
School of Medicine
University of Colorado – Denver
Aurora, CO
USA

Sir Richard Doll DM Dsc FRCP FRS
Honorary Member, Clinical Trial Service Unit and
Epidemiological Studies Unit
Nuffield Department of Clinical Medicine
University of Oxford
Oxford
UK

Charlotte Foley BM BCh MA MRCS
Department of Urology
Barnet and Chase Farm Hospitals NHS Trust
Barnet General Hospital
Barnet
UK

Desmond Chia Chin Gan MBBS BMedSci
Department of Dermatology
St Vincent's Hospital
Melbourne
Australia

Allan Gaw MD PhD
Director, Clinical Trials Unit
Glasgow Royal Infirmary
Glasgow, Scotland
UK

Rod Griffiths CBE
Past President
Faculty of Public Health
London
UK

David Haslam MD
General Practitioner
Watton Place Clinic
Watton
Physician in Obesity Medicine
Centre for Obesity Research
Luton & Dunstable Hospital
Luton
and Clinical Director
National Obesity Forum
UK

Feng J He
Blood Pressure Unit
Cardiac and Vascular Sciences
St George's, University of London
London
UK

Paul K Hegarty
Department of Urology
University of Texas MD Anderson Cancer Center
Houston, TX
USA

Nick Hervey
South London and Maudsley Hospital
London
UK

Simon AV Holmes MB MS FRCS(Urol)
Consultant Urologist
St Mary's Hospital
Portsmouth
UK

J Slade Hubbard MD
Division of Urology
University of North Carolina at Chapel Hill
Chapel Hill, NC
USA

Robert Huddart
Institute of Cancer Research
and The Royal Marsden Hospital Trust
The Bob Champion Unit
Sutton
UK

Ben Hughes MBBS FRCS
Clinical Research Fellow in Urology
St George's Hospital
London
UK

Adam Humphries MBBS BSc MRCP
Department of Histopathology
London Research Institute, Cancer Research
and Department of Gastroenterology
St Mary's Hospital, Imperial College
Healthcare NHS Trust
London
UK

Simon Kimm MD
Urology Resident
Stanford University
Stanford, CA
USA

Michael G Kirby
Visiting Professor
University of Hertfordshire and the Prostate
Centre
London
UK

Roger S Kirby MA MD FRCS(Urol) FEBU
Director
The Prostate Centre
London
UK

Karl J Kreder MD MBA
Professor and Vice Chair
Department of Urology
University of Iowa
Iowa City, IA
USA

Louis Kuritzky MD
Family Medicine Residency Program
University of Florida
Gainesville, FL
USA

Dominique LeTouze
Southwark Primary Care Trust
Southwark
UK

Lionel S Lim MBBS MPH FACP FACPM
Assistant Clinical Professor of Medicine
Griffin Hospital
Derby, CT
USA

Graham A MacGregor
Blood Pressure Unit
Cardiac and Vascular Sciences
St George's, University of London
London
UK

Jack W McAninch MD FACS
Professor and Vice Chairman
Department of Urology
University of California
San Francisco General Hospital
San Francisco, CA
USA

Donald R McCreary PhD
Adjunct Professor of Psychology
York University
Toronto, ON
and Brock University
St Catherines, ON
Canada

Phillip H McKee MD
Director, Division of Dermopathology
Brigham and Women's Hospital
Boston, MA
USA

Tom McNicholas MB BS FRCS FEBU
Consultant Urological Surgeon
Visiting Professor, University of Hertfordshire
Lister Hospital
Hertfordshire
UK

Randall B Meacham MD
Division of Urology
School of Medicine
University of Colorado – Denver
Aurora, CO
USA

Martin M Miner MD
Co-Director Men's Health Center
The Miriam Hospital
and Associate Clinical Professor of
Family Medicine
The Warren Alpert School of Medicine
Brown University School of Medicine
Providence, RI
USA

Andrew M Moon
Kilimanjaro Christian Medical Centre
Duke University Collaboration
Moshi
Tanzania

Clare Moynihan
Research Associate and Senior Research Fellow
Academic Department of Radiotherapy
Institute of Cancer Research
and The Royal Marsden Hospital Trust
The Bob Champion Unit
Sutton
UK

David Sutherland Muckle MD FRCS
Consultant Surgeon in Trauma and Orthopaedics
Medical Adviser to FIFA, UEFA, and The FA.
Examiner, Royal College of Surgeons
Edinburgh
and Park View Medical Clinic
Middlesbrough
UK

Moira MB Mungall MB
Clinical Research Fellow
Glasgow Royal Infirmary
Glasgow, Scotland
UK

J Curtis Nickel MD FRCSC
Professor of Urology
Canada Research Chair in Urologic Pain and
Inflammation
Queen's University
Kingston General Hospital
Kingston, ON
Canada

Craig S Niederberger MD
Department of Urology
University of Chicago at Illinois
Chicago, IL
USA

John Northover MS FRCS
Professor of Intestinal Surgery
Imperial College
London
UK

RTD Oliver MD FRCP
Professor Emeritus in Medical Oncology
Institute of Cancer Research
St Barts and The London Medicine School
Queen Mary University of London
London
UK

Hitendra RH Patel BMSC PhD BM MRCS FRCS(Urol)
Honorary Clinical Lecturer in Urology
Senior Specialist Registrar
Institute of Urology
University College London
London
UK

Sean Preston BSc (Hons) PhD MBBS MRCP
Department of Gastroenterology
Barts and The London NHS Trust
London
UK

Alan Pringle RGN RMN PhD
Lecturer in Mental Health Nursing
School of Nursing
University of Nottingham
Sutton-in-Ashfield
UK

Henry Purcell MB PhD
Senior Fellow in Cardiology
Royal Brompton Hospital
London
UK

Daniel Rosenstein MD FACS FRCSC(Urol)
Associate Chief, Division of Urology
Santa Clara Valley Medical Center
and Clinical Instructor
Stanford University Department of Urology
Palo Alto, CA
USA

Richard Sadovsky MD
Associate Professor of Family Practice
State University of New York
Health Science Center at Brooklyn
Brooklyn, NY
USA

Majid Shabbir MBBS MD FRCS
Higher Surgical Trainee in Urology
St George's Hospital
London
UK

Roy J Shephard
Faculty of Physical Education and Health
and Department of Public Health Sciences
Faculty of Medicine
Toronto, ON
Canada

Rodney Sinclair MBBS MD FACD
Professor of Dermatology
University of Melbourne
Director, Department of Dermatology
St Vincent's Hospital
Melbourne
Australia

Karen E Smith MD
Fellow Associate
Department of Urology
University of Iowa
Iowa City, IA
USA

Hemant Solomon BSc(Hons) MRCP
The Southeastern Heart and Vascular Center
Greensboro, NC
USA

David A Swanson
Department of Urology
University of Texas MD Anderson Cancer Center
Houston, TX
USA

Tatum Tarin MD
Urology Resident
Stanford University
Stanford, CA
USA

Justin Varney MBBS FFPH MSc
Assistant Director of Health Improvement
NHS Barking and Dagenham
Barking
UK

Nick Watkin MA MChir FRCS(Urol)
Consultant Urological Surgeon
Department of Urology
St George's Hospital
London
UK

Brian Wells FRCPsych
Consultant Psychiatrist
and Director
Leading Health Care International (LHCI)
London
UK

Alan White PhD RN
Centre for Men's Health
Faculty of Health
Leeds Metropolitan University
Leeds
UK

Angus HN Whitfield
Reading Hospital
Reading
UK

Hugh N Whitfield FRCS
London
UK

Klaus KA Witte MB MRCP
Specialist Registrar and Lecturer in Cardiology
Leeds General Infirmary
and Department of Cardiology
University of Hull
Castle Hill Hospital
Kingston-upon-Hull
UK

Christopher RJ Woodhouse MB FRCS FEBU
Professor of Adolescent Urology
The Institute of Urology
and Honorary Consultant Urologist
The Hospital for Children
London
UK

Foreword

Life expectancy continues to extend, but inequitably. Women live longer than men; richer men live longer than their counterparts who are less well off.

In developed nations, mortality rates from the major killers are falling and the pattern of disease is changing, so that, in general, there are better outcomes and more long-term survivors.

Attitudes to health between the sexes vary, as does their willingness to seek medical help. Women tend to seek help earlier and are more likely to confide in friends and relatives, whereas men stick it out, keep mum and hope for the best.

Why should these differences remain prominent when so much more can be done to alter risk and improve outcomes? Should the medical profession be more proactive in seeking out the younger and middle-aged men in order to help them confront their demons? Should the screening programs currently offered to women, such as breast and cervical screening, be developed for similar key conditions in men? Should men be offered advice and lifestyle interventions in a more proactive fashion?

Many questions remain unanswered, but clearly an important first step is to ensure that medical and other health professionals are fully educated in the specific issues relating to men's health. This third edition of *Men's Health* provides a commendable step in that direction, covering specific conditions as well as the important issues of lifestyle and well-being.

Roger Boyle CBE
November 2008

Preface

Ten years ago, as we put together the first edition of *Men's Health*, we asked an important question: 'Why do men die on average five years younger than women?' A decade later, although we now have at least a partial answer, namely that men look after themselves less well than women, the so-called gender gap still persists. The key issue then for readers of the third edition of this book is what can be done to narrow this gap, thereby allowing men to live longer and healthier lives. This is precisely the problem that we have asked each of our authors to address. Accordingly, the third edition of this book provides practical information that will help physicians to close the gap.

All three editions of *Men's Health* have been inspired by, and dedicated to, the memory of the father of two of the editors, namely Professor Ken Kirby FRS, who died prematurely from heart disease in 1967 aged 49. Unfortunately, middle-aged men continue to suffer sudden, and often fatal, cardiac events, even though our knowledge about the ways and means of reducing cardiovascular risk has increased in leaps and bounds. The problem lies mainly in the difficulty in persuading men to make the necessary modifications in their lifestyle that can dramatically reduce their cardiovascular risk. Their current attitude towards their health is 'If it ain't broke don't fix it'. Somehow we have to effect a sea-change in their attitude to a more pro-active 'If you look after it, it doesn't break' mentality. Unfortunately, if anything, the situation has deteriorated recently with an ever-increasing incidence of obesity, diabetes, and hypertension, both in the developed and under-developed world. Although the number of men who smoke has fallen in the United States and many European countries, sadly the smoking habit in men continues to rise in developing countries, with an inevitable increase in lung cancer deaths. Clearly there is still much to be done.

The third edition of *Men's Health* has been extensively revised and rewritten, with many new chapters. In particular, each of our authors has addressed the problem of the gender gap, especially in terms of cancer care and cardiovascular disease. The book is aimed not only at primary care practitioners, who need to encourage their male patients to visit them more often and to embrace preventative strategies for their health, but also at specialists, who too often focus too narrowly on their own areas of expertise, ignoring other potentially remedial problems, such as central obesity and unhealthy lifestyles, rather than tackling them pro-actively. We hope most sincerely that this new edition of our book will help to narrow the 'gender gap' and pro-actively prevent some of the premature deaths and illnesses afflicting men that tragically affect so many families, with such long-lasting negative impact.

Roger S Kirby, Culley Carson,
Michael G Kirby, and Alan White
October 2008

Men and cancer

CHAPTER 1

Men and cancer (epidemiology)

Alan White

Introduction

The new Cancer Reform Strategy for the UK has specifically noted that of the 10 commonest cancers that affect both men and women, age standardized mortality rates are in every case higher in men.[1] A recent expert symposium on men and cancer highlighted that, though there were assumptions as to why this may be the case, it was not yet clear as to the exact mechanisms and that there was a need for more research into how sex impacts on the risk of developing and dying from cancer.[2] This chapter outlines the scale of the issues facing men and some of the possible causes of their increased susceptibility.

The significance of cancer with regard to men's generally high rate of premature death has changed over the past 30 years. The incidence rate for all cancers (excluding non-malignant skin cancer) for Great Britain has risen from 353.7 per 100 000 in 1975 to 408.2 per 100 000 in 2004 (Fig. 1.1); however, the overall mortality has dropped from 284.1 per 100 000 in 1976 to 215.9 per 100 000 in 2005 (Fig. 1.2),[3,4] suggesting that, though the overall number has increased, the advances in treatment have resulted in more people surviving their cancer.

Prostate cancer

The rising trend in cancer incidence rates for men can in part be attributed to the aging population and the increasing diagnosis of prostate cancer, which has risen from 35.2 per 100 000 in 1975 to 97.9 per 100 000 in 2004 (Fig. 1.3).[5] Whilst the death rate has risen it is predominately in the over-85-year-olds (Fig. 1.4) and therefore it has not overly affected the overall falling cancer mortality trend.

Burden of cancer as a cause of mortality

In 2004 there were 71 878 male deaths from cancer in England and Wales and 66 576 female deaths from cancer, which account for 29.5% of total male mortality and 24.7% of total female mortality (calculated from figures produced by the Office for National Statistics).[6] Nevertheless, when the burden of death is calculated for different age groups (see Fig. 1.5) it can be seen that cancer does tend to account for a greater proportion of younger female deaths than it does for men.

When the rate ratios of male to female deaths are calculated (Table 1.1), it is seen that there is a slightly higher rate of death for men (with a male: female ratio of 1.14) across all ages, but that this drops to about parity in the 15–64 year age range before rising to nearly a 50% higher rate of death in men over the age of 65 years. Predominately the cancer deaths that women succumb to in their early years are those related to the breast and

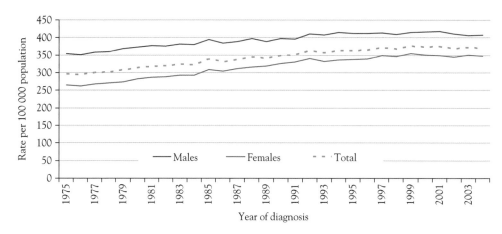

Figure 1.1. *Age-standardized (European) incidence rates for all cancers excluding non-malignant skin cancers, by sex, Great Britain, 1975–2004.*[3]

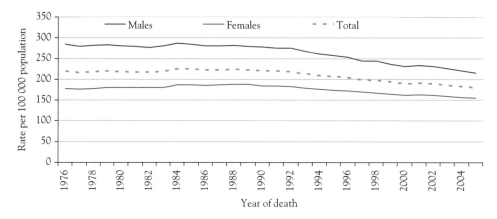

Figure 1.2. *Age-standardized (European) mortality, all cancers, by sex, Great Britain, 1976–2005.*[4]

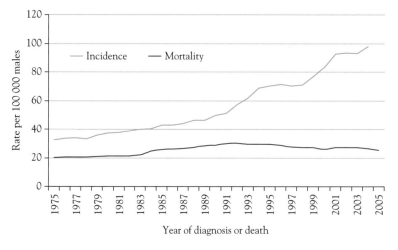

Figure 1.3. *Age-standardized (European) incidence and mortality rates, prostate cancer, males, Great Britain, 1975–2005.*[5]

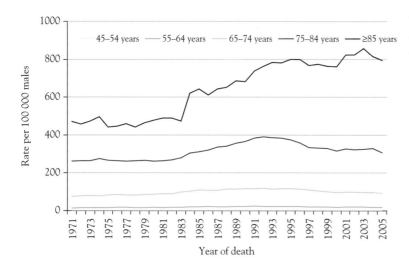

Figure 1.4. *Age-specific mortality rates, prostate cancer, males, UK, 1971–2005.*[5]

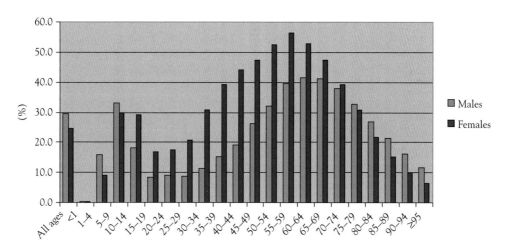

Figure 1.5. *Cancer deaths as a proportion of total deaths by age and by sex, England and Wales, 2004.*[6]

genital organs (27.6% overall and over 50% in the 35–44 year age range) (calculated from figures produced by the Office for National Statistics).[6] For men there are no significant numbers of deaths that can be attributed to a sex-specific cause, such that if the rate ratios are calculated when breast cancer and those cancers that can be seen to be unique to men or women are excluded a different picture emerges, with over 60% more men in the 15–64 year age range succumbing to cancers that should be affecting men and women equally. This increased risk is seen across a broad range of principal cancers.

When the incidence data are considered (Table 1.2),[7] it can be seen that there are more women registered with cancer in England and Wales in the 15–64 year age range (with a male:female ratio of 0.83), but again when breast cancer and the cancers relating to genital organs are removed from the equation a greater number of men are seen to be at risk of the non-sex-specific cancers. This tendency is seen across the cancers listed in Table 1.2, with the exception of skin cancer, where more women are registered, but as can be seen from Table 1.1, more men actually die from the condition.

Table 1.1. *Rate ratio of male to female deaths, England and Wales, 2004*[6]

ICD-10 code	Site description	Rate ratios, male to female		
		All ages	15–64 years	≥65 years
C00–C97	All cancers	1.14	1.03	1.49
C00–C97 excluding C50, C51–C58, C60–C63	All cancers excluding breast and sex-specific cancers	1.37	1.61	1.65
C15	Esophagus	1.90	3.34	2.06
C16	Stomach	1.68	1.90	2.08
C18–C21	Colon and rectum	1.20	1.55	1.43
C22	Liver	1.50	1.93	1.73
C25	Pancreas	0.97	1.26	1.14
C33–C34	Lung	1.53	1.45	1.97
C43	Malignant melanoma of skin	1.31	1.34	1.61
C64	Kidney	1.65	2.15	1.89
C67	Bladder	2.02	2.36	2.53
C71	Brain	1.55	1.69	1.76
C82–C85	Non-Hodgkin's lymphoma	1.16	1.68	1.29
C90	Multiple myeloma	1.17	1.45	1.43
C91–C95	Leukemia	1.30	1.51	1.59

The increased risk of premature male death is seen clearly when the years of life lost and the mean age of death are considered (Table 1.3),[9] with 112 000 years of life being lost by men for the portfolio of cancers as opposed to 73 000 years of life being lost by women in the age bracket 15–64 years, and the median age of death being 71 years for men and 74 for women.

A development of this UK analysis was undertaken by White in 2007 for the Congresso Nacional de Epidemiologia, which focused on 'An Epidemiological Perspective of Men's Health' as part of the Portuguese Presidency of the European Union (Fig. 1.6).[10] An examination of the data for a broad span of countries held on the World Health Organization Mortality Database explored if there were similarities relating to the increased risk of the non sex-specific cancers. The countries from which data were examined were Argentina (data from 2001), Australia (2001),

Austria (2002), Brazil (2000), Denmark (1999), Estonia (2002), Hungary (2002), Japan (2002), Portugal (2002), Spain (2001), Sweden (2001), Thailand (2000), the UK (2002), and the USA (2000).

The median rate ratio was calculated by age from the 14 countries for all cancers and for cancers excluding the available data on breast cancer and genital cancer. The picture for all cancers showed that the age groups 25–34 years and 35–44 years had a median rate ratio below 1, indicating that more women were dying, but when breast cancer and the cancers relating to genitalia were omitted (Figure 1.7) then the median rate ratio rose to 1.4 in these age groups and was higher in other age groups.

What seems to be emerging is that men are at greater risk of developing and dying from those cancers that should be seen to affect men and women equally.

Table 1.2. *Rate ratio of male to female registrations, England[7] and Wales,[8] 2004*

ICD-10 code	Site description	Rate ratios male to female		
		All ages	15–64 years	≥65
C00–C97	All cancers	1.10	0.83	1.59
C00–C97 excluding C50, C51–C58, C60–C63	All cancers excluding breast and sex-specific cancers	1.34	1.35	1.68
C15	Esophagus	1.93	3.19	2.05
C16	Stomach	1.80	2.27	2.15
C18–C21	Colon and rectum	1.25	1.42	1.51
C22	Liver	1.52	2.10	1.71
C25	Pancreas	0.99	1.23	1.17
C33–C34	Lung	1.52	1.45	1.96
C43	Malignant melanoma of skin	0.85	0.75	1.26
C64	Kidney	1.69	1.91	1.99
C67	Bladder	2.60	2.96	3.21
C71	Brain	1.53	1.61	1.77
C82–C85	Non-Hodgkin's lymphoma	1.18	1.30	1.37
C90	Multiple myeloma	1.26	1.48	1.49
C91–C95	Leukemia	1.42	1.50	1.75

Causes of cancer

For a cell to mutate and become carcinogenic, changes have to occur at the level of the DNA; these changes can be seen to be either as a result of a germline (or inherited) factor or through some sort of somatic event (acquired during life). Examination of the different causes of cancer highlight that the reasons that men seem to be so much more at risk of developing and prematurely dying of cancers are not as clear-cut as perhaps previously thought.

Germline factors

There is much known about germline risks for women with regard to breast cancer and the other sex-specific cancers, but it is less well known that the same changes also have implications for male cancers. The life-time breast cancer risk for men with BRCA2 mutations is between 2.8% and 6.9%,

and these mutations have been shown to increase the risk of prostate cancer by 7.5%.[11]

Another example of a germline link can be found in the association between prostate cancer and the Y-chromosomal haplogroups. For instance, the incidence rate of prostate cancer in African–American males is twice as high as the incidence rate in Caucasian men and ten times higher than the incidence rate in Japanese men.[12] The CHEK2 mutation doubles the risk of prostate cancer and quadruples the risk in men with a family history of the condition.[13]

With regard to testicular cancer, the standardized incidence ratios for familial risk were 3.8-fold higher when a father has had testicular cancer and 7.6-fold higher when a brother had it. Moreover, there is an association between testicular cancer and leukemia, distal colon and kidney cancer, melanoma, connective tissue tumors, and lung cancer in families.[14]

Table 1.3. *Total number of deaths, mean age at death, and years of life lost for selected cancers, England and Wales, 2004*[9]

		Total deaths (n)	Mean age at death (years)	Working life (age 15–64 years)	Total life (to age 85 years)
				Years lost (000s)	Years lost (000s)
Malignant neoplasm of esophagus	Male	4071	71	10	58
	Female	2227	77	3	21
Malignant neoplasm of stomach	Male	3144	74	5	36
	Female	1954	77	3	19
Malignant neoplasm of colon, rectum, and anus	Male	7575	73	13	93
	Female	6596	77	10	63
Malignant neoplasm of liver and intrahepatic bile ducts	Male	1370	70	4	21
	Female	951	74	2	11
Malignant neoplasm of pancreas	Male	3036	72	6	41
	Female	3258	75	5	35
Malignant neoplasm of trachea, bronchus, and lung	Male	16 862	73	27	216
	Female	11 466	73	21	145
Malignant melanoma of skin	Male	890	66	5	17
	Female	707	68	4	13
Malignant neoplasm of kidney, except renal pelvis	Male	1816	70	6	28
	Female	1144	72	3	15
Malignant neoplasm of bladder	Male	2840	77	2	25
	Female	1461	80	1	10
Malignant neoplasm of brain	Male	1798	61	15	44
	Female	1205	63	9	27
Non-Hodgkin's lymphoma	Male	2075	70	8	33
	Female	1863	74	4	21
Multiple myeloma and malignant plasma cell neoplasms	Male	1208	74	2	14
	Female	1071	76	1	11
Leukemia	Male	2126	70	9	32
	Female	1702	73	7	23

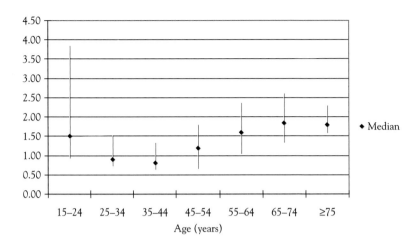

Figure 1.6. *The median rate ratio, male to female, for cancer mortality for 14 countries, for all malignant neoplasms.*[10]

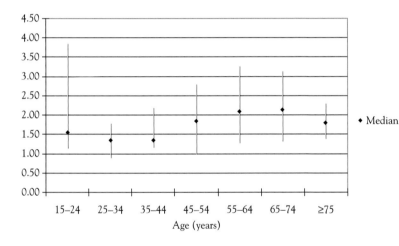

Figure 1.7. *The median rate ratio, male to female, for cancer mortality for 14 countries, for all malignant neoplasms, excluding breast and the principal sex-specific cancers.*[10]

Somatic causes of cancer

A key study by Danaei et al. identified that more than a third (37%) of all risk-factor attributable deaths are from:[15]

- Smoking
- Alcohol use
- Diet
- Overweight and obesity
- Physical inactivity
- Urban air pollution
- Indoor smoke – in the developing world
- Unsafe sex for women (cervical cancer)
- Contaminated injections – in the developing world.

The first six of these factors are explored below to demonstrate how men's lifestyles adversely affect their chances of developing cancer.

Influence of tobacco on cancer

Tobacco accounts for about 29% of the attributable risk for cancer in the UK and causes most cases of lung cancer, in addition it increases risk of developing the following cancers:[16]

- Oral cavity
- Nasal cavity and sinuses
- Larynx
- Pharynx
- Esophagus
- Stomach

- Kidney
- Bladder
- Pancreas
- Myeloid leukemia.

The greater the duration and intensity of smoking the higher the risk of developing lung cancer (Fig. 1.8). When the data on smoking are considered, despite the increase in smoking among young women, it is still predominately men who smoke (Fig. 1.9). Data from the Office for National Statistics in the UK showed that, in 2004–2005, 26% of men and 23% of women were cigarette smokers, compared with the early 1970s when around 50% of men and 40% of women smoked. Male smokers smoked more cigarettes a day on average than female smokers. In each year since 1998–1999, men smoked on average 15 cigarettes a day compared with 13 for women.[18]

Influence of alcohol on cancer

Alcohol is now recognized as a significant factor in both the cause and development of cancer. Animal studies suggest that alcohol stimulates angiogenesis, increasing blood supply to cancers.[19] Ethanol converts to the toxic, mutagenic, and carcinogenic acetaldehyde, which can interact with polyamines within the cell, leading to damaged DNA, with the alcohol effect magnified by smoking.[20]

Consumption of alcohol increases the risk of cancers of the oral cavity and pharynx, esophagus, larynx, and liver, even at low levels of consumption (up to two drinks per day); at higher levels, the incidence of cancers of the colon and rectum, stomach, and prostate are also seen to be raised (Table 1.4).[21]

When the data on men and drinking are considered it can be seen that there is an increased prevalence of men abusing alcohol. Binge drinking

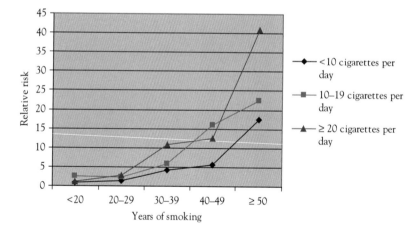

Figure 1.8. *Relative risk of lung cancer according to duration and intensity of smoking, men.*[16]

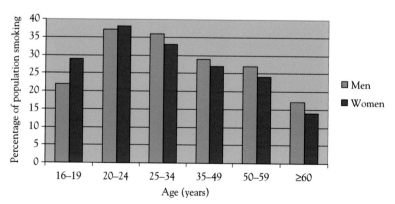

Figure 1.9. *Percentage of population cigarette smoking by age and sex, England and Wales, 2002.*[17]

Table 1.4. *Relative risks of alcohol consumption for each cancer site*[21]

Cancer site	Cases	Relative risk		
		25 g/day	50 g/day	100 g/day
Oral cavity and pharynx	7954	1.8	2.9	6.0
Esophagus	7239	1.5	2.2	4.2
Larynx	3759	1.4	1.9	4.0
Liver	2294	1.2	1.4	1.9
Colon and rectum	11296	1.1	1.2	1.4
Stomach	4518	1.1	1.2	1.3
Prostate	4094	No association	1.1	1.2

accounts for 40% of all drinking occasions by men and 22% of those by women, with 24% of men and 13% of women having engaged in binge drinking at least once in the past week.[22] There are also differences that should be noted for men from different backgrounds, which raises the need for more targeted health advice, since single men are more likely than married men to drink heavily, and alcohol consumption is higher than average among divorced and separated men.[23]

Influence of diet on cancer

There is now a substantial body of evidence that demonstrates the influence of diet on the development of cancer, with the EPIC study, covering some 500000 people in 10 European countries showing that dietary fiber has a strong protective effect against bowel cancer, that a high intake of red or processed meat increases the risk of stomach and bowel cancer, and that a high intake of fruit may reduce the risk of lung cancer.[24] An exploration of men's dietary habits suggests that men are increasing their cancer risk through a tendency to have lower levels of dietary fiber and higher levels of red or processed meat.[25]

Influence of obesity on cancer

About 10% of all non-smoking-related deaths in men are a result of obesity.[26] The male form of obesity with the tendency to lay down visceral fat within the abdomen, giving the characteristic apple shape to men, is a more dangerous form than the

Box 1.1. *Secretions from visceral fat cells*

- Leptin
- Tumor necrosis factor-alpha
- Adiponectin
- Interleukin-6
- Inducible nitric oxide synthase
- Macrophage migration inhibitory factor
- Transforming growth factor-p
- Insulin-like growth factor-1

gynoid fat distribution of hip and thigh fat found in women. The visceral fat is linked to the metabolic syndrome, which comprises hyperinsulinemia leading to diabetes, hypertension, hyperlipidemia, and in addition to the fat-related cancers. The cause of these problems can be traced to both the male-form central obesity increasing the secretion of 'fat toxins' (Box 1.1) and to the mechanical consequences of the mass of fat within the abdomen in overweight men – for instance, acid reflux increases the risk of esophageal cancer,[27] disruption to gall bladder function increases the risk of gall bladder cancer, and a high girth measurement has been found to increase the risk of pancreatic cancer. A relationship has also been found between being overweight or obese and the risk of kidney cancers, and reduced plasma levels of sex-steroid-binding globulin increases the risk of prostate cancer.[28] Calle et al. have also found that category 1 obese men [with a body mass index (BMI) of 30.0–34.9 kg/m^2] were 20% more likely to die from prostate cancer than normal-weight men (with a BMI of 18.5–24.9 kg/m^2), whereas men who were category 2 obese (with a BMI of 35.0–39.9 kg/m^2) were 34% more likely to die from prostate cancer than lean controls.[29]

Influence of physical activity and inactivity on cancer

Exercise has been found to be independently related to cancer risk, with the risk of colon cancer being significantly reduced in men by regular aerobic exercise,[30] and moderately vigorous activity in middle aged men being associated with a reduced risk of total cancers, prostate cancer, upper digestive, and stomach cancer.[31] Exercise appears to have its own effects, but to date the exact processes are still unidentified. However, it appears that the following are implicated.[31]

- Alterations to steroid hormones, with excess exercise in young men being linked to increased risk of prostate and testicular cancer as a result of altered androgen synthesis
- Immune modulation; again, both too much and too little exercise have been found to influence the body's response to cancer, a notable finding being the decrease in cancer mortality in the active older person as a result of attenuation of the immune senescence that usually occurs with aging
- Alterations in free radical generation – over-exercise can create excess oxygen free radicals that swamp the body's normal homeostatic mechanisms, thus leaving lipids, protein and DNA at risk of damage
- Alterations to insulin and insulin-like growth hormones – insulin is recognized as a promoter of carcinogenesis, and exercise results in increased insulin insensitivity, decreased insulin concentrations, decreased C-peptide, and increased glucagon, and thus has a protective effect
- Changes in energy balance and body composition – obesity is known to cause cancer, but there is a greater protective effect in achieving energy balance through exercise than by dieting alone

- Direct effects on tumors – exercise training has been found to result in smaller tumors and a reduction in their growth rate, but the exact reason for this remains unknown.

All of this has wide implications for men, since these effects are seen both in those who over-exercise and in those who lead a sedentary lifestyle.

Effect of urban air pollution on cancer

The risk of lung cancer increases significantly if there is a high exposure to urban air pollution, but in addition to this risk, it is possible to extend this category to include environmental risks in general.

The US National Cancer Institute review of cancer and the environment highlighted that we are in constant interaction with a potentially hostile 'environment', which the body has to react to.[32] Any changes within the defense mechanisms or exposure to environmental carcinogens (Box 1.2) can increase the possibility of developing cancer. The working environment for many men employed in industry, the farming trade, the building trade, and the motor trade increases exposure to many of these risk factors.

Influence of other factors on cancer

There are other risks that increase the chance of men developing cancer. For instance, diabetes was found to be associated with a 27% increase in total

---

Box 1.2. *Environmental carcinogens*

- Ultraviolet radiation
- Viruses and bacteria
- Ionizing radiation
- Pesticides
- Medical drugs
- Solvents
- Fibers, fine particles, and dust
- Dioxins
- Polycyclic aromatic hydrocarbons
- Metals
- Diesel exhaust particles
- Toxins from fungi
- Vinyl chloride
- Benzidine

cancer in men, with a high hazard ratio for cancer of the liver, pancreas, and kidney and a moderately increased risk of colon cancer and an increased risk of borderline significance for stomach cancer. In women, a different picture was seen, with a borderline significant increase in risk for the incidence of total cancers, while statistical significance was observed for the incidence of stomach cancer and liver cancer and borderline significance was observed for the incidence of ovarian cancer.[33] Anal cancer, which is caused by human papillomavirus, is rare in men but the numbers dying increase rapidly in men who have sex with men or have HIV infection.[34]

Women, cancer, and their immune response

A suggestion has been made that the reason for greater numbers of men developing and dying of cancers is that women have a higher humoral immunity.[35] This is suggested by the fact that women seem to have:

- higher immunoglobulin levels than men;
- more vigorous antibody responses to exogenous antigens than men;
- a higher cellular immunity than men;
- a lower incidence of tumors than men;
- a better resistance against viral and parasitic infections than men; and
- an ability to reject allograft more rapidly than men.

The case of colorectal cancer

Colorectal cancer is the third biggest cause of cancer death in men. Figures 1.10 and 1.11 show that there are more men than women registered with this cancer and that more die at an earlier age.

It is suggested that genetic factors are involved in the development of 35% of cases of colorectal cancer, with hereditary non-polyposis colorectal cancer being implicated in 3–5% of cancers. Moreover, having a first-degree affected relative increases the risk between two- and four-fold, and there may also be recessive genes, pathogenic mutations of low penetrance, and complex gene–gene and gene–environment interactions involved in the process.[36] Fearon and Vogelstein also suggest that cancer development is aggravated by mutations in APC, p53, k-ras, and MSH2 genes.[37]

In addition, the risk of developing colorectal cancer is increased by factors that have already been alluded to as being problematic for some men:

- A diet low in fruit and vegetables
- A high intake of red and processed meat
- Low levels of physical activity
- Alcohol
- Smoking
- Diabetes
- Obesity.

Using the case of colorectal cancer demonstrates that with these multiple factors implicated it is less surprising that men have an increased chance of

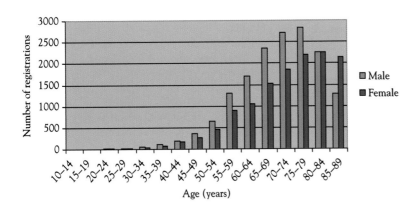

Figure 1.10. *Registrations of newly diagnosed cases of malignant neoplasm of the colon and rectum, England, by age and sex, 2004.*[7]

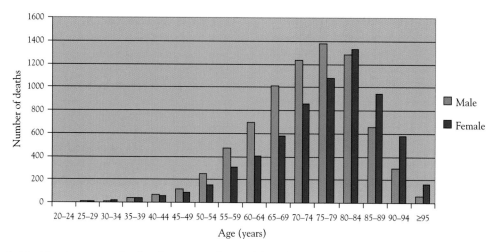

Figure 1.11. *Deaths as a result of malignant neoplasm of the colon, rectum, and anus, by age and sex, 2004 for England and Wales.*[6]

developing this condition and to perhaps show that it is not straightforward in deciding what can be done to decrease their susceptibility.

Conclusion

There have been concerns that men's high rate of premature death from cancer may be due to delay in seeking medical help.[2,38,39] It is necessary to see this as a factor, especially since the screening uptake for men for bowel cancer suggests that though they are at greater risk they are less likely to be tested.[2] However, this cannot be the sole reason because the picture seems much more complex, with increased risk, and reduced chance of survival.[40]

The causes of cancer are many and varied, both inherited and acquired. There are both biological and lifestyle factors that seem to make men specifically vulnerable to developing and dying prematurely from cancers that should affect men and women equally. Despite this there are no systematic studies of men's increased risk and little publicity aimed at men to highlight that lifestyle choices can have such a profound effect on their health and the necessity to have early diagnosis for maximal effect.

Acknowledgments

With thanks to: Professor David Forman, Professor of Cancer Epidemiology, University of Leeds, UK, and Director, Northern and Yorkshire Cancer Registry and Information Service; David Wilkins, Policy Officer, The Men's Health Forum; and Dr Lesley Farley, Senior Medical Statistician, Northern and Yorkshire Cancer Registry and Information Service – for their help, advice, and comments on my earlier work on men and cancer.

References

1. Cancer Reform Strategy. London: Department of Health, 2007.
2. Wilkins D. Tackling the Excess Incidence of Cancer in Men: Proceedings of the Expert Symposium. London: Men's Health Forum, 2006.
3. Trends in UK Cancer Mortality Statistics. Cancer Research UK, 2007 [available at: http://info.cancerresearchuk.org/cancerstats/mortality/timetrends/; data accessed November 2008].
4. Trends in UK Cancer Incidence Statistics. Cancer Research UK, 2007 [available at: http://info.cancerresearchuk.org/cancerstats/incidence/trends/; data accessed November 2008].

5. CancerStats Key Facts on Prostate Cancer. Cancer Research UK, 2007.
6. Mortality Statistics: Cause DH2 No 31 ONS 2004. London: Office for National Statistics [available at: http://www.statistics.gov.uk; data accessed November 2008].
7. Cancer Statistics: Registrations MB1 No 35, ONS 2004. London: Office for National Statistics [available at: http://www.statistics.gov.uk].
8. Cancer Incidence in Wales 2000–2004. Cardiff: Welsh Cancer Intelligence and Surveillance Unit (WCISU) Annual Publication, No SA6/01, 2006.
9. Mortality Statistics: General DH 1 No 37 ONS 2004. London: Office for National Statistics [available at: http://www.statistics.gov.uk].
10. White AK. The State of Men's Health: a Global Perspective. Presented at An Epidemiological Perspective of Men's Health, Congresso Nacional de Epidemiologia, Lisbon, Portugal, 14 November, 2007.
11. Levy-Lahad E, Friedman E. Cancer risks among BRCA1 and BRCA2 mutation carriers. Br J Cancer 2007; 96: 11–15.
12. Ewis AA, Lee J, Naroda T et al. Prostate cancer incidence varies among males from different Y-chromosome lineages. Prostate Cancer Prostatic Dis 2006; 9: 303–9.
13. Cybulski C, Wokolorczyk D, Huzarski T et al. A large germline deletion in the Chek2 kinase gene is associated with an increased risk of prostate cancer. J Med Genet 2006; 43: 863–6.
14. Hemminki K, Bowang C. Familial risks in testicular cancer as aetiological clues. Int J Androl 2006; 29: 205–10.
15. Danaei G, Lawes CMM, Vander Hoorn S, Murray CJL, Ezzati M. Causes of cancer in the world: comparative risk assessment of nine behavioural and environmental risk factors. Lancet 2006; 366: 1784–93.
16. Tobacco and Cancer Risk. Cancer Research UK, 2005 [available at: http://info.cancerresearchuk.org/cancerstats/causes/lifestyle/tobacco/?a=5].
17. Smoking. Living in Britain, General Household Survey 2002. London, Office for National Statistics, 2002.
18. Smoking Habits in Great Britain. General Household Survey, National Statistics Omnibus Survey. London, Office for National Statistics, 2006 [available at: http://www.statistics.gov.uk/cci/nugget.asp?id=313].
19. Raloff J. Alcohol spurs cancer growth. Sci News 2006; 169: 238.
20. O'Hanlon LH. Studies seek molecular clues on alcohol's role in cancer. J Natl Cancer Inst 2005; 97: 1563–4.
21. Bagnardi V, Blangiardo M, La Vecchia C et al. Alcohol consumption and the risk of cancer. Alcohol Res Health 2001; 25: 263–70.
22. Health Related Behaviour: Alcohol: More Men than Women Exceed Recommended Daily Limit. London: Office for National Statistics, 2007 [available at: http://www.statistics.gov.uk/CCI/nugget.asp?ID=1894&Pos=&ColRank=2&Rank=224].
23. Drinking. Living in Britain, General Household Survey 2002. London: Office for National Statistics, 2002.
24. Diet, Alcohol and Cancer in the UK. Cancer Research UK, 2008 [available at: http://info.cancerresearchuk.org/cancerstats/causes/lifestyle/diet/?a=5441].
25. Diet and Nutrition: Only 14% of Men Consume Five a Day. London: Office for National Statistics, 2006 [available at: http://www.statistics.gov.uk/CCI/nugget.asp?ID=739&Pos=2&ColRank=1&Rank=208].
26. Haslam D, James W. Obesity. Lancet 2005; 366: 1197–209.
27. Calle EE, Rodriguez C, Walker-Thurmond K, Thun MJ. Overweight, obesity, and mortality from cancer in a prospectively studied cohort of US adults. N Engl J Med 2003; 348: 1625–38.
28. Bodyweight and Risk of Cancer in the UK. Cancer Research UK, 2006 [available at: http://info.cancerresearchuk.org/cancerstats/causes/lifestyle/bodyweight/?a=5441].
29. Chung WK, Leibel RL. The links between obesity, leptin, and prostate cancer. Cancer J 2006; 12: 178–81.
30. McTiernan A, Yasui Y, Sorensen B et al. Effect of a 12-month exercise intervention on patterns of cellular proliferation in colonic crypts: A randomized controlled trial. Cancer Epidemiol Biomarkers Prev 2006; 15: 1588–97.
31. Wannamethee SG, Shaper AG, Walker M. Physical activity and risk of cancer in middle-aged men. Br J Cancer 2001; 85: 1311–16.
32. Cancer and the Environment. Np: National Cancer Institute, 2003.
33. Inoue M, Iwasaki M, Otani T et al. Diabetes mellitus and the risk of cancer: results from a large-scale population-based cohort study in Japan. Arch Intern Med 2006; 166: 1871–7.
34. Welton ML, Winkler B, Darragh TM. Anal-rectal cytology and anal cancer screening. Semin Colon Rectal Surg 2005; 15: 196–200.

35. Bouman A, Schipper M, Heineman MJ et al. Gender difference in the non-specific and specific immune response in humans. Am J Reprod Immunol 2004; 52: 19–26.

36. Mitchell RJ, Farrington SM, Dunlop MG et al. Mismatch repair genes hMLH1 and hMSH2 and colorectal cancer: a HuGE review. Am J Epidemiol 2002; 156: 885–902.

37. Fearon E, Vogelstein B. A genetic model for colorectal tumorigenesis. Cell 1990; 61: 759–67.

38. Smith LK, Pope C, Botha JL. Patients' help-seeking experiences and delay in cancer presentation: a qualitative synthesis. Lancet 2005; 366: 825–31.

39. Evans RE, Brotherstone H, Miles A et al. Gender differences in early detection of cancer. J Mens Health Gend 2005; 2: 209–17.

40. Verdecchia A, Francisci S, Brenner H et al. Recent cancer survival in Europe: a 2000–02 period analysis of EUROCARE-4 data. Lancet Oncol 2007; 8: 784–96.

CHAPTER 2

Ignorance and uncertainty regarding cancer and cancer genetics in men

Clare Moynihan, Robert Huddart

The challenge for practitioners and policy makers is both to recognize and to respond to individual practice where structural and everyday constraints interacting with social values, shape and are shaped by the human experience of health, its maintenance and its loss.

(J. Watson p 30[1])

Introduction

Men are thought to be dangerous to their health. In recent years the topic of men's health has given rise for concern. The United Kingdom Department of Health,[2] scientific journals,[3] popular magazines and awareness campaigns[4] have all commented on the ways in which men are 'at risk'. Others have commented on how underrepresented men are in terms of research in general[5] and psychosocial cancer research in particular.[6]

In this chapter we will look at the assumptions that we make about men and women in the context of health and illness and how they can lead to negative outcomes. I will convey the ways in which we expect men to follow conventional 'rules' regarding health and disease while at the same time withholding information from them. I will also argue for the importance of 'seeing' differences and similarities between and within men and women who are ill in a quest for equal delivery of health services. Finally, we will highlight the urgency of listening to men's beliefs, needs and ways of understanding

cancer and genetic cancer in particular, in the context of their everyday lives.

Men are shown to live shorter lives than women.[5] Social class differences are thought to account for the inverse social gradient for mortality. Men in lower socioeconomic groups are likely to die earlier than their upper class counterparts.[7] Studies in health and illness indicate an excess of female morbidity compared to males despite the difference in longevity.[8] Women apparently access all health services more readily including information services,[9] while men do not.[10] Men are said to be inexpressive; avoiding intimacy[11] while leaving 'health work' to women.[12]

The reasons for these differences have taken several perspectives. The Public Understanding of Science lobby would have us believe that a lack of involvement in science including medicine, rests on a deficit model of lay understanding. There is an assumption that knowledge will be assimilated through uniform educational programs delivered in ways that 'the' public will comprehend.[13] This, however, assumes homogeneity and fails to address the ways that men (and women) jettison (or include) information according to their social context and the ways in which health educationalists deliver information in the first place.

'Men' versus 'Women'

A biomedical perspective observes differences in morbidity and mortality as the product of biologically based inherited risks. For example, Nathanson points to the ways in which explanations for women's greater access to medical support rests on their destiny as child bearers, although when reproduction is excluded in analyses, women continue to have higher rates than men for all indices of illness experience.[14] Men on the other hand, are thought to be less 'biologically durable' than women.[15] This one-dimensional 'blanket' approach fails to address the many methodological, conceptual and theoretical problems and issues inherent in investigations regarding sex differences in health and illness. For example the *meanings* that certain points in the life course may hold in relation to health are almost never investigated.[16,17]

Sociobiologists have turned to 'social role' theory to explain the ways that men and women are assigned and acquire behavior that is linked to their 'roles'. For example, men are socialized to negate expression while the 'stiff upper lip' is encouraged from a very early age. Stoicism is fostered in the face of 'work orientation' and a refusal to admit weakness,[11] leading them into stressful and risky situations in order to 'prove' their masculinity.[18] These so-called 'masculine' traits are said to 'block' an engagement with medicine[19] leading to earlier death.[5] Women on the other hand are socialized to being mothers; they are expected to be expressive, compliant, emotionally labile[20] and nurturing as they seek medical advice for themselves and their families.[14]

These ways of explaining morbidity, mortality and health behavior are 'essentialist'.[6] It assumes that we are 'born' with certain characteristics and obligatory 'roles' that relate to biological sex. Difference is a static trait; ambiguity is never acknowledged.[20] However, when we look at 'gender' as opposed to 'sex',[21] men and women are no longer what they *are* but what they *do* and *achieve* in relations with others or with institutions including medicine.[20] A man may wish to cry while holding a teddy bear but does so in secret in the context of a hospital ward for fear of appearing a 'wimp', the same man may be stoical in his relations with doctors provoking awe; women may exhibit masculine traits in the context of ill health but may be considered 'pathological'. Some men may actively seek out health information and behave in a wholly

'responsible' way regarding health and illness some or part of the time while some men are constrained.[20]

This negation of ambiguity and similarity *as well as* difference between and within the sexes helps to conjure up conflicting findings,[9] and overall patterns of morbidity or the sex difference between mortality and morbidity are never fully explained.[9] As Verbrugge points out, the salience of any given hypothesis tends to vary with the outcome measure under consideration.[22] Added to this is the sex bias that exists in medicine creating inequality in many aspects of health care.[6,22] In the field of cancer and especially psychosocial care, women have taken center stage in terms of research.[6] The work that has shown that ways of coping affect outcome and even survival have been carried out in women with breast cancer.[6] Indeed breast disease has become the exemplar of all other cancer journeys despite the many different types of cancer that may in themselves impact on responses.[6] Clinicians are known to treat men and women in differing ways for no apparent reason other than their sex[23] as they hold onto stereotypical assumptions and values in their working lives.[6,20] This is dangerous in that it will lead to unequal and less than optimal services but it also helps to direct attention away from structural issues that underlie the quality of health care and the possible reasons why men seem to appear 'irresponsible' with regard to their health.[6] It should never be forgotten that the institution of medicine may itself foster health behaviors. Consider how hospitals are imbued with so-called masculine traits of competitiveness,[20] stoicism and an ability to create a chasm between doctors and their patients in relation to emotions and behaviors.[24] While creating a 'nest' of inexpressiveness, men who are ill are expected to adhere to the stiff upper lip image while women are expected or 'allowed' to express emotion.[20] At the same time a hierarchical order between the 'expert' and 'lay man' is established; the latter seldom being privy to the full knowledge base of medicine.[25] This is notwithstanding the advances in communication technology that enables some lay people access to details about cancer, however out of date and however unreliable.

Despite all these caveats the search for innate differences between the sexes continues unabated even though important research findings have shown striking similarities in terms of individual attributes.[26] In health and illness men have been shown to act in ways that would surprise the essentialists.[27] The inherent 'head in the sand' approach often used to describe men's attitudes towards their health is undermined by the ways, for example, men with colorectal cancer, are more likely to want to hear their prognosis.[25] No differences have been found between the sexes in respect to ignoring symptoms, or the ways that they take care of themselves when employment status, marital status and age are adjusted.[9] An analysis of general practice consultations for common chronic conditions reported in early and late mid life shows that women are no more likely to consult than men at a given level of reported severity for a given condition type, except in the case of mental health problems.[28] However, there appears to be one particular area in which men and women differ; that is in the utilization of medical services for conditions that are not considered to be 'serious'. Men do not, apparently, seek support readily.[9,29]

Younger men

This is corroborated in the context of testicular cancer. Young men, in 'good' health, have been shown to wait up to 3 years before presenting symptoms to their doctor who are also known to delay in referring to specialist care.[30] Men's ignorance, and the rarity of the disease may provoke the patient's delay and the doctor's uncertainty in making a diagnosis.[28] Be that as it may, it may also be that doctor's prevarication rests on assumptions that are easily made regarding young men. Virility and youth do not commonly go hand in hand with a life-threatening illness, making it difficult for the doctor to 'see' beyond this and to take a young man's presenting symptoms seriously.[6] In turn young men speak about their propensity to shyness and embarrassment and a feeling that they are often ridiculed by physicians for wasting time, while being devoid of information regarding the disease.[31]

Older men

As a result of the paucity of research regarding older prostate cancer patients, not enough is known about how factors may predispose them to seek help and information or how medical professionals will respond to them regarding symptoms. We do know, however, that disease-free men are self-confessedly 'clueless' about cancer and specifically about prostate (and testicular) disease.[29] Men in general, and older men in particular, have also been found to be less likely to access cancer help centers when compared with women.[32] We know too, that many of the needs of prostate cancer patients are unmet including emotional support.[33,34] Elusive information about the disease, brochures about services and benefits, and 'a series of talks by staff members on aspects of cancer' have been requested.[34] All have been perceived to be lacking.

On close analysis, age is a determinant of men's enquiries, the kinds of information sought and possibly the ways in which they adjust to their illness. When 70-year-old retired prostate cancer patients were compared with employed men below 59 years of age and men 60 years and above, the latter were more likely to request emotional support than the first two groups.[25] It is difficult to predict the reasons why this should be the case, largely as a result of the methods used that preclude ways that might elicit *meaning*[6] but it may conceivably be due to a man's self-perception at a certain stage in life. In any case it highlights the importance of taking age and other life factors into account when talking about the ways in which men respond in the context of cancer. Older men with cancer apparently feel more helpless and hopeless than younger ones.[35] This is likely to be nothing to do with an innate propensity to so-called 'helplessness' in older men, but perhaps more to do with a perception that they are made 'invisible' in the context of illness. Lack of resources may lead to an underfunding of services, but it may also be the case that we make gender assumptions regarding older men in that they are likely to have established relationships with people who will possibly do 'health work' for them,[12] or that they do not require support, including information,[36] in their quest to maintain a veneer of stoicism.

So far, we have illustrated the ways in which men (and women) are depicted in Western society; how they are *expected* to behave, particularly in the context of medicine and how conceptual differences between the sexes hold sway despite evidence to the contrary, leading to unequal services. We have indicated how we as health professionals make assumptions about gender that may impact on health behavior. While important work has been carried out that indicates the ways in which context is important when assessing the ways in which men respond to illness (and health) and the differing conclusions this research engenders[1,21] few investigations have been carried out in the field of cancer that are grounded in men's everyday lives and how the latter may impact on their knowledge regarding cancer and specifically genetic disease.

Men's beliefs and needs regarding genetic cancer

> We men don't know anything about cancer, 100% we don't. … I think it (information) would be welcomed with open arms by men if it was just basically written.
>
> (35-year-old shop owner with father with prostate cancer[31])

We want to turn briefly to work where an indepth interview and qualitative analysis were deployed to explore men's understanding of cancer in general and genetic prostate and testicular disease in particular.[31] No genes have been found for these two cancers, but there is an increased risk for unaffected men with first- or second-degree relatives with the diseases. Most prostate cancers develop in men above the age of 65 years while testicular tumors are most likely to be found in men between the ages of 25 and 35 years. Both cancers are treatable, the latter having an overall 97% cure rate if caught early.[37,38]

The sample consisted of 30 white predominately middle class men who were married with children, and who had (i) a relative in a higher-risk prostate or testicular cancer group or (ii) a relative in a lower-risk group or (iii) no cancer in the family.[31] The mean ages for the 2 groups were 49 and 34 years, respectively – the very ages that will be a focus of interest in a genetic clinic.

Ignorance and uncertainty

Self confessed 'ignorance' and uncertainty regarding cancer cut across age and disease groups and permeated almost all aspects of the men's talk. This was despite their high educational status, and a striking interest in healthy lifestyles. Men with cancer in the family tended to be slightly better informed than those who had never experienced the illness but it was superficial knowledge. Signs, symptoms and management of the cancers were often unheard of or forgotten and body parts strangely 'ungendered'. Some men wondered whether women too had a prostrate while cross-gendered cancer was hard to conceptualize. Cancer was perceived to be a global concept and a terminal disease.

When testicular cancer had been heard of, it was usually in the context of a corporate endeavor such as a football team inspection or when office colleagues had 'let the cat out of the bag'. A few had practised self-examination at the time of their relative's diagnosis but it was performed in a rudimentary way and then forgotten about or practised intermittently 'when the panic was over'. The link between an enlarged testicle and a possible cancer was almost never made. Instead a swelling might symbolize a healthy virility and even a worrying signal that the adjacent testicle might have diminished in size.

Targeted information was perceived as sorely lacking both by older and younger men especially when their situation was compared to women who were thought to be overloaded with facts and figures regarding cancer, especially breast and cervical disease. The majority, younger and older, ruminated about the reasons as to why a national screening campaign had not been set up for them regardless of whether they would actually have participated or not. 'Left out' feelings only reinforced the absence of conventional health practices, and a determination to keep fit by living healthy lifestyles in order that their families were subsidized.

Causes of cancer

> No it's not the gene that dictates . . . there is the environment and there is the outside influence and the internal influence and it's a mixture that puts you in a higher or lower risk . . . at the end it could come down to chance . . .
>
> (<28-year-old man with no cancer in the family[31])

When men were asked to talk about genetic cancer, aspects of their accounts reflected 'scientific' knowledge and the uncertainties inherent in the latter. This was as a result of its accessibility in the popular press including films such as *Jurassic Park* and television programs. However, this knowledge extended itself to the causes of cancer and not to the intricacies of molecular genetics. Causes were thought to revolve equally around heredity and the environment, the former being linked to visibility of clustering patterns both in and outside families, but also to collective habits and social background such as living in the same street, drinking the same water, having the same education, and even watching the same television programs; the latter being akin to receiving identical health messages. Genes were often thought to be embedded within everyone, sometimes developing over time and triggered by stress, food and chemicals or weak bodies as opposed to strong ones, the former being inherited, not the disease.

Risk perceptions

Risk? Me? I don't know, one in 20 ... and testicular cancer ... one in twenty, one in thirty, one in forty maybe one in fifty even ... I don't know anyone or even read about it ... I haven't got a clue ... so why do people get it? Is cancer linked to anything else?

(22-year-old professional footballer with no cancer in the family[31])

I don't feel susceptible to cancer because all the family on my father's side have been very old when they died ... and of other diseases.

(52-year-old company director in high-risk prostate group[31])

Genetic transmission was thought to be linear passing through same-sex family members. Sometimes transmission of cancer was thought to depend on individual traits such as personality, the latter being more likely to be inherited than cancer itself. By what means genes were passed on was not known and not relevant. Perhaps it is not surprising that population and individual risk was under- or overestimated even amongst men whose relative had been in a high-risk group. This often depended on family

longevity, or another life-threatening or chronic illness 'eclipsing' cancer in the family. Sometimes this ignorance depended on biographical factors such as the perceived frailty of a family member and a fear that he might collapse if told bad news; the ways that AIDS had overshadowed all other concerns, or men's preoccupation with a cancer in the family that he was unlikely to be at risk of getting, because of his age.

Respectful silence

I wouldn't talk to anybody about cancer ... it's a very private thing, a very personal thing ... telling them about (a gene) might mark the end of comfortable relationships.

(32-year-old banker with no cancer in the family[31])

Sometimes ignorance relied on the fact that men and their relatives had not spoken about their cancer. Indeed men recounted their dislike of talking about health matters and especially cancer to people in general and especially other men including fathers, sons, brothers and friends. When cancer had been discussed within the family the latter was described as 'talkative' and/or 'close' and in any case even then, details were often whitewashed or forgotten after the initial spate of inquisitiveness, usually after a family member had received a diagnosis of cancer. This silence did not always follow the stereotypical reticence that is supposed to be inherent in men, however. While masculinity, culture, stigma and taboo played their part, reticence concerning cancer was more likely to be about a notion of privacy and a mindfulness that respect was important when it came to telling or asking about bodily details. This 'respect' was extended to men who worked with the opposite sex and who were concerned that talking about men's matters might intrude on women's privacy. In almost all cases, non-communication or silence regarding cancer, was a way of preventing splintered relationships.

Screening

I'd go for genetic screening if they could tell me at what age I was likely to get the gene or the disease ... if someone was to say that is what's going to cause it, then I wouldn't do it ... wouldn't eat it, wouldn't drink it. . .

> (28-year-old man with no cancer in the family[31])

While men bemoaned the ways in which they were exempt from national screening programs, their interest in testing for a gene or screening for a cancer was by no means uniform. Indeed when interest was voiced, it depended on access to knowledge concerning the date of onset of cancer and/or the ways in which advice might be given to stave away disease. Despite the possible anxiety it may cause, having a gene was perceived as a way of paving the way for future life plans for themselves and their families. This especially related to younger men who talked about the heavy onus of family responsibility and the 'relevance' of given information. Single men and those who could not countenance a disease without an illness, revealed the uselessness of knowing that they owned a gene; that other more pressing needs engulfed their daily lives such as work.

Information

> There are a lot more important things to be doing (than looking for cancer information) like making enough money to take the family down to Bognor.
>
> (35-year-old banker with brother with testicular cancer[31])

Ignorance regarding genetics (and other aspects of cancer) was often a deliberate choice. Leisure, work and families separated men from the details of disease while the women in the family were, in these situations, used to disseminating health information. However a renewed inquisitiveness regarding cancer and cancer genetics was contingent on life events such as a marriage or the birth of a baby but they too might be overshadowed by the ways in which the responsibilities of family life took precedence over concerns regarding disease. Rather, responsibility lay in 'keeping fit' in preference to reading health leaflets and taking time off work to go to the doctor over seemingly trivial matters. Long-lasting ailments would indeed be taken to a general practitioner (GP), but only when symptoms were made sense of in terms of

their seriousness. But first, they had to know what 'serious' meant.

> You lot have got to bring the message into the social aspects of young men's lives
>
> (30-year-old night club manager with no cancer in the family[31])

During the interviews men became their own health strategists, musing over and suggesting ways in which much wanted information might be successfully transmitted to them. A 30-year-old night club manager advised that young people's lives were enveloped by 'smoking, drinking, sex and having a good time'. He opined that health educationalists might target them in their relevant social environments although he warned that they had other things to think about besides cancer. A 50-year-old business man suggested the work environment as being a place where health education regarding prostate cancer might be promoted, and where a more serious approach might be taken. A 47-year-old foreman of a factory, suggested that his young male workforce were 'too interested in sex to think about cancer'. He advised that health messages be placed in pornographic magazines that would inevitably 'be read in a lunch break'. Many younger men thought that the GP's surgery didn't necessarily work for them as a repository for information, since they rarely went to one. Older men in the prostate group suggested that their GPs, to whom they looked to for advice, were sometimes unable or too busy to answer questions and seemed to have preferences when it came to testing for prostate cancer, although they were more likely to use primary care services more readily than younger men. One grateful 57-year-old man spoke about a pinned-up message in a toilet in an M1 motorway service break that had provided information regarding colorectal cancer. The place in which that information had been provided, was, he said, 'entirely appropriate!' In any case, time and place were important pointers in terms of 'health work' regardless of age.

Both younger and older men spoke of the ways in which 'bad news' made more impact than bland, uniform information although they preferred the straightforward truth. However, the men were concerned about being patronized, and felt that information should center on basic, plainly written facts but only if they were relevant to their everyday lives. Leaflets and brochures were often read superficially and/or simply 'binned' when they bore no relevance to a man's situation or when they were written in a way that they found they could not understand. This did not depend on educational status but was more likely to be linked to events in their daily lives and the difficulty of believing unreliable and contradictory health messages given by a health profession that induced cynicism and mistrust. Many men, but by no means all, spoke of the internet as a means of information, but often described as 'overload' and out of date. A few subscribed to men's health magazines but found them generally unhelpful in terms of cancer.

Responsibility regarding their health was evident, but always in the wake of perceived exclusion from scientific discourse. This was seen in the striking ways in which the men continually asked questions concerning prostate and testicular disease as they spoke to the interviewer.

Discussion

There are limitations to the study referred to above. Men from lower socioeconomic groups and those from ethnic minorities are conspicuously absent. More research is required that will shed light on these groups as well as families and the perceptions of health professionals in the context of caring for men and especially in the domain of genetic cancer. Nevertheless the study highlights the ways that men's so-called 'irresponsible' approach to their health is far from being a global truth and does not wholly rely on women to orchestrate health matters in the family. The relatively young sample of men in our study showed a striking display of responsibility towards their jobs and families. Like men in other samples and in other contexts,[1] all were aware of the dangers of smoking, the consumption of alcohol, eating too much and exercising too little and where possible, they had adhered to these health messages. As Watson[1] points out, it is not always entirely clear as to whether these messages have been taken on board as a result of assimilating knowledge or

changes in structural factors such as the environment, community facilities, work situations or social factors such as becoming a father or a husband (pp 142–3). It is likely to be (at least in part) about the latter if we consider how men explained their interest in cancer genetics in the light of life events as 'triggers' to action.

The ideology of a stereotypical masculinity was evident, in, for example, the ways that men were mindful of 'keeping well' in order to do their jobs; the latter being symbolic of their roles as breadwinners. This focus on employment is substantiated by others when they illustrate the ways that men live out 'masculinities' in the public realm of work.[11,20] It was also about the *meaning* of being a family man. Men's relationship to medicine relied on gender relations and to the ways in which the constraints of life helped to dictate their responses and behaviors. This reveals a much more complicated picture of men's relationship with health and illness than is given in the mainstream literature.

It may be a reality that aspects of the life course help to obscure or illuminate the importance of risk for illness and disease. This will make men *seem* like selfish risk takers when they are not perceived as responsible punters. It is as well to remember again that these were men in upper socioeconomic groups but it would not be surprising if social class and masculinity were conflated in the sense that men's ways of 'doing' health work construes altruism as *gendered* practice.[1] Interestingly however, similar ways of displaying a moral obligation to look after families by working have also been found to be the case amongst single mothers and in the context of genetic cancer.[39]

While so called 'ignorance' and uncertainty is palpable amongst this UK sample, it is also found in other populations outside Britain.[40,41] Ignorance is not, however, confined to men. Studies have shown the ways in which women mistake their risk[42] and their knowledge of cancer genetics is known to be at 'odds' with Mendelian theory[43] but nevertheless has its own internal rationality.[44] Indeed 'ignorance' is a misnomer in this context. Those who do not take ignorance at its face value mirror our questioning of the concept, but in other populations where people perceive themselves to be excluded in terms of relevant facts concerning science.[13] In this sample, cancer information was found to be elusive and when it was available, it was confusing or irrelevant.

Information is not necessarily passed on by family members and this also lends itself to a seeming withdrawal from matters relating to health and illness and in this case cancer genetics. In our sample, men were hesitant about talking to each other about this and other diseases partly as a result of masculine ideology, but also because of their need for privacy and respect. This so-called silence is crucial in the context of genetic disease where, at least in the early stages, communication between families is a prerequisite for testing. This reticence has, however, been reported elsewhere[45] and has been found to be the case amongst women who also have difficulty in 'selecting' people with whom they want to share their cancer talk.[46] Communication between family members in the light of genetics, requires very careful thought. People's wishes and the difficulties of disclosure must be taken into consideration and respected. Health professionals would do well to think through the options that might alleviate these difficulties and to provide choice to would-be consumers.

Where cancer and genetic disease are concerned, health professionals need to be alert to the ways in which they may be absenting men from relevant facts about all aspects of cancer; that there are many similarities in women's responses in this context,[39,42,46] and yet men's voices are seldom heard.[1,6] We cannot know about men's practices, needs and understanding and they, in turn, cannot be expected to meet conventional rules of assessing care, if we leave them out of research and at the same time make assumptions that help to legitimate the withholding of information. Information giving is, however, by no means a simple exercise.[36] Men in the sample indicated that not only would the assimilation of information depend on context, but interest in screening and cancer genetic testing would be precipitated by advice concerning prevention and age of disease onset. This kind of expectation requires clarification, as do many other aspects regarding cancer and cancer genetics. The assimilation of knowledge will, however, depend on transparency and clarity, *as well as* relevancy,

tailored to specific groups of men in order that the 'noise' surrounding them at specific time points in their lives is taken into account. By doing so we will be closer to giving men equal delivery of health services and opportunities to make choices that will possibly be conducive to healthier outcomes for everyone.

Acknowledgments

First, we would like to thank the men who have spoken to us about their understanding regarding cancer and cancer genetics. Second, we would like to thank our funders, Cancer Research UK and the Bob Champion Cancer Trust. Last but not least, we would like to acknowledge our colleagues, both in the Academic Department of Radiotherapy and the Department of Psychological Medicine, although we take full responsibility for the argument set forward here.

References

1. Watson J. Male Bodies, Health, Culture and Identity. Buckingham, Philadelphia: Open University Press, 2000.
2. Department of Health. On the State of the Public Health. The Annual Report of the Chief Medical Officer of the Department of Health. London: HMSO, 1992.
3. Men's Health. BMJ 2001; 323.
4. Everyman Campaign. Institute of Cancer Research. London: Sutton UK.
5. Lloyd T. Men's Health Review. London: Royal College of Nursing, 1996.
6. Moynihan C. Men, women, gender and cancer. Eur J Cancer Care 2002; 11: 166–72.
7. Griffiths S. Inequalities in men's health. In: Davidson N, Lloyd T (eds). Promoting Men's Health: A Guide for Practitioners. London: Bailliere Tindall, 2001.
8. Waldron I. Sex differences in illness incidence, prognosis and mortality: Issues and evidence. Soc Sci Med 1983; 17: 1107–11.
9. Kandrack M, Grant K, Segall A. Gender differences in health related behaviour: some unanswered questions. Soc Sci Med 1991; 32: 579–90.

10. Health Education Authority. Men's attitudes to health checks and awareness of male-specific cancers. London: Health Education Authority, 1996.

11. Seidler VJ. Men, heterosexualities and emotional life. In: Pile S, Thrift N (eds). Mapping the Subject: Geographies of Cultural Transformation. London: Routledge, 1996; 170–91.

12. Northcross W, Ramirez C, Palinkas L. The influence of women on health care seeking behaviour of men. J Fam Pract 1960; 43: 475–80.

13. Michael M. Knowing ignorance and ignoring knowledge: discourses of ignorance in the public understanding of science. In: Irwin A, Wynne B (eds). Misunderstanding Science? The Public Reconstruction of Science and Technology. Cambridge University Press, 1996; 107–26.

14. Nathanson CA. Illness and the feminine role: a theoretical review. Soc Sci Med 1975; 57–60.

15. Waldron I. Sex differences in human mortality: the role of genetics. Soc Sci Med 1983; 17: 321–6.

16. MacIntyre S, Hunt K, Sweeting H. Gender differences in health: are things really as simple as they seem? Soc Sci Med 1996; 42: 617–24.

17. Verbrugge LM. Role burdens and physical health of women and men. Women Health 1986; 11: 47–77.

18. Doyal L. Sex, gender and health: the need for a new approach. BMJ 2001; 323: 1061–3.

19. Harrison J, Chin J, Ficarrotto T. Warning: masculinity may damage your health. In: Kimmel M, Messner M (eds). Men's Lives. New York: Macmillan, 1992.

20. Moynihan C. Theories in health care and research. Theories of masculinity. BMJ 1998; 317: 1072–5.

21. Schofield T, Connell R, Walker L et al. Understanding men's health and illness: a gender relations approach to policy, research and practice. J Am Coll Health 2000; 48: 247–58.

22. Verbrugge LM. Gender and health: an update on hypotheses and evidence. J Health Soc Behav 1985; 26: 156–82.

23. Marshall JR, Funch DP. Gender and illness behaviour among colorectal cancer patients. Women Health 1986; 11: 67–82.

24. Ramirez AJ, Graham J, Richards M, Cull A, Gregory W. Mental health of hospital consultants: the effects of stress and satisfaction at work. Lancet 1996; 347: 724–8.

25. Stacey M. The Sociology of Health and Healing. University of Warwick: Routledge, 1991.

26. Sayers J. Sexual contradictions: psychology, psychoanalysis and feminism. London: Tavistock. In: Watson J (ed). Male Bodies: Health, Culture and Identity. Buckingham, Philadelphia: Open University Press, 2000: 35.

27. Boudioni M, McPherson K, Moynihan C et al. Do men with prostate or colorectal cancer seek different information and support from women with cancer? Br J Cancer 2001; 85: 641–8.

28. Hunt K, Ford G, Harkins L, Wyke S. Are women more ready to consult than men? Gender differences in family practitioner consultation for common chronic conditions. J Health Serv Res Policy. 4: 96–100.

29. Bradlow J, Coulter A, Brooks P. Patterns of referral. Oxford: Health Services Research Unit, 1992.

30. Chilvers C, Saunders M, Bliss J et al. Influence of delay in diagnosis on prognosis in testicular cancer. Br J Cancer 1989; 89: 126–8.

31. Moynihan C, Burton S, Huddart R et al. Men's Understanding of Genetic Cancer with Special Reference to Testicular and Prostate Disease. London: Cancer Research UK, 1999.

32. Slevin M, Terry, Hallett N et al. BACUP – the first two years: evaluation of a national cancer information service. BMJ 1988; 297: 699–72.

33. Gray R, Fitch M, Davis C et al. Interviews with men with prostate cancer about their self help group experience. J Palliat Care 2000; 13: 15–21.

34. Lintz K, Moynihan C, Steginga S et al. Prostate cancer patients' support and psychological care needs: survey from a non-surgical oncology clinic. Psychooncol 2003; 12: 769–83.

35. Akechi T, Okamura H, Yamawaki S, Uchitomi Y. Predictors of patients' mental adjustment to cancer: patient characteristics and 'social support'. Br J Cancer 1998; 77: 2381–3.

36. Leydon GM, Boulton M, Moynihan C et al. Cancer patients' information needs and information seeking behaviour: in depth interview study. BMJ 2000; 320: 909–13.

37. Cancer Research Campaign. Cancer of the prostate. Fact-sheet. 1994; 20: 1–6.

38. Cancer Research Campaign. Testicular Cancer UK Fact-sheet. 1998; 16: 1–6.

39. Hallowell N. Doing the right thing: genetic risk and responsibility. Sociol Health Illness 1999; 597–621.

40. Fitzpatrick P, Concoran N, Fitzpartick J. Prostate cancer: how aware is the public? Br J Urol 1998; 82(1): 43–8.

41. Brett T. Patients' attitudes to prostate cancer. Aust Fam Phys 1998; 27: 584–8.

42. Evans D, Burnell L, Hopwood P, Howell A. Perception of risk in women with a family history of breast cancer. Br J Cancer 1993; 67: 612–14.

43. Richards M. The new genetics: some issues for social scientists. Sociol Health Illness 1993; 15(5): 567–86.

44. Horton R. African traditional thought and Western science. In: Marwick M (ed). Witchcraft, Sorcery and Magic. Harmondsworth: Penguin, 1971.

45. Arar N, Thompson I, Sarosdy M et al. Risk perceptions among patients and their relatives regarding prostate cancer and its heredity. Prostate Cancer Prostatic Dis 2000; 176–185.

46. Julien-Reynier C, Eisinger FA, Vennin P et al. Attitudes towards cancer predictive testing and transmission of information to the family. J Med Genet 1996; 33: 731–6.

CHAPTER 3

Prostate cancer

Roger S Kirby

Introduction

Prostate cancer is the most enigmatic of the common malignancies. Second only to lung cancer as a killer of men beyond middle age, it clearly warrants much more attention than it currently receives from governments, researchers, and particularly the general public worldwide. One major reason for this neglect is the observation that the majority of men as they age harbor small foci of adenocarcinoma within their prostate that often never become clinically significant.[1] As a consequence, worries about over-diagnosis and over-treatment have surfaced and turned many doctors away from the task of identifying and treating earlier the more aggressive lesions that so commonly cause significant morbidity and mortality.

In fact, the time has come to abandon the prevalent attitude of nihilism about prostate cancer, because, potentially, much morbidity could be avoided and many lives saved. A number of new ways are becoming available to distinguish the higher-risk 'tigers' from the low-risk 'pussy cats'. Sequential, rather than one-off, prostate-specific antigen (PSA) determination allows an analysis of PSA kinetics, and new gene-based tests, such as measurements of PCA3 and other molecular markers, look promising as predictors of tumor behavior. Better staging of cancer by magnetic resonance imaging (MRI) now allows us to identify more accurately those patients who are either likely or unlikely to benefit from surgery. Advances in technology, with for example the da Vinci robot, have improved the patient experience of radical prostatectomy. And finally, at last new approaches to the management of hormone-relapsed prostate cancer look increasingly promising. This chapter aims to analyze some of these new developments and set them against the background of what is already established about this very common cause of morbidity and mortality among men.

Risk factors

Despite the high incidence of prostate cancer, relatively little is known about the fundamental causes of the disease. However, a number of risk factors have been established.

Aging
Age is the greatest factor influencing the development of prostate cancer. Clinical disease is rather rare in men under the age of 50 years, and the incidence increases markedly in men aged over 60 years of age. As the population of the world continues to age, this disease seems certain to increase in its impact.

Race
There are marked geographical and ethnic variations in the incidence of clinical prostate cancer.

The risk is highest in North America and northern European countries, and lowest in the Far East. In the USA, the risk is higher in blacks than in whites, and blacks also appear to develop the disease earlier. Chinese and Japanese races show the lowest incidence of prostate cancer. The incidence of latent disease, however, is similar in all populations studied. In migration studies, the incidence of prostate cancer in men who have emigrated from a low-risk area to a high-risk area increases to that of the local population within two generations. This suggests that environmental influences such as diet and nutrition may have marked effects either on the development of prostate cancer or on the progression of histological cancer to a clinically detectable cancer.

Family history

Approximately 9% of all cases of prostate cancer have a genetic basis.[2] A number of hereditary prostate cancer genes have been localized; the first was on the short arm of chromosome 1. Others have been localized to 1q42.2–43, Xq27–28, p36, 20q13, 16q23, 8p22–23, 17p11 and 22q. Testing for these genes is not yet routinely available but may become so soon. The risk of a man developing prostate cancer if he has a first-degree relative affected is increased approximately 2.5-fold. Currently there is interest in the possibility of modifying prostate cancer risk factors with 5-alpha-reductase inhibitors such as finasteride and dutasteride.[3] Dietary modification by reducing the intake of saturated fats may also be important.

Histological features

Most prostate cancers turn out to be an adenocarcinoma on histological analysis and to arise in the peripheral zone of the gland (>70%). Approximately 5–15% arise in the central zone and the remainder in the transition zone, which is where benign prostatic hyperplasia (BPH) also develops, and tumors there can be difficult to detect.

Microscopic foci of 'latent' prostate cancer are a common autopsy finding and may appear very early in life; approximately 30% of men over 50 years of age have evidence of so-called latent disease. Because of the very slow growth rate of these microscopic tumors, many never progress to clinical disease. Beyond a certain size, however, these lesions progressively de-differentiate, owing to clonal selection, and become increasingly invasive. A tumor that has a volume greater than $0.5\,cm^3$ or that is anything other than well differentiated is generally regarded as clinically significant.

The Gleason system

The Gleason system is the most widely used system for grading prostate cancer. It recognizes five levels of increasing aggressiveness.

- Grade 1 tumors consist of small, uniform glands with minimal nuclear changes.
- Grade 2 tumors have medium-sized acini, still separated by stromal tissue, but more closely arranged.
- Grade 3 tumors, the most common finding, show marked variation in glandular size and organization, and generally show infiltration of stromal and neighboring tissues.
- Grade 4 tumors show marked cytological atypia with extensive infiltration.
- Grade 5 tumors are characterized by sheets of undifferentiated cancer cells.

Because prostatic cancers are often heterogeneous, the numbers of the two most widely represented grades are added together to produce the Gleason score (e.g. 3+4). This score (or sum) provides useful prognostic information; Gleason scores above 4 are associated with a progressive risk of more rapid disease progression, increased metastatic potential, and decreased survival. A meta-analysis of patients being managed by active surveillance, for example, found that the annual rate of developing metastases was 2.1% in patients with Gleason scores of less than 4, compared with 5.4% in patients with scores between 5 and 7, and 13.5% in patients with scores above 7. The chance of relapse after radical prostatectomy has also been shown to be directly proportional to the percentage of Gleason grade 4 and 5 cancer in the specimen.

Prostate cancer screening and presentation

The past decade has seen a significant downward shift in the stage at presentation of prostate cancer in most countries. Historically, most men with significant disease presented with a combination of weight loss, bone pain, lethargy, and bladder outflow obstruction, features attributable to locally advanced or metastatic disease. Increasingly, however, the disease is being diagnosed incidentally by prostate cancer screening in younger, asymptomatic patients or as an incidental histological finding following a transurethral resection of the prostate (TURP) for benign obstructive symptoms. This earlier presentation of prostate cancer has posed difficult dilemmas for clinicians and patients concerning management, and the increasing life expectancy of patients underscores the need for effective, evidence-based diagnosis and treatment regimens.

Early detection of prostate cancer

In general, the earlier prostate cancer is detected, the better the outlook for the patient in terms of cure or arresting cancer progression. Most patients in whom prostate cancer is suspected are identified on the basis of abnormal findings on digital rectal examination (DRE) or, more commonly now, by raised PSA levels. An increasing majority of patients present simply with an isolated increase in PSA or a change in PSA kinetics.

Digital rectal examination
DRE is the simplest, safest, and most cost-effective means of detecting prostate cancer, provided that the tumor is posteriorly situated and is sufficiently large to be palpable. The test can be performed with the patient either in the left lateral position or standing and leaning forwards; with either approach only the posterior portion of the gland is palpable. In addition to providing information on the size of the prostate, DRE can reveal a number of features that may indicate prostate cancer. However, only around one-third of suspicious prostatic nodules are actually confirmed as malignant when analyzed histologically after transrectal biopsy.

Prostate-specific antigen
PSA is a glycoprotein responsible for liquefying semen. PSA measurement is the most effective single screening test for early detection of prostate cancer; in fact, it can detect more than twice as many prostate cancers as DRE. However, the predictive value is increased further if the measurement is combined, as it always should be, with DRE. PSA determinations may also be useful in the staging of prostate cancer and evaluating the response to therapy.

Approximately 25% of men with PSA levels above the normal range ($\geq$4 ng/mL) have prostate cancer, and the risk increases to more than 60% in men with PSA levels above 10 ng/mL.[4] A recent study in prostate cancer prevention, in which all men in the placebo group received a biopsy, reported that the incidence of prostate cancer in men with PSA less than 4 ng/mL and normal DRE was high.[5] The median PSA and 95th percentile values for the 'normal' population at each age group have been determined. A significant percentage of men with PSA values below the 95th percentile will harbor prostate cancer. There is no clear agreement on the best PSA cut-off at which men should be biopsied. A cut-off of 4.0 ng/mL has been used, but it has been shown that a cut-off at 2.5 ng/mL will double the cancer detection rate from 18% to 36% in men younger than 60 years, and will have a minimal negative effect on specificity.

It is clear that PSA is by no means a perfect test, as many men with mildly elevated PSA values do not have prostate cancer. As a result, several different concepts have been developed over the past few years to improve the clinical value of the test in detecting early prostate cancer. These so-called PSA derivatives include PSA density, PSA velocity, age-specific reference ranges, and differential assay of the different molecular forms of serum PSA. All of these have been proposed in an attempt to enhance the utility of PSA with regard to detecting early prostate cancer at a curable stage and to reduce the number of negative transrectal biopsies. In practical terms, only the molecular forms (free:total PSA ratio) and PSA velocity calculation are clinically useful, since they can help the physician and patient to decide whether and when to proceed to a transrectal biopsy.

Prostate-specific antigen density

PSA density is calculated by dividing the total PSA by the prostate volume. A PSA density above 0.15 ng/mL has been shown to increase the specificity of the PSA test. This modification does, however, have many potential sources of error, such as volume calculation, assay variability, and sampling bias.

Prostate-specific antigen

PSA velocity refers to the rate of PSA change with time, usually over 1 or 2 years, with a minimum of three readings. A velocity above 0.75 ng/mL/year has been used to predict the presence of prostate cancer. More recent studies have shown that the average PSA velocity of men without prostate cancer is 0.03 ng/mL/year compared with 0.4 ng/mL/year in men ultimately diagnosed with prostate cancer. Problems associated with PSA velocity include inaccuracy of velocity calculation over short time periods and insufficient numbers of measurements. However the rate of rise in PSA prior to diagnosis has been linked to risk of eventual death from prostate cancer.[6]

Molecular forms

PSA exists in the serum in several molecular forms; most of it is bound to protein, but some is unbound or 'free'. Studies show that patients with BPH but not prostate cancer have a higher amount of free PSA, while men with prostate cancer appear to have a greater amount of PSA complexed with α_1-antichymotrypsin. Measuring the concentration of these different molecular forms in the serum is a clinically useful way to distinguish men who have BPH from men with early prostate cancer. The currently accepted cut-off point of the ratio of free: total PSA is 0.15. Men with ratios below this should be considered for further investigation, including transrectal prostatic biopsies.

PCA3 testing and other markers

One particular test showing promise is the PCA3 test. This test detects the mRNA in voided urine of the PCA3 gene, which is highly over-expressed in prostate cancer. The levels are then compared with PSA mRNA in the urine. At a sensitivity of 50%, this test has a specificity of 76%, which is substantially better than PSA. Other promising new bio-markers include the tissue methylation markers *GSTP1* and *APC*, as well as serum marker proPSA and *EPCA-2*. However, trials in large populations are required to determine their true utility.

Screening

The value of screening asymptomatic men for prostate cancer is controversial. As mentioned, there is a great discrepancy between the incidence of clinically significant disease and the prevalence of microscopic disease, and identification of those men in whom disease progression is probable remains inexact. Two randomized trials testing the ability of prostate cancer screening to reduce mortality have several years to run before reporting.[7] Until the results are available, the practice of screening remains controversial. Prostate cancer screening potentially has the greatest benefit in younger men, who have a greater life expectancy. Groups that advocate screening generally suggest screening between the ages of 50 and 70 years – earlier if the patient has a family history. Screening is generally not beneficial in elderly men, or men with significant comorbidities, who have reduced life expectancy and are likely to die from other causes.

The family physician has an important role in assessing the likely benefits and risks for individual patients according to their age and life expectancy; appropriate counseling of the patient and his immediate family is an essential element of this process.

Clinical symptoms

Patients with prostate cancer may present with a variety of symptoms.

Localized cancer

When the cancer is localized, it is generally asymptomatic. The man presents with symptoms of BPH, in which the benign prostatic tissue compresses and obstructs the urethra, resulting in frequency, hesitancy, and poor flow. Prostate cancer may present as an 'incidental' finding after TURP; nowadays, less than 10% of men undergoing TURP for BPH are found to have microscopic foci of prostate cancer.

Locally advanced cancers

Locally advanced cancers (usually palpable by DRE) may cause symptoms resulting from local extension of the tumor, such as irritative symptoms (frequency, urgency) caused by invasion of the bladder trigone and pelvic nerves. Involvement of the perineal or suprapubic nerves can lead to pain, and thus the possibility of prostate cancer should be considered in the investigation of prostatitis-like symptoms.

Hematuria can occur from erosion of the cancer into the urethra or bladder. Loin pain can occur because of ureteric obstruction and hydronephrosis. Symptoms of bladder outlet obstruction can occur when a large prostate cancer obstructs the bladder outlet, as occurs in BPH. Invasion of the urethral sphincter or surgery itself may cause urinary incontinence. It is important to exclude the possibility that incontinence is a result of chronic urinary retention with overflow, which may be amenable to treatment with procedures such as TURP.

Metastatic disease

The most common presenting symptom is pain resulting from bony metastases, particularly in the pelvis and lumbar spine. Thus the sudden onset of progressive low back or pelvic pain is an important diagnostic feature of metastatic prostate cancer. Pathological fractures may also occur, particularly affecting the neck of the femur. Metastases within the vertebrae, sometimes leading to spinal cord compression, are not uncommon and may produce backache or neurological symptoms in up to 12% of affected men.

Metastasis into the lymph nodes may result in lymph node enlargement. Intra-abdominal lymph node metastasis usually begins in the obturator and internal iliac nodes and spreads to the iliac nodes and beyond; it may, with local tumors, result in obstruction of the ureters. In advanced disease, lymphatic involvement may extend to the thoracic, cervical, inguinal, and axillary nodes. Lymph node metastases may produce a number of symptoms, including palpable swellings, loin pain or anuria caused by obstruction of the ureters, and swelling of the lower limbs as a result of lymphedema.

Systemic metastases in the liver, lungs, or elsewhere may produce non-specific symptoms, such as lethargy resulting from anemia or uremia, weight loss, and cachexia.

Management of localized disease

The aim of treatment in patients with localized prostate cancer is usually cure – whether eliminating the tumor or preventing death from prostate cancer (as opposed to death with prostate cancer). As men with localized disease often do not experience significant disease-related morbidity for several years after diagnosis, and curative treatment itself may result in some morbidity, those with a shorter life expectancy are likely to benefit least from radical treatment.

Radical prostatectomy

Radical prostatectomy involves surgically removing the entire prostate, the seminal vesicles, and a variable amount of adjacent tissue. It is appropriate for men for whom it is believed the tumor can be removed completely by surgery. The procedure is most commonly performed via the retropubic route, though the perineal approach can also be used. The major advantage of radical prostatectomy is that it excises all prostatic tissue and provides precise histological information and definitive cure in patients in whom the tumor is specimen-confined. Thus, the patient's anxiety is relieved during the postoperative period; given that prostate cancer has a long natural history, this is an important consideration in terms of the patient's quality of life. Long-term studies have shown normal life expectancies in those with complete excision of specimen-confined disease. Ten-year survival for men with clinically localized disease treated with radical prostatectomy is 98%, 91%, and 76% for Gleason scores 2–4, 5–7, and 8–10, respectively. Moreover, the procedure also offers definitive treatment of concomitant BPH.

The principal adverse events associated with radical prostatectomy are persistent urinary incontinence (<2–3%) and erectile dysfunction (>50%); the latter is age-related, tends to improve with time, and can be minimized by nerve-sparing approaches.

Moreover, erectile dysfunction after surgery can now be treated effectively.

Radical prostatectomy, by whichever means achieved, is believed by many urologists to offer the best opportunity for cure in patients with localized prostate cancer. A randomized study from Sweden showed that at a median 8.2 years' follow-up, radical prostatectomy decreased prostate-cancer-related mortality by 44% and overall death by 26% when compared with watchful waiting.[8] The difference was largest in men under 65 years of age. Because the total number of prostate-cancer-related deaths was low, it would require 20 men to undergo prostatectomy to save one man from death. A similar study known as the PIVOT trial is fully recruited in the USA, and results will be available in 2009. Meanwhile, it seems reasonable to discuss the option of radical prostatectomy with younger men with clinically localized disease and no significant cardiovascular or pulmonary comorbidity.

Laparoscopic and robotically assisted radical prostatectomy

Laparoscopic and robotically assisted radical prostatectomy has recently been developed. It can be facilitated by robotic assistance. The results of the procedure to date appear broadly equivalent to open radical prostatectomy. The operating time is usually longer, but blood loss and length of hospital stay are reduced. The advent of the da Vinci robot has made the technically demanding process of laparoscopic radical prostatectomy much quicker and easier to learn (Fig. 3.1).[9] The 10-fold magnification and three-dimensional vision allows very precise nerve sparing and a much more accurate anastomosis between the bladder and urethra.[10] Debate is ongoing about whether eventual outcomes will be improved by these innovations.

External-beam radiotherapy

External-beam radiotherapy is widely used in the treatment of localized prostate cancer; it offers a particular advantage in patients who are unsuitable for surgery because of comorbidity or evidence of extraprostatic extension of cancer. The treatment generally involves a 7-week course of radiotherapy. Ten-year survival of patients undergoing external-beam radiation for clinically localized, prostate cancer with Gleason scores 2–4, 5–7, and 8–10 is reported to be approximately 89%, 74%, and 52%, respectively.

The principal side effects are due to bladder, urethra, and rectal damage from the radiation scatter. Urinary frequency and urgency are common. In its severe form, urinary bleeding and pain may occur in 2–3% of patients. Rectal side effects consist of urgency, frequency, and tenesmus. If severe, rectal bleeding, pain, or fistula may very occasionally require a colostomy. Erectile dysfunction due to damage to the neurovascular supply to the corpora cavernosa can also occur, typically over a 6–18-month period.

A number of studies have shown better cancer control for men with intermediate- or high-risk prostate cancer if the radiation dose is escalated to 78 Gy or higher. The advent of intensity-modulated radiotherapy (IMRT) allows more precise targeting of the prostate, with less radiation scatter to surrounding organs. As a consequence, higher doses can be given to men without a significant increase in local toxicity. Several studies have confirmed that the outcomes are improved by the use of adjuvant androgen ablation for 3 months prior to irradiation therapy and during the therapy,[11] especially in higher-risk, locally advanced cases.

Low-dose brachytherapy

Low-dose brachytherapy involves placing either iodine-125 or palladium-103 seeds into the prostate via the transperineal route, using a template and transrectal ultrasound (TRUS) guidance.[12] The results of seed brachytherapy in low-risk men (PSA <10 ng/mL, Gleason score <7 and ≤ cT2b) is equivalent to radical prostatectomy at 10 years, but they are highly dependent on the quality of seed placement. The results in patients with intermediate risk are worse, however, with freedom from recurrence approximately 66% at 10 years. The method is gaining popularity, particularly in the USA, because of its low morbidity – the side effects are similar in nature to those of external-beam radiotherapy, but they also include voiding dysfunction caused by swelling of the prostate after treatment, resulting in obstruction.

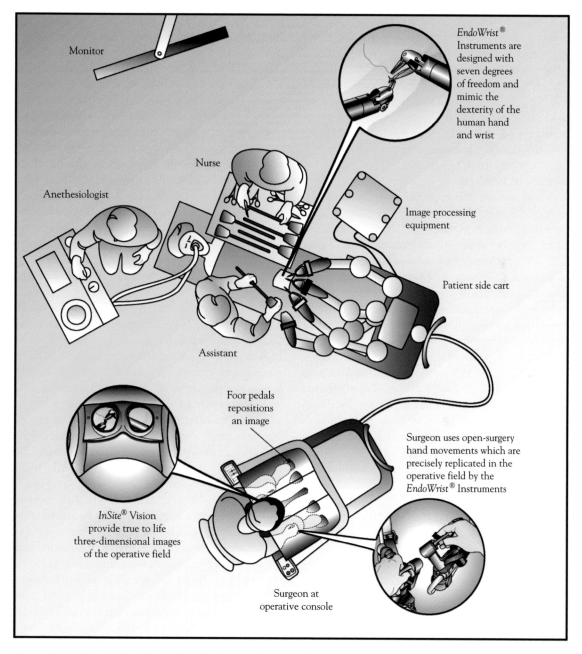

Figure 3.1. *The da Vinci Surgical Robot in a urology procedure setting.*

Active surveillance

Active surveillance is traditionally reserved for men with small-volume and low-to-moderate-grade prostate cancer, who have a low risk of death from prostate cancer. These men would be eligible for curative therapy, but this option is deferred until objective signs of biological activity are observed. This approach means the majority of men are spared the side effects of curative therapy when they do not require it.[13]

During active surveillance, men are followed closely with repeated PSA measurements and DREs and regular prostate biopsies, as well as MRI scans. If the cancer appears to change significantly, curative therapy is initiated before the cancer becomes incurable.[14] While men avoid the physical side effects of cancer treatment, they have to live with the psychological effects of having an untreated cancer; however, this does not seem to be too troublesome.

Watchful waiting

Watchful waiting differs from active surveillance in that it is utilized for men who are older or who have shorter life expectancy and who have prostate cancer that is unlikely to shorten their life. These men are counseled, and reviewed regularly with clinical examination and PSA measurements. When disease progression is identified, instead of having curative therapy, palliative androgen deprivation is initiated. This is continued until death. In a recent meta-analysis, the development of metastatic disease during watchful waiting was reported to be 2.1% per year in patients with well-differentiated tumors (Gleason scores 2–4) and 13.5% per year in patients with aggressive tumors (Gleason scores 7–10). In another study, patients with low-grade tumors treated with watchful waiting had a 92% disease-specific survival at 10 years compared with 76% and 43% for moderate-grade and high-grade tumors, respectively.

High-intensity focused ultrasound

High-intensity focused ultrasound (HIFU) technology has been developed to treat localized prostate cancer. A specially designed probe delivers HIFU transrectally to the prostate and achieves focal tissue destruction. Early results are promising, with 94% of men reported to be disease free at 3 years' follow-up.[15] HIFU can also be used for the treatment of cancer recurrence after radiotherapy. Urinary incontinece as well as fistulae have been reported as a result of this treatment. The method should currently be regarded as experimental and restricted to clinical studies.

Cryoablation

Freezing temperatures can be used to destroy prostatic tissue. Under TRUS guidance, a number of cryogenic probes are inserted into the prostate via the perineum. Liquid nitrogen is then circulated through the probes, producing 'ice balls' with a temperature of approximately $-180°C$ that disrupt cell membranes, thereby destroying the surrounding tissue. The urethra is protected by circulating warm (44°C) water through a catheter. Although some studies have reported outcomes comparable with those achieved by radical prostatectomy, others have reported a significant incidence of complications such as rectal and urethral damage.[16] No long-term, randomized, controlled trials have yet compared cryoablation with more established treatments, and most still regard it as investigational.

Management of metastatic disease

Although there is an increasing trend towards earlier detection of prostate cancer, many men still present with metastatic disease. In countries where PSA testing is not widely used, around 30% of patients present with localized disease, 40% with locally advanced disease, and the remaining 30% with metastases. In contrast to localized or locally advanced disease, metastatic prostate cancer is associated with high mortality – approximately 70% within 5 years. Androgen deprivation, which has become the mainstay of treatment, effectively reduces intraprostatic dihydrotestosterone (DHT) concentration by over 80%, resulting in reduced androgen receptor stimulation and increased prostate cancer apoptosis. Androgen deprivation can be achieved by orchidectomy or treatment with luteinizing hormone-releasing hormone (LHRH) analogs, and the value of adding an antiandrogen (maximal androgen blockade) is still debated. Pure LHRH antagonists are currently under investigation, but are not yet approved by regulatory authorities.

Orchidectomy

Bilateral orchidectomy or bilateral subcapsular orchidectomy is performed through a midline scrotal incision under local, regional, or light general anesthesia. The procedure is simple and is associated with little morbidity. The principal adverse events that may occur after orchidectomy are local complications such as hematoma and wound infections, together with general complications of androgen deprivation such as loss of libido, erectile dysfunction, and hot flashes. Clinical responses (decreased bone pain and reduced PSA concentration) are obtained in more than 75% of patients. Because of the psychological and cosmetic impact of orchidectomy, however, most patients prefer reversible non-surgical treatment with LHRH analogs.

Luteinizing hormone-releasing hormone analogs

LHRH analogs, such as goserelin acetate, buserelin, and leuprolide, are highly potent LHRH agonists (superagonists). After administration, there is a transient initial increase in luteinizing hormone (LH) secretion, and hence in testosterone secretion; this is followed by desensitization (downregulation), resulting in a fall in LH and testosterone secretion. These agents can be delivered via 1-, 3-, or 6-monthly depot preparations administered subcutaneously or intramuscularly. A potential side effect is tumor 'flare', which 8–32% of patients experience as a result of the initial transient increase (140–170%) in testosterone. This may result in increased bone pain or worsening of symptoms of bladder outflow obstruction; spinal metastases may also be stimulated, increasing a risk of spinal cord compression. Tumor flare can be avoided by prior and concomitant administration of an antiandrogen during the first 6 weeks of treatment. Comparative trials have shown that the response rates obtained with LHRH analogs are equivalent to those obtained after orchidectomy in terms of time to progression and overall survival.

Luteinizing hormone-releasing hormone antagonists

Recently, pure LHRH antagonists have been developed and tested. These peptides inhibit LHRH release without the initial stimulation seen with LHRH analogs by blocking pituitary receptors, and thus they are not associated with a surge in testosterone ('flare'). This results in a more rapid achievement of the castrate state. More rapid return of testosterone with intermittent application is potentially an additional benefit. However, none of these agents is currently licensed for clinical use.

Antiandrogens

Antiandrogens are taken in tablet form, and do not alter the levels of circulating androgens. Instead, they inhibit the androgen receptor where testosterone or DHT binds. There are two classes of these drugs. The steroidal antiandrogens (e.g. cyproterone acetate) also have a central testosterone-lowering effect and can be taken as monotherapy instead of castration. The non-steroidal antiandrogens inhibit the androgen receptor only and cannot be taken as monotherapy for metastatic disease.[17]

Intermittent hormonal therapy

It has been suggested that continuous androgen ablation therapy may, in fact, increase the rate of progression of prostate cancer to an androgen-independent state. For this reason, attention is currently focused on the use of intermittent hormonal therapy which also has the potential advantage of decreasing the side effects of therapy. In this approach, hormone therapy is initially given for approximately 9 months. Intermittent therapy becomes an option for men in whom there is a response to therapy with PSA levels becoming normalized, and their LHRH analog therapy is temporarily discontinued, the so-called 'hormone holiday'.

Hormone therapy is resumed when the serum PSA concentration returns to pre-treatment levels in patients who had a PSA at diagnosis of <20 ng/mL, or when PSA increases to >20 ng/mL in patients with an initial PSA above this. Such a regimen allows serum testosterone to return to normal, thereby stimulating atrophic cells and rendering them more sensitive to androgen ablation. The use of a pure LHRH antagonist, which blocks the receptor without initial stimulation, could be advantageous in this setting owing to the absence of 'flare' and potentially a more rapid restoration of testosterone level after cessation of therapy. In some studies of intermittent hormonal therapy, up to five treatment cycles have been given before evidence of androgen independence has appeared and during this time men have spent approximately 50% of the time off therapy.

Management of hormone-refractory disease

In most cases, advanced prostate cancers treated with any form of androgen deprivation eventually begin to progress, a phenomenon known as hormone-refractory or androgen-independent disease. This is probably due either to clonal selection of androgen-independent cell lines or to increased ligand-independent activation of androgen receptors. Thus, an increase in PSA level after initially successful androgen deprivation almost inevitably indicates impending clinical progression. This group is, however, quite heterogeneous, and includes men with PSA rises only and no demonstrable metastases as well as men who have many bone and visceral metastases, pain, and poor functional status; survival can range from only a few months to 4 years. Historically, therapy had little impact beyond modest palliation; however, treatments that may delay the progression of symptoms and reduce serum PSA as well as increase survival are becoming available.

Antiandrogen manipulation

When the serum PSA level rises after a period of androgen deprivation therapy alone, an initial move may be to add an anti-androgen to the treatment. This may have an effect in reducing PSA, but after some time the PSA will start rising again. At this time, withdrawal of the anti-androgen treatment may also result in a favorable PSA response (in approximately 40% of men). This phenomenon (which also occurs in breast cancer treated with anti-estrogens) has been ascribed to a mutation of androgen receptors in malignant tissue that renders the anti-androgen an agonist rather than an antagonist in effect. This response may last for a few months, after which the PSA will start to rise again.[18]

Estrogens

Estrogen treatment may benefit some men with androgen-independent prostate cancer. Such treatment appears to have two effects:

- inhibition of pituitary gonadotropin secretion; and
- direct cytotoxic effect on the tumor.

The synthetic estrogen diethylstilbestrol (DES) has been used in prostate cancer, but its use as first-line therapy is limited by side effects such as gynecomastia, deep-vein thrombosis, and other cardiovascular complications. Combination of DES with aspirin or warfarin may reduce the thrombotic and cardiovascular toxicity that can be hazardous in men of this age.

Cytotoxic therapy

Mitoxantrone plus prednisone

Mitoxantrone plus prednisone was the first chemotherapy combination to be tested in a randomized fashion in advanced prostate cancer.[19] This combination was shown to be very well tolerated and to reduce PSA levels significantly. The combination has been shown to more than double the time of palliation response compared with prednisone alone and to improve the quality of life of men with androgen-independent prostate cancer. In asymptomatic men with metastases, it also prolongs the time to disease progression. This combination has not, however, been shown to increase survival time.

Docetaxol

Docetaxol, another chemotherapy agent, which is a member of the taxoid family, induces apoptosis in cells through microtubule depolymerization. It has recently been tested in a randomized trial against mitoxantrone plus prednisone in men with androgen-independent prostate cancer. The results of this study (TAX-327) were reported in 2004 and showed docetaxol, given in a 3-week schedule, to be superior to mitoxantrone plus prednisone in terms of decreasing disease progression, improving PSA response, and improving pain.[20] In addition, docetaxol significantly improved survival from a median of 16.4 months for mitozantrone plus prednisone to 18.9 months for 3-weekly docetaxol, which translates into a 24% reduction in death rate.

The side effects associated with docetaxol include neutropenia, skin reactions, and gastrointestinal problems. In the trial described, the incidence of these side effects was higher in the group receiving docetaxol than in the group receiving mitoxantrone plus prednisone. However, docetaxol is generally well tolerated, and overall quality of life was better for the men who had received docetaxol compared with those who had received mitozantrone plus prednisone.

Management of bone metastases

Bone pain is one of the most intractable problems associated with androgen-independent prostate cancer, and conventional analgesics may not always provide adequate relief.

Palliative radiotherapy

Men with hormone-naïve disease will initially be managed by androgen-deprivation therapy. But some men will not get full pain resolution or may have painful bone metastases in the setting of androgen-independent prostate cancer. For these men, focal external-beam radiotherapy is a well-established treatment, and up to 80% of treated men will experience rapid improvement in pain. Treatment can be given as a single fraction or as multiple fractions over 2–3 weeks. There are very few side effects associated with this type of irradiation.

Bisphosphonates

There is now evidence that some patients benefit symptomatically from treatment with bisphosphonates, which suppress bone resorption and demineralization. A study involving over 600 patients with androgen-independent prostate cancer compared zoledronic acid, given as an intravenous infusion over 15 minutes every 3 weeks, with placebo.[21] There was a significant reduction in the number of patients with skeletal-related events, and the first such event was significantly delayed in the bisphosphonate-treated arm. It would, however, require 10 men to be treated to save one from a skeletal-related event. Side effects include renal deterioration and, rarely, jaw necrosis.

Conclusions

There has never been a time of greater focus on prostate cancer as a major issue in men's health.

This is the result of the aging of the population and the successful treatment advances in areas such as cardiovascular disease, which have resulted in men surviving longer and therefore becoming more susceptible to this highly age-dependent disease. Prominent personalities who have been affected by the disease, such as Arnold Palmer and Bob Monkhouse, have been prepared to speak out, and government agencies such as the National Institute for Health and Clinical Excellence (NICE) in the UK have produced guidelines.[21] The charity sector is also playing an increasing role as a prostate cancer lobby develops akin to one that breast cancer sufferers and their supporters created some years ago. Of course prostate cancer research and treatment suffers compared with breast cancer from the traditional reluctance of men to pay attention to their own health and from the previous lack of interest in men's health. Fortunately these issues are now finally being addressed and it seems certain that in the future the toll taken by prostate cancer will be reduced as diagnosis, staging, and treatments all continue to improve.[22]

References

1. Albertsen PC, Hanley JA, Fine J. 20-year outcomes following conservative management of clinically localized prostate cancer. JAMA 2005; 293: 2095–101.
2. Johns LE, Houlston RS. A systematic review and meta-analysis of familial prostate cancer risk. BJU Int 2003; 91: 789–94.
3. Thompson IM, Goodman PJ, Tangen CM et al. The influence of finasteride on the development of prostate cancer. N Engl J Med 2003; 349: 215–24.
4. Catalona WJ, Partin AW, Slawin KM et al. Use of the percentage of free prostate-specific antigen to enhance differentiation of prostate cancer from benign prostatic disease: a prospective multicenter clinical trial. JAMA 1998; 279: 1542–7.
5. Thompson IM, Pauler DK, Goodman PJ et al. Prevalence of prostate cancer among men with a prostate-specific antigen level < or =4.0 ng per milliliter. N Engl J Med 2004; 350: 2239–46.
6. D'Amico AV, Chen MH, Roehl KA, Catalona WJ. Preoperative PSA velocity and the risk of death from prostate cancer after radical prostatectomy. N Engl J Med 2004; 351: 125–35.

7. de Koning HJ, Liem MK, Baan CA et al. Prostate cancer mortality reduction by screening: power and time frame with complete enrollment in the European Randomised Screening for Prostate Cancer (ERSPC) trial. Int J Cancer 2002; 98: 268–73.

8. Bill-Axelson A, Holmberg L, Ruutu M et al. Radical prostatectomy versus watchful waiting in early prostate cancer. N Engl J Med 2005; 352: 1977–84.

9. Tewari A, Peabody J, Sarle R et al. Technique of da Vinci robot-assisted anatomic radical prostatectomy. Urology 2002; 60: 569–72.

10. Dasgupta PD, Patil K, Anderson C, Kirby RS. Transition from open to robotic-assisted radical prostatectomy. BJU Int 2008; 101: 667–8.

11. Bolla M, Collette L, Blank L et al. Long-term results with immediate androgen suppression and external irradiation in patients with locally advanced prostate cancer (an EORTC study): a phase III randomised trial. Lancet 2002; 360: 103–6.

12. Blasko JC, Mate T, Sylvester JE et al. Brachytherapy for carcinoma of the prostate: techniques, patient selection, and clinical outcomes. Semin Radiat Oncol 2002; 12: 81–94.

13. Klotz L. Active surveillance for prostate cancer: for whom? J Clin Oncol 2005; 23: 8165–9.

14. Klotz L. Low-risk prostate cancer can and should be managed by active surveillance and selected delayed intervention. Nat Clin Pract Urol 2008; 5: 2–3.

15. Gelet A, Chapelon JY, Bouvier R et al. Transrectal high intensity focused ultrasound for the treatment of localized prostate cancer: factors influencing the outcome. Eur Urol 2001; 40: 124–9.

16. Zisman A, Pantuck AJ, Cohen JK, Belldegrun AS. Prostate cryoablation using direct transperineal placement of ultrathin probes through a 17-gauge brachytherapy template-technique and preliminary results. Urology 2001; 58: 988–93.

17. Tyrrell CJ, Denis L, Newling D et al. Casodex™ 10–200 mg daily used as monotherapy for the treatment of patients with advanced prostate cancer. An overview of the efficacy, tolerability and pharmacokinetics from three phase II dose-ranging studies. Casodex Study Group. Eur Urol 1998; 33: 39–53.

18. Scher HI, Kelly WK. Flutamide withdrawal syndrome: its impact on clinical trials in hormone-refractory prostate cancer. J Clin Oncol 1993; 11: 1566–72.

19. Kantoff PW, Halabi S, Conaway M et al. Hydrocortisone with or without mitoxantrone in men with hormone-refractory prostate cancer: results of the cancer and leukemia group B 9182 study. J Clin Oncol 1999; 17: 2506–13.

20. Petrylak DP, Tangen CM, Hussain MH et al. Docetaxel and estramustine compared with mitoxantrone and prednisone for advanced refractory prostate cancer. N Engl J Med 2004; 351: 1513–20.

21. National Institute for Health and Clinical Excellence. Prostate Cancer: Diagnosis and Treatment, issued February 2008. http://www.nice.org.uk/guidance/index.jsp?action=byID&o=11924

22. Saad F, Gleason DM, Murray R et al. A randomized, placebo-controlled trial of zoledronic acid in patients with hormone-refractory metastatic prostate carcinoma. J Natl Cancer Inst 2002; 94: 1458–68.

CHAPTER 4

Testicular cancer

RTD Oliver

Introduction

Today nowhere is it more apparent that conservative management is critical to the safety than in the treatment of men with testis cancer, in which the cure of allcomers is in excess of 97% at 10 years (Fig. 4.1), though this is at a considerable price for a minority of patients. This chapter reviews this success; explains what is known about causation; discusses what men, by learning about this relatively rare disease, can do to try to reduce its occurrence and the delays in diagnosis that still occur because of the late detection of these tumors; and discusses what is being done today to reduce the late sequelae of treatment.

Definition

Most growth of tissues is regulated by switching on and off tissue regulating 'hormones' that are specific for each tissue. The most graphic illustration of this is what happens if a surgeon either operating on an experimental animal or a patient with a liver tumor or major liver trauma removes more than half the liver: it re-grows to precisely the same volume as before. Positive growth is produced by switching on factors that stimulate cell division and inhibit cell death while negative regulators of tissue growth (controlled by so-called suppressor genes) inhibit replication and enhance cellular maturation to enable organs to function. Understanding the way these hormones or growth regulators work is increasingly important in cancer, because mutation in the set of genes called cellular oncogenes (so called because mutated forms of these genes were found in cancer-causing oncogenic viruses) leads to uncontrolled growth of cancers, as do deletions of DNA material controlling suppressor genes.[1]

More than 90% of malignant tumors that arise in the testicle develop from sperm precursor cells that have at some stage in their development been altered by environmental factors thought to be acting while they were developing *in utero* but have lain dormant until after puberty when the sex hormones cause them to grow. Known collectively as germ cell cancers (GCC), there are two main groups. Seminomas are so called because they consist of sheets of cells looking like sperm precursor cells. The second group, non-seminomas, lack seminoma cells but have a characteristically large number of different embryonal (primitive) cells from any part of the normal developing embryo. As well as glands, cartilage, and nerves, these cells may include some that function like placental cells and secrete human chorionic gonadotropin (hCG), the hormone responsible for giving a positive pregnancy test in women. Measurement of hCG, with α-fetoprotein (normally produced by fetal liver) as tumor markers enables rapid assessment of whether there is any disease[2] and whether it is sensitive to treatment.

It is now more than 30 years since Atkin studying the chromomal content of GCC first showed

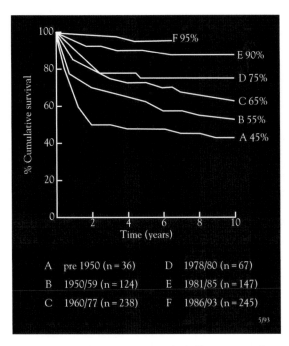

Figure 4.1. *Changes in survival of all patients with testicular germ cell tumors presenting to the Royal London Hospitals (1950–1993).*

that non-seminomas had less DNA than seminomas.[3] Subsequently the pre-cancerous cells in testis biopsies were found to have a higher chromosome number and DNA content than both seminomas and non-seminoma tumors, and a minority of tumors containing both seminoma and non-seminoma elements had a gradient in DNA content between carcinoma *in situ*, seminoma, and non-seminoma components.[4] This led to the conclusion that loss of DNA coded suppressor genes played a part in this increasing malignant behavior that was characteristic of non-seminomas[5] and that for all parameters examined including age and extent of metastases, patients with combined seminoma/non-seminoma were intermediate between those of pure seminoma and pure non-seminoma.

Diagnosis of testicular germ cell cancers

Most testicular cancers present with a painless hard lump, which is usually 1–2 cm in size before it is detected, but it can reach as much as 10–12 cm – if the patient is in denial or does not have access, through poverty or fear, to medical services as my group has recently experienced amongst refugees in the UK.[6] The larger the tumor the more likely it is that spread has occurred to other organs, starting with local draining lymph glands at the back of the abdomen, moving next to glands in the chest and neck, before getting into the blood stream and landing in the lungs. If there is further delay or the tumor is resistant to treatment a second wave of spread occurs to the liver or to the brain (Fig. 4.2), though rarely to both sites; and even rarer is spread to the bone, which is in marked contrast to prostate cancer, in which bone involvement is nearly universal with the first wave of spread.

For about one-third of patients developing testicular cancer, the tumor is not painless but exhibits a varying degree of pain that can fluctuate but is usually not much more than a dull ache. However, very occasional patients have a tumor that grows so fast or in such a disorganized way that it blocks its own blood supply and presents with acute severe pain. Much more common are patients with fluctuating testicular pain and tenderness who do not have a testicular cancer. These patients often include patients who have had one testis removed and also probably represent people in the population who have had a past viral infection affecting the testis, such as mumps, that has persisted. These people often need to have an ultrasound to convince them that they don't have cancer, though this may find evidence of 'micro-calcification'.[7] This is a form of excessive scar formation from a previous episode of inflammation or past trauma, and it is enhanced by our increasingly sedentary life style.

The final category of presentation, which occurs in one in 10 patients, who often have considerable difficulty in getting diagnosed, is presentation with lumps or symptoms from a site of metastasis outside the testis that have been biopsied and have suggested a testis GCC primary. In such patients, testis ultrasound usually makes the diagnosis since the patient has either a scar from a burnt out primary or an extremely small primary tumor, the so-called Azzopardi–Hoffbrand syndrome.[8] These patients seem to have had a primary tumor that has been

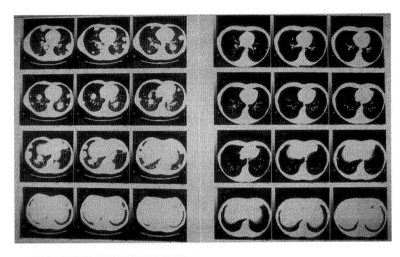
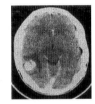
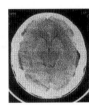
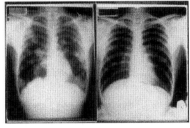

Figure 4.2. *Chest X rays, chest CT and brain scans showing distribution and response of primary BEP chemotherapy-resistant metastases to salvage chemotherapy.*

completely or partially rejected while the metastases have grown considerably. They have usually been complaining of a longstanding backache keeping them awake at night and are only comfortable rolling up into a ball on the side, though occasionally the patient has persistent abdominal pain instead.

Such patients often have prolonged delay in diagnosis[9] since they are unaware they have a problem in the testis and are seen in orthopedic (Fig. 4.3) or gastroenterology departments (Fig. 4.4). Others present to chest physicians, who investigate for chronic cough or hemoptysis for prolonged periods, thinking it to be tuberculosis (Fig. 4.5), to neurologists for investigation following an epileptic fit (see Fig. 4.2), or to ENT surgeons for biopsy of an enlarged lymph node in the neck.

The final group of rarer presentations are those presenting to endocrinologists complaining of enlargement of the breast tissue, so called gynecomastia. It is common for men at the start of puberty to develop some thickening of breast tissue during the first year until the body has adjusted to making

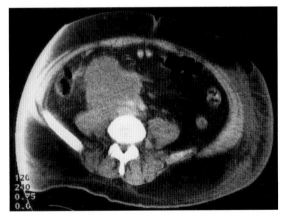

Figure 4.3. *CT scan from a patient presenting after prolonged delay with large retroperitoneal lymph node metastases causing backache.*

the correct ratio of male and female sex hormones. However, about one-fifth of patients with testicular cancer present with thickening and tenderness of the nipples because of raised hCG levels. As there

41

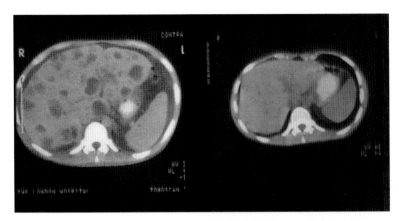

Figure 4.4. *CT of liver before and after chemotherapy from a patient presenting with unexplained abdominal pain from slowly progressive tumor thrombosis in the vena cava leading to presentation with renal and liver failure due to extension of the thrombosis.*

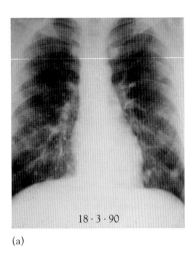

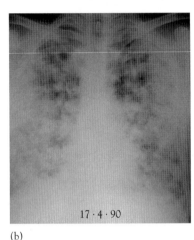

(a)   (b)

Figure 4.5. *(a) Chest X ray at presentation to a chest physician of a heroin addict who presented with hemoptysis and was admitted for exclusion of TB and pneumocystis crinii; (b) Chest X ray when admitted to cancer center one month later with a strong positive urinary pregnancy and died before treatment could be started.*

are multiple other rare causes of these symptoms, such as liver disease, infertility leading to increased estrogen production, rare side effects of some drugs, and even 'joggers nipple', these patients are occasionally misdiagnosed unless a urinary pregnancy test is performed.[2]

Etiology

The causation of testicular cancer has been reviewed in a number of publications.[3,10,11]

One of the problems with getting a true perspective on the cause of cancer, is that if one listens to the media one is overwhelmed by the fact that there are too many, not too few, suspected causes of cancer. Despite this, when one actually meets someone who has cancer it is rarely clear what caused it to develop at the time it occurred. However, what science has now proved beyond all doubt is that all of the known causes of cancer act by either leading to damage to DNA, by reducing the body's ability to repair DNA, or by reducing the body's ability to reject the early stages of malignant development. Furthermore, as illustrated by the increased susceptibility of people with ginger hair to skin cancer from sun exposure, the risks of any given carcinogenic influence are modified by the genetic inheritance of the individual person and the multiplicity of hits with carcinogen.

The consequence of this is that even smoking, the most closely examined cause of cancer, is associated with fewer than 20% of regular users developing cancer after more than 40 years' use.

This is one of the facts that contributes to why many youngsters fail to heed the message. However, the most telling message about smoking is not being emphasized – namely, that it is the number of cigarettes smoked per year during the body's pubertal growth phase before the age of 18 that is most important in predicting the later risk of getting cancer by the age of 50–60.[12] Though this is partially due to faster-growing tissues having less time to repair DNA damage, getting the growing brain exposed to the addictive substance by the age of 18 is as relevant in inducing addiction to nicotine as it is to alcohol and other addictive drugs such as heroin and cannabis. However, even though for smokers it is the first few years that are the most important individually, it is the total number of years that ends up making the real difference, and so any time spent as a non-smoker helps to reduce the risk, and the longer the better.[12]

Though neither testicular cancer[3] nor prostate cancer is primarily caused by smoking, there is some evidence that both behave in a more malignant way in heavy smokers.

Safe sex and good diet in prostate and testicular cancer

For testicular cancer, there is increasing evidence that an early onset of puberty increases the risk,[13,14] though the exact mechanism of this is not clear. As discussed below, under the effects of exercise, it is thought to be mediated in part via an effect of the body's sex hormones, although there is also evidence that an early onset of sexual activity increases the risk of sexually acquired infection, contributing to the increase in risk. Similar evidence in prostate cancer patients also suggests that early onset of puberty increases the risk, and here there is now beginning to be a more clear-cut explanation.[15] Recent work has suggested that it is because at a younger age men are more prone to damage their prostates by developing an asymptomatic form of 'honeymoon prostatitis' (which is the equivalent of the honeymoon cystitis that women often experience when they first begin sexual activity). It is now known that 40% of men will get at least one attack before the age of 50. In some people who are more susceptible, this may lead to a lifetime's hidden persistence of mild infection, which is

amplified by repeat exposures. Inadequate vitamin A and D levels may facilitate this persistent infection by reducing function of immune cells and phagocytes. This chronic damage to the prostate seems to encourage DNA mutations to accumulate and prostate cancer ultimately develops 25–50 years later. A similar mechanism is suspected to explain the contribution of sexually transmitted infection to causes of testis cancer.

These observations have led to the hypothesis that a possible late effect of the anti-AIDS safe sex campaign of the early 1980s may be a contribution to the recent unexplained decline of prostate cancer deaths in the late 1990s in the UK before there was any major degree of screening for prostate-specific antigen. Reports that 6 months of condom use can lead to regression of the early stages of cervix cancer[16] raise the question as to whether education about the risks of early sex and importance of using barrier contraception such as condoms will have a major impact on risks of later development of prostate and testis cancer. With recent evidence that the 1980s safe sex message is being forgotten by today's youth, there is a need to represent this message from a different perspective.

How can regular exercise prevent testis and prostate cancer?

While it has long been known that exercise reduces risks of heart disease, the message that exercise is good for prevention of several types of cancer,[17] such as breast, bowel, testis[13] and prostate cancer, is less well known.

For testis cancer there are thought to be two mechanisms that may be acting together. Firstly, lack of exercise leads to a greater sedentary existence. Sitting down, particularly in tight underpants, heats up the testicle and this is known to damage the sperm cells from which testis cancers develop (Table 4.1).[18] The second mechanism is that regular exercise has a beneficial effect on regulation of sex hormones that control puberty[19] and this leads to a more gradual development of puberty, thus reducing the deleterious effects of an early puberty. It is a similar mechanism that is thought to be a factor in why exercise, particularly in schools, is beneficial in reducing later risks of prostate cancer, though it may also be that those

Table 4.1. *Impact of testicular heating on sperm count*

	Technique 1 (n=3)	Technique 2 (n=6)
Pre-treatment mean sperm count ($\times 10^6$)	50.2	40.2
Time in sperm count nadir	11 months	3 months
Sperm count nadir (8–36 months) ($\times 10^6$)	1.86	0.12
Cycles of contraceptive use (pregnancies)	42 (1)	117 (0)
Post treatment (0–6 months) ($\times 10^6$)	51	26.5
Post treatment (7–18 months) ($\times 10^6$)	98.7	36.3

Technique 1, less tight scrotal support technique; Technique 2, tighter scrotal support technique. From reference 18.

who take more exercise have more sun exposure and better vitamin D levels (see below). As with heart disease prevention, it is by no means certain that exercise has to be excessive. The critical thing is developing a regular pattern and maintaining it over a lifetime.

Safe sun and men's cancers

The Chinese philosophy of yin and yang recognizes that there is good and bad in everything and nowhere is this clearer than in the effects of the sun on development of cancer. The sun keeps us warm but burns the skin if the dose is excessive. If you burn your skin excessively, and particularly as a child, and get blisters, you increase your risk of getting melanoma,[20] which can kill people as young as 20–30 years of age. If you have 50–60 years of chronic sunburn you end up with

a different type of skin cancer, squamous cell cancer. Though this is less malignant it can keep recurring all over the sunburnt areas and can be quite disfiguring.

However, there is now new evidence emerging that sun can have important life-time benefits as well. It has long been known that sunlight reduces the risk of tuberculosis and helps it heal. This is now known to be due to the sun stimulating the body to make vitamin D,[21] which helps the body's scavenging phagocytes to resist the tuberculosis infection.[22] (Decreased outdoor sports, and more indoor computer games and clubbing, as well as increased immigration from areas where skin phenotype or cultural behavior results in less vitamin D synthesis,[21] could be unsuspected factors adding to the resurgence of tuberculosis in the UK.) It is now emerging that a lifetime's regular low level sun exposure may be helping to reduce the risk of prostate, breast, colon (but not rectal), and lung cancer,[23] possibly by the same mechanism since the scavenging phagocytes are as effective at eliminating early stages of cancer as they are at eliminating tuberculosis bacteria. There is as yet no study with enough patients with testis cancer to know if regular low level sun exposure reduces testis cancer, though there is emerging evidence that vitamin D could benefit some causes of infertility.[24] As there is increasing recognition of links between declining sperm count and rising testis cancer (see below) this issue needs further exploration.

Partial commonality of causation between infertility and testis cancer[11]

Two-thirds of men with testis cancer when they are diagnosed have a sub-fertile sperm count and some have had problems with infertility that have led to the diagnosis of testis cancer. A similar proportion of testis cancer patients have evidence of damage to their testicles, having 'microcalcification' and other pathological changes of inflammation and scarring when the testicle is examined pathologically. This is reflected by the discovery that about 40% of patients have raised levels of the pituitary hormone follicle stimulating hormone, which regulates sperm count levels, a finding in common between infertile patients and those at increased risk of testis cancer (Table 4.2).[25] The final observation has been reports

Table 4.2. *Follicle stimulating hormone levels and risk of contralateral tumor after unilateral orchidectomy: proportion of patients with elevated follicle stimulating hormone*

Hoff Wanderas et al.[25]	Cases (n)	Elevated follicle stimulating hormone level
Patients with second germ cell carcinoma	13	77%
Control (no second germ cell carcinoma)	26	15%
Oliver et al.[37]	Cases (n)	Median follicle stimulating hormone level (IU/L)
Patients with second germ cell carcinoma	12	19.9
Control (no second germ cell carcinoma)	985	9.3

showing that the rising incidence of testis cancer has been correlated with evidence of a declining sperm count, particularly in those parts of the world where the incidence of testis cancer is high. The exact cause of this and of the few exceptions is not known in detail though it is likely to be the accumulation of multiple effects. There are clues implicating multiple chemical exposures such as plastics and pesticides, viruses such as mumps, and an increasingly sedentary lifestyle. It is the latter whose direct effect has been most convincingly demonstrated (as explained in the discussion of Table 4.1 above).

Landmarks in the progress from 90% lethality to 90% cure of metastatic germ cell cancer[26]

Prior to 1970, less than 5% of metastatic non-seminomas became long-term cures. However the next two steps, the achievement of 25% durable cure with high-dose bleomycin and vinblastine in the mid-1970s and then the 64% durable cure with three-drug combination of bleomycin, vinblastine, and cisplatin (BVP) in 1978, became established because of such leaps in cure rate that nobody doubted they were advances. The final step in the onward progress with increasing cure was demonstrated only when Einhorn's team undertook a randomized trial and demonstrated that bleomycin, etoposide, and cisplatin (BEP) produced 80% lasting cure compared with 70% that was then being achieved with BVP.[27] Since that landmark trial was reported in 1988 there has been no improvement in the chemotherapy of producing primary cure of metastatic germ cell cancer. However, increasing awareness amongst young men of the importance of early diagnosis of testis cancer, in part led by such campaigns as Orchid's 'Know Your Balls … Check Them Out' targeted at young adolescents, has decreased the size of tumors from 4.2 cm to 2.6 cm in the past 20 years (Fig. 4.6).[28] As well as reducing the extent of metastasis, this has produced a drift upwards in overall cure,[30] so that most centers report rates of 85–90%. BEP remains standard despite testing up to seven-drug regimens and much higher doses requiring stem cell transplantation to prevent deaths from bone marrow failure. There has, however, been considerable progress in developing regimens to cure BEP failures,[31] and cure rates have gone from 5% to 60% over the past 15 years.

Progress in reducing toxicity of treatment[26]

Initially in the 1960s those rare cures were maintained on oral chemotherapy for 2–5 years. However, as the cure rate got higher and the toxicity got worse, maintenance was progressively reduced from 2 years to 1 year, as was the duration of induction (from 12 months to 6 months and then 3 months, which became the first standard with BEP).[27] All the reduction of treatment times was achieved without any randomized trial, though Einhorn's group used randomized trials to establish that there was no gain from 12 months' maintenance vinblastine and then that BEP was superior

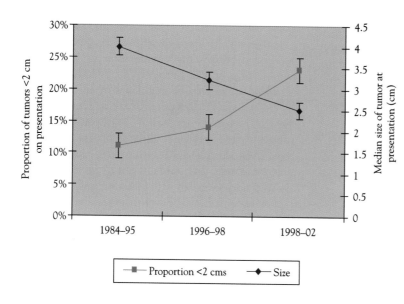

Figure 4.6. *Increase in proportion of men presenting with testis tumors small enough for testis conservation. From reference 29.*

Table 4.3. *Overview of trials in good-risk patients*[26]

Trial	Number of trials	Number of cases	Progression-free (%)
Platinum combination with bleomycin	4	434	86
without bleomycin	4	425	77
Combination plus			
cisplatin	3	256	91
carboplatin	3	240	79
Number of courses			
BEP×4	2	502	90
BEP×3	2	494	91
BEP, bleomycin plus etoposide plus cisplatin			

to PVB. Even so, toxicity from 3 months' induction was considerable and, as recorded by Lance Armstrong, the testis cancer patient who won the Tour de France, in his memoirs *It's Not about the Bike*, it took him 2 years to get to full fitness after his treatment (which I would think is within the norm of 18–24 months).

Reducing this toxicity further has proved more difficult, with risking a loss of cure for men with a 40-year life expectancy making trials difficult (Table 4.3). The first attempt at reduction was to

drop bleomycin because of a 5% incidence of treatment-related mortality from lung toxicity. Meta-analysis of three such trials showed that there were 9% fewer cures without bleomycin. The second attempt was to test a non-nephrotoxic analog of cisplatin, carboplatin, which proved to be 15% less effective, a fact that took nearly 10 years to discover in a trial of 600 patients. The third trial established the safety of using 9 weeks rather than 12 weeks of induction treatment and 3-day rather than 5-day cycles of therapy.

Changes in adjuvant treatments for stage 1 germ cell cancer[32–34]

Stage 1 non-seminoma

The toxicity of cisplatin-based combination treatment was initially so bad that it was not thought safe to use it as adjuvant treatment for early-stage disease and it very soon became evident that relapse following radiation increased risk of toxic death from BVP treatment. As a result, centers using radiation rather than surgery for early-stage non-seminoma rapidly learnt to use tumor marker and computed tomography (CT) radiological surveillance for these patients. They detected most of the 35% of patients who relapsed at a very early stage so that overall survival was identical to those who had retroperitoneal lymph node surgery and suffered a long-known but little discussed complication of surgery, loss of ejaculation. However, the surgeons did provide important information of the inaccuracy rate of the first generation CT scans, with 40% of negative scans proving to have histologically positive nodes and, more significantly, 25% of early stage 2 cases found to have false-positive scans. They also demonstrated that two courses of adjuvant treatment would eliminate a 50% risk of relapse, and this ushered in the era of adjuvant chemotherapy without surgery for stage 1 patients with a high risk of relapse, which produced similar overall survival.

The surgeons meanwhile went on to improve their technique and identify the nerves responsible for ejaculation and performed nerve-sparing operations that enabled preservation of ejaculation in most, but not all, patients. Some also began to use laparoscopy and the da Vinci robot to diminish the morbidity of surgery, and they continued to prove the inaccuracy of even second- and third-generation CT scans (Table 4.4). Medical oncologists, increasingly aware of this inaccuracy, learnt to defer treatment in such stage 2 patients as they had done for stage 1 patients until it was clear that the patient had active disease, and they treated only when serial scans or rising tumor markers showed progression. In addition, they demonstrated in pilot studies in high-risk patients that one course of BEP may produce as good relapse-free survival as retroperitoneal lymph node dissection;[35] and this is now being further investigated.

Stage 1 seminomas[26]

In the early 1930s radiotherapists demonstrated the differential radio-sensitivity between seminoma and non-seminoma, with 3000 cGy producing 50% cure of stage 2 disease while 4500 cGy only produced 25% cure of stage 2 non-seminomas. Less has been done to clarify whether a similar degree of differential sensitivity to chemotherapy exists, though the clearest evidence in favor of this view was the comparative response rate to single-agent cisplatin. The initial report in 1974 showed that 10% of non-seminoma achieved durable complete remission with single-agent cisplatin, while 10 years

Table 4.4. *Open versus laparoscopic RPLND for clinical stage I and II non-seminoma[42,43]*

Open RPLND	Number of cases	Pathological stage II (% of patients)	Overstaging
Clinical stage I	308	29	Nil
Clinical stage II	145	67	37%
Laparoscopic RPLND			
Clinical stage I	320	22.2	Nil
Clinical stage II	11	64	33%

RPLND, retroperitoneal lymph node dissection

later a small study of 12 patients with metastatic seminoma reported 83% durable cure rates after single-agent cisplatin, and a more recent report has shown that with dose escalation, in excess of 90% can be cured with single-agent carboplatin and that these cures may be predicted on the basis of changes in positron emission tomography 72 hours after starting treatment.

At that time there was increasing evidence for the development of late second malignancies after adjuvant radiotherapy in up to 20% of stage 1 patients followed for 15–20 years. In an attempt to reduce this, oncologists initially began surveillance studies as they had done with non-seminoma. However, late relapse up to 8 years after orchidectomy, which in occasional patients led to invasion of the spinal canal and paralysis, led to a divergence of opinion worldwide. Some authors, preferring to limit adjuvant studies to those with a high risk of relapse, thought that this was not highly discriminatory. Others sought to reduce the amount of radiation (Table 4.5). My group, encouraged by the low toxicity and higher cure rate of carboplatin than radiation, began studies in 1986 of two courses then one course of the single-agent platinum analog, carboplatin (Table 4.6). Last year, in a

randomized trial involving 1477 patients comparing one course carboplatin and radiation, a similar relapse rate of 3% was achieved.[36] However, more unexpectedly, there was a 72% reduction of 5-year risk of second tumors in the contralateral testis. This, taken with the results from a pilot study of using chemotherapy to preserve the primary testis in 28 patients with tumors in a solitary testis,[37] which achieved 75% successful testis preservation and recovery of fertility using chemotherapy with or without lumpectomy with 7 years follow-up, has opened the possibility that in the long term testis preservation could be as safe as breast preservation.

Conclusions and future directions

In the past 30 years the treatment of testis cancer has been changed dramatically and the cure is so good that some people question the need to spend any more money on this rare cancer. Much of this success has been achieved without any massive increase in cost of treatment, since today the savings achieved from reducing the average treatment from 20 days to 9 days has more than covered the cost of the new salvage treatment of the 10–15% of

Table 4.5. *Randomized trials of potential new standards for stage 1 seminoma*[26]

	ARM A		ARM B		Median follow-up (years)
	Cases (n)	Relapse rate	Cases (n)	Relapse rate	
MRC TE10 (1989–1993) Dog-leg vs PA strip	242	3%	236	4%	4.5
MRC TE18 (1995–1998) 30 Gy vs 20 Gy (88% PA st)	313	3%	312	4%	5.1
MRC TE19 (1996–2001) 30 Gy vs 20 Gy (87% PA st)	289	5.9%	289	2.1%	4.0
MRC TE19 (1996–2001) Radiation vs Carboplatin (x1)	904	4%	573	5%	4.0

Dog-leg field irradiation includes both PA and ipsilateral iliac lymph nodes. MRC, Medical Research Council; PA, para-arotic.

Table 4.6. *Phase II studies in metastatic and stage I seminoma (1984–2005)*

Metastatic seminoma[44]	Cases (n)	Relapse-free survival rate	Overall survival (median follow-up)
Carboplatin dose phase II studies			
Carboplatin AUC × 10 q21 × 3–4	24	93%	100%
Carboplatin AUC × 7/8 q21 × 4	17	88%	94%
Carboplatin 450 mg/m² q21 × 4	19	79%	95%
Stage I seminoma[45]			
Carboplatin dose phase II studies			
Carboplatin 400 mg/m² q28 × 2	644	98.5%	98.3% (3.8 years)
Carboplatin 400 mg/m² × 1	116	91.4%	99% (4 years)
Carboplatin AUC × 7 (564 mg/m² × 1)	274	98.2%	99%
		0%	(7.5 years)

AUC, area under the curve; method for calculating dose.

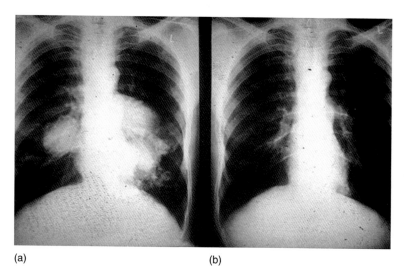

(a) (b)

Figure 4.7. *(a) Patient with mediastinal metastases from seminoma causing bilateral bronchial obstruction and inability to walk more than ten yards without sitting; (b) The same patient twenty-one days later after a single dose of cisplatin, having been able to be discharged forty-eight hours after treatment and return home by public transport.*

patient in whom treatment fails (of whom 60% are cured today).

The past 10 years has seen exciting developments in surgery, chemotherapy, and imaging that make it possible that treatment of testis cancer could become as simple as that of breast cancer.

More than 40 years ago, most breast cancer patients underwent radical mastectomy, a treatment that required masterful surgery to remove the breast and most of the muscles of the chest wall and lymph glands in the axilla. Today, lumpectomy and sentinel lymph node sampling followed by 2–5 years of an anti-estrogen not only achieves results as good but it also reduces by more than two-thirds the occurrence of new tumors that would normally occur in the contralateral breast.[38] By contrast, although the first active drugs that produced long-term disease cure of testis cancer were discovered in the early 1960s and today 97% of all patients become long-term cures, 99% or more of patients still undergo radical orchidectomy and the gold standard for lymph node staging (retroperitoneal lymph node dissection, still a standard of care in the USA though rarely performed in the UK), requires a large incision from pubis to xiphisternum and takes several hours. Furthermore for the one patient in 20 who develops a second primary cancer in the other testicle, total castration is the only standard of care despite it now being 10 years since the first reports that it was possible to conserve testes and recover spermatogenesis using chemotherapy. As an increasing number of patients are being diagnosed with testis tumors small enough for testis conservation, there is now a need for a carefully controlled study to validate the long-term safety of such a procedure for all patients. This will require follow-up for at least 20 years because of the persistence of functional but *in utero* sensitized spermatogonia at heightened risk of developing further malignancy. Such a study if it were to demonstrate a delay of andropause and reduction of cardiac deaths could have major lasting impact beyond the field of testis cancer.

The reason for this is that late follow-up studies are demonstrating an excess of cardiac deaths in all stages of testis cancer. These men also had increased weight gain, raised serum cholesterol, and diabetes,[39] suggesting that they had an increased risk of premature development of metabolic syndrome. This syndrome has increasingly been recognized as a manifestation of declining Leydig cell function with age, the so-called 'andropause'. Observations of increased incidences of osteopenia and osteoporosis within this population have lent additional support to this theory.[40,41] Epidemiological studies demonstrating that testis cancer patients have lower sperm counts and increased Leydig cell dysfunction[11] suggest that these patients are prone to developing premature andropause.[25] Setting up a testis conservation study with patient-preference-based consent could provide important understanding for this increasingly significant area of all men's health.

References

1. Vogelstein B, Fearon ER, Hamilton SR et al. Genetic alterations during colorectal-tumor development. N Engl J Med 1988; 319: 527–32.
2. Caulfield MJ, Dilkes MG, Iles RK, Handel BT, Oliver RTD. Rapid diagnosis of testicular choriocarcinoma by urinary pregnancy tests. Lancet 1990; 355: 1230.
3. Oliver RTD. Clues from natural history and results of treatment supporting the monoclonal origin of germ cell tumours. Cancer Surv 1990; 9: 332–68.
4. Oosterhuis JW, Gillis AJM, van Putten WJL, de Jong B, Looijenga LHJ. Interphase cytogenetics of carcinoma in situ of the testis. Eur Urol 1993; 23: 16–22.
5. Oliver RTD, Leahy M, Ong J. Combined seminoma/non-seminoma should be considered as intermediate grade germ cell cancer (GCC). Eur J Cancer 1995; 31A: 1392–4.
6. Steele JP, Oliver R. Testicular cancer: perils of very late presentation [comment]. Lancet 2002; 359: 1632–3.
7. Otite U, Webb JA, Oliver RT, Badenoch DF, Nargund VH. Testicular microlithiasis: is it a benign condition with malignant potential? Eur Urol 2001; 40: 538–42.
8. Azzopardi JG, Hoffbrand AV. Retrogression in testicular seminoma with viable metastases. J Clin Pathol 1965; 18: 135.
9. Oliver RTD. Factors contributing to delay in diagnosis of testicular tumour. BMJ 1985; 290: 356.
10. Oliver RTD. Atrophy, hormones, genes and viruses in aetiology of germ cell tumours. Cancer Surv 1990; 9: 263–8.
11. Oliver R. Epidemiology of testis cancer. In: Vogelzang N, Shipley W, Scardino P, Debruyne F, eds. Comprehensive Textbook of Genitourinary Oncology, 3rd edn. Philadephia: Lippincott Williams and Wilkins, 2006: 547–8.
12. Vineis P. Epidemiological models of carcinogenesis: the example of bladder cancer. Cancer Epidemiol Biomarkers Prev 1992; 1: 149–53.
13. Forman D, Chilvers CED, Oliver RTD, Pike MC. The aetiology of testicular cancer: association with congenital abnormalities, age at puberty, infertility and exercise. BMJ 1994; 308: 1393–9.

14. Chilvers C, Forman D, Oliver RTD et al. Social, behavioural and medical factors in the aetiology of testicular cancer – results from the UK study. Br J Cancer 1994; 70: 513–20.

15. Oliver T, Lorincz A, Cuzick J. Prostate Cancer Prevention: Rationale Behind the Design of Trials. Heidelburg: Springer, 2008.

16. Richardson AC, Lyon JB. The effect of condom use in squamous cell cervical intra-epithelial neoplasia. Am J Obstet Gynaecol 1981; 140: 909–13.

17. Wannamethee SG, Shaper AG, Walker M. Physical activity and risk of cancer in middle-aged men. Br J Cancer 2001; 85: 1311–16.

18. Mieusset R, Bujan L. Testicular heating and its possible contributions to male infertility: a review. Int J Androl 1995; 18: 169–84.

19. Oliver RTD. Screening for colorectal cancer. Lancet 1993; 341: 1033.

20. Wartman D, Weinstock M. Are we overemphasizing sun avoidance in protection from melanoma? Cancer Epidemiol Biomarkers Prev 2008; 17: 469–70.

21. Clemens TL, Adams JS, Henderson SL, Holick MF. Increased skin pigment reduces the capacity of skin to synthesise vitamin D3. Lancet 1982; 1: 74–6.

22. Liu PT, Stenger S, Li H et al. Toll-like receptor triggering of a vitamin D-mediated human antimicrobial response. Science 2006; 311: 1770–3.

23. van der Rhee HJ, de Vries E, Coebergh JW. Does sunlight prevent cancer? A systematic review. Eur J Cancer 2006; 42: 2222–32.

24. Lackner JE, Herwig R, Schmidbauer J et al. Correlation of leukocytospermia with clinical infection and the positive effect of antiinflammatory treatment on semen quality. Fertil Steril 2006; 86: 601–5.

25. Hoff Wanderas E, Fossa SD, Heilo A, Stenwig AE, Norman N. Serum follicle stimulating hormone – predictor of cancer in the remaining testis in patients with unilateral testicular cancer. Br J Urol 1990; 66: 315–17.

26. Oliver T. Conservative management of testicular germ-cell tumors. Nat Clin Pract Urol 2007; 4: 550–60.

27. Williams SD, Birch R, Einhorn LH et al. Treatment of disseminated germ-cell tumours with Cisplatin, Bleomycin, and either Vinblastine or Etoposide. N Engl J Med 1987; 316: 1435–40.

28. Bhardwa JM, Powles T, Berney D et al. Assessing the size and stage of testicular germ cell tumours: 1984–2003. BJU Int 2005; 96: 819–21.

29. Powles T, Bhardwa J, Shamash J, Mandalia S, Oliver T. The changing presentation of germ cell tumours of the testis between 1983 and 2002. BJU Internat 2005; 95: 1197–200.

30. Ravi R, Oliver RT, Ong J et al. A single-centre observational study of surgery and late malignant events after chemotherapy for germ cell cancer. Br J Urol 1997; 80: 647–52.

31. Shamash J, Oliver R, Ong J et al. 60% salvage rate for germ cell tumours using sequential m-BOP, surgery and ifosfamide based chemotherapy. Ann Oncol 1999; 10: 685–92.

32. de Wit R, Fizazi K. Controversies in the management of clinical stage I testis cancer. J Clin Oncol 2006 10; 24: 5482–92.

33. Freedman LS, Parkinson MC, Jones WG et al. Histopathology in the prediction of relapse of patients with stage 1 testicular teratoma treated by orchidectomy alone. On behalf of MRC Testicular Tumour Subgroup (Urological Working Party). Lancet 1987; ii: 294–8.

34. Oliver R, Ong J, Ravi R et al. Long term follow up of Anglian Germ Cell Cancer Group surveillance versus adjuvant chemotherapy treated stage 1 nonseminoma patients. Urology 2004; 63: 556–61.

35. Albers P, Siener R, Krege S et al. Randomized phase III trial comparing retroperitoneal lymph node dissection with one course of bleomycin and etoposide plus cisplatin chemotherapy in the adjuvant treatment of clinical stage I nonseminomatous testicular germ cell tumors: AUO trial AH 01/94 by the German Testicular Cancer Study Group. J Clin Oncol 2008; 26: 2966–72.

36. Oliver RTD, Mason MD, Mead GM et al. Radiotherapy versus singe-dose carboplatin in adjuvant treatment of stage 1 seminoma: a randomised trial. Lancet 2005; 366: 293–300.

37. Oliver RTD, Ong J, Berney D et al. Testis conserving chemotherapy in germ cell cancer: Its potential to increase understanding of the biology and treatment of carcinoma-in-situ. Acta Pathologica, Microbiologica et Immunologica Scandinavica 2003; 111: 86–92.

38. Howell A, Cuzick J, Baum M et al. Results of the ATAC (Arimidex, Tamoxifen, Alone or in Combination) trial after completion of 5 years' adjuvant treatment for breast cancer. Lancet 2005; 365: 60–2.

39. Nuver J, Smit AJ, Wolffenbuttel BH et al. The metabolic syndrome and disturbances in hormone levels in long-term survivors of disseminated testicular cancer. J Clin Oncol 2005; 23: 3718–25.

40. Willemse PPM. Bone abnormalities in male germ-cell cancer survivors. J Clin Oncol 2007; 25(Proc Amer Soc Clin Oncol): 248 abst. 5053.

41. Mardiak J. Damage of bone metabolism and osteoporosis in testicular cancer patients. J Clin Oncol 2007; 25 (Proc Amer Soc Clin Oncol): 248 abst. 5052.

42. Stephenson AJ, Bosl GJ, Motzer RJ et al. Retroperitoneal lymph node dissection for nonseminomatous germ cell testicular cancer: impact of patient selection factors on outcome. J Clin Oncol 2005; 23: 2781–8.

43. Steiner H, Peschel R, Janetschek G et al. Long-term results of laparoscopic retroperitoneal lymph node dissection: a single-center 10-year experience. Urology 2004; 63: 550–5.

44. Oliver RTD, Shamash J, Powles T, Somasundram U, Ell PJ. 20 year phase 1/2 study of single agent carboplatin in metastatic seminoma: could it have been accelerated by 72 hour PET scan response? J Clin Oncol 2004; 23: 445 (Suppl; abstr. 4763).

45. Oliver TD, Steiner K, Skoneczna H. I. Pooled analysis of phase II reports of 2 vs. 1 course of Carboplatin as adjuvant for Stage 1 Seminoma. J Clin Oncol 2005; 23(Proc Amer Soc Clin Oncol): 395s abst. 4572.

CHAPTER 5

Bladder cancer

David A Swanson, Paul K Hegarty

Introduction

Cancer of the bladder is the fourth most common cancer in men in the USA, ranking behind only prostate cancer, cancers of the lung and bronchus, and colon and rectal cancers in incidence.[1] Ironically, it may also be one of the most preventable cancers, owing to the well-documented, strong etiologic influence of smoking and, to a lesser extent, of exposure to some industrial chemicals. Bladder cancer has a broad range of behavior, which dictates different treatments and offers far different prognoses. Superficial bladder cancer is almost an entirely different disease from invasive bladder cancer. As our understanding of this disease evolves, there are increasing opportunities to tailor our treatments based on risk of progression. The future is even brighter, because laboratory research has already made great strides in dissecting molecular pathways and finding novel therapeutic targets for this cancer. We present herein a brief overview of bladder cancer.

Epidemiology

According to the American Cancer Society, there will be 67 160 new cases in the US in 2007, just over 50 000 in men and 17 120 in women.[1] Death due to bladder cancer will occur in 9630 males and 4120 females. In the UK, there were 5800 new cases of bladder cancer in men registered in England in 2004, 661 in Wales, 559 in Scotland, and 148 in Northern Ireland.[2] The comparable numbers in women for 2004 were 2337, 253, 273, and 62, respectively.

Bladder cancer has the highest recurrence rate of any cancer. Patients who get one bladder tumor are at high risk of developing another, which demands rigorous follow-up and surveillance tests.[3] Autopsy studies show that undiagnosed cases of bladder cancer are rare in comparison with other tumors such as prostate or renal cancer, which is a more common unexpected finding at autopsy because the cancers had not been diagnosed *ante mortem*.[4] This has a number of implications:

1. The incidence of patients diagnosed with bladder cancer represents close to the true incidence of the disease.
2. The difference in observed incidence between men and women is a genuine phenomenon and not a result of bias in investigation of symptoms.
3. Most people with bladder cancer are diagnosed before death.
4. The lead-time between developing bladder cancer and its diagnosis is generally short.
5. Virtually all cases of bladder cancer are clinically significant.

Etiology

The main risk factors for developing bladder cancer are smoking tobacco and exposure to certain organic chemicals. Smoking accounts for about 50% of cases, with the risk proportional to the amount and duration of smoking exposure.[3] Also, it is estimated that up to 25% of cases may be ascribed to occupational exposure to chemicals such as benzene derivatives and arylamines. Chronic infection with schistosomiasis is associated with the development of squamous cell carcinoma of the bladder, particularly in countries where that disease is endemic, such as in Egypt. Clearly, work and lifestyle factors are central to modifying the risk of developing the disease. The influence of family history is controversial. An Icelandic study suggested a slightly increased incidence among family members of patients with bladder cancer; however, the risk was greater for second- and third-degree relatives than for primary relatives. Furthermore, such studies cannot control for exposure to smoking or for clustering of families in particular occupations.[5]

Staging classification

Bladder cancers are staged according to the joint American Joint Committee on Cancer/International Union against Cancer TNM system (Table 5.1).[6] Using physical examination, endoscopy, and cross-sectional imaging, about one-third of cases are understaged when compared with pathological specimens following extirpative surgery. This makes comparison of different clinical series difficult, especially when non-operative regimens are considered and results based on clinical stage are compared with those based on pathological stage. It is important, therefore, that all reported stages be noted as clinical (e.g. cT1) after endoscopic or radiographic evaluation, or pathological following adequate biopsy or excisional surgery (e.g. pT1).

Pathology

Over 90% of bladder cancers in the UK and the USA are urothelial carcinomas (formerly known as transitional cell carcinoma). About one-third of

Table 5.1. *AJCC–UICC staging system according to primary tumor (T), nodes (N), and metastasis (M)*

Stage	Features
Tis	Carcinoma *in situ* (flat, non-invasive, high-grade cancer)
Ta	Confined to epithelium (papillary tumor)
T1	Invasion of lamina propria
T2a	Superficial invasion of muscularis propria
T2b	Deep invasion of muscularis propria
T3a	Microscopic transmural invasion into perivesical fat
T3b	Macroscopic transmural invasion into perivesical fat
T4a	Invasion of pelvic viscera
T4b	Invasion of pelvic sidewalls or abdominal muscle
N0	Lymph nodes clear
N1	Single lymph node <2 cm diameter involved
N2	Lymph node 2–5 cm, or multiple nodes <5 cm involved
N3	Lymph node >5 cm in diameter involved
M0	No identifiable metastasis
M1	Metastases

urothelial cancers have elements of squamous cell carcinoma or adenocarcinoma, or they may have undergone sarcomatoid dedifferentiation. More rarely, these variant histologies occur as pure forms. Squamous cell carcinoma usually arises in a background of chronic inflammation, such as caused by bladder stones or by schistosomiasis, which is endemic in the Middle East, where squamous cell carcinoma of the bladder is common. Adenocarcinoma commonly arises in a persistent urachus, typically at the dome of the bladder, although it can occur without urachal carcinoma. This chapter discusses only urothelial (transitional cell) carcinoma.

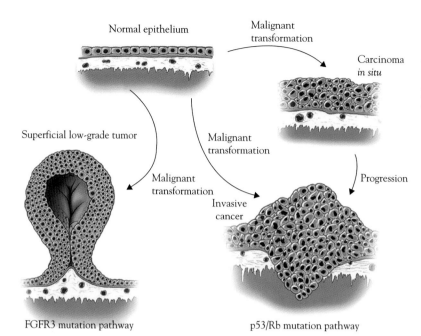

Normal epithelium

Malignant
transformation

Carcinoma
in situ

Superficial low-grade tumor

Malignant
transformation

Malignant
transformation

Invasive
cancer

Progression

FGFR3 mutation pathway

p53/Rb mutation pathway

Figure 5.1. *Different bladder cancer phenotypes arise from different molecular pathways. FGFR3, fibroblast growth factor receptor-3; Rb, retinoblastoma gene.*

In the broadest sense, there are two types of bladder cancer (Fig. 5.1). About 70% of cases are characterized by low-grade papillary cancers, which have a propensity to recur elsewhere in the urinary tract, but mostly within the bladder. This leads, potentially, to multiple interventions over many years, which helps to explain the high cost of managing this cancer. Despite the risk of recurrence, the progression of disease (i.e. progression of grade or stage) is far less common, and prognosis for this type is excellent, provided that patients comply with surveillance protocols. Few patients will die of the superficial low-grade type of bladder cancer.

The remaining 30% of patients have a more aggressive type of cancer that is high-grade and has the capacity to invade and metastasize, even when the initial cancer is carcinoma *in situ* (CIS). Also, as many as 50% of patients with high-grade, muscle-invasive bladder cancer have lymph node involvement at presentation and have an inherently poorer prognosis. Such cases require more than surgical therapy alone.

Molecular pathways

Despite common etiologies, the two types of bladder cancer appear to have distinct pathways of pathogenesis (see Fig. 5.1). About 75% of low-grade superficial bladder cancers have a mutation of fibroblast growth factor receptor-3 (FGFR3), which is encoded on chromosome 9.[7] FGFR3 is one of four fibroblast growth factor receptors that are all transmembrane tyrosine kinases. By phosphorylating intracellular proteins, FGFR3 regulates several cellular functions, including differentiation, proliferation, migration, wound healing, and angiogenesis. In the human embryo, mutations that cause constant activation induce lethal skeletal abnormalities. Mutation later in life is associated with the development of cancer such as of the bladder or cervix. The most common mutation in superficial bladder cancer is S249C (a mutation of the 249th codon exchanging the amino acid serine for a cysteine residue), found in 60% of cases, which means the receptor is constantly active and driving cellular function to favor survival of the cancer cell.[8] The authors examined the genetic changes found in 81 different cases of bladder cancer, and the expression of FGFR3 mutations by stage were 71%, 30%, 0%, and 5% for pTa, pT1, CIS, and pT2–4, respectively. Thus, with advancing stage, fewer tumors demonstrate mutation of FGFR3. CIS has expression similar to the more invasive tumor types, confirming that it is not a precursor of pTa disease.

The intracellular protein p53 has a molecular weight of 53 000 D and functions as a transcription factor that regulates several genes. Its gene is encoded on chromosome 17. Wild-type (normal) p53 regulates the cell cycle and allows repair of damaged cells. If the cell is irreparable, it induces apoptosis (programmed cell death). Mutation of p53 allows the cell to survive despite accumulating abnormalities of its genes, leading to more aggressive types of cancer. In a series of 216 bladder tumors, 65% of CIS showed an accumulation of mutated p53.[9] This mutation is common in CIS and invasive bladder cancer and supports the idea that CIS is a precursor for invasive bladder cancer, rather than the superficial low-grade cancer type. Furthermore, when controlled for stage, tumors with this mutation have a higher risk of recurrence. The two mutations – FGFR3 and p53 – are nearly mutually exclusive, occurring simultaneously in less than 4% of tumors.[8]

Another gene involved in the invasive type of bladder cancer is the retinoblastoma gene (Rb). Knudson was the first to hypothesize the existence of genes that inhibit the formation of cancer, and loss of function of such a tumor suppressor gene was subsequently shown to lead to cancer.[10] Mutations are found in up to 20% of non-invasive tumors, but have been reported to occur in 36% of invasive cancers.[11] Patients with a T1 tumor and a mutation of either Rb or p53, or both, have a significantly greater risk of progression.[12]

Because a small proportion of patients presenting with superficial bladder cancer do eventually go on to develop invasive cancer, there may be some genetic or epigenetic events common to both pathways that have yet to be defined. For this reason, among others, patients with superficial tumors still need to be closely followed on surveillance programs.

There are two main benefits to profiling tumors by their genetic fingerprint. First, it provides more information on prognosis and may lead to better selection of the optimal therapy. Second, these genetic abnormalities provide potential targets for novel therapies, such as blocking an overactive pathway or replacing a mutated gene. This approach of individualized medicine is already in clinical trials for bladder cancer.

Clinical presentation

The cardinal presenting complaint of bladder cancer is hematuria, either seen by the patient (gross hematuria) or found during routine urinalysis (microscopic hematuria). The hematuria is typically painless; however, dysuria plus microscopic hematuria is a hallmark of CIS. Also, if the bleeding is sufficient to form clots, acute urinary retention may occur, which is indeed painful. The differential diagnosis is often cystitis, and patients may give a history of being treated for a urinary tract infection. However, no organism is detected in many of such cases, or symptoms do not resolve with antibiotics. All patients with frank (gross) hematuria should undergo evaluation to exclude cancer of the urinary tract, as should patients with microscopic hematuria if over 40 years old. Owing to the local symptoms associated with bladder cancer, it is rare for a patient to present initially with symptoms of metastatic disease only.

Evaluation

A complete evaluation of men with hematuria can often be delivered in a single visit to a urologist, who performs a complete history and physical examination, integrated with the disciplines of radiology, laboratory studies, endoscopy (occasionally with biopsy), and possibly even a point-of-care tumor marker evaluation like nuclear matrix protein-22 (NMP22) (see below).

The history should be full, documenting the presenting complaint and associated symptoms, but also focusing on risk factors for bladder cancer. For smokers, the intensity and duration of exposure (e.g. number of packs smoked per day for how many years) are recorded. Starting to smoke at a younger age is likely to increase the risk of developing bladder cancer.[3] Exposure to organic chemicals at work or in hobbies should also be recorded. Men diagnosed with bladder cancer ought to be made aware of its potential association with current or past occupation. This can be the starting point for helping the patient to manage lifestyle factors, which have implications not just for bladder cancer but also for overall health.

The physical examination should rule out a palpable bladder, kidneys, liver, or spleen, as well as checking for lymphadenopathy, especially in the supraclavicular basin. The external meatus should be inspected for blood on genital examination. The foreskin, if present, should be retracted to inspect it and the glans, because the rare disease penile cancer may present with hematuria or a painless discharge. Digital rectal examination is mandatory. The evaluation has several stages to it, and explaining the findings as one goes along, and what remains to be done, may help to minimize anxiety.

Tests

Midstream urine is collected and may be divided into aliquots for examination to determine whether the hematuria is initial, total, or terminal. First, apply the urine to a dipstick. Once all portions are wet, hold the stick horizontally to prevent mixing of reagents on the stick. Blood is detected through the peroxidase-like activity of hemoglobin. Urine containing myoglobin may give a false-positive result for blood. Dipstick analysis is more than 90% sensitive for blood, but it tells us nothing about whether malignancy is the source. NMP22 is a point-of-care test on urine that can reveal the presence of cancer, even when the tumor is low-grade and superficial.[13] Other positive reagent tests in the urine (e.g. for protein and nitrites) may point to a non-malignant etiology for the hematuria.

Microscopic analysis of the urine looks for the presence of intact erythrocytes, leukocytes, micro-organisms, casts, and crystals. Hemolyzed blood or the presence of casts in the urine suggests a nephrological diagnosis.

Cytology looks for the presence of abnormal urothelial cells, which line the urinary tract. High-grade malignancy, including CIS, is more likely to shed epithelial cells into the urine. Thus, a negative cytology does not exclude urothelial cancer, particularly low-grade disease. An infection in the urinary tract also causes shedding of transitional epithelial cells, which may be difficult to distinguish from dysplastic or malignant cells. Patients may, in fact,

require multiple serial investigations based on abnormal cytology only. Mentioned above, NMP22 has been shown to improve diagnostic accuracy compared with cytology alone, and is more likely to be positive even when the tumor is low-grade and superficial.[13] Unlike cytology, it also has the distinct advantage of providing a result during the patient's visit.

The upper urinary tract is imaged by ultrasound, intravenous pyelography (IVP, also called excretory urography), or computed tomography (CT) urogram. Ideally, upper tract evaluation is performed prior to cystoscopy. High-grade invasive bladder tumors need more extensive staging with CT or magnetic resonance imaging (MRI), and imaging of the lungs by either plain X-ray or CT. Note, however, that CT scans performed *after* transurethral resection of a bladder tumor commonly show abnormalities of the bladder wall that should not be interpreted as invasion into or through the bladder wall. Skeletal isotope scintigraphy (bone scan) is used for patients who have known metastasis or who have symptoms or abnormal biochemistry, such as an elevated serum calcium or alkaline phosphatase.

Although endoscopy of the urinary tract has been practiced for over a century, there have been many substantial improvements in optics and image processing in recent decades. The flexible cystourethroscope, widely available today, facilitates office-based endoscopy. To perform a flexible cystourethroscopy, local anesthetic is instilled into the urethra and kept in place by pinching off the distal urethra. Sufficient dwell time helps to minimize discomfort and anxiety. Passage of the endoscope through the prostatic urethra in the male patient is often uncomfortable, so encourage him to relax his sphincter at this stage, if possible. Once the cystoscope has reached the bladder, the procedure is usually more comfortable, provided that the bladder does not become overfilled. It is possible to retroflex the flexible cystourethroscope for inspection of the bladder neck from inside the bladder. An enlarged intravesical lobe of the prostate may obscure small tumors near the bladder neck if a rigid cystourethroscope is used. A patient who is awake may be curious to learn the anatomy, and modern cameras and viewing screens make this possible. It should be explained that any tumor will appear magnified.

Although frightening for some patients, seeing a tumor in the bladder may help the patient to comply with prescribed treatment, lifestyle management, and recommended follow-up. Biopsy forceps can perform a biopsy in the office, even without anesthesia, which may be appropriate to confirm the diagnosis prior to scheduling a procedure in the operating room, although the diagnosis and plan may be obvious without a biopsy. In selected patients, the urologist may be able to remove in its entirety a small, low-grade or superficial-looking tumor (or tumors) in the office, and fulgurate the tumor base.

Management of superficial bladder cancer

The extent of disease dictates management of bladder cancer. The care pathways are based on algorithms that frequently require multidisciplinary contributions, especially for advanced bladder cancer. However, even superficial bladder cancer may be optimally treated by adding intravesical therapy to surgical control.

The cornerstone of management of superficial bladder cancer is a transurethral resection (TUR). The goal is to remove all visible tumor, making sure the resection carries into the bladder wall deeply enough to determine depth of invasion (if any) in order to stage the disease accurately. Any suspicious areas should also be biopsied. Patients with superficial tumors around the bladder neck (or apparently invasive tumors) should also undergo biopsy of the prostatic urethra with the resectoscope to look for involvement of the prostatic ducts, with or without invasion of the prostatic stroma. Because non-invasive tumor (Ta) lesions frequently recur, close surveillance is warranted looking for *new* tumors (based on the premise that the TUR totally eradicated the original tumor).

Following complete resection of superficial bladder tumors, a single dose of intravesical chemotherapy will reduce the incidence of recurrences and should be administered. Several agents, including mitomycin C, thiotepa, doxorubicin, and epirubicin, have produced similar results. It is best to administer the chosen agent within 6 hours of resection, to avoid irrigation of the bladder, and to limit urine production during dwell time of the agent.

Intravesical therapy has two other proven roles. It can successfully ablate superficial, low-grade tumors as primary therapy, particularly when they are relatively small and few in number. Many chemotherapeutic agents have been tried. Mitomycin C is popular because of its favorable toxicity profile (it is a large molecule and is not absorbed through the bladder mucosa). Immunotherapy with bacille Calmette–Guérin (BCG) can also ablate untreated tumor and is so successful in treating primary CIS that this is a primary indication for its use.

The other role for intravesical therapy lies in the patient who has demonstrated a pattern of frequent or rapid recurrences, and in whom a protracted course of intravesical chemotherapy or BCG immunotherapy can reduce the number of tumor recurrences and increase the interval between tumor recurrences. Investigators have shown that mitomycin C is even more effective when given as a 40 mg dose in 20 mL of sterile water with pharmokinetic manipulations to increase drug concentration, instilled for 2 hours each week.[14] Compared with a 20 mg dose and no pharmokinetic manipulations, the optimized intravesical mitomycin C increased the median time to recurrence from 11.8 months to 29.1 months, and the recurrence-free rate at 5 years from 24.6% to 41%. BCG seems to be far more successful for high-grade tumors and tumors with associated CIS than intravesical chemotherapy (e.g. mitocycin C). Whilst intravesical therapy reduces the risk of recurrence, no randomized study has demonstrated a reduction in the rate of disease progression.

This fact becomes particularly pertinent when dealing with younger patients with high-grade tumor or patients with high-grade T1 tumors, especially with coexisting CIS, because the favorable impact of BCG has been reported to be less beneficial at 10–15 years.[15] Thus, more aggressive management of T1 tumors or CIS may be appropriate, especially when coexisting, and particularly in the younger patient, and these patients should be considered for early radical cystectomy.[16] The case for early cystectomy is supported by the well-known problem of understaging T1 tumors by clinical examination and TUR, with up to 40% of cases found to have a higher stage at subsequent cystectomy.[17] Patients who present with T1 tumors should always undergo early repeat transurethral resection to help to minimize understaging. Finally, patients who get a T1 recurrence after adequate BCG therapy should undergo radical cystectomy.[18]

Because of the strong predilection for recurrence of superficial bladder cancer, follow-up of patients is very important. Fortunately, the likelihood of recurrence of superficial bladder tumors can be largely predicted by findings on initial cystourethroscopy and pathology of the bladder lesion, supplemented by the clinicopathological findings at 3 months (Table 5.2).[19] Many different follow-up schedules, based on the estimated risk of developing a recurrence, have been proposed. One proposed schedule is presented in Table 5.3.[19] In a multi-center prospective study of 668 consecutive patients with a diagnosis of bladder cancer who were undergoing surveillance, Grossman et al. reported that cystourethroscopy alone detected only 91.3% of all tumors.[13] The addition of urinary cytology produced a non-significant increase in sensitivity to 94.2%, whereas cystourethroscopy combined with NMP22 had a sensitivity of 99.0%. Seven of the additional nine cases identified by NMP22 were high-grade malignancies.[13]

Management of invasive bladder cancer

Patients with tumor invasion of the muscularis propria of the bladder wall (T2 and T3) are usually treated with radical cystectomy and urinary diversion, although high-dose radiation therapy may be offered, often in conjunction with systemic chemotherapy for both modalities. Transurethral resection may be recommended for selected patients with T2 tumors, and partial cystectomy may be appropriate for highly selected patients with T2 or T3 tumors.

Radical cystectomy
Radical cystectomy denotes removal of the intact bladder *en bloc* with the urachus, plus removal of

Table 5.2. *Influences on recurrence-free rate for pTa and pT1 bladder tumors*

Risk factor	Recurrence-free rate at 2 years
Number of tumors	Solitary, 69%; Multiple, 42%
Grade of tumor	Grade 1, 64%; Grade 2, 62%; Grade 3, 30%
Stage	pTa, 63%; pT1, 56%
Maximum diameter of largest tumor	<2.5 cm, 71%; 2.5–4.9 cm, 51%; >5.0 cm, 38%
Tumor located on posterior wall	No, 69%; Yes, 56%
Negative 3-month cystourethroscopy	Yes, 66%, No, 30%

Table 5.3. *Recommended follow-up protocols based on risk of recurrence*

Group	Findings	Recurrence-free rate at 1 year	Follow-up protocol
1	Single tumor and no recurrence at 3 months	78–81%	At 3 months, then yearly
2	Multiple tumors or recurrence at 3 months	60–69%	Every 3 months for 1 year, then every 6 months for 1 year, then yearly
3	Multiple tumors and recurrence at 3 months	8–29%	Every 3 months for 2 years, then yearly

the regional lymph nodes. In the male, the prostate has traditionally been removed, although there are proponents who now argue that the prostate may be preserved if the prostate and urethra are clear on staging and the patient is a suitable candidate for an orthotopic neobladder. This is not yet standard therapy. In the female patient, the reproductive organs and anterior wall of the vagina have traditionally been removed, although here again, surgical modifications are being proposed and evaluated.

Pelvic lymph node dissection up to at least the level of the bifurcation of the iliac vessels is standard, as it improves staging; many argue that it should go up just above the aortic bifurcation. Furthermore, removal of 10 or more lymph nodes predicts for achieving clear surgical margins and better 5-year survival and local control, independent of stage or whether or not patients received adjuvant therapy.[20]

Historically, the most common urinary diversion was the ileal conduit; however, orthotopic neobladders that permit the patient to void 'naturally', constructed from ileum as described by Studer or Hautmann, are being created with ever-increasing frequency in both men and women.[21] Alternatively, one can construct an internal reservoir with a continent cutaneous stoma, such as an Indiana pouch, which the patient empties by self-catheterization.

Progress in minimally invasive surgery now permits selected surgeons to perform laparoscopic and robot-assisted laparoscopic radical cystectomy.[22] Following removal of the specimen through a small lower abdominal incision, some surgeons create the ileal conduit or ileal neobladder outside the abdominal cavity, whereas others are now performing the entire procedure intracorporally, which does prolong operative time. The main advantages of these minimally invasive surgical approaches include reduced blood loss, reduced analgesic requirements, shorter hospital stay, and earlier return to full normal activity.[22]

Historically, radical cystectomy was associated with a high mortality rate. However, with refinements in surgery, anesthesia, and perioperative care, centers performing a high volume of cystectomies now report a mortality rate as low as 0.54%, compared with centers performing fewer than 50 cases per annum, which have a mortality of 2.70%.[23]

Large retrospective studies account for most of the data on outcomes following cystectomy. Data from a series of over 1054 cases demonstrated recurrence-free survival rates of 68% and 66% at 5 and 10 years, respectively.[24] The same authors report that node-negative patients with pT0 and pT1 tumors had 5-year survival rates of 92% and 83%, respectively; 10-year survival rates were 86% and 78%, respectively. Patients with node-negative, organ-confined, muscle-invasive cancers had 5- and 10-year survival rates ranging from 89% to 76%. Twenty-four percent of patients had positive lymph nodes, with 35% and 34% surviving 5 and 10 years, respectively.

Most recurrences (local, urethral, upper tract, and metastatic) occur in the first 2 years after surgery. Follow-up strategies are based on the likely time and location of recurrence.[25] However, metabolic complications such as vitamin B12 deficiency, hyperchloremic acidosis, or renal impairment demand lifetime follow-up. Urethral recurrence occurs in less than 10% of cases, usually in men with prostatic urethral, prostatic ductal, and prostatic stromal involvement. For this reason, the presence of urothelial cancer in these sites provides a strong relative, if not absolute, contraindication for an orthotopic diversion, and suggests, instead, the need for urethrectomy at the time of cystoprostatectomy. Nonetheless, the risk of urethral recurrence has been reported to be lower in patients with an orthotopic neobladder (2–4%) compared with an ileal conduit (4–8%). It is unclear if this observation is due to patient selection or, possibly, the potentially beneficial effect of urine flowing through the urethra.[26]

Radiotherapy

Radiotherapy may also be used as definitive local treatment of invasive bladder cancer, although its efficacy versus radical cystectomy has never been tested by a randomized trial. A recent retrospective non-randomized trial showed similar 5-year survival rates for radiotherapy-treated patients compared with patients treated with surgery, albeit with poorer local control in the radiotherapy group.[27] Data from the Princess Margaret Hospital in Toronto show

10-year cancer-specific survival of 35% for organ-confined, node-negative bladder cancer.[28] Comparisons of radiotherapy with cystectomy are hampered by the inaccuracies of clinical staging and patient selection, because patients with fewer comorbidities tend to undergo surgery. One advantage of radiotherapy is that it is suited for patients who are not fit for surgery. Radiotherapy can be combined with chemotherapy (particularly cisplatin and 5-fluorouracil) following TUR, which, it is argued, improves local control and treats some micrometastases. Despite some reports of patients with muscle-invasive or high-risk T1 disease who have a 5-year cancer-specific survival rate as high as 82%, of whom 82% had an intact bladder,[29] side effects after chemoradiation can be severe, and this approach is not widely practiced. Radiotherapy may be used in some patients with metastases or locally advanced tumors, such as T4b, for local consolidation following a response to systemic chemotherapy if the patients are not candidates for surgical consolidation. Finally, symptomatic bone metastases may be palliated by external beam radiotherapy.

Bladder preservation

Following TUR of the bladder tumor about 15% of patients have no tumor (pT0) in the cystectomy specimen, rising to 38% in those who have received neoadjuvant chemotherapy.[30] This seems almost to invite the development of strategies for preserving the bladder in selected cases if we could be sure of achieving the same rate of cancer control as cystectomy, while maintaining bladder function and quality of life. However, several facts argue against the routine use of this approach. Recent improvements in perioperative care and the development of orthotopic ileal neobladders and minimally invasive surgical techniques tend to favor early cystectomy by reducing morbidity and the negatives of having an ileal conduit. The high rates of clinical understaging by TUR of the bladder and available imaging studies also argue against conservative therapy. During counseling, it must be stressed that only about 50% of those in the conservative therapy group will keep an intact bladder permanently. Patients who want to preserve their bladders must agree to close surveillance and early repeat cystoscopy with biopsies. Patients with no residual disease

may have a 10-year survival of up to 82%, compared with 57% if they have residual disease determined by re-resection of the tumor and its bed.[31] Patients who seem to be better candidates for bladder preservation by endoscopic management have lower stage disease, especially if a single tumor less than 3–5 cm in diameter that is not palpable by bimanual examination, and no hydronephrosis, although these features have yet to be confirmed by prospective randomized clinical trials.

About 5% of patients who require extirpative surgery for bladder cancer may be appropriate candidates for definitive therapy with partial cystectomy. To be suitable for this approach, patients should have a solitary lesion without CIS that is located within the bladder where it is possible to get a surgical margin of at least 2 cm. Perhaps even more important, given the history of failure of this approach as a result of recurrent tumor, this should be the *initial* tumor (i.e. patients should have no history of prior bladder tumors).[32] Even so, patients must commit to lifetime follow-up, because life-threatening tumor may recur even after many years in the bladder remnant. One advantage of partial cystectomy compared with endoscopic management is the inclusion of a lymph node dissection, which, if it reveals positive nodes, permits timely adjuvant chemotherapy.

Finally, chemoradiation as definitive therapy for invasive bladder cancer has been labeled a 'bladder-preservation' strategy, which accounted for some of its short-lived popularity. As discussed earlier, however, progression-free survival with an intact functioning bladder has not been good enough to outweigh the intensity of therapy and potential for long-term side effects, many of which are severe.

Chemotherapy

Several different chemotherapy regimens are available to treat urothelial (transitional cell) carcinoma of the bladder, and they can be very effective. There is no doubt that we achieve optimal results in patients with advanced bladder cancer when chemotherapy is integrated with surgery, either before surgery (neoadjuvant) or after surgery (adjuvant).

The goal of neoadjuvant therapy is to treat micrometastatic disease present at the time of diagnosis, although reducing the size of the primary tumor is an additional benefit. Because there is less risk that a surgical complication or poor recovery by the patient will delay or even prevent all courses from being given, giving chemotherapy before the cystectomy ensures a greater likelihood of receiving what is recommended and planned. Following surgery, the response to chemotherapy can then be accurately assessed in both the bladder specimen and the involved lymph nodes, which indicates tumor sensitivity to that particular regimen. Potential disadvantages of this approach are that surgery may be delayed and the incidence of surgical complications may be higher.

There is no doubt that neoadjuvant chemotherapy is effective, however, and it is considered to have risen to be the gold standard for muscle-invasive bladder cancer by many experts. In a prospective randomized clinical trial that compared 153 patients treated with neoadjuvant MVAC chemotherapy (methotrexate, vinblastine, adriamycin and cisplatin) and cystectomy with 154 patients who underwent cystectomy alone, the first treatment (chemotherapy plus cystectomy) increased the median survival time from 46 months to 77 months and the 5-year survival rate from 43% to 57%.[30] The proportion of patients with complete response (pT0 in the cystectomy section) appears to drive the differences. In the combination group, 38% of patients had a complete response compared with only 15% in the cystectomy alone group; patients with complete response in both groups had similar 5-year survival rates of 85% and 82%, respectively. The main disadvantage of neoadjuvant chemotherapy was that one-third of patients developed severe neutropenia. A meta-analysis of randomized cisplatinum-based trials indicates a 5% survival advantage to neoadjuvant chemotherapy, mostly in cases of pT3 disease.[33]

Some clinicians recommend adjuvant chemotherapy to patients following cystectomy if they have gross extravesical extension or positive lymph nodes, hoping to delay recurrence and extend survival. This approach permits immediate surgery for all patients, including those who might not respond to chemotherapy and who would be placed at a disadvantage if there were tumor growth. If cystectomy is performed first, chemotherapy can be recommended (or not) on the basis of pathological stage, which means that some patients overstaged by clinical evaluation may be spared potentially unnecessary chemotherapy. Furthermore, cystectomy may relieve hydronephrosis caused by ureteral obstruction by tumor and so improve renal function and tolerance of chemotherapy. The potential disadvantages of giving adjuvant chemotherapy after the cystectomy are delayed treatment of occult metastatic disease while the primary is being treated surgically, especially if there is a delay longer than expected because of protracted recovery from surgery. Furthermore, patients may find it more difficult to tolerate chemotherapy following major surgery, even more so if rehabilitation has been slow. There have been several retrospective trials that have suggested a benefit to adjuvant chemotherapy, but virtually no randomized studies of adjuvant chemotherapy confirm this observation. A number of international trials are currently under way to try to clarify the value of this approach, with an emphasis on selecting according to prognostic markers such as mutant p53 expression.[33]

There is clear benefit, however, to giving combination chemotherapy, such as MVAC, to patients with metastases. Patients with measurable lesions have reported response rates of 76%, with 36% showing complete response and some patients achieving long-term survival.[34] Patients with lymph node metastases respond better than those with visceral metastases. Multiple effective regimens are currently available; one regimen may work when another one doesn't, and one may be better tolerated than another. Gemcitabine and cisplatin produce similar responses to MVAC with less toxic side effects.[35] Other regimens include taxanes (either as a single agent or in combination with other agents), dose escalation of MVAC with granulocyte colony-stimulating factor support, and substitution of carboplatin for cisplatin in unfit patients.

Palliative care

Some patients with locally advanced bladder cancer (T4), with or without metastatic disease, are unlikely to be cured, even with multimodality therapy. In this clinical setting, symptom control and strategies for palliation become paramount. Patients may receive benefit from transurethral resection, systemic chemotherapy, radiation therapy, and even – in highly selected cases – radical cystectomy. We have observed palliative radical cystectomy to be well tolerated in selected patients with hormone-refractory prostate cancer, and it has controlled local disease for more than 2 years before problems with systemic disease become prominent.[36] A dedicated palliative care team can best manage pain, gastrointestinal symptoms, and end-of-life issues. It is essential to use a holistic approach with focus on the patient's wishes, and to make care available either at home or in a hospice.

References

1. Jemal A, Siegel R, Ward E et al. Cancer Statistics, 2007. CA Cancer J Clin 2007; 57: 43–66.
2. Cancer Research UK. http://info.cancerresearchuk. org/cancerstats/types/bladder/incidence. Accessed October 29, 2007.
3. Pashos CL, Botteman MF, Laskin BL et al. Bladder cancer: epidemiology, diagnosis, and management. Cancer Pract 2002; 10: 311–22.
4. Kishi K, Hirota T, Matsumoto K et al. Carcinoma of the bladder: a clinical and pathological analysis of 87 autopsy cases. J Urol 1981; 125: 36–9.
5. Kiemeney LA, Moret NC, Witjes JA et al. Familial transitional cell carcinoma among the population of Iceland. J Urol 1997; 157: 1649–51.
6. Sobin LH, Wittekind C. Urinary bladder. International Union Against Cancer (UICC). In Greene FL, Page DL, Fleming ID et al., eds. AJCC Cancer Staging Manual, Sixth Edition. New York: Springer-Verlag, 2002: 335–8.
7. Billerey C, Chopin D, Aubriot-Lorton MH et al. Frequent FGFR3 mutations in papillary non-invasive bladder (pTa) tumors. Am J Pathol 2001; 158: 1955–9.
8. Bakkar AA, Wallerand H, Radvanyi F et al. FGFR3 and TP53 gene mutations define two distinct pathways in urothelial cell carcinoma of the bladder. Cancer Res 2003; 63: 8108–12.
9. Spruck CH 3rd, Ohneseit PF, Gonzalez-Zulueta M et al. Two molecular pathways to transitional cell carcinoma of the bladder. Cancer Res 1994; 54: 784–8.
10. Knudson AG Jr. Mutation and cancer: statistical study of retinoblastoma. Proc Natl Acad Sci U S A 1971; 68: 820–3.
11. Miyamoto H, Shuin T, Torigoe S et al. Retinoblastoma gene mutations in primary human bladder cancer. Br J Cancer 1995; 71: 831–5.
12. Grossman HB, Liebert M, Antelo M et al. p53 and RB expression predict progression in T1 bladder cancer. Clin Cancer Res 1998; 4: 829–34.
13. Grossman HB, Soloway M, Messing E et al. Surveillance for recurrent bladder cancer using a point-of-care proteomic assay. JAMA 2006; 295: 299–305.
14. Au JL, Badalament RA, Wientjes MG et al. Methods to improve efficacy of intravesical mitomycin C: results of a randomized phase III trial. J Natl Cancer Inst 2001; 93: 597–604.
15. Cookson MS, Herr HW, Zhang ZF et al. The treated natural history of high risk superficial bladder cancer: 15-year outcome. J Urol 1997; 158: 62–7.
16. Bianco FJ Jr, Justa D, Grignon DJ et al. Management of clinical T1 bladder transitional cell carcinoma by radical cystectomy. Urol Oncol 2004; 22: 290–4.
17. Soloway MS, Lopez AE, Patel J et al. Results of radical cystectomy for transitional cell carcinoma of the bladder and the effect of chemotherapy. Cancer 1994; 73: 1926–31.
18. Herr HW, Badalament RA, Amato, DA et al. Superficial bladder cancer treated with bacillus Calmette-Guerin: a multivariate analysis of factors affecting tumor progression. J Urol 1989; 141: 22–9.
19. Parmar MK, Freedman LS, Hargreave TB et al. Prognostic factors for recurrence and followup policies in the treatment of superficial bladder cancer: report from the British Medical Research Council Subgroup on Superficial Bladder Cancer (Urological Cancer Working Party). J Urol 1989; 142: 284–8.
20. Herr HW, Faulkner JR, Grossman HB et al. Pathologic evaluation of radical cystectomy specimens: a cooperative group report. Cancer 2004; 100: 2470–5.
21. World Health Organization (WHO) Consensus Conference on Bladder Cancer. Hautmann RE, Abol-Enein H, Hafez K et al. Urinary diversion. Urology 2007; 69(Suppl 1): 17–49.
22. Aron M, Colombo JR Jr, Haber GP et al. Laparoscopic radical cystectomy. BJU Int 2007; 100: 455–76.
23. Barbieri CE, Lee B, Cookson MS et al. Association of procedure volume with radical cystectomy outcomes in a nationwide database. J Urol 2007; 178: 1418–22.
24. Stein JP, Lieskovsky G, Cote R et al. Radical cystectomy in the treatment of invasive bladder cancer: long-term results in 1,054 patients. J Clin Oncol 2001; 19: 666–75.

25. Bochner BH, Montie JE, Lee CT. Follow-up strategies and management of recurrence in urologic oncology bladder cancer: invasive bladder cancer. Urol Clin North Am 2003; 30: 777–89.

26. Stein JP, Clark P, Miranda G et al. Urethral tumor recurrence following cystectomy and urinary diversion: clinical and pathological characteristics in 768 male patients. J Urol 2005; 173: 1163–8.

27. Kotwal S, Choudhury A, Johnston C et al. Similar treatment outcomes for radical cystectomy and radical radiotherapy in invasive bladder cancer treated at a United Kingdom specialist treatment center. Int J Radiat Oncol Biol Phys 2008; 70: 456–63.

28. Chung PW, Bristow RG, Milosevic MF et al. Long-term outcome of radiation-based conservation therapy for invasive bladder cancer. Urol Oncol 2007; 25: 303–9.

29. Weiss C, Engehausen DG, Krause FS et al. Radiochemotherapy with cisplatin and 5-fluorouracil after transurethral surgery in patients with bladder cancer. Int J Radiat Oncol Biol Phys 2007; 68: 1072–80.

30. Grossman HB, Natale RB, Tangen CM et al. Neoadjuvant chemotherapy plus cystectomy compared with cystectomy alone for locally advanced bladder cancer. N Engl J Med 2003; 349: 859–66.

31. Herr HW. Transurethral resection of muscle-invasive bladder cancer: 10-year outcome. J Clin Oncol 2001; 19: 89–93.

32. Kassouf W, Swanson D, Kamat AM et al. Partial cystectomy for muscle invasive urothelial carcinoma of the bladder: a contemporary review of the M. D. Anderson Cancer Center experience. J Urol 2006; 175: 2058–62.

33. Sternberg CN, Donat SM, Bellmunt J et al. Chemotherapy for bladder cancer: treatment guidelines for neoadjuvant chemotherapy, bladder preservation, adjuvant chemotherapy, and metastatic cancer. Urology 2007; 69: 62–79.

34. Sternberg CN, Yagoda A, Scher HI et al. Methotrexate, vinblastine, doxorubicin, and cisplatin for advanced transitional cell carcinoma of the urothelium. Efficacy and patterns of response and relapse. Cancer 1989; 64: 2448–58.

35. von der Maase H, Hansen SW, Roberts JT et al. Gemcitabine and cisplatin versus methotrexate, vinblastine, doxorubicin, and cisplatin in advanced or metastatic bladder cancer: results of a large, randomized, multinational, multicenter, phase III study. J Clin Oncol 2000; 18: 3068–77.

36. Leibovici D, Kamat AM, Pettaway CA et al. Cystoprostatectomy for effective palliation of symptomatic bladder invasion by prostate cancer. J Urol 2005; 174: 2186–90.

CHAPTER 6

Colorectal cancer

John Northover

Introduction

Colorectal cancer is very common in Western countries, being the second most prevalent malignancy in men after lung cancer. In non-smoking males it is the major cause of cancer mortality. Globally, colorectal cancer is fourth in the league of cancers causing death;[1] in 1996, there were 510 000 colorectal cancer deaths worldwide, which represented 7.2% of all cancer deaths. In the UK, there are around 36 000 new cases annually, of whom nearly 16 000 are destined to die of the disease. In many Western countries, colorectal cancer is even more common than this, and in many developing countries, the incidence, and hence the importance as a public health issue, is increasing.

Pathogenesis

Understanding of the pathogenesis of colorectal cancer at the molecular level has increased over the past 20 years. Unlike the other common cancers, colorectal cancer usually passes through an orderly sequence – the adenoma–carcinoma sequence (ACS). Normal mucosa first becomes dysplastic, then small benign adenomas develop. These usually become raised, making them visible macroscopically.[2] A proportion of adenomas go on to become larger adenomas, while others may undergo malignant change, ultimately metastasizing

to lymph nodes and distant sites.[3] Probably less than 1% of adenomas progress to malignancy.[4]

Several genetic alterations are causally related to the macroscopic stages of the ACS.[5] These mostly occur during life as a result of damage caused by environmental factors, but some are inherited. In a small proportion of people, perhaps around 5%, dominantly inherited mutations induce a high risk of colorectal cancer at an early age (Fig. 6.1).[6–8]

Both the carcinoma and its precursor lesion, the adenoma, have a predilection for the distal third of the large bowel – 75% of colorectal neoplasms occur in this segment, with the cecum as the next most prevalent site, harboring around 10% of tumors. In the latter part of the 20th century there was a rightward shift in sub-site distribution, more apparent in women than in men.[9]

Trends in incidence and mortality

Within a generation bowel cancer has become both more common and less frequently fatal in the UK and most other Western countries.[10,11] In 1975 about 68% of male patients died, compared with 43% in 2004, while during the same period there has been a 20% increase in the number of cases. While the fall in the death rate has been steady and continues, the rise in incidence flattened out around 1995. The US began to see a fall in incidence and mortality much earlier: in the short period 2002–2004, the death rate there fell a full 5% in men.[12]

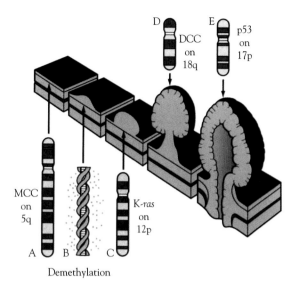

Figure 6.1. *The adenoma-carcinoma sequence and its associated gene mutations.*

Predispositions: sex, race, and social deprivation

The most comprehensive data on sex differences in colorectal cancer incidence and mortality are available from the US. Data derived from the Surveillance, Epidemiology and End Results (SEER) Program indicate that there are significant differences in age-adjusted colorectal cancer mortality between men and women, and that blacks are more frequently affected than whites.[13] The SEER data indicate that the incidence of colorectal cancer increased in male patients in the period 1950–1984, while falling slightly in female patients. From the mid-1980s in the US, though not in the UK, there has been a steady decline in incidence in both sexes.[14]

There are enormous variations in colorectal cancer incidence between countries, with a 20-fold variation in the incidence of rectal cancer and a six-fold variation in that of colon cancer in men worldwide (Figs. 6.2 and 6.3).[15] Japanese men in Hawaii, the descendants of migrants, are twice as likely to develop rectal or colon cancer as their cousins in Japan. These classic observations were part of the evidence that environmental factors and,

in particular, diet play a major part in the etiology of colorectal cancer. Although worldwide, colon cancer affects the sexes equally, in countries with the highest incidence (in North America and in Australasia) and those with a rapidly increasing incidence (Japan and Italy), there is an age-adjusted 20% excess in males; this difference is less marked in the UK. The greatest male–female difference is seen in Hawaiian Polynesians (28 and 14 cases per 100 000, respectively).[16] In general, there is a tendency for colon cancer to be more common in women than in men below the age of 50, but more common in men after that age.[17] For whatever reason, in the UK there appears to be a 25% higher incidence of rectal cancer amongst men in the most socially deprived group compared with the most affluent.[18] Social deprivation is also associated with a 5–9% survival advantage for the most affluent compared with the most deprived. It has been reckoned that if outcomes were uniformly at the level of the most affluent, 2000 deaths would be avoided annually.

Etiology

Diet

Fiber
High fiber intake appears to be generally protective, although cereal intake appears proportionately related to cancer risk in Italy and Japan.[17] The EPIC study is looking at dietary habits in more than 500 000 people in 10 countries, and it has found that those with the highest fiber intake are 40% less likely to develop bowel cancer than those with the lowest.[19]

Fruit and vegetables
Data on the protective effects of fruit and vegetables are more limited.[1] The most consistent dietary observation is that vegetable consumption is inversely proportional to the risk of colorectal cancer.[20] EPIC-Spain, covering about 60 000 people, reports a 25% advantage in death rates from a range of chronic diseases, including cancer, in high fruit and vegetable eaters compared with the lowest. Other collected studies have supported this.[21,22]

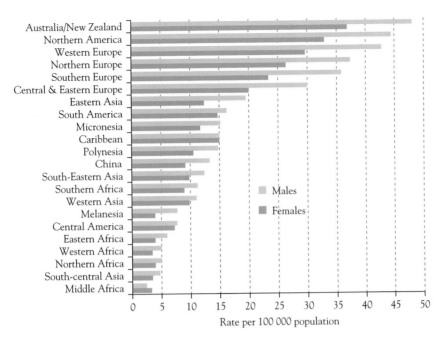

Figure 6.2. *Bowel cancer incidence, men and women, world regions, 2002 estimates.*

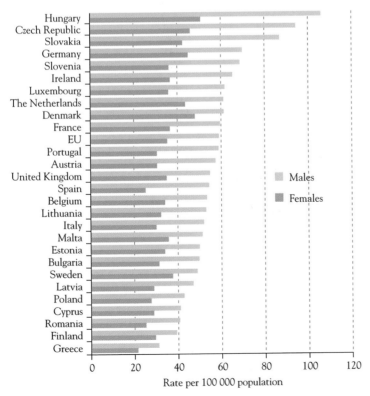

Figure 6.3. *Bowel cancer incidence, men and women, Europe, 2005 estimates.*

Meat

Animal protein consumption is generally associated with a risk of colorectal cancer, although fish and seafood consumption may be inversely related.[20] The specific mechanisms whereby animal protein predisposes to colorectal cancer are unclear; however, the presence of fat, as well as processing and cooking methods, may be factors.[1,23] Heavily browned meat, with a consequent excess of mutagenic heterocyclic amines, may be an important meat-related factor.[24] On the other hand, EPIC has reported that those taking >80g fish per day have a 30% lower risk of bowel cancer.[25]

Micronutrients

Evidence about calcium and vitamin D intake has been conflicting. The intake of various micronutrients, such as selenium and the carotenoids, has been said to be protective, but current evidence is not conclusive.[17]

Genetic predisposition

Around 5% of bowel cancers arise in families with a strong predisposition to bowel cancer; this subject is covered in more detail later in the chapter. In many more people their 'genetic makeup' may make them more sensitive to some of the environmental factors that can give rise to the disease.

Physical activity

Regular physical activity apparently protects against some cancers. Regular exercise helps maintain a 'healthy' body weight, while being overweight and obese can greatly increase the risk of cancer. Exercise itself is also reported to have a protective effect, independent of its effects on body weight.[26–28] People with the lowest cancer risks are those who have healthy body weights and who engage in the most physical activity (all other risk factors being equal).

Over 50 scientific studies around the world have shown that physical activity can reduce the risk of bowel cancer, and the largest of these studies agree that people who are physically active can halve their risk, especially if they also keep a healthy body weight. People who are involved in active jobs are less likely to develop bowel cancer.

Occupation

Certain occupations may expose workers to specific substances that produce an increased risk of colorectal cancer. Asbestos, with a two-fold colon cancer risk excess, is the best documented; pesticide and herbicide exposure may also carry some risk. Painters, printers, railway workers, and wood, metal, and car workers have all been shown to be at increased risk of colorectal cancer.[17]

Smoking

Cigarette smoking has not been implicated in colon cancer, whereas cigar and pipe smoking have been shown to be more common in case control studies.[17]

Alcohol

Of 19 population studies, the slight majority has shown a positive correlation between colon cancer risk and alcohol intake.[17] Beer consumption appears to be more positively correlated with rectal cancer in men than in women. It is likely that the association is related to total ethanol intake rather than to the type of drink.[1,29] The EPIC study has addressed this question also, and has found that 2 units of alcohol daily is associated with a 10% increase in the risk of bowel cancer. A recent American study showed that heavier drinkers (5–6 units daily) have a 40% increase in the risk of bowel cancer.[30]

Caffeine

The few studies in this area have produced conflicting data.[17] Taken together, evidence suggests that coffee may decrease colorectal cancer risk.[1]

Clinical presentation

Symptoms

Colorectal cancer often causes symptoms late in the evolution of the disease: in some series, as many as 50% of cases were manifestly beyond cure by the time that symptoms compelled sufferers to seek help. In part, this is due to the lack of symptoms until an advanced disease stage; however, it is also due to a delay in presentation after symptom onset. The symptoms of colorectal cancer may be mistaken for those of more minor conditions, such as hemorrhoids or irritable bowel syndrome, leading to further delay.[31,32] The most common symptoms are bleeding, change of bowel habit, mucous discharge, and tenesmus; any of these symptoms should lead the patient, particularly the middle-aged and elderly, to seek medical advice. Symptom combinations – bleeding, change of bowel habit, anal symptoms – combined with age allow very reliable predictions of cancer risk in general practice populations.[33]

Change of bowel habit

Change of bowel habit may be a minor alteration in frequency or timing of defecation, with or without an unexplained change in the consistency of the stool. This symptom has been shown to be the best diagnostic discriminator in an influential case control study.[34]

Bleeding

Blood may be mixed with the motion or separate from it. Various shades of color of the blood may be seen: it is often plum-colored if the tumor is proximal or bright red if the tumor is in the rectum, but no shade is truly site-specific. In people at and beyond middle age, rectal bleeding has a positive predictive value for cancer of at least 10%.[35,36]

Mucous discharge

Mucous discharge may be a prominent feature, particularly in distal tumors, often stained by stool or blood.

Tenesmus

A rectal tumor can give a sensation of incomplete evacuation, as the 'malignant stool' remains firmly attached to the rectal wall.

Anemia

Classically, anemia may be the only clinical feature of right-sided colonic tumors, inducing shortness of breath, angina, or even heart failure. Colorectal cancer is an important differential diagnosis of anemia of unknown origin, especially after the age of 55.

Acute complications

Around 30% of all bowel tumors present as emergencies with obstruction or peritonitis,[37,38] though this high proportion is improving in some countries, perhaps related to early diagnosis through screening.

Physical signs

General signs of anemia or weight loss should be sought. Abdominal examination may reveal a mass, particularly in the presence of a large sigmoid or cecal tumor. The liver may be enlarged, owing to metastasis. As the predominant anatomical site of colorectal cancer is the distal segment, digital examination should always be a part of the examination of a patient presenting with any of the above symptoms. Rectal tumors up to 10 cm from the anus may be palpable as a firm, sometimes ulcerated, mass arising from the rectal wall. Even if the tumor is not palpable, blood or mucus on the glove may provide a clue. Rigid sigmoidoscopy is a routine part of the outpatient examination, permitting the distal 25 cm to be examined.

Investigations

The decision whether symptoms and signs require investigation may be difficult for the general practitioner. In general terms, if the clinical picture requires investigation, the general practitioner should assume that the whole length of the rectum and colon needs examination, although the surgeon to whom the patient is referred may feel that this can be avoided in some cases. The two major methods of investigation in cases of suspected colorectal cancer are endoscopy and radiology.

Endoscopy

Colonoscopy is widely available. It allows biopsy of any lesion identified and is more sensitive than the time-honored barium enema X-ray (still widely used in the UK) in the detection of small cancers and adenomas, particularly in the sigmoid colon, where convolution and the presence of diverticular disease can make radiological interpretation difficult. A small proportion of cancers is identified as malignant polyps on endoscopy and may be treated definitively by endoscopic polypectomy (Figure 6.4). Colonoscopy carries a small but definite morbidity and mortality risk. In patients with 'left-sided' symptoms (principally fresh bleeding), the shorter

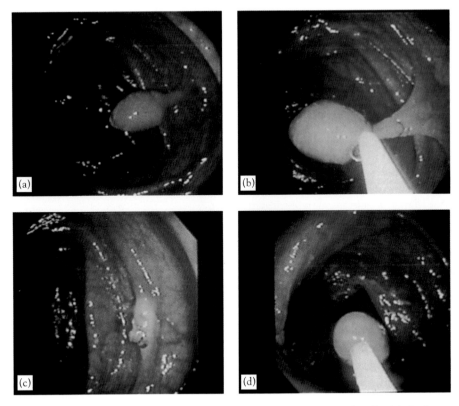

Figure 6.4. *Colon polyp at endoscopy: (a) stalked polyp; (b) snare paced around stalk; (c) diathermied stalk base after polyp excision; (d) excised polyp held in snare for transanal retrieval.*

flexible instrument, the flexible sigmoidoscope, may be used instead.

Radiology

Barium enema
Double-contrast barium enema is still widely used in the UK (Fig. 6.5), at least in part because of waiting list problems in colonoscopy. It provides the least information – compared with cross-sectional imaging – since it can only display luminal deformities.

Cross-sectional imaging
Computed tomography (CT) scanning provides comprehensive data on the local stage of a primary tumor, and it is sensitive in the detection of metastatic spread. Magnetic resonance scanning is mandatory in the assessment of rectal tumors, providing highly predictive data on the local extent of the tumor, and hence informing decisions on the need for preoperative adjuvant radiotherapy (see below).

Ultrasound scanning
Ultrasound scanning can be used to examine rectal tumors, particularly 'early' tumors, to provide reliable evidence regarding degree of spread through the rectal wall.[39]

CT colonography ('virtual colonoscopy')
The technique of CT colonography is becoming more widely used, particularly in patients whose general health makes the bowel preparation required for optical colonoscopy a concern. Using modern computer reconstruction techniques it is possible to use data derived by CT scanning to produce images closely resembling those seen in optical colonosopy – but without 'invading' the patient (Fig. 6.6).

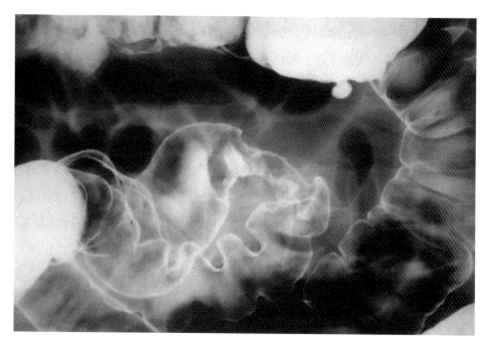

Figure 6.5. *Colon cancer on double contrast barium enema. Irregular 'apple core' stricture due to carcinoma of the sigmoid colon.*

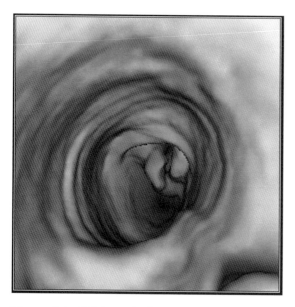

Figure 6.6. *CT 'virtual colonoscopy'. Computerized reconstruction of scan data produces image resembling optical colonoscopy. A cancer is seen in the 'distance'.*

Surgical treatment

Rectal cancer

There are three main categories of potentially curative surgery for rectal cancer:

- *anterior resection (AR)*, which involves radical removal of the involved segment of bowel followed by joining ('anastomosis') of the two bowel ends; if the operation is technically difficult a temporary diversion of the bowel (ileostomy) into a bag on the abdominal surface protects the anastomosis. If X-rays show the join to be healthy 2 months later, the ileostomy is closed and the rectum returns to anatomically normal function. There is much evidence that the quality of surgery affects the risk of local recurrence and survival; in particular there must be meticulous dissection and removal of the fatty tissue surrounding the rectum (the 'mesorectum'), into which the tumor may spread outwards from the primary tumor;[40,41]

- *abdominoperineal excision (APER)*, which is used for the 10–20% of patients in whom the tumor is so low in the rectum that it is impossible to remove the cancer without also removing the anal sphincter muscles, which maintain continence. The operation therefore requires formation of a permanent colostomy; and
- *transanal local excision (LE)*, which involves 'simple' removal (via the anus) of the disc of rectal wall harboring the tumor. This operation is reserved for small tumors in which investigations show no evidence of spread beyond the bowel wall.

In some cases, the choice is obvious. With a small tumor in the upper rectum in a fit man, treatment is usually by AR, whereas the very low, bulky, aggressive tumor, particularly in the unfit or obese man, is best treated by APER. A small proportion (around 5%) of small, early tumors close to the anus may be suitable for LE. In many cases, however, the choice of procedure is less clear-cut and is more likely to depend on the surgeon's experience and inclinations.

Complications of rectal cancer surgery

Perhaps more than any other type of non-genital cancer surgery, that for rectal cancer carries a threat to sexual function, particularly in men.[42,43] The nerve supply of the bladder and of sexual function lies in close proximity to the planes of surgical dissection. These comprise the sympathetic nerves in the hypogastric plexus and the sacral parasympathetic supply in the nervi erigentes (Fig. 6.7).[44] Damage to these nerves may result in disorders of bladder emptying and failure of penile erection and ejaculation. Throughout much of the 20th century, many surgeons were fatalistic about nerve damage during such surgical procedures; rates of up to 50% were reported. In recent times, as the anatomy of the nerves has become better understood and as the pattern of dissection and the methods of achieving it have been refined, the risk has fallen dramatically. Unless the nerves are actually invaded by the tumor or the anatomy of the patient is such as to make

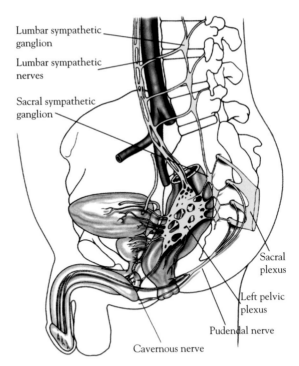

Figure 6.7. *Anatomy of pelvic autonomic nerve supply.*

visualization of the area at risk very difficult, it is usually possible to avoid these complications.

Nerve damage may be partial or complete, in terms of both the anatomy of the injury and the extent of functional deficit. If injury does occur, it is unlikely to recover completely. Methods of dealing with partial or complete erectile dysfunction are beyond the scope of this chapter, and are dealt with elsewhere in this book (see Chapter 14).

Colon cancer

In principle, the operations for tumors in different parts of the colon are similar: the affected segment and its lymphatic drainage are isolated by an appropriate dissection and then removed; subsequently, the two bowel ends are joined, usually using a hand-sutured technique.

Laparoscopic surgery

Known sometimes as 'keyhole surgery', this revolutionary approach avoids the conventional long abdominal incision. First the abdominal cavity is inflated via a cannula inserted through the

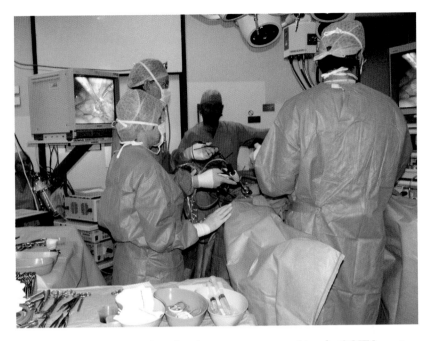

Figure 6.8. *Laparoscopic colon surgery. Note that the surgeons are watching the CCTV monitor, not the patient, in order to direct the procedure.*

abdominal wall. A high-resolution telescope (the laparoscope) is inserted next to the umbilicus. Then several 'ports' are placed through the abdominal wall to allow special instruments to be introduced to hold, dissect, and cut the bowel (Fig. 6.8). A relatively small incision is needed to allow delivery of the resected bowel, and to make anastomosis easier and quicker. As a result of avoiding the long incision, postoperative recovery is usually quicker, allowing earlier discharge from hospital, and a more speedy return to normal activities.

Although not the routine operative method in the UK yet, laparoscopic surgery is being used ever more widely. There is good evidence that the results are as good as in open surgery, at least in colon cancer, and probably also in the rectal cancer.[45]

Postoperative follow-up

Most colorectal cancer patients are reviewed for 5 years after surgery. Most surgeons see their patients 3 monthly for the first 2 years and 6 monthly thereafter until 5 years after surgery. This is based on two tenets: that the majority of the risk of recurrence has dissipated after 2 years, and that the survival becomes parallel with the general population curve (and hence the risk of recurrence has gone) at 5 years.

The process of follow-up after cancer surgery has several aims, including:

- the identification of postoperative complications;
- the provision of patient reassurance;
- audit of the surgeon's performance;
- detection of new primary tumors; and
- detection of recurrent cancer.

Criticism of these objectives is based on the following observations:

- most postoperative complications, except perhaps incisional hernia, manifest themselves within the first year;
- many patients are alarmed rather than reassured by an impending outpatient follow-up visit;
- few surgeons make proper use of follow-up data to review, criticize, and alter their cancer management strategies; and

- only around 5% of colorectal cancer patients develop a new primary cancer.

Consequently, detection of recurrent cancer should be the main reason for follow-up in most cases.

Reflecting the high cost and low evidence base for effectiveness of colorectal cancer follow-up, a large UK multicenter randomized trial (the FACS trial) is being conducted to try to determine the most cost-effective program.

Clinical assessment

Clinical assessment is likely to be offered according to the schedule stated earlier. It includes enquiry after symptoms, general physical examination, and – particularly after rectal cancer surgery – rigid sigmoidoscopic examination. Various investigations may be used in addition.

Colonoscopy

Colonoscopy should have been performed peri-operatively to exclude a second primary cancer and associated adenomata. Depending on the presence of associated neoplasia, the age of the patient, and the enthusiasm of the clinician, repeated colonoscopy may be offered every 3–5 years in perpetuity after primary treatment.

Scanning procedures

As the liver and lungs are the most frequently affected distant sites for metastasis, examination may be performed using ultrasound or CT scanning, particularly in the first few years after surgery. The possibility of cure by resection of localized liver or lung recurrence is quite high (in the region of 30%).[46,47] MR scanning is the preferred method to look for local recurrence after rectal cancer surgery. Whether pre-symptomatic diagnosis by regular scanning increases the proportion cured remains another area for debate in the controversy surrounding follow-up practice.

Serum marker assay

Positive evidence is emerging slowly for the usefulness of the serum carcinoembryonic antigen (CEA) assay, not just for early diagnosis but crucially also for translating CEA assay findings into potentially curative re-operation in some cases.[48] The FACS trial is addressing this question also.

Adjuvant therapy

Overall, surgery alone is curative in around 60% of operated colorectal cancer cases. Although improvements in outcome may be possible through improvements in surgical technique, most effort to increase the cure rate has gone into adjuvant therapy – the addition of radiotherapy, chemotherapy, or immunotherapy to surgery, before, during, or after the operation. Today there is no doubt that at least some forms of adjuvant therapy can improve the outlook in this disease, although which patients are most likely to benefit and which modes or regimens of treatment should be used remain the focus of debate and widespread clinical research. Radiotherapy is essentially a loco-regional modality, aimed mainly at reducing the risk of local recurrence in rectal cancer cases, whereas chemotherapy is seen as a means of improving the chance of survival through the prevention of distant metastasis.

Radiotherapy

Radiotherapy is used mainly in the management of rectal cancer. It may be delivered preoperatively or postoperatively; in a few centers, though none in the UK, it can be delivered to the precise site at risk of recurrence during surgery after removal of the primary tumor. Given preoperatively, radiotherapy has been shown in randomized trials to downstage the disease.[49] Regimens range from high-dose therapy (4000–5000 cGy total dose, delivered over 4–5 weeks, followed by a 6-week rest prior to surgery) to short-course therapy (2500 cGy in the week immediately prior to surgery).[50] Preoperative radiotherapy is generally given in combination with chemotherapy; patients to be offered this treatment are those with rectal cancer in whom MR scanning indicates that the tumor is sufficiently advanced for there to be a significant risk of leaving some tumor tissue behind at surgery.

Postoperative radiotherapy is used in those rectal cancer patients who, having undergone surgery without preoperative treatment, are found by the pathologist to have cancer at or very close to the surface of the operative specimen, indicating a high risk of residual tumor and hence of later, life-threatening recurrence. The major disadvantage of postoperative therapy is small bowel radiation damage, made more likely by operation-induced adhesions that cause the small bowel to be held inevitably in the field of treatment. This leads to significant morbidity, and occasional mortality, in around 5% of cases.

Finally, trials in Sweden and the Netherlands and most recently in the UK have yielded evidence that the unselected use of short-course preoperative therapy in all rectal cancer cases decreases the risk of local recurrence overall.[50,51]

Bladder and sexual dysfunction after pelvic radiotherapy

As mentioned earlier, nerve damage can occur during pelvic dissection during rectal cancer surgery. Adjuvant radiotherapy, either before or after surgery, may sometimes induce similar problems, particularly in men.[42,52]

Chemotherapy

Adjuvant chemotherapy for colon and rectal cancer has been investigated for more than 40 years, and has involved mainly the use of 5-fluorouracil (5-FU), either alone or in combination with other drugs. Until around 1990 the results were uniformly quite disappointing; however, a series of trials that published their results from 1990 onwards has led to much wider use of adjuvant chemotherapy. As a rule patients found to have involvement of lymph nodes in the operative specimen in cases both of colon and of rectal cancer are offered postoperative chemotherapy. Today the standard regimen includes a combination of 5-FU, folinic acid, and oxaliplatin.[53] Other combinations are being investigated, including a whole new family of substances,

known colloquially as 'biologicals' – the common characteristic of these drugs is that they are antibodies that act in various ways such as blocking the formation of blood vessels supplying the tumor (bevacizumab) or preventing the action of substances ('growth factors') that drive the growth of cancer cells (cetuximab).[54]

Prognosis

Pathologists are able to provide information on the degree of risk of recurrence through their examination of the operative specimen. The main staging system for colorectal cancer is Dukes' classification. This is based on the depth of invasion by the primary tumor and lymph node involvement. Dukes' classification and its prognostic significance are shown in Table 6.1. Unfortunately, although this and other systems can predict a high or low risk of recurrence in around 50% of patients, the other 50% are rather left in limbo, with a predicted risk of recurrence no more accurate than a toss of a coin. Many institutions today use the tumor–nodes–metastasis (TNM) staging system, which merely describes these crucial parts of the clinicopathological picture.[55]

Prevention

Diet

A large proportion of colorectal cancer risk appears to be associated with dietary and other environmental and lifestyle factors. Consequently, a corresponding proportion of cases ought to be

Table 6.1. *Dukes' classification system*

Dukes' classification	Criteria	Cases (%)	5-year survival (%)
A	▪ Confined to bowel wall ▪ Lymph nodes clear	10	90
B	▪ Penetrates bowel wall ▪ Lymph nodes clear	45	60
C	▪ Lymph nodes involved	45	30

preventable by suitable alterations in diet and lifestyle. In order to provide evidence upon which to base dietary advice, various randomized controlled trials (RCTs) have been, or are being, performed. Because of the relative rarity of colorectal cancer in the general population (prevalence around 1 in 500 at any one time), and despite its prominence in the league table of killing cancers, dietary RCTs using cancer incidence or mortality as the end-point are very difficult to conduct, and it is therefore difficult to produce robust dietary advice from the findings of RCTs. Instead, adenoma incidence or recurrence have been generally used as measures of effect. The Women's Health Initiative in the US, involving 63 000 randomized persons, is the largest study on lifestyle indicators using cancer itself as the measured end-point.[56] Within the next decade there should be evidence upon which to develop preventive dietary advice, applicable to men as well as to women!

Screening

Screening is a process by which an intervention is made in a defined population in order to improve the population outcome for the target disease. The intervention must be cost effective, and should cause minimum population harm as a nevertheless necessary cost for the beneficial effect.

Rigorous research over the past 25 years has shown conclusively that fecal occult blood testing (FOBT) is just such a test in bowel cancer. Several major RCTs have concurred in showing that population screening in the population aged 60 and above produced a 15–20% decrease in bowel cancer deaths. One important, and fairly obvious, requirement for successful screening is sufficient take up ('compliance') in the target population; research has consistently shown that women are more compliant in this regard than men. This test involves submitting several small stool samples to the screening center; these are tested for minute amounts of blood that may have been shed by a tumor. If the test is positive there is a 10% chance that the person being screened has bowel cancer. Those found to have a positive result are therefore invited for colonoscopy. The majority of cancers thus detected are at a very early stage of development, and are

therefore most likely to be cured. The UK national screening program is well under way, and by 2009 the test should have been offered to the whole population aged 60 and over.[57] Public education must be an integral part of the program if it is to be successful.[58]

Other screening tests are being evaluated, most notably flexible sigmoidoscopy, in which the rectum and lower part of the colon are examined with a 60 cm flexible scope. This is the segment of the bowel most predisposed to cancer. The test has the added advantage that it can be cancer-preventive by identifying and removing pre-malignant adenomas. A very large trial soon to be completed in the UK is likely to show that this test too can decrease mortality by around 15–20%. It is likely that the test will need to be performed only once in ten years to produce this effect – unlike FOBT, which has to be repeated twice yearly. The trial result is awaited, after which it will be necessary to decide how it might be added into the national program to best effect.[59]

High-risk groups

Certain groups are at increased risk of colorectal cancer, primarily those with an inheritable predisposition and those with longstanding inflammatory bowel disease.

Inherited predisposition

There are two principal dominantly inherited conditions predisposing to colorectal cancer: familial adenomatous polyposis (FAP) and hereditary non-polyposis colorectal cancer (HNPCC) syndrome. Both are rare, accounting for no more than 5% of all colorectal cancers between them. Neither condition is sex-linked, nor is there evidence of significant geographical variation.

FAP is characterized by the development in the teenage years of large numbers of adenomas on the colorectal mucosa, some of which progress to malignancy by age 40 years if left untreated.[60] Associated lesions in affected people include duodenal adenomas, desmoid tumors (mainly affecting the abdomen), and various incidental abnormalities, such as benign osteomas, skin cysts, and retinal pigmentation. FAP is caused by mutations in a gene located on the long arm of chromosome 5. Cancer-preventive measures involve the removal of the bulk of the large intestine in affected people in their mid- to late teens.[60] Chemoprevention is an area of considerable research.[61]

HNPCC syndrome produces a less obvious clinical picture: there is no carpet of adenomas to betray the diagnosis. There is, however, a predilection for right-sided tumors, occurring at a younger average age, and more frequently with multiple primary tumors.[62] The condition is caused by mutations in the mismatch repair genes that 'police' the process of cell division, usually identifying and rectifying chance mutations in the genome.[8,63] The resulting deficiency in the process leads to the accumulation of the somatic mutations that underlie the development of malignancy. In families harboring this condition, regular colonoscopic surveillance is offered in order to identify and remove any adenomas before they progress to frank malignancy.

Certain families harbor an inheritable risk, but do not possess the currently understood predisposing mutations. If a family pedigree gives rise to sufficient suspicion of a predisposition, even in the absence of an identified genetic explanation, colonoscopic surveillance should be offered.

Inflammatory bowel disease

Colorectal cancer occurs more frequently in patients with ulcerative colitis (UC) or Crohn's disease than in the general population. The cancer risk is small in patients with Crohn's disease, and in those with anatomically limited UC or UC of recent onset. In those who have UC of 10 years' or more duration and in whom the disease affects the majority of the large bowel, cancer risk rises sharply. In those with extensive UC of more than 20 years' duration, the cancer risk exceeds 20%. Cancer is usually preceded by the development of dysplastic mucosal lesions; regular (1–2 yearly) colonoscopy to try to identify these pre-malignant lesions may lead to effective preventive surgical treatment, but debate continues over the efficacy of such surveillance programs.[64,65]

References

1. Potter J. Colon, rectum. In: Potter J, ed. Food, Nutrition and the Prevention of Cancer: A Global Perspective. Washington, DC: American Institute for Cancer Research, 1997.
2. Muto T, Bussey H, Morson B. The evolution of cancer of the colon and rectum. Cancer 1975; 36: 2251–70.
3. Gutman M, Fidler I. Biology of human colon cancer metastasis. World J Surg 1995; 19: 226–34.
4. Hamilton S. Pathology and biology of colorectal neoplasia. In: Young GP, Rozen P, Levin B, eds. Prevention and Early Diagnosis of Colorectal Cancer. London: Saunders, 1996: 321.
5. Fearon E, Vogelstein B. A genetic model for colorectal tumorigenesis. Cell 1990; 61: 759–67.
6. Bodmer W, Bailey C, Bodmer J et al. Localization of the gene for familial adenomatous polyposis on chromosome 5. Nature 1987; 328: 614–16.
7. Fishel R, Lescoe M, Rao M. The human mutator gene homologue MSH2 and its association with hereditary nonpolyposis colon cancer. Cell 1993; 75: 1027–38.
8. Bronner C, Baker S, Morrison P. Mutation in the DNA mismatch repair gene homologue hMLH1 is associated with hereditary nonpolyposis colon cancer. Nature 1994; 368: 258–61.
9. Butcher D, Hassanein K, Dudgeon M et al. Female gender is a major determinant of changing subsite distribution of colorectal cancer with age. Cancer 1985; 56: 714–16.
10. Coleman M, Babb P, Damiecki P. Cancer Survival Trends in England and Wales. 1971–1995: Deprivation and NHS Region. London: TSO, 1999.
11. Cancer Research UK, CancerStats: Survival-England and Wales, 2004.
12. Ries LAG, Melbert D, Krapcho M et al. SEER Cancer Statistics Review. 1975–2004. Bethesda, MD: National Cancer Institute, based on November 2006 SEER data, posted to the SEER website 2007.
13. Schottenfeld D. Epidemiology. In: Cohen A, Winawer S, eds. Cancer of the Colon, Rectum and Anus. New York: McGraw Hill, 1995: 1124.
14. Chu K, Tarone R, Chow W et al. Temporal patterns in colorectal cancer incidence, survival and mortality from 1950 through 1990. J Natl Cancer Inst 1994; 86: 997–1006.
15. Parkin D, Muir C, Whelan S et al. Cancer Incidence in Five Continents, vol. VI. Lyon: International Agency for Research on Cancer, 1992.

16. Parkin D, Muir C, Whelan S. Cancer Incidence in Five Continents, vol V. Lyon: International Agency for Research on Cancer, 1987.

17. Potter J. Epidemiologic, environmental and lifestyle issues in colorectal cancer. In: Young GP, Rozen P, Levin B, eds. Prevention and early detection of colorectal cancer. London: WB Saunders, 1996: 23–43.

18. Coleman M, Rachet B, Woods LM et al. Trends on socioeconomic inequalities in cancer survival in England and Wales up to 2001. Br J Cancer 2004; 90: 1367–73.

19. Bingham SA, Day NE, Luben R et al. Dietary fibre in food and protection against colorectal cancer in the European Prospective Investigation into Cancer and Nutrition (EPIC): an observational study. Lancet 2003; 361: 1496–501.

20. Potter J, Slattery M, Bostick R, Gapstur S. Colon cancer: a review of the epidemiology. Epidemiol Rev 1993; 15: 499–545.

21. Norat T, Riboli E. Fruit and vegetable consumption and risk of cancer of the digestive tract: meta-analysis of published case-control and cohort studies. IARC Sci Publ 2002; 156: 123–5.

22. Agudo A, Cabrera L, Amiano P et al. Fruit and vegetable intakes, dietary antioxidant nutrients, and total mortality in Spanish adults; findings from the Spanish cohort of the European Prospective Investigation into Cancer and Nutrition (EPIC-Spain). Am J Clin Nutrition 2007; 85: 1634–42.

23. Navarro A, Osella AR, Muñoz SE et al. Meat cooking habits and risk of colorectal cancer in Cordoba, Argentina. Nutrition 2004; 4: 873–7.

24. Gerhardsson-de-Verdier M, Hagman U, Peters R. Meat, cooking methods and colorectal cancer: a case-referent study in Stockholm. Int J Cancer 1991; 49: 520–5.

25. Norat T, Bingham S, Ferrari P et al. Meat, fish and colorectal cancer risk: the European Prospective Investigation into Cancer and Nutrition. J Natl Cancer Inst 2005; 97: 906–16.

26. Hou L, Ji BT, Blair A et al. Commuting physical activity and risk of colon cancer in Shanghai. Am J Epidemiol 2004; 160: 806–67.

27. Slattery M, Edwards SL, Ma KN et al. Physical activity and colon cancer: a public health perspective. Ann Epidemiol 1997; 7: 137–45.

28. Giovannucci E, Ascherio A, Rimm EB et al. Physical activity, obesity, and risk for colon cancer and adenoma in men. Ann Intern Med 1995; 122: 327–34.

29. Cho E, Smith-Warner SA, Ritz J et al. Alcohol intake and colorectal cancer: a pooled analysis of 8 cohort studies. Ann Intern Med 2004; 140: 603–13.

30. Wei EK, Giovannucci E, Wu K et al. Comparison of risk factors for colon and rectal cancer. Int J Cancer 2004; 108: 433–42.

31. Holliday H, Hardcastle J. Delay in diagnosis and treatment of symptomatic colorectal cancer. Lancet 1979; 1: 309–11.

32. Crosland A, Jones R. Rectal bleeding: prevalence and consultation behaviour. BMJ 1995; 311: 486–8.

33. Thompson MR, Perera R, Senapati A, Dodds S. Predictive value of common symptom combinations in diagnosing colorectal cancer. Br J Surg 2007; 94: 1260–5.

34. Curless R, French J, Williams G, James O. Comparison of gastrointestinal symptoms in colorectal carcinoma patients and community controls with respect to age. Gut 1994; 35: 1267–70.

35. Goubston K, Dent O. How important is rectal bleeding in the diagnosis of bowel cancer or polyps? Lancet 1986; 2: 261–5.

36. Fitjen G, Starmans R, Muris J et al. Predictive value of signs and symptoms for colorectal cancer in patients with rectal bleeding in general practice. Fam Pract 1995; 12: 279–86.

37. Chester J, Britton D. Elective and emergency surgery for colorectal cancer in a district general hospital: impact of surgical training on patient survival. Ann R Coll Surg Engl 1989; 71: 370–4.

38. Waldron R, Donovan I, Drumm J et al. Emergency presentation and mortality from colorectal cancer in the elderly. Br J Surg 1986; 73: 216.

39. Hildebrandt U, Feifel G. Preoperative staging of rectal cancer by intrarectal ultrasound. Dis Colon Rectum 1995; 28: 42–6.

40. Heald RJ, Ryall RD. Recurrence and survival after total mesorectal excision for rectal cancer. Lancet 1986; 1: 1479–82.

41. Quirke P. Training and quality assurance for rectal cancer: 20 years of data is enough. Lancet Oncol 2003; 4: 695–702.

42. Hendren SK, O'Connor BI, Liu M et al. Prevalence of male and female sexual dysfunction is high following surgery for rectal cancer. Ann Surg 2005; 242: 212–23.

43. Shah EF, Huddy SPJ. A prospective study of genito-urinary dysfunction after surgery for colorectal cancer. Colorectal Dis 2001; 3: 122–5.

44. Scholefield J, Northover J. Surgical management of rectal cancer. Br J Surg 1995; 82: 745–8.

45. Buchanan GN, Malik A, Parvaiz A, et al. Laparoscopic resection for colorectal cancer. Br J Surg 2008; 95: 893–902.

46. Garden OJ, Rees M, Poston G et al. Guidelines for resection of colorectal liver metastases. Gut 2006; 55 (Suppl 3): iii, 1–8.

47. Khatri VP, Chee KG, Petrelli NJ. Modern multimodality approach to hepatic colorectal metastases: solutions and controversies. Surg Oncol 2007; 16: 71–83.

48. Renehan AG, Egger M, Saunders MP, O'Dwyer ST. Impact on survival of intensive follow up after curative resection for colorectal cancer: systematic review and meta-analysis of randomised trials. Br Med J 2002; 324: 813.

49. Nicholls RJ, Tekkis PP. Multidisciplinary treatment of cancer of the rectum: a European approach. Surg Oncol Clin N Am 2008; 17: 533–51.

50. Swedish Rectal Cancer Group. Improved survival with preoperative radiotherapy in rectal cancer. N Engl J Med 1997; 336: 980–7.

51. Srinivasaiah N, Joseph B, Mackey P, Monson JR. How do we manage early rectal cancer? A national questionnaire survey among members of the ACPGBI after the preliminary results of the MRC CR07/NCIC CO16 randomized trial. Colorectal Dis 2008; 10: 357–62.

52. Konish T, Watanabe T, Kiyomatsu T, Nagawa H. Perioperative radiation for rectal cancer and sexual dysfunction after TME: cause and effect? Ann Surg 2007; 245: 155.

53. National Institute for Health and Clinical Excellence (NICE). Colorectal cancer (advanced) – irinotecan, oxaliplatin and raltitrexed (review). TA 93. London: National Institute for Health and Clinical Excellence, 2005.

54. National Institute for Health and Clinical Excellence (NICE). The use of bevacizumab and cetuximab for the treatment of metastatic colorectal cancer. Final Protocol. London: National Institute for Health and Clinical Excellence, 2005.

55. Moran B, Brown G, Cunningham D, Daniels I, Heald R, Quirke P, Sebag-Montefiore D. Clarifying the TNM staging of rectal cancer in the context of modern imaging and neo-adjuvant treatment: 'y"u' and 'p' need 'mr" and 'ct'. Colorectal Dis 2008; 10: 242–3.

56. Roussouw J, Finnegan L, Harlan W. The evolution of the Women's Health Initiative: a perspective from the NIH. J Am Med Womens Assoc 1995; 50: 50–5.

57. Tappenden P, Chilcott J, Eggington S et al. Option appraisal of population-based colorectal cancer screening programmes in England. Gut 2007; 56: 677–84.

58. Woodrow C, Watson E, Rozmovits L, Parker R, Austoker J. Public perceptions of communicating information about bowel cancer screening. Health Expect 2008; 11: 16–25.

59. Atkin WS, Edwards R, Wardle J et al. Design of a multicentre randomised trial to evaluate flexible sigmoidoscopy in colorectal cancer screening. J Med Screen 2001; 8: 137–44.

60. Bussey H. Familial polyposis coli. Family studies, histopathology, differential diagnosis, and results of treatment. Baltimore: The Johns Hopkins University Press, 1975.

61. Arber N, Levin B. Chemoprevention of colorectal neoplasia: the potential for personalized medicine. Gastroenterology 2008; 134: 1224–37.

62. Lynch H, Kimberling W, Albano W et al. Hereditary nonpolyposis colorectal cancer (Lynch syndromes I and II). I. Clinical description of resource. Cancer 1985; 56: 934–8.

63. Parsons R, Li GM, Rao M. Hypermutability and mismatch repair deficiency in RER+ tumor cells. Cell 1993; 75: 1227.

64. Hodgson SV, Bishop DT, Dunlop MG et al. Suggested screening guidelines for familial colorectal cancer. J Med Screen 1995; 2: 45–51.

65. Lennard-Jones J, Morson B, Ritchie J, Williams C. Cancer surveillance in ulcerative colitis. Experience over 15 years. Lancet 1983; ii: 149–52.

CHAPTER 7

Penile cancer and associated dermatoses

Majid Shabbir, Ben Hughes, Nick Watkin

Introduction

Penile skin conditions can be difficult to diagnose. Lesions can range from simple benign to pre-malignant and malignant conditions requiring a more specialized approach. Surprisingly, men's natural tendency to defer self-referral is even more prevalent with penile lesions. Given the easily detectable and visible nature of penile tumors compared with other malignancies, such as prostate cancer, one has to wonder why such delays in seeking help occur. Likely factors include embarrassment, fear, ignorance, and being single. The subsequent late presentation of serious conditions can often render a simple treatable lesion into one requiring a more invasive and dramatic surgical approach.

Part of the problem in distinguishing the spectrum of penile dermatoses from cancer lies with the relative inexperience of the treating physician. Penile cancer is an uncommon malignancy, affecting approximately 1 in 100 000 men per year in Europe and the USA, with most professionals seeing only one or two cases in their career. Approximately 350 men are diagnosed with this condition every year in the UK, and up to 20% of cases are in men aged less than 40 years. Early recognition and diagnosis of malignant lesions is necessary to improve prognosis and allow for penis-preserving surgery, thus avoiding the devastating psychosexual effects of emasculating radical surgery.

Risk factors

The risk factors for penile cancer are listed in Table 7.1.

Human papillomavirus infection (condylomata acuminata)

Human papillomavirus (HPV) infection presents as an exophytic wart in the genital region. While clinically obvious lesions are seen in approximately 1% of the population, HPV DNA can be detected in up to 50% of penile tumors.[1] While several types of HPV have been identified in malignant lesions, types 16 and 18 are the most common, with the former being found in up to 70% of cases (Fig. 7.1). The risk of developing penile cancer has been reported as being six times greater in men with a history of genital warts. In almost all cases transmission is through sexual contact.

Classical lesions are often multiple, and typically occur on the coronal sulcus and the frenulum, but can also be found as flat lesions on the penile shaft. Extension into the anterior urethra is occasionally seen, although extension into the posterior urethra and bladder is usually seen only in immunocompromised patients. Often the appearance can be difficult to distinguish from pre-malignant conditions or verrucous carcinoma (Bushke–Löwenstein tumor). Biopsy is recommended if the lesion is unusually large or atypical, or resistant to treatment.

Visible lesions often regress spontaneously, and no treatment is required in such cases. Persistent or

Table 7.1. *Risk factors for penile cancer*

Non-circumcision	
Phimosis and poor hygiene	
Human papillomavirus (HPV 16, 18)	
Smoking	
Immunosuppression (including that due to HIV infection)	
Pre-malignant dermatoses:	Bowen's disease (shaft)
	Erythroplasia of Queyrat (glans)
	Bowenoid papulosis

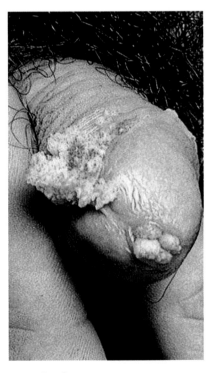

Figure 7.1. *Penile warts.*

symptomatic lesions can be treated with topical podophyllin, or with liquid nitrogen cryotherapy. Surgical excision is reserved for persistent or suspicious lesions and for urethral lesions requiring endoscopic removal. All treatments have similar efficacy with recurrences seen irrespective of the treatment modality. As with all cases of sexually transmitted infection, contact tracing is essential.

Smoking

Cigarette smoking has been shown to be associated with a four- to five-fold increased risk of developing invasive penile cancer.[2] This risk is dose-dependent, and is independent of the co-existence of phimosis.[3]

Phimosis, hygiene and neonatal circumcision

Circumcision remains a contentious issue. While the majority of circumcisions worldwide are performed for religious or cultural reasons, neonatal circumcision has been proposed as a protective measure against penile cancer. The original theory stemmed from the belief that smegma, the by-product of bacterial action on desquamated cells within the preputial sac, was irritative and led to chronic inflammation and subsequent malignancy. This is mirrored by the fact that penile cancer is rare in circumcised men. Studies have shown that phimosis is linked to an increased risk of developing invasive penile cancer, whereas neonatal circumcision is protective.[4] No definitive evidence has established a carcinogenic role for human smegma, and the inevitable poor hygiene associated with an abnormal phimotic foreskin may be a more relevant etiological factor.

Studies have clearly shown that circumcision reduces the incidence of infections, including sexually transmitted HPV and HIV, risk factors themselves for penile cancer.[5,6] It has also been shown to protect against inflammatory dermatoses, including balanitis xerotica obliterans (BXO).[7] Numerous studies have subsequently concluded that neonatal circumcision reduces the relative risk of developing penile cancer by a factor of approximately 3.[1,8]

While good evidence exists to promote the wider benefits of neonatal circumcision, its benefit specific to the prevention of penile cancer is more difficult to establish given the low incidence of this malignancy and the large number of circumcisions needed to prevent one tumor. This may explain the observation of a low incidence of penile cancer in communities where circumcision is rare,[9]

81

suggesting a more multifactoral pathogenesis than circumcision status alone.

Although the controversy of prophylactic circumcision continues, there remains no doubt as to the benefit of circumcision in the treatment of pre-malignant and malignant penile conditions.

Benign penile dermatoses

Benign penile dermatoses can occur in isolation in the genital region, or be associated with widespread dermatological changes. They can range from simple contact dermatitis to psoriasis and lichen planus. Patients with extensive dermatological changes are best reviewed in conjunction with a dermatologist. Only localized, common benign genital dermatoses, which can cause diagnostic confusion with malignant penile conditions, are discussed in this chapter. In all cases, lesions should be distinguishable by examination or biopsy if necessary.

Zoon's balanitis

Otherwise known as plasma cell balanitis, Zoon's balanitis is an idiopathic chronic inflammation of the glans and inner prepuce. The classical appearance is of a bright red, well-demarcated, solitary moist patch occurring on the glans and matched to a mirror image lesion on the inner prepuce,

where the skin has been in close ('kissing') contact. These lesions are clinically different from balanitis seen with candidal infections, which is characterized by a diffusely erythematous glans with small pustules or erosions.

The natural history of Zoon's balanitis is chronic, with episodes of relapse and remission. While the condition itself is not pre-malignant, it can be difficult to distinguish it clinically from erythroplasia of Queyrat when it has been present for some time. In cases of uncertainty, biopsy is recommended. Histology classically reveals skin with a marked plasma cell infiltrate, which is diagnostic. Definitive treatment is by circumcision.

Balanitis xerotica obliterans

BXO is a genital variant of lichen sclerosus et athrophicus, and occurs almost exclusively in uncircumcised men. It presents most commonly in men in their third and fourth decades. The exact etiology remains unclear, but is thought to be multifactoral. Clinical presentation ranges from asymptomatic disease with mild phimosis to severe scarring and a non-retractile foreskin that has become adherent to the underlying glans. Typically, patients present with white, atrophic patches over the prepuce and glans, with a progressive loss of compliance of the foreskin. They often describe a history of chronic irritation with splitting of the frenulum and prepuce, eventually leading to a

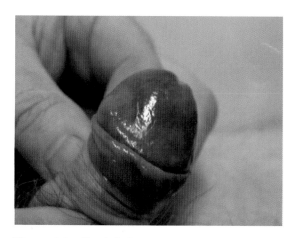

Figure 7.2. Zoon's balanitis.

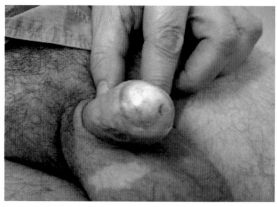

Figure 7.3. Balanitis xerotica obliterans.

complete inability to retract the foreskin. Occasionally, the disease can affect the urethral meatus, leading to meatal stenosis and stricture formation.

Occasionally, topical treatment with corticosteroid cream can be effective in controlling this condition, but failure of medical therapy necessitates surgical intervention by circumcision. This leads to complete remission of glans BXO in over 90% of patients. More advanced cases may require extensive glans resurfacing procedures, depending on the extent of the disease. This may have to be combined with meatotomy and urethral stricture repair to correct the severe damage seen in some patients. Patients with extensive lichen sclerosus can also develop oral lesions. This can make urethral stricture repair more challenging since the quality of the buccal mucosa, the most common graft harvest site, is poor.

BXO does have an association with malignancy. It is a common associated finding in penile cancer specimens (25%), and penile cancer has been reported to occur in up to 5% of BXO cases.[10] While no causal relationship has been shown, the development of persistent skin lesions or chronic inflammation in patients with BXO should be monitored closely and any such lesions biopsied to ensure no concurrent cancer exists.

Pre-malignant dermatoses

Bowen's disease and erythroplasia of Queyrat

Bowen's disease and erythroplasia of Queyrat are both pre-malignant, squamous cell carcinomas *in situ* (CIS). Histologically they are difficult to distinguish from each other, the main difference being that Bowen's disease tends to occur on the penile shaft, whereas the presence of the same lesion on the glans and inner prepuce is referred to as erythroplasia of Queyrat. Clinically, the lesions are red patches with an irregular edge, measuring approximately 1–1.5 cm in diameter. As Bowen's disease occurs on keratinized epithelia, these lesions can occasionally have a scaly appearance. Typically, they have been present for some time and have failed to respond to courses of antifungal creams and topical corticosteroids.

As with all chronic penile dermatoses, biopsy is recommended. Excision biopsy should be performed whenever possible, especially since invasive malignancy is found in approximately 25% of cases.

Bowenoid papulosis

Bowenoid papules are slow-growing warty papules that tend to occur on the penile shaft; they are another form of penile CIS. They are distinguishable from simple condylomata acuminata in that they are more pigmented (often black) and less papillomatous, with a smoother, velvety surface. Lesions can be pruritic but are often asymptomatic. As with all unusual and refractory warty lesions, they are best removed surgically to establish a diagnosis. While the histological changes can resemble the atypia seen in Bowen's disease, Bowenoid papulosis has a low risk of progression to invasive cancer.

Treatment of carcinoma *in situ*

The non-invasive nature of CIS makes it amenable to curative penis-preserving therapies. In the absence of invasive carcinoma, first-line treatment is topical chemotherapy using 5% 5-fluorouracil (5-FU) cream, with reported sustained response rates of 100% at 5 years.[11] The topical use of chemotherapy has been shown to be safe, with low

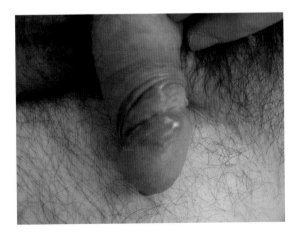

Figure 7.4. *Carcinoma in situ (erythroplasia of Queyrat).*

morbidity and minimal systemic absorption. Carbon dioxide and Nd:YAG lasers have also been used as first-line therapy with equally good response rates.[12] Intractable or recurrent disease is best managed by surgical excision, with extensive lesions often requiring additional skin grafting. Oncological and cosmetic results from such surgery are excellent.

Penile carcinoma

Over 95% of penile cancers are squamous cell carcinomas (SCC), with the remaining rare tumors being melanomas, sarcomas, or basal cell carcinomas.

Verrucous carcinoma

Verrucous carcinoma, also known as Bushke–Löwenstein tumor, is a low-grade SCC of the penis, accounting for approximately 5% of all cases of penile carcinoma. Clinically it presents as an exophytic, rapidly growing, cauliflower-like growth, usually arising from the preputial sac. The appearance can be difficult to distinguish from large condylomata, and excision biopsy is recommended if there is any uncertainty. While this type of tumor has a low risk of metastasis, it can invade local structures such as the urethra. Treatment is by surgical excision and reconstruction accordingly.

Invasive penile carcinoma

SCC of the penis can present in a variety of ways, ranging from an innocuous painless ulcer or red patch to phimosis or a large exophytic, warty growth. Suspicion should always be raised with any chronic lesion or one that persists after treatment. Deep biopsies should always be taken to allow for diagnosis and assessment of invasion, to stage the disease accurately. Examination of the patient should always include assessment of the inguinal region, which is the primary site of lymph node metastasis.

The standard treatment options for patients with penile cancer are radical radiotherapy or surgery. While radiotherapy allows oncological control with preservation of the penis, local recurrence has been reported in up to 40% of cases.[13] In addition, despite preservation, the penis never looks or functions the same again. Recurrence after radiotherapy can be difficult to detect and difficult to treat, with the development of an 'unstable penis', which is a challenge to manage effectively without radical surgery.

Although oncological control with primary radical surgery has stood the test of time, it is not without its own problems. Classically, primary penile lesions were 'over-treated' with a more radical dissection of the primary lesion than was necessary. The previously held belief that a 2 cm clear margin was necessary for adequate clearance has been challenged.[14] While total penectomy is essential in cases

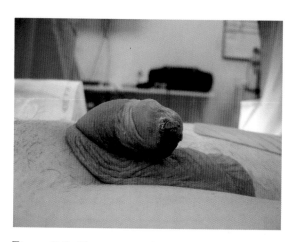

Figure 7.5. *Verrucous carcinoma.*

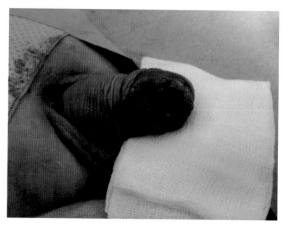

Figure 7.6. *Invasive squamous cell carcinoma of the penis.*

where tumors invade extensively into the corpora or down the penile shaft close to the scrotum, such surgery carries huge social and psychosexual consequences. In the UK, only approximately 15% of tumors invade deeply into local structures such as the corpora at presentation, making the vast majority suitable for penis-preserving surgery.

Penis-preserving surgery

The choice of surgery depends on the grade and stage of disease. Small distal tumors of low grade and stage are most amenable to organ-sparing surgery.[15] However, patient selection and careful follow-up are vital to ensure that local recurrences are detected early and treated accordingly.

Surgical options range from wide local excision combined with circumcision for small glans tumors to complete glansectomy for larger tumors confined to the glans and prepuce. Glansectomy involves complete excision of the glans penis from the corpora cavernosa, with the subsequent formation of a new urethral meatus at the tip of the shaft. The shaft skin is sutured 2 cm down from the tip, with the remaining tips of the corporal heads covered with a split skin graft taken from the thigh. The procedure can be used for patients with up to stage T2 disease, and allows effective oncological control with an excellent cosmetic and functional result. In recent studies, 96% of patients had no

signs of recurrence after a mean follow-up of 27 months,[16] and return to normal sexual function has been reported 1 month postoperatively.[17]

The prognosis of penile cancer is stage-dependent. Low-stage disease (Ta, T1, T2pN0) has a good prognosis, with a 5-year survival rate of 80–90%. However, in the presence of lymph node metastases, this is reduced to 20–40%.[18]

Management of involved lymph nodes

Delay in assessment and diagnosis of penile cancer can often lead to presentation with palpable lymph nodes. Further assessment is with computed tomography scanning and fine needle aspiration cytology of the groins. Up to 50% of patients with palpable nodes at presentation have lymphadenopathy due to secondary infection. Nodes are therefore reassessed after excision of the primary penile tumor and treatment with antibiotics. Persistence of palpable nodes necessitates *en bloc* groin dissection.

Inguinal lymph node dissection (ILND) is associated with significant morbidity, primarily in the form of penoscrotal and lower limb lymphedema. Routine prophylactic ILND for impalpable groin nodes therefore creates a dilemma in that treatment can cause more harm than good. Of the 50% of patients with intermediate- and high-risk penile cancer who have no palpable nodes at presentation, approximately 25% harbor occult disease within

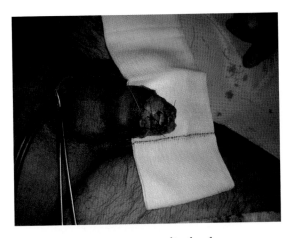

Figure 7.7. *Appearance immediately after glansectomy and split skin graft for squamous cell carcinoma of the penis.*

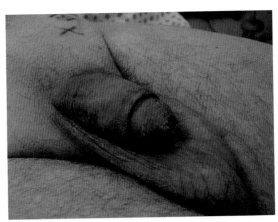

Figure 7.8. *Delayed appearance after glansectomy and resurfacing procedure.*

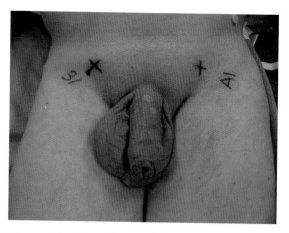

Figure 7.9. *Sentinel inguinal lymph nodes marked on skin for sampling after lymphoscintigraphy.*

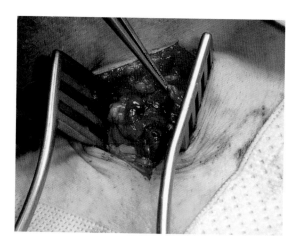

Figure 7.10. *Sentinel lymph node detected intra-operatively using a gamma probe with visual confirmation of a blue node.*

their nodes. The remaining 75% would therefore undergo invasive ILND for no added oncological control or survival benefit.

In this subgroup of patients, dynamic sentinel lymph node sampling can be used to detect micro-metastases. This technique involves using lympho-scintigraphy to detect the first draining lymph node following injection of a radio-labeled tracer around the primary tumor. A further injection of patent blue dye is given in the operating theater, and a gamma probe is used to help identify the sentinel

draining node. The blue dye further aids detection of the sentinel node intra-operatively, which is excised and examined for micro-metastases. Complete ILND is then performed only if the sentinel node is found to contain tumor. In a recent study, only 15% of 143 groins had a tumor-positive sentinel node, and of these only 3 (17%) had further positive nodes on completion of ILND.[19] Only one false-negative result was found in 143 groins, and only 6% of patients had minor complications. Long-term oncological control is also good, with reported 5-year disease-specific survival rates of 96% in patients with benign sentinel nodes.[20]

Conclusions

The early detection and treatment of malignant penile lesions is essential to ensure a good outcome. Increased awareness among both patients and clinicians can help overcome this problem. Most malignant lesions are obvious, but for the more subtle presentations, early and adequate biopsy is recommended. The use of penis-preserving surgical techniques, in conjunction with dynamic sentinel lymph node sampling, has dramatically improved the management of this rare malignancy, with more acceptable cosmetic and functional results, as well as excellent oncological control. Close follow-up and early detection of tumor recurrence is essential to ensure favorable long-term outcomes.

References

1. Maden C, Sherman KJ, Beckmann AM et al. History of circumcision, medical conditions, and sexual activity and risk of penile cancer. J Natl Cancer Inst 1993; 85: 19–24.
2. Daling JR, Madeleine MM, Johnson LG et al. Penile cancer: importance of circumcision, human papillomavirus and smoking in in situ and invasive disease. Int J Cancer 2005; 116: 606–16.
3. Hellberg D, Valentin J, Eklund T, Nilsson S. Penile cancer: is there an epidemiological role for smoking and sexual behaviour? BMJ 1987; 295: 1306–8.
4. Tsen HF, Morgenstern H, Mack T, Peters RK. Risk factors for penile cancer: results of a population-based case-control study in Los Angeles County

(United States). Cancer Causes Control 2001; 12: 267–77.

5. Castellsagué X, Bosch FX, Muñoz N et al. Male circumcision, penile human papillomavirus infection, and cervical cancer in female partners. N Engl J Med 2002; 346: 105–12.

6. Sahasrabuddhe VV, Vermund SH. The future of HIV prevention: control of sexually transmitted infections and circumcision interventions. Infect Dis Clin North Am 2007; 21: 241–57.

7. Mallon E, Hawkins D, Dinneen M et al. Circumcision and genital dermatoses. Arch Dermatol 2000; 136: 350–4.

8. Schoen EJ, Oehrli M, Colby C, Machin G. The highly protective effect of newborn circumcision against invasive penile cancer. Pediatrics 2000; 105: E36.

9. Frisch M, Friis S, Kjaer SK, Melbye M. Falling incidence of penis cancer in an uncircumcised population (Denmark 1943–90). BMJ 1995; 311: 1471.

10. Depasquale I, Park AJ, Bracka A. The treatment of balanitis xerotica obliterans. BJU Int 2000; 86: 459–65.

11. Goette DK, Elgart M, DeVillez RL. Erythroplasia of Queyrat. Treatment with topically applied fluorouracil. JAMA 1975; 232: 934–7.

12. Shirahama T, Takemoto M, Nishiyama K et al. A new treatment for penile conservation in penile carcinoma: a preliminary study of combined laser hyperthermia, radiation and chemotherapy. Br J Urol 1998; 82: 687–93.

13. McLean M, Akl AM, Warde P et al. The results of primary radiation therapy in the management of squamous cell carcinoma of the penis. Int J Radiat Oncol Biol Phys 1993; 25: 623–8.

14. Hoffman MA, Renshaw AA, Loughlin KR. Squamous cell carcinoma of the penis and microscopic pathologic margins: how much margin is needed for local cure? Cancer 1999; 85: 1565–8.

15. Gotsadze D, Matveev B, Zak B, Mamaladze V. Is conservative organ-sparing treatment of penile carcinoma justified? Eur Urol 2000; 38: 306–12.

16. Smith Y, Hadway P, Biedrzycki O et al. Reconstructive surgery for invasive squamous carcinoma of the glans penis. Eur Urol 2007; 52: 1179–85.

17. Hatzichristou DG, Apostolidis A, Tzortzis V et al. Glansectomy: an alternative surgical treatment for Buschke-Löwenstein tumors of the penis. Urology 2001; 57: 966–9.

18. Sarin R, Norman AR, Steel GG, Horwich A. Treatment results and prognostic factors in 101 men treated for squamous carcinoma of the penis. Int J Radiat Oncol Biol Phys 1997; 38: 713–22.

19. Hadway P, Smith Y, Corbishley C, Heenan S, Watkin NA. Evaluation of dynamic lymphoscintigraphy and sentinel lymph-node biopsy for detecting occult metastases in patients with penile squamous cell carcinoma. BJU Int 2007; 100: 561–5.

20. Kroon BK, Horenblas S, Meinhardt W et al. Dynamic sentinel node biopsy in penile carcinoma: evaluation of 10 years experience. Eur Urol 2005; 47: 601–6.

CHAPTER 8

Cutaneous melanoma

Keliegh S Culpepper, Phillip H McKee

Introduction

Melanoma arises from melanocytes, which are derived from the neural crest and migrate to the skin during embryonic development. Their primary function is to generate melanin pigment, which contributes to skin color and provides protection from the sun. Aggregates of melanocytes within the skin form nevi, and malignant degeneration of melanocytes, either de novo or within nevi is the origin of melanoma. This chapter focuses on cutaneous melanoma, although a small percentage of melanoma arises from extracutaneous sites. The study of melanoma is broad, with entire textbooks dedicated to the topic. General principles will be addressed in this discussion, and the reader is referred to more comprehensive texts for more detailed information.

Epidemiology

The worldwide incidence of melanoma has escalated over the past several decades.[1] Australia has the highest incidence;[2] from 1980 to 1987 the incidence rate of melanoma in Australian men peaked at 55.8/100 000. In contrast, the peak incidence in Scotland was significantly lower (6.4/100 000) during the same time period,[3] and incidence in Germany was similar to Scotland.[4]

The majority of all deaths from skin cancer can be attributed to melanoma.[5] Recent data from the USA for the years 1969–1999 show significant increases in melanoma mortality in men aged 45 to 64 years (by 66%) and significantly, a 157% increase in mortality in men aged 65 years and above.[6] In contrast, mortality decreased by 29% in men age 20–44 years. This difference is thought to be due to the increase in the diagnosis of lesions at an earlier stage in the younger population.[7] The incidence of melanoma in men is also increasing, however, this rate of increase may be stabilizing.[7,8] In Scotland, mortality from melanoma has been decreasing over the last two decades, an improvement which is attributed to earlier diagnosis.[3]

The most common site for melanoma in men is on the trunk, and for women the extremities.[9] Melanoma in whites has been estimated to be at least 10 times greater than in blacks. Black men are more likely to present with cutaneous melanoma than black women. One study showed that acral lesions were the most commonly diagnosed site, followed by mucosal melanoma. Overall survival time of African Americans with melanoma was approximately one-third of Caucasians included in that study.[10]

Risk factors

An individual's risk for melanoma is multifactorial, and the overall risk for each individual is likely a result of the combination of genetic susceptibility and lifestyle factors. Fair skin, blue eyes and blond or red hair have traditionally been regarded as risk factors for melanoma. These features may in fact serve as a marker for the four risk factors identified by MacKie and Hole:[11]

- the presence of benign melanocytic nevi
- the presence of freckles or lentigines
- a history of three or more blistering sunburns, and
- the presence of atypical nevi.

The sun plays a role in each of these four features, however, the contribution of sun exposure is complex, and patients with intermittent bursts of sun exposure (such as outdoor recreational or holiday exposure) appear to be more at risk for melanoma than those with chronic daily exposure.[12,13] As a corollary, higher socioeconomic status is associated with an increased risk for melanoma; in contrast, lower socioeconomic groups are more likely to die from their melanoma.[14] The role of sun exposure also varies with the clinical subtype of melanoma. Lentigo maligna is associated with chronic sun exposure and presents on areas such as the face or neck, whereas superficial spreading melanoma affects the trunk and extremities, which tend to have less cumulative sun exposure. The role of ultraviolet radiation as a risk for melanoma is well illustrated by xeroderma pigmentosum. Patients with xeroderma pigmentosum have an inability to repair DNA damage caused by ultraviolet light, and develop multiple skin cancers at an early age, including melanoma. In one recent study, the majority of melanomas were of the lentigo maligna type, and xeroderma pigmentosum has been proposed as a model for lentigo maligna melanoma induction.[15] Albinos also are at risk for melanoma due to the inability to synthesize melanin, however this risk is less than that of xeroderma pigmentosum.

Patients with a personal history of melanoma are at increased risk of a second primary melanoma[16] and this risk is greater than for individuals in the general population.[17] Patients with a prior history of melanoma have their second melanomas detected earlier,[18] and this is largely due to improved patient awareness and follow-up.[19]

Several studies have documented an elevated risk of melanoma in individuals with a large number of common melanocytic nevi. This risk appears to increase as the number of nevi increases.[20] Patients with dysplastic (atypical) nevi[21] have an even greater risk for melanoma. Dysplastic nevi occur sporadically or may run in families (dysplastic nevus syndrome) in which affected individuals may have hundreds of clinically atypical nevi. The tendency to develop dysplastic nevi serves as a marker of melanoma risk (rather than solely a precursor lesion) since melanoma is more likely to arise de novo, rather than in a preexisting nevus.[22]

Melanoma can cluster in families, and approximately 5% of patients with melanoma will have at least one affected first-degree relative. Several genes have been linked to melanoma, including CDKN2A (p16),[23] CDK4,[24] and the melanocortin 1 receptor gene.[25] Twenty percent of melanoma patients with a family history of melanoma have a mutation in the CDKN2A gene.[26] Extensive research of these genes is currently underway, however, clinical applications are limited at this time.

Clinical evaluation

As part of the clinical history, assessment of risk factors and family history should be obtained. In particular, a history of blistering sunburns, prior mole removal and personal or family history of melanoma should be obtained. It is also important to establish whether any family members have an abundance of moles.

The full body skin examination is the best screening tool for melanoma. Although patients and their family members detect the majority of melanomas, studies have shown that physicans are more likely to detect thinner melanomas.[18] Of more concern is that men are less likely than women to detect their own melanoma.[27] The following are guidelines for the skin exam, and patients should be encouraged to do this themselves on a regular basis.

Ideally, the examination room should be well lit, with the patient undressed and wearing an examination gown. Under these circumstances, a visual inspection of the skin is a quick and efficient way to gather information, both about the presence of a lesion suspicious for melanoma, and also to assess a patient's overall risk by the detection of numerous nevi, freckles, skin type, etc. Particular attention should be paid to the back, chest and extremities. Nails, mucous membranes and scalp should also be examined.

Assessing nevi

The American Cancer Society developed screening criteria to determine the likelihood of an individual nevus being diagnosed as melanoma by biopsy, a system known as the ABCDs of melanoma.

A – asymmetry of the nevus
B – border irregularity
C – variegated color
D – diameter greater than 6 mm.

These criteria are most applicable to common acquired nevi. In general, common nevi are less than 6 mm in diameter, and are symmetrical and evenly colored, with smooth borders. One caveat is that not every melanoma is greater than 6 mm in diameter; some may be smaller.[28]

The revised British seven-point check list differs from the ABCD technique by emphasizing changes within a mole as the major criteria in the checklist.

Major criteria:

- change in shape of a previously pigmented lesion
- change in size of a previously pigmented lesion
- change in color of a previously pigmented lesion.

Minor criteria:

- size greater than 6 mm
- inflammation
- oozing or crusting
- mild itch.[29]

Lesions that fulfill either one major or two minor criteria should be regarded as suspicious, and referral to a dermatologist or biopsy considered. One study suggests that the seven-point checklist is slightly more sensitive than the ABCD technique, although both are clinically useful.[30]

Many non-melanocytic cutaneous lesions may mimic melanoma, such as seborrheic keratoses and pyogenic granuloma, and these lesions should not be evaluated by these assessment systems. The practitioner may find it useful to have a photo atlas of common skin lesions available in the clinic for comparison.

Congenital nevi

Congenital nevi are usually present at birth, or appear within the first year of life and affect 1% of infants. These nevi are divided into groups based upon size: small (<1.5 cm in diameter), medium (1.5–20 cm in diameter) (Fig. 8.1), and large or giant (>20 cm in diameter).[31] Congenital nevi are circumscribed hyperpigmented plaques that may have terminal hairs and a cobblestone-like surface. Pigmentation is usually fairly uniform, but may be mottled. The nevus tends to increase in size in proportion to the growth of the child[32] and by adulthood, the size should be stable. Risk of malignant degeneration in small congenital nevi is low, while that of large nevi is very high (5–20%).[33] In a study by Swerdlow et al the largest risk of melanoma was in patients whose nevi covered

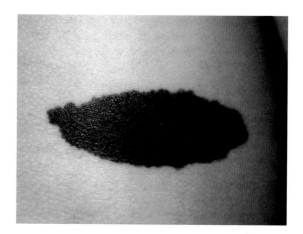

Figure 8.1. *Congenital nevus with mildly cobblestoned surface. (Photo credit: Bernard Cohen, MD. © Dermatlas; http://www.dermatlas.org.)*

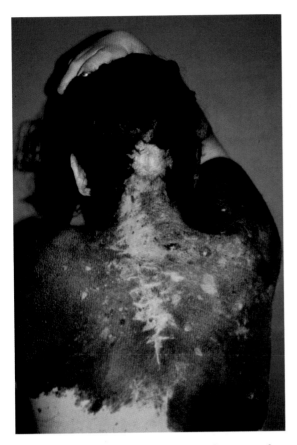

Figure 8.2. *Giant congenital nevus with variegated color on the back of a young woman. A scar is present from a partial excision. (Photo credit: Adrienne Rencic, MD, PhD.)*

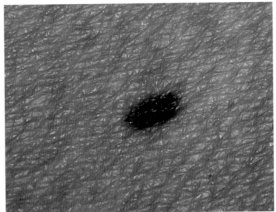

Figure 8.3. *Junctional nevi are pigmented macules with even color. (Photo credit: Adrienne Rencic, MD, PhD.)*

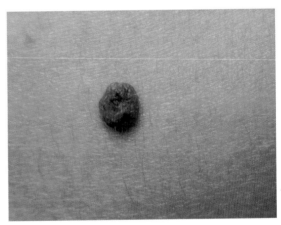

Figure 8.4. *Compound nevus with little pigmentation. (Photo credit: Adrienne Rencic, MD, PhD.)*

more than 5% of their body surface.[32] The majority of melanomas arising in giant congenital nevi do so prior to adulthood, however, malignant degeneration appears to be bimodal, with 30% of melanomas occurring later in life.[34] Many patients undergo surgical excision of intermediate and larger lesions prior to adulthood (Fig. 8.2). Small-sized lesions may be followed using the same criteria outlined above.

Common acquired nevi

Common nevi arise in early childhood and new nevi may continue to develop until the fourth decade, after which they slowly begin to disappear. Nevi are generally less than 5 mm in size, and the total number of nevi is variable.[35] The development of new nevi in an elderly patient is uncommon and a new 'nevus' should be regarded with suspicion for melanoma.

There are three types of acquired nevus: junctional, compound and dermal. These designations have both clinical and histologic relevance. Junctional nevi are flat (macular) and pigmented with nevus cells confined to the epidermis (Fig. 8.3). Compound nevi are often raised (papule), and may be pigmented or pink in color (Fig. 8.4). Histologically, the nevus cells are present both

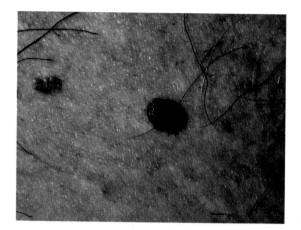

Figure 8.5. *Dermal nevus. Note similarity to Figure 8.4; often the distinction between compound and dermal nevi is only possible with microscopy. (Photo credit: Adrienne Rencic, MD, PhD.)*

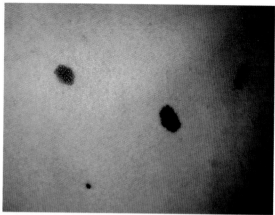

Figure 8.6. *Dysplastic nevi are large in size and demonstrate variable morphology. (Photo credit: Bernard Cohen, MD. © Dermatlas; http://www.dermatlas.org.)*

in the epidermis and the dermis. Dermal nevi are also papules, and are often non-pigmented (Fig. 8.5). As the name implies, nevus cells are confined to the dermis.

Dysplastic nevi

Dysplastic nevi were first described by Wallace Clark in 1978.[36] Although these nevi were initially described in families with melanoma, they also occur sporadically in 5% of the population.[37] In contrast to common acquired nevi, dysplastic nevi begin to appear during puberty and patients may continue to develop new ones throughout life. Patients with dysplastic nevus syndrome may have hundreds of moles. Several authors have recommended diagnostic criteria for the clinical diagnosis of dysplastic nevi.[38–40]

These nevi appear clinically atypical and, by ABCD criteria, fit the profile for a 'suspicious' lesion. They are usually greater than 6 mm in diameter, asymmetrical, and have irregular pigmentation and fuzzy borders (Fig. 8.6). Occasionally mild erythema is present, lending a pink hue. The nevi are usually slightly raised and may have a central papule giving the overall appearance of a 'fried egg'. These nevi may be present anywhere on the body, and particular attention should be given to the scalp and bathing trunk region.

Major melanoma subtypes

There are four main subtypes of melanoma: superficial spreading melanoma, nodular melanoma, lentigo maligna melanoma and acral lentiginous melanoma.

Superficial spreading melanoma is the most common type of melanoma in whites, and accounts for approximately 70% of melanomas in this group. Although superficial spreading melanoma may arise at any site, in men the back is the most frequent location.[41] This site may be difficult for the patient to see, thus leading to a delay in diagnosis. About one half may arise in a pre-existing nevus and patients will notice a change in color or size. The remaining superficial spreading melanomas arise de novo, and patients may complain of a new mole. Clinically, lesions may be macules or papules, and have an irregular border and variable pigmentation (Fig. 8.7). White areas often develop within the lesion and are a sign of regression.

Microscopically, atypical melanocytes are present singly and in nests scattered through the epidermis. The cells may migrate up in the epidermis towards the stratum granulosum, in a pattern known as pagetoid spread. If no invasion is present, the histology is that of melanoma in situ. From the epidermis, cells invade into the dermis and may be detected as

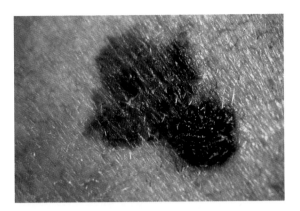

Figure 8.7. *Superficial spreading melanoma. The lesion is asymmetric, with variable color. (Reprinted from PH McKee. Pathology of the Skin with Clinical Correlations, 2nd edn, 1996, with permission from Elsevier Science.[42])*

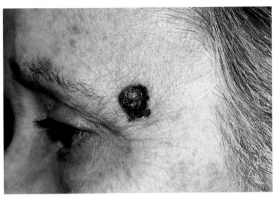

Figure 8.8. *Pigmented nodular melanoma. (Reprinted from PH McKee. Pathology of the Skin with Clinical Correlations, 2nd edn, 1996, with permission from Elsevier Science.[42])*

a few atypical cells, or as an expansile population within the dermis.

Nodular melanoma is the second most frequently encountered melanoma, and affects all ages, with a peak incidence in the 50 year age range.[43] The lesion is usually a pigmented papule or nodule on the skin, and may resemble a traumatized hemangioma (Fig. 8.8). In 5% of cases, these lesions may be amelanotic[44] and can mimic dermal nevi or other benign lesions, and therefore a high index of suspicion must be maintained for dermal nevi in the older patient. In men, nodular melanomas may be present on the head/neck region, anterior trunk, or even the lower extremity.[45] As the age of presentation increases, so does thickness of the melanoma.

Nodular melanoma is characterized by rapid growth. Unlike superficial spreading and lentigo maligna melanoma, there is no prolonged horizontal (radial) growth phase, and the nodular clinical appearance corresponds to vertical invasion into the dermis. Thus, these lesions are usually deeper and have a poor prognosis at the time of diagnosis.

Histologically, nodular melanoma appears as a nodular aggregate of cytologically atypical cells with variable pigmentation. In contrast to superficial spreading melanoma, there is no overlying pagetoid proliferation of atypical melanocytes.

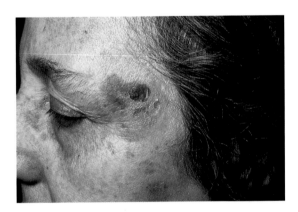

Figure 8.9. *Lentigo maligna melanoma on the temple. The variegated color is typical. (Reprinted from PH McKee. Pathology of the Skin with Clinical Correlations, 2nd edn, 1996, with permission from Elsevier Science.[42])*

Lentigo maligna melanoma is found in older patients on light-exposed skin, usually the face and neck. The lesion begins as a pigmented macule that slowly increases in size. There may be variegated color (Fig. 8.9). The non-invasive (in situ) phase is prolonged, but once invasive, palpable nodular areas may develop within the lesion.

Like superficial spreading melanoma, lentigo maligna melanoma also has an in situ phase. The epidermis is atrophic, with underlying sun damage of the dermal connective tissue. Along the basal layer of the epidermis is a single-file (lentiginous) proliferation of atypical melanocytes. Some atypical melanocytes may form nests. This in situ phase is known as lentigo maligna. Once the cells invade into the dermis, the lesion is considered lentigo maligna melanoma. The invasive melanoma may be nested, desmoplastic or neurotropic. Desmoplastic melanoma is characterized by spindle-shaped melanoma cells that infiltrate through a sclerotic stroma. Lentigo maligna is usually present in the epidermis above the tumor. In neurotropic melanoma, the melanoma cells infiltrate and extend along the cutaneous nerves. Both desmoplastic and neurotropic melanoma sometimes occur in the absence of any overlying epidermal pigmentation, and are often deeply invasive at the time of diagnosis.

Acral lentiginous melanoma affects the soles, palms and subungual areas in older individuals. Although the incidence of this form of melanoma is similar for all ethnic groups, this type of melanoma affects blacks and Asians in proportionally higher numbers, due to the lower incidence of melanomas on other skin surfaces within these groups.[46,47]

Acral lentiginous melanoma begins as a pigmented macule on the foot, hand, or under the nail, that slowly increases in diameter. Similar to lentigo maligna, the color may be variegated (Fig. 8.10). Delay in diagnosis of this type of lesion may be prolonged due to the unusual site. Subungual melanomas may be mistaken for traumatic bruises. If undetected, the lesion may attain a large size, develop nodular areas, and ulcerate or bleed.

Histologically, acral lentiginous melanoma demonstrates a lentiginous proliferation of atypical and pleiomorphic melanocytes, and pagetoid spread may be present. This type of melanoma is often invasive at the time of biopsy, and the invasive tumor cells can be spindled or epitheloid in shape. Desmoplastic variants may occasionally be encountered.

Biopsy

Lesions suspicious for melanoma are easily assessed by skin biopsy with local anesthesia. In general, it is best to remove the entire lesion for histologic

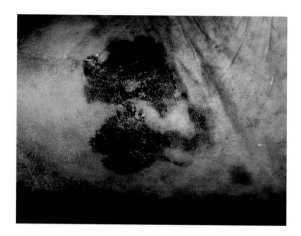

Figure 8.10. *Acral melanoma. The white area represents focal regression of melanoma. (Photo credit: Bernard Cohen, MD. © Dermatlas; http://www. dermatlas.org.)*

analysis. The biopsy should include a 2 mm margin of normal-appearing skin, to ensure complete removal. An excisional biopsy is preferred. Some dermatologists favor a shave biopsy, utilizing the 'scoop' shave technique but this should be discouraged. The caveat of the scoop shave is that there is a risk of transecting the lesion at the level of the dermis. This may result in difficulty in establishing the diagnosis and determining the precise thickness of the melanoma.

Occasionally, lesions may be quite large (as in lentigo maligna or a large superficial spreading melanoma). In these cases, selected punch biopsies of the darkest or most nodular areas may be performed to confirm the diagnosis and establish thickness of the melanoma. Full excision may be deferred to the time of sentinel node biopsy or until appropriate surgical excision is arranged. Although this sampling approach is practical for the larger lesions, there is a risk of sampling error leading to an underestimation of the precise thickness of the tumor.

Staging/prognosis

In 2002, the American Joint Committee on Cancer (AJCC) (Table 8.1) adopted a revised melanoma staging system that used data from 30 450 melanoma patients.[48] The staging system correlates well with

Table 8.1. *AJCC TNM classification for melanoma**

T classification	Thickness (mm)	Ulceration status
T1	≤1.0	a: without ulceration and level II/III b: with ulceration or level IV/V
T2	1.01–2.0	a: without ulceration b: with ulceration
T3	2.01–4.0	a: without ulceration b: with ulceration
T4	>4.0	a: without ulceration b: with ulceration
N classification	**No. of metastatic nodes**	**Nodal metastatic mass**
N1	One lymph node	a: micrometastasis[a] b: macrometastasis[b]
N2	2–3 lymph nodes	a: micrometastasis[a] b: macrometastasis[b] c: in transit met(s)/satellite(s) without metastatic nodes
N3	4 or more metastatic lymph nodes, matted lymph nodes, or combinations of in-transit met(s)/ satellite(s) and metastatic lymph node(s)	
M classification	**Site**	**Serum lactate dehydrogenase**
M1a	Distant skin, subcutaneous, or lymph node mets	Normal LDH
M2b	Lung metastases	Normal LDH
M3c	All other visceral metastases Any distant metastasis	Normal LDH Elevated LDH

[a]Micrometastases are diagnosed after sentinel or elective lymphadenectomy.
[b]Macrometastases are defined as clinically detectable nodal metastases confirmed by therapeutic lymphadenectomy or when nodal metastasis exhibits gross extracapsular entension.
*Source: Balch CM, Buzaid AC, Soong SJ, et al: Final Version of the American Joint Committee on Cancer Staging System for Cutaneous Melanoma. J Clin Oncol 2001; 19(16): 3635–48. Reprinted with permission from the American Society of Clinical Oncology.

prognosis,[49] and the study established several features that are major determinants of prognosis in patients with melanoma. This staging system has also been recomended for use in the United Kingdom (UK).[50]

Thickness

Breslow thickness is the strongest predictor of prognosis in localized early melanomas. The thickness is measured in whole integers and is assessed by measuring from the granular cell layer of the epidermis to the deepest point of invasion within the dermis. In the past, the Clark level (anatomic location of the deepest point of invasion) was considered important, however, this is only relevant in melanomas which are less than 1 mm thick and have a deeper level of invasion (Clark IV or V).

Ulceration

One of the most important factors to emerge with the new classification system is the presence of ulceration of localized primary melanoma. This is considered second only to the thickness of the primary melanoma in its effect on prognosis. For a given melanoma thickness, the presence of ulceration upstages the patient in the classification scheme. As might be expected, the thicker the melanoma (and the more rapidly it is growing), the more likely the tumor is to ulcerate. Interestingly, the presence of ulceration of the primary melanoma is the only feature of the primary tumor that is associated with poor prognosis for patients with stage III disease. The breadth of the ulcer is recorded in millimeters.

Node status

The presence of nodal metastasis of melanoma, when present, imparts a poor prognosis. Significant predictors of outcome in node-positive patients include the number of metastatic nodes and tumor burden within a node (clinically detectable versus microscopic).

Other variables

Older age, site of the primary melanoma (extremities versus axial location), level of invasion and gender are all statistically significant factors related to prognosis, however, the risk ratios are all much lower than those for thickness and ulceration.

Evaluation for metastases

Once the initial diagnosis of melanoma is established, a full physical exam with particular attention to lymph nodes should be performed. For patients with melanoma in situ, no other evaluation for metastatic disease is currently recommended.

All patients with invasive melanoma should have routine blood tests (complete blood count, serum chemistries and liver function tests) performed. Elevated serum lactate dehydrogenase (LDH) levels have been shown to be associated with poorer survival[51] in patients with metastatic disease. Indeed, LDH is considered a parameter for stage IV patients in the new AJCC staging system. Therefore, in patients with invasive melanoma the staging bloodwork should also include an LDH level. Should the LDH be elevated the AJCC recommends a second test be performed due to the possibility of falsely elevated tests from hemolysis of the blood sample, or other causes of elevated LDH.[48]

Patients with invasive melanoma up to 1 mm in thickness should have a chest radiograph in addition to the routine blood tests. For those with melanomas greater than 1 mm in thickness, computed tomography (CT) scan of the chest/abdomen and pelvis is warranted.[52] Patients with thick melanomas may also benefit from a magnetic resonance imaging (MRI) scan of the brain, and possibly positron emission tomography (PET). PET scans are a newly emerging staging tool for melanoma. Current recommended use of PET scans in melanoma patients is limited to evaluation for recurrence.[53] However, recent studies have suggested that the greater sensitivity and specificity of PET over CT scan may favor this modality for initial staging of patients with thick melanomas in the future.[54]

Surgical management

Surgery is the mainstay of melanoma therapy, and may be curative for thin lesions. Once the diagnosis is made, the melanoma should be re-excised. For melanoma in situ the current recommended excision margin is 0.5 cm.[52] A 1 cm surgical margin is recommended[55] to excise melanomas less than 1 mm in thickness. For melanomas of intermediate thickness (1–4 mm) a 2 cm radial margin of excision is recommended.[56] For thicker melanomas (>4 mm), a similar 2 cm margin is recommended since disease-free and overall survival are not increased by a larger margin of excision.[57] Since the recurrence risk in thick melanomas is primarily vascular and lymphatic, no added benefit is achieved with a wider primary excision. These excision recommendations are similar to the UK guidelines.[50]

Elective lymph node dissection and sentinel lymph node biopsy

Elective lymph node dissection is the removal of the lymph node basin draining the region of the primary invasive melanoma. Patients usually have no clinically apparent adenopathy. The rationale is that for patients at risk for metastases, metastatic melanoma cells would first travel to the draining lymph node basin, and from there to the rest of the body. When these micrometastases in lymph nodes are surgically removed, perhaps further metastatic spread could be prevented. Despite the potential therapeutic benefits,[58] whether this procedure improves overall survival of patients remains controversial.[59–61] In addition, the procedure is not without risk of morbidity. Potential complications include wound infections, lymphedema, thrombophlebitis, and rarely pulmonary embolism.[62]

Nonetheless, evaluation of the lymph nodes is essential for staging purposes and survival estimates. The sentinel lymph node technique initially described by Morton et al.[63] and subsequently modified uses a vital dye and radioactive probe to identify the first draining lymph node(s) within the basin draining the primary tumor. The dye is injected intradermally around the tumor site, and a gamma probe is used intraoperatively to identify the node(s). The node is removed, and examined microscopically. Immunohistochemical stains for S100, MART-1 or HMB-45 may be used to further enhance the detection of metastatic melanoma cells in the lymph node.[64,65] By selectively removing the sentinel node, and avoiding a formal dissection, many of the complications of elective lymph node dissection may be avoided while still providing important staging information. Only those with a positive sentinel node then undergo regional lymph node dissection. One recent retrospective study indicates possible survival advantage of performing elective lymph node dissection in patients with positive sentinel nodes and melanomas greater than 1 mm in thickness.[66]

Medical management

The primary treatment of melanoma is surgical. Patients with metastatic disease have a poor prognosis, and no single intervention has been consistently shown in clinical trials to be of benefit. As a result, there are numerous studies underway to better define the appropriate therapeutic interventions.

Patients with advanced disease should be referred to an oncologist specializing in melanoma, or to a hospital center that serves a large number of advanced-stage patients. Treatments that may be offered include chemotherapy, limb perfusion, interferon or vaccine therapy.

Follow-up

Following a diagnosis of melanoma, patients should have regular follow-up for the remainder of their lifetime. The benefit of follow-up can be appreciated by the decreased thickness of a second melanoma in patients with regular follow-up following the diagnosis of their first primary tumor.[67] There is no established algorithm, however, in general, patients should have a full skin examination every 3 months for the first 2 years, and then twice yearly after that. Inquiry should be made as to new skin lesions, swelling of lymph nodes, sun protection measures, and a general review of systems including headaches, visual changes or back pain. At each visit, a full skin examination should be performed with particular attention to the surgical scar and regional lymph nodes. The physician should maintain a low threshold for biopsy of new or changing lesions.

Patients with numerous nevi may benefit from full body photographs, since detecting subtle changes in countless moles (and identifying new ones) can be a difficult task. Patients use a set of photos at home to follow their nevi, and physicians can use them at subsequent visits to evaluate for changes in existing nevi and to detect new nevi.[68]

Prevention and early detection

Assessment of risk factors and a full skin exam should be part of the general check-up for each patient. Patients must be educated about self skin examinations, appropriate use of sunscreens and sun protective clothing. Primary care physicians are in a unique position to encourage the practice of self skin examinations, and one study concluded that patients who were advised of their own risks for melanoma were more likely to perform self skin examinations.[69] Because females are 7.5 times more likely to detect melanomas in their husbands than husbands detect their wives',[27] spouses should be encouraged to examine their husbands (and vice versa). Pamphlets with the ABCDs of melanoma or similar evaluation schemes may be obtained and distributed, so patients have guidelines for self skin examinations. Screening programs targeting middle-aged and older men will increase the likelihood of earlier diagnosis of melanoma in this high-risk population.[70]

Since individuals with a history of skin cancer have a risk of developing a second cancer (including basal cell carcinoma, squamous cell carcinoma and melanoma), the benefits of general sun protection precautions have extended benefits in that they not only serve to protect against melanoma, but other non-melanoma skin cancers as well.[71] Many companies now manufacture bathing suits and clothing with sun protection factor (SPF). In the USA, a product called TINOSORB™ FD adds temporary SPF protection to clothing during laundering. Patients should be encouraged to wear sunscreen on a daily basis, even in winter. The sunscreen should be at least SPF 15, and block both UVA and UVB. Hats with a 5 cm brim should be encouraged.

Finally, patients with children should be educated regarding protecting their children from the sun in order to limit their future risk of melanoma.

Conclusion

Although melanoma is one of the most frightening diagnoses for a patient, with early diagnosis, surgical treatment can be curative. Middle-aged and older men are the most at-risk group, and intensive screening and education programs are necessary to diagnose melanoma at an early stage. New advances in medical treatments for more advanced stage melanoma are underway and will hopefully provide more effective therapy and longer disease-free survival time. Concurrent advances in the genetic study of melanoma may effectively further stratify at-risk patients, and contribute a better understanding of the pathogenesis of melanoma.

References

1. Armstrong BK, Kricker A. Cutaneous melanoma. Cancer Surv 1994; 20: 219–40.
2. MacLennan R, Green AC, Mcleod GR, Martin NG. Increasing incidence of cutaneous melanoma in Queensland, Australia. J Natl Cancer Inst 1992; 84: 427–32.
3. MacKie RM, Bray CA, Hole JD et al. Incidence of and survival from malignant melanoma in Scotland: an epidemiological study. Lancet 2002; 360: 587–91.
4. Stang A, Stang K, Stegmaier C, Hakulinen T, Jockel KH. Skin melanoma in Saarland: incidence, survival and mortality 1970–1996. Eur J Cancer Prev 2001; 10: 407–15.
5. Anonymous. Deaths from melanoma – United States 1973–1992. MMWR Morb Mortal Wkly Rep 1995; 44: 343–7.
6. Geller AC, Miller DR, Annas GD, Demierre M. Melanoma incidence and mortality among US whites, 1969–1999. JAMA 2002; 288: 1719–20.
7. Jemal A, Devesa SS, Hartge P, Tucker MA. Recent trends in cutaneous melanoma incidence among whites in the United States. J Natl Cancer Inst 2001; 93: 678–83.
8. Hall HI, Miller DR, Rogers JD, Bewerse B. Update in the incidence and mortality from melanoma in the United States. J Am Acad Dermatol 1999; 40: 35–42.
9. Dennis LK, White E, Lee JAH. Recent cohort trends in malignant melanoma by anatomic site in the United States. Cancer Causes Control 1993; 4: 93–100.
10. Bellows CF, Belafsky P, Fortgang IS, Beech DJ. Melanoma in African-Americans: trends in biological behavior and clinical characteristics over two decades. J Surg Oncol 2001; 78: 10–16.
11. MacKie RM, Hole D. Clinical audit of public education campaign to encourage earlier detection of malignant melanoma. BMJ 1992; 304: 1012–15.
12. Zanetti R, Rossos R, Martinez C et al. The multicentre South European study Helios. I: skin characteristics and sunburns in basal and squamous cell carcinomas of the skin. Br J Cancer 1996; 73: 1440–4.
13. Elwood JM. Melanoma and sun exposure: contrasts between intermittent and chronic exposure. World J Surg 1992; 16: 157–65.
14. Lee JAH, Strickland D. Malignant melanoma, social status and outdoor work. Br J Cancer 1980; 41: 757–63.

15. Spatz A, Giglia-Mari G, Benhamou S, Sarasin A. Association between DNA repair-deficiency and high level of p53 mutations in melanoma of Xeroderma pigmentosum. Cancer Res 2001; 61: 2480–6.

16. Tucker MA, Boice JD, Hoffman DA. Second cancer following cutaneous melanoma and cancers of the brain, thyroid, connective tissue, bone and eye in Connecticut, 1935–82. Natl Cancer Inst Monogr 1985; 68: 161–89.

17. Scheibner A, Milton GW, McCarthy WH et al. Multiple primary melanoma – a review of 90 cases. Aust J Dermatol 1982; 23: 1.

18. Schwartz JL, Wang TS, Hamilton TA et al. Thin primary cutaneous melanomas – associated detection patterns, lesion characteristics, and patient characteristics. Cancer 2002; 95: 1562–8.

19. Oliveria SA, Christos PJ, Halpern AC et al. Patient knowledge, awareness, and delay in seeking medical attention for malignant melanoma. J Clin Epidemiol 1999; 52: 1111–16.

20. Sverdlow AJ, English J, MacKie RM et al. Benign melanocytic naevi as a risk factor for melanoma. BMJ 1986; 292: 1555–9.

21. NIH Consensus Development Conference. Diagnosis and treatment of early melanoma. Presented at the NIH Consensus Development Conference. January 27–29, 1992; 10: 1–25.

22. Ackerman AB, Mihara I. Dysplasia, dysplastic melanocytes, dysplastic nevi, the dysplastic nevus syndrome, and the relation between dysplastic nevi and malignant melanomas. Hum Pathol 1985; 16: 87–91.

23. Piepkorn M. Melanoma genetics: an update with focus on the CDKN2A/ARF tumor receptors. J Am Acad Dermatol 2000; 42: 705–22.

24. Zuo L, Weger J, Yang Q et al. Germline mutations in the p16INK4A binding domain of CDK4 in familial melanoma. Nat Genet 1996; 12: 97–9.

25. Palmer JS, Duffy DL, Box NF et al. Melanocortin 1 receptor polymorphism and risk of melanoma: is the risk explained solely by pigmentation phenotype? Am J Hum Genet 2000; 66: 176–86.

26. Haluska FG, Hodi FS. Molecular genetics of familial cutaneous melanoma. J Clin Oncol 1998; 16: 670–82.

27. Brady MS, Oliveria SA, Christos PJ et al. Patterns of detection in patients with cutaneous melanoma. Cancer 2000; 89: 342–7.

28. Bono A, Bartoli C, Moglia D et al. Small melanomas: a clinical study on 270 consecutive cases of cutaneous melanoma. Melanoma Res 1999; 9: 583–6.

29. MacKie RM. Malignant Melanoma. In: Skin Cancer. St. Louis: Mosby, 1996: 199.

30. Healsmith MF, Bourke JF, Osborne JE, Graham-Brown RA. An evaluation of the revised seven-point checklist for the early diagnosis of cutaneous malignant melanoma. Br J Dermatol 1994; 130: 48–50.

31. Precursors to Malignant Melanoma. NIH Consensus Statement Online, 1983; 4: 1–14. (Consensus.nih.gov, accessed 12/7/02).

32. Swerdlow AJ, English JSC, Qiao Z. The risk of melanoma in patients with congenital nevi: a cohort study. J Am Acad Dermatol 1995; 32: 595–9.

33. Rhodes AR, Albert LS, Weinstock MA. Congenital nevomelanocytic nevi: proportionate area expansion during infancy and early childhood. J Am Acad Dermatol 1996; 34: 51–62.

34. Marghoob AA. Congenital melanocytic nevi: evaluation and management. Dermatol Clin 2002; 20: 607.

35. Kanzler MH, Mraz-Gernhard S. Primary cutaneous malignant melanoma and its precursor lesions: diagnostic and therapeutic overview. J Am Acad Dermatol 2001; 45: 260–76.

36. Clark WH JR, Reimer RP, Greene M, Ainsworth AM, Mastrangelo JH. Origin of familial malignant melanoma from heritable melanocytic lesions: the B-K mole syndrome. Arch Dermatol 1978; 114: 732–8.

37. Crutcher WA, Sagebiel RW. Prevalence of dysplastic nevi in a community practice. Lancet 1984; 1: 729.

38. Elder DE, Green MH, Guerry IV D et al. The dysplastic nevus syndrome: our definition. Am J Dermatopathol 1982; 4: 455–60.

39. Kelly JW, Yeatman JM, Regalia C et al. A high incidence of melanoma found in patients with multiple dysplastic naevi by photographic surveillance. Med J Aust 1997; 167: 191–4.

40. Tucker MA, Halpern A, Holly EA et al. Clinically recognized dysplastic nevi. A central risk factor for cutaneous melanoma. JAMA 1997; 277: 1439–44.

41. Hall HI, Miller DR, Rogers JD, Bewerse B. Update in the incidence and mortality from melanoma in the United States. J Am Acad Dermatol 1999; 40: 35–42.

42. McKee PH. Pathology of the Skin with Clinical Correlations. 2nd edn. St Louis, MO: Elsevier Science, 1996.

43. Clark WH Jr, Elder DE, Van Horn M. The biologic forms of malignant melanoma. Hum Pathol 1986; 17: 443.

44. Langley RGB, Fitzpatrick TB, Sober AJ. In: Cutaneous Melanoma. Balch CM, Houghton AN, Sober AJ, Soong S (eds). St Louis: Quality Medical Publishing, Inc, 1998: 81–101.

45. Chamberlain AJ, Fritschi L, Giles GG, Dowling JP, Kelly JW. Nodular type and older ages as the most significant associations of thick melanoma in Victoria, Australia. Arch Dermatol 2002; 138: 609–14.

46. Reintgen DS, McCary KM Jr, Cox E, Seigler HF. Malignant melanoma in black American and white American populations. A comparative review. JAMA 1982; 248: 1856–9.

47. Stevens NG, Liff JM, Weiss NS. Plantar melanoma: is the incidence of melanoma of the sole of the foot really higher in blacks than whites? Int J Cancer 1990; 45: 691–3.

48. Balch CM, Buzaid AC, Soong SJ et al. Final version of the American Joint Committee on cancer staging system for cutaneous melanoma. J Clin Oncol 2001; 19: 3635–48.

49. Balch CM, Soong SJ, Gershenwald JE et al. Prognostic factors analysis of 17 600 melanoma patients: validation of the American Joint Committee on cancer melanoma staging system. J Clin Oncol 2001; 19: 3622–34.

50. Roberts DLL, Anstey AV, Barlow RJ et al. UK Guidelines for the management of cutaneous melanoma. Br J Dermatol 2002; 146: 7–17.

51. Manola J, Atkins M, Ibrahim J, Krikwood J. Prognostic factors in metastatic melanoma: a pooled analysis of Eastern Cooperative Oncology Group trials. J Clin Oncol 2000; 18: 3782–93.

52. Shapiro RL. Surgical approaches to malignant melanoma: practical guidelines. Dermatol Clin 2002; 20: 681.

53. Swetter SM, Carrol LA, Johnson DL, Segall, GM. Positron emission tomography is superior to computed tomography for metastatic detection in melanoma patients. Ann Surg Oncol 2002; 9: 646–53.

54. Prichard RS, Hill ADK, Skehan SJ, O'Higgins NJ. Positron emission tomography for staging and management of malignant melanoma. Br J Surg 2002; 89: 389–96.

55. Cascinelli N. Margin of resection in the management of primary melanoma. Semin Surg Oncol 1998; 14: 272–5.

56. Balch CM, Soong SJ, Smith T et al. Investigators from the Intergroup Melanoma Surgical Trial. Long-term results of a prospective surgical trial comparing 2 cm versus 4 cm excision margins for 740 patients with 1–4 mm melanomas. Ann Surg Oncol 2001; 8: 101–8.

57. Heaton KM, Sussman JJ, Gershenwald JE et al. Surgical margins and prognostic factors in patients with thick (>4 mm) primary melanoma. Ann Surg Oncol 1998; 5: 322–8.

58. Balch CM, Soong SJ, Bartolucci AA et al. Efficacy of an elective regional lymph node dissection of 1 to 4 mm thick melanomas for patients 60 years of age and younger. Ann Surg 1996; 224: 255–66.

59. Piepkorn M, Weinstock MA, Barnhill RL. Theoretical and empirical arguments in relation to elective lymph node dissection for melanoma. Arch Dermatol 1997; 133: 995–1002.

60. Sim FH, Taylor WF, Pritchard DJ, Soule EH. Lymphadenectomy in the management of stage I malignant melanoma: a prospective randomized study. Mayo Clin Proc 1986; 61: 697–705.

61. McCarthy WH, Shaw HM, Cascinelli N, Santinami M, Belli F. Elective lymph node dissection for melanoma: two perspectives. World J Surg 1992; 16: 203–13.

62. Balch CM, Cascinelli N, Sim FH et al. In: Balch CM, Houghton AN, Sober AJ, Soong S (eds). Cutaneous Melanoma 3rd edn. St Louis: Quality Medical Publishing, 1998.

63. Morton DL, Wen DR, Wong JH et al. Technical details of intraoperative lymphatic mapping for early stage melanoma. Arch Surg 1992; 127: 392–9.

64. Yu LL, Flotte TJ, Tanabe KK et al. Detection of microscopic melanoma metastases in sentinel lymph nodes. Cancer 1999; 86: 617–27.

65. Baisden BL, Askin FB, Lange JR, Westra WH. HMB-45 immunohistochemical staining of sentinel lymph nodes: a specific method for enhancing detection of micrometastases in patients with melanoma. Am J Surg Path 2000; 24: 1140–6.

66. Dessureault S, Soong SJ, Ross MI et al. Improved staging of node-negative patients with intermediate to thick melanomas (>1 mm) with the use of lymphatic mapping and sentinel lymph node biopsy. Ann Surg Oncol 2001; 8: 766–70.

67. Johnson TM, Hamilton TA, Lowe L. Multiple primary melanomas. J Am Acad Dermatol 1998; 39: 422–7.

68. Kanzler MH, Mraz-Gernhard S. Primary cutaneous malignant melanoma and its precursor lesions: diagnostic and therapeutic overview. J Am Acad Dermatol 2001; 45: 260–76.

69. Robinson JK, Rigel DS, Amonette RA. What promotes skin self-examination? J Am Acad Dermatol 1998; 38: 752–7.

70. Geller AC, Sober AJ, Zhang Z et al. Strategies for improving melanoma education and screening for men age >50 years. Cancer 2002; 95: 1554–61.

71. Czarnecki D, Sutton T, Czarnecki C, Culjak G. A 10-year prospective study of patients with skin cancer. J Cutan Med Surg Online, 29 August 2002.

Cardiovascular risk reduction and men

CHAPTER 9

Coronary heart disease in men

Henry Purcell

Introduction

The recently published and appropriately entitled *Why Men Die First* puts it very succinctly. 'Coronary artery disease looms larger than any other illness on the horizon that threaten men in the prime of their lives. It claims more lives every year than any other in both sexes, but it begins at least a decade earlier in men than women.'[1] This short review looks a little more closely at the reasons men succumb to coronary heart disease (CHD) in such large numbers and often comparatively early in their lifespan and at the steps that we might take to prevent heart disease developing in both men and women.

Background

Cardiovascular disease (CVD) is the world's largest killer, claiming 17.5 million lives a year. Ischemic heart disease, or coronary heart disease (CHD), and stroke comprise most of the burden, with almost half of all cardiovascular deaths being due to CHD and one quarter to stroke. Men tend to be over-represented with one in four dying from myocardial infarction (MI) compared with one in six women.[2] Not surprisingly, the incidence and prevalence of CHD increases proportionally with advancing age in both sexes. The risk of premature heart disease is even greater in some ethnic groups, particularly South Asian males living in the UK. Atherosclerosis

is endemic, beginning in early childhood, and the lifetime risk of developing CHD at age 40 is one in two for men and one in three for women. Even at 70 years these odds become one in three and one in four for men and women, respectively.

Because CVD is multifactorial, many risk factors conspire, along with age and genotype, to cause premature CHD, arbitarily defined as evidence of coronary disease before the age of 65. Data from the Framingham Heart Study and other epidemiological studies have identified the major modifiable risk factors for CHD which include:

- Smoking
- Dyslipidemia
- Hypertension.

These and many more factors, such as obesity and type 2 diabetes, commonly co-exist, and therefore strategies to prevent cardiovascular disease and its complications should ideally address the 'global' cardiovascular risk.

Cardiovascular risk factors

Smoking is the single largest cause of preventable death in our society. It is also one of the major underlying determinants of health inequalities. Latest data from the Health Survey for England 2006[3] show that 24% of men and 21% of women

105

are identified as current cigarette smokers. The highest prevalence – 34% – is in males aged between 25 and 34 years. About 30% of cancer deaths and 20% of CHD deaths are directly attributable to smoking, and the British government is committed to getting rates below 26% in manual occupations and to below 21% overall by 2010. On quitting, the risk of MI falls to about 50% of that of a non-smoker by 1 year and to the same level as someone who has never smoked by 15 years. The lesson for patients therefore is, 'it's never too late to quit'. This is particularly true in patients who have suffered an MI or who have undergone coronary artery bypass surgery. A wide range of nicotine replacement therapies and other new pharmacological and psychological support is available to assist smoking cessation. It is hoped that quit rates are also likely to be improved with the implementation of smoke-free legislation in England in 2007 and in other countries such as Ireland, where it was introduced several years earlier.

Hypertension and dyslipidemia are covered in detail below. It is important to highlight other significant cardiovascular risk factors including:

- Sedentary lifestyle
- Obesity
- Type 2 diabetes.

Obesity has become a major problem, in that currently one in five people is clinically obese and some 70% of the population is overweight. Many of these people will develop type 2 diabetes. Obesity increases risk of developing diabetes 80-fold. Diabetes has become an enormous public health issue with an estimated 194 million people affected worldwide, with numbers increasing at an alarming rate. The vast majority suffer from type 2 diabetes. Data from 2008 from Diabetes UK estimate that there are about 2.3 million people in the UK with diabetes, and a further half a million are believed to be undiagnosed. Patients with type 2 diabetes are at greater risk of stroke and peripheral arterial disease and are between two and four times more likely to develop CVD than patients without it. The largest cause of mortality in diabetic patients is from macrovascular events such as MI and stroke. Risk is further amplified when diabetes occurs as part of the

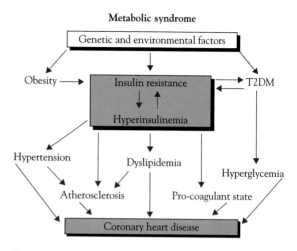

Figure 9.1 *Inter-relationship of components of metabolic syndrome resulting in increased cardiovascular risk. Adapted from Campbell IW, Purcell H.[30]*

metabolic syndrome, where there is clustering of risk factors including central (visceral) obesity, hypertension, insulin resistance, and lipid abnormalities (Fig. 9.1).

Hypertension

Hypertension increases a person's risk of cardiovascular disease about two- to three-fold.[4] Indeed there is a continuum of risk across levels of blood pressure. Chronically high blood pressure causes adaptive changes in the cerebral circulation and it is an important risk factor for stroke and transient ischemic attack (TIA). Stroke is the third-greatest killer in our society and the leading cause of chronic disability. Approximately 150 000 strokes occur in the UK each year. Between 20 and 30% of those who have a stroke die within 1 month. In the USA, 780 000 people experience a new or recurrent stroke each year, where in adults aged >55 years, the lifetime risk of stroke is greater than one in six. Interestingly, women have a higher risk than men.[5] A study from the Netherlands[6] has shown that roughly 10 years after suffering a TIA or minor ischemic stroke, about 60% of patients had died and 54% had experienced at least one new vascular attack. Because of the high prevalence of hypertension in the general population, and its sizable risk ratio, it is estimated that approximately 35% of atherosclerotic events may be attributable to high blood pressure.[7] The prevalence of hypertension (generally considered to be a blood pressure ≥140/90 mmHg) among adults across different world regions is estimated to have been a staggering 26.4% in the year 2000.[8] This is expected to rise above 29% by the year 2025. This is in line with estimates in the UK that suggest that overall about 30% of men and women have hypertension – that is, approximately 16 million Britons. Nine out of 10 middle-aged and older adults are likely to develop hypertension over their remaining lifetime. Worryingly, around one-third do not know they have hypertension. Rates rise dramatically with age and some 70% of older people will have hypertension,[9] the majority having isolated systolic hypertension. The predominance of high systolic blood pressure (SBP) over diastolic blood pressure (DBP) is now well established.[10]

As well as increasing risk of stroke, uncontrolled hypertension leads to greater likelihood of developing MI, heart disease, renal failure and peripheral arterial disease. The effect of blood pressure on the heart is dramatic, and the incidence of all aspects of CHD, including not only MI but also angina and sudden cardiac death, is increased; the risk is proportional to the severity of the prior hypertension. For reasons that remain unclear, hypertension predisposes to unrecognized or 'silent' MI. In men with hypertension, some 35% of MI's go unrecognized; in women the figure is 45%. Chronic hypertension also predisposes to the development of left ventricular hypertrophy (Fig. 9.2), which greatly increases risk of ventricular ectopy and sudden cardiac death.

'High normal' blood pressure (SBP 130–139 mmHg or DBP 85–89 mmHg) and 'normal' blood pressure (SBP 120–129 mmHg or DBP 80–84 mmHg) have been shown in the Framingham Heart Study[11] to progress frequently to hypertension over a period of a mere 4 years, especially in older adults. Patients with these 'high-normal' pressures had higher rates of cardiovascular events than those with 'optimal' blood pressures (SBP <120 mmHg and DBP <80 mmHg).[12] One mechanism that may contribute to the association between blood pressure levels and atherosclerotic events is endothelial

dysfunction, where there is reduced availability of vasoactive dilatory substances such as nitric oxide (NO) from endothelial cells (see Male-specific factors, below). Such findings would support the idea that patients with 'high-normal' pressures should be monitored annually. The Framingham Study also tells us that midlife blood pressures continue to affect the future risk of stroke, not only over a short span such as 4–5 years, but also over more prolonged periods, up to 30 years. Therefore, optimal prevention of late-life stroke is likely to require control of midlife blood pressure.[13]

While all antihypertensives have similar long-term efficacy and safety, calcium-channel blockers may be especially effective in stroke prevention[14] and angiotensin converting enzyme (ACE) inhibitors appear to have the edge in terms of preventing CHD events.[15] Another major message from clinical trials is that the majority of patients with hypertension will require several drugs, a cocktail, in order to achieve treatment goals.

Dyslipidemia

There is now substantial and conclusive evidence that increased serum cholesterol is an important cause of CHD and that lowering serum cholesterol reduces the risk.[16]

There is a strong and continuous relationship between average serum cholesterol and CHD mortality. On average, out of a total serum cholesterol (TC) of about 6.0 mmol/l in Western populations (in the UK it is about 5.5 mmol/l), two-thirds is low density lipoprotein (LDL) cholesterol and one-quarter is high density lipoprotein (HDL) cholesterol. The predominant atherogenic particle is LDL cholesterol. Estimates for different World Health Organization regions in developed countries showed that about two-thirds of CHD can be attributed to TC levels >3.8 mmol/l, and that there are an estimated 3.6 million deaths worldwide attributable to non-optimal TC levels (>3.8 mmol/l). Cholesterol-lowering drugs, notably the hydroxymethyl-glutaryl coenzyme A reductase inhibitors (the statins), can lower LDL cholesterol by 30–60% and reduce the risk of heart attack, stroke, and revascularization by about one-third.

There is a linear relationship between TC lowering and CHD risk reduction. Clinical trials,

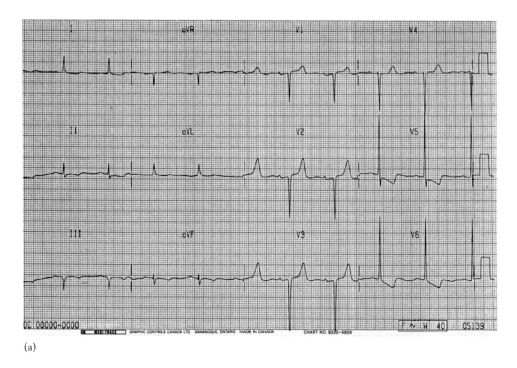

(a)

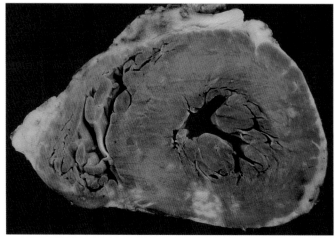

(b)

Figure 9.2 *Target organ damage in hypertension. (a) Electrocardiographic changes in left ventricular hypertrophy (LVH). The QRS amplitude is increased. Other changes of LVH include QRS prolongation, left axis deviation, and ST–T changes, as shown here. (b) Post-mortem heart of an obese male patient showing a dramatic example of left ventricular hypertrophy. (Courtesy of Dr M Sheppard.)*

conducted predominantly in men, and epidemiological studies have shown that benefits extend to both men and women such that, for every 0.025 mmol/l reduction in LDL cholesterol, the relative risk of CHD is reduced by 1%.[17] A recent meta-analysis of data from 90 056 participants in 14 randomized trials of statins[18] has shown that statin therapy can reduce the 5-year incidence of major coronary events, coronary revascularization, and stroke by about one-fifth per mmol/l reduction in LDL cholesterol, largely irrespective of the initial lipid profile or other presenting characteristics. This translates into 48 participants having fewer major vascular events per 1000 participants among those with pre-existing CHD at baseline compared with 25 per 1000 among participants with no such history.

A further meta-analysis of cardiovascular outcome trials in stable CHD or acute coronary syndromes[19] has shown that intensive lipid lowering with high-dose statin therapy provides a significant benefit over standard-dose therapy for preventing non-fatal cardiovascular events, including stroke, with a trend towards decreasing cardiovascular mortality as well. European guidelines[20] recommend that, in patients with clinically established cardiovascular disease and diabetes, TC should be <4.5 mmol/l and that LDL cholesterol should be <2.5 mmol/l. Recommendations from the Joint British Societies are that these treatment goals are <4.0 mmol/l and <2.0 mmol/l, respectively.[21]

Since cardiovascular risk factors also interact with each other, moderate reductions in several risk factors can be more effective than major reductions in one.[22] Non-adherence to medication remains a major barrier to achieving control of high blood pressure and lipids. A possible aid to improving adherence to antihypertensive treatment is to select 'more forgiving' drugs[23] that either do not depend on their half-life for full efficacy or that have an inherently long duration of action. Similarly, prescribers may be able to improve adherence significantly by initiating antihypertensive and lipid-lowering therapy concomitantly and by reducing pill burden,[24] although there does not yet seem to be universal support for the concept of the 'polypill'.

Male-specific risk factors

So far, this chapter has focused on some of the key cardiovascular risk factors that are common to men and women. There are, however, a number of male-specific factors that appear to influence the risk of heart disease independently. There is now an extensive literature that suggests that there is a clear link between erectile dysfunction (ED) and CVD. Atherosclerosis accounts for nearly half of all cases of ED in men aged over 50, and not only is it a marker of occult CVD, but the degree of ED also correlates with the severity of vascular disease.[25] The common link between ED and CVD appears to be endothelial dysfunction,[26] which results from reduced availability of NO which, when released from endothelial cells, causes smooth muscle relaxation and vasodilatation. It is also an important neurotransmitter, which mediates penile tumescence. It has been suggested therefore that ED, like diabetes, should be considered a 'cardiovascular equivalent', and that it should be screened for (via a comprehensive medical history and generalized vascular disease investigations) in all men with established or a high suspicion of CVD.

Further observations have shown that men with coronary heart disease have significantly lower concentrations of bioavailable testosterone than men with normal coronary angiograms. Similarly, the prevalence of hypogonadism in men with CHD is about twice that seen in the general population. Testosterone causes dose-dependent vasodilatation when administered into coronary arteries, and hypotestosteronemia is associated with an atherogenic lipid profile, hypercoagulation, and other metabolic dysfunction such as insulin resistance and hyperinsulinemia. Whether, however, the 'male menopause' (andropause) exists is controversial. Likewise it remains to be established whether testosterone replacement therapy might have beneficial effects in treatment of CHD, without increasing reciprocal risk of prostate cancer.[27]

Prevention

There are reasons to be optimistic about cardiovascular disease reduction in the UK and other countries. CHD rates have been declining since the 1970s. Over the two decades between 1980 and 2000, CHD rates in England and Wales fell by 62% in men and 45% in women aged 25–84 years. More than half the reduction in the CHD mortality rate was due to reductions in major risk factors, principally smoking, but also in blood pressure and lipids.[28] This emphasizes the importance of a comprehensive strategy to promote both primary and secondary prevention of CHD in both men and women in our population.

A factor that has contributed greatly to the further decline in cardiovascular morbidity and mortality within the UK in recent years is the introduction of the National Service Framework (NSF) for CHD, a strategy laid out by the Department of Health that involves interactions between hospital and primary care in order to achieve staged milestones of disease prevention and treatment.[29] Similarly, the revised General Medical Services contract, along with the Joint British Societies' guidelines on prevention of cardiovascular disease in clinical practice, are likely to have made the goals set out in the NSF standards more achievable.[21]

The Joint British Societies' guidelines (JBS-2),[21] produced by the British Cardiovascular Society, the British Hypertension Society, Diabetes UK, HEART UK, the Primary Care Cardiovascular Society, and the Stroke Association, recommend that statins should be prescribed to a much wider group of patients, including all those with existing CVD, those at high risk of developing the disease, and most people with diabetes.

They recommend significantly lower cholesterol targets than previous guidance did, with a target for TC of 4.0 mmol/L and for LDL cholesterol of 2.0 mmol/L for those at high risk. The blood pressure target has also been reduced to 140/85 mmHg.

Who should be targeted?

The guidelines, which aim to promote a consistent multidisciplinary approach to the management of people with established CVD and those at high risk of developing symptomatic atherosclerotic disease, recommend that prevention efforts should focus equally on three main groups:

- people with established atherosclerotic disease;
- people with diabetes mellitus; and
- apparently healthy people at high risk of developing symptomatic atherosclerotic disease (deemed to be those with an estimated multifactorial CVD risk >20% over 10 years).

In addition, the guidelines note that other people with particularly elevated single risk factors also require some intervention. These include:

- those with blood pressure >160 mmHg systolic or >100 mmHg diastolic, or lesser degrees of blood pressure elevation with target organ damage;
- those with an elevated TC to HDL cholesterol ratio >6.0 mmol/L; and
- those with familial dyslipidemias.

Finally, people with a family history of premature CVD should be assessed and then managed appropriately.

Who should be screened?

The guidelines recommend that all adults over the age of 40 who are not already known to be at high risk of developing heart disease should be considered for an opportunistic comprehensive CVD risk assessment in primary care. Younger adults with a family history of premature atherosclerotic disease should also have their cardiovascular risk factors measured.

A risk prediction chart is available to estimate total risk of developing CVD (CHD and stroke) over 10 years. A CVD risk >20% over 10 years is defined as 'high risk' and requires professional lifestyle intervention and, where appropriate, drug therapies to achieve the lifestyle and risk factor targets. Those who are not found to be at high risk should have their risk assessment repeated, ideally within 5 years. For people with established atherosclerotic CVD, hypertension with target organ damage, familial dyslipidemias such as familial hypercholesterolemia, or diabetes, formal risk estimation is not necessary, since all these people are already at high total CVD risk.

Lifestyle and intervention targets

The guidelines remind clinicians that lifestyle intervention to discontinue smoking, make healthier food choices, increase aerobic physical activity, and achieve optimal weight is central to CVD prevention. Targets for blood pressure, lipid levels, and blood glucose levels are also recommended, and advice is given on who should receive cardiovasular protective drug therapy, such as antithrombotics, beta-blockers, ACE inhibitors, calcium-channel blockers, diuretics and lipid-lowering therapy.

They advise that, as a general guide, a total CVD risk of more than 20% of developing CVD over the next 10 years justifies drug treatment if targets have not been achieved. However, a final decision about using drug therapy will also be influenced by other factors such as co-existent non-vascular disease and life expectancy.

For apparently healthy people with a 10-year total CVD risk of less than 20%, appropriate life-style advice should still be given, but drug treatment by physicians is usually not required. Care of people with CVD should be integrated between hospital and general practice through the use of agreed protocols designed to ensure optimal long-term lifestyle, risk factor, and therapeutic management. First-degree blood relatives of people with prema-ture CVD are screened in primary care and first-degree relatives of those affected by familial dyslipidemia should also be screened and specialist care provided through a lipid clinic.

Conclusion

This chapter has reviewed the growing challenge of cardiovascular disease worldwide. While overall rates are diminishing in developed countries, this is not true in the developing world, where CVD, mainly heart attacks and strokes, is rising exponen-tially. Even within the UK, CHD continues to be the most common cause of premature death, repre-senting about one-fifth (20%) of early deaths in men and one-ninth (11%) in women. Recent evi-dence also suggests that CHD rates in women may actually be increasing relative to those in men. CVD risk factors are well recognized, and they rarely occur in isolation. Because of the co-existence of multiple risk factors it becomes increasingly important to treat the 'global' cardiovascular risk – a process of implementing lifestyle change and optimal medical treatment, frequently with several drugs. Equally importantly, however, public health measures should be started early in life, in order to prevent the burden of heart disease developing when patients are in their forties and fifties (or younger) in the future.

References

1. Legato MJ. Why Men Die First. New York, Basingstoke, UK: Palgrave Macmillan, 2008.
2. Purcell H, Daly C, Petersen S. Coronary heart disease in men (reversing the 'descent of man'). In: Kirby RS, Carson CC, Kirby MG, Farah RN, eds. Men's Health, 2nd ed. London: Taylor and Francis, 2004: 101–9.
3. Health Survey for England 2006. Leeds, UK: The Information Centre, 2008.
4. Padwal R, Straus SE, McAlister FA. Cardiovascular risk factors and their effects on the decision to treat hypertension: evidence based review. BMJ 2001; 322: 977–80.
5. AHA statistical update: heart disease and stroke statistics – 2008 update. Dallas: American Heart Association, 2008.
6. van Wijk I, Kappelle LJ, van Gijn J et al. Long-term survival and vascular event risk after transient ischaemic attack or minor ischaemic stroke: a cohort study. Lancet 2005; 365: 2098–104.
7. Kannel WB. Blood pressure as a cardiovascular risk factor. JAMA 1996; 275: 1571–6.
8. Kearney PM, Whelton M, Reynolds K et al. Global burden of hypertension: analysis of worldwide data. Lancet 2005; 365: 217–23.
9. Williams B, Poulter NR, Brown MJ et al. Guidelines for management of hypertension: report of the fourth working party of the British Hypertension Society, 2004 – BHS IV. J Hum Hypertens 2004; 18: 139–85
10. Wang J-G, Staessen JA, Franklin SS, Fagard R, Gueyffier F. Systolic and diastolic blood pressure lowering as determinants of cardiovascular outcome. Hypertension 2005; 45: 907–13.
11. Vasan RS, Larson MG, Leip EP et al. Assessment of frequency of progression to hypertension in non-hypertensive participants in the Framingham Heart Study: a cohort study. Lancet 2001; 358: 1682–6.
12. Vasan RS, Martin MG, Leip EP et al. Impact of high-normal blood pressure on the risk of cardiovas-cular disease. N Engl J Med 2001; 345: 1291–7.
13. Seshadri S, Wolf PA, Beiser A et al. Elevated midlife blood pressure increases stroke risk in elderly persons. Arch Intern Med 2001; 161: 2343–50.
14. Stassen JA, Wang J-G, Thijs L. Cardiovascular protection and blood pressure reduction: a meta-analysis. Lancet 2001; 358: 1305–15.
15. Verdecchia P, Reboldi G, Angeli F et al. Angiotensin-converting enzyme inhibitors and calcium channel blockers for coronary heart

disease and stroke prevention. Hypertension 2005; 46: 386–92.

16. Law MR, Rodgers A. Lipids and cholesterol. In: Marmot M, Elliott P, eds. Coronary Heart Disease Epidemiology. From Aetiology to Public Health, 2nd ed. Oxford: Oxford University Press, 2005: 174–86.

17. Grundy SM, Cleeman JI, Merz CNB et al. Implications of recent trials for the National Cholesterol Education Program Adult Treatment Panel III Guidelines. Circulation 2004; 110: 227–39.

18. CTT Collaborators. Efficacy and safety of cholesterol-lowering treatment: prospective meta-analysis of data from 90,056 participants in 14 randomised trials of statins. Lancet 2005; 366: 1267–78.

19. Cannon CP, Steinberg BA, Murphy SA, Mega JL, Braunwald E. Meta-analysis of cardiovascular outcomes trials comparing intensive versus moderate statin therapy. J Am Coll Cardiol 2006; 48: 438–45.

20. De Backer G, Ambrosioni E, Borch-Johnsen K et al. European Guidelines on Cardiovascular Disease. Third Joint Task Force of European and other Societies on Cardiovascular Prevention in Clinical Practice. Eur J Cardiovasc Prev 2003; 10(Suppl 1): S1–78.

21. British Cardiac Society, Diabetes UK, HEART UK, Primary Care Cardiovascular Society, The Stroke Association. JBS 2: Joint British Societies' Guidelines

on prevention of cardiovascular disease in clinical practice. Heart 2005: 91(Suppl V): v1–52.

22. Jackson R, Lawes CMM, Bennett DA et al. Treatment with drugs to lower blood pressure and blood cholesterol based on an individual's absolute cardiovascular risk. Lancet 2005; 365: 434–41.

23. Osterberg L, Blaschke T. Adherence to medication. N Engl J Med 2005; 353: 487–97.

24. Chapman RH, Benner JS, Petrilla A et al. Predictors of adherence with antihypertensive and lipid-lowering therapy. Arch Intern Med 2005; 165: 1147–52.

25. Kirby M. ED as a marker for cardiovascular disease. Br J Diabetes Vasc Dis 2002; 2: 239–41.

26. Solomon H, Man JW, Jackson G. Erectile dysfunction and the cardiovascular patient: endothelial dysfunction is the common denominator. Heart 2003; 89: 251–4.

27. Channer KS, Jones TH. Cardiovascular effects of testosterone: implications of the 'male menopause'? Heart 2003; 89: 121–2.

28. Unal B, Critchley JA, Capewell S. Explaining the decline in coronary heart disease mortality in England and Wales between 1981 and 2000. Circulation 2004; 109: 1101–7.

29. National Service Framework (NSF) for Coronary Heart Disease. London: Department of Health, 2000.

30. Campbell IW, Purcell H. The silent sextet. Br J Diab Vasc Dis 2001; 1: 3–6.

CHAPTER 10

Raised blood pressure: the biggest cause of premature death and disability in men?

Graham A MacGregor, Feng J He

Introduction

Men die before women. In the UK, average life expectancy in women is approximately 5 years longer than men. Until recently it was thought that this was due to some genetic or hormonal difference between men and women, but it has become clear over the past decade that the reason why men have a lower life expectancy is largely due to their different lifestyle and diet.

Cardiovascular disease

Cardiovascular disease (i.e. strokes, heart attacks, and heart failure) is the leading cause of death and disability in the UK and worldwide. It is well established that the major causes of cardiovascular disease are raised blood pressure, cholesterol, and smoking. Importantly, when looking at blood pressure and cholesterol, the risk is not solely confined to those with elevated levels (e.g. a blood pressure greater than 140/90 mmHg), but exists throughout the range.[1] Although the risk is less for people with blood pressure in the upper range of normal, the number of strokes and heart attacks attributable to blood pressure in this range is greater than in those with high blood pressure, since the majority of the population have blood pressure in the upper range of normal.

This chapter focuses on the importance of blood pressure; however, when one looks at other known risk factors for cardiovascular disease, men come out worse than women. For instance, at least historically, men smoke more than women. However, this trend is now being reversed and will take some years to have its full impact, and if continued, it may narrow the gap in life expectancy between men and women. Men, particularly at a younger age, tend to have a diet that is higher in saturated fat, eat more salt, consume less fruit and vegetables, and drink more alcohol. At the same time, they are more likely to get abdominal obesity and this puts them at risk of the metabolic syndrome and diabetes. It is perhaps not surprising, therefore, that more men die prematurely from cardiovascular disease. Indeed, most of those who die from cardiovascular disease before the age of 65 (i.e. an age when they are still productive) are men.

Blood pressure

Raised blood pressure throughout the range, starting at a systolic pressure of 115 mmHg, is a major risk factor for cardiovascular disease.[1] Raised blood pressure accelerates the deposition of atheroma and, very importantly, destabilizes plaques, and it is one of the major factors leading to either ulceration or fissuring of plaques, which lead to most of the manifestations of atheromatous disease, particularly heart attacks and many thrombotic strokes. At the same time, raised blood pressure has direct effects, causing cerebral hemorrhage or, more commonly,

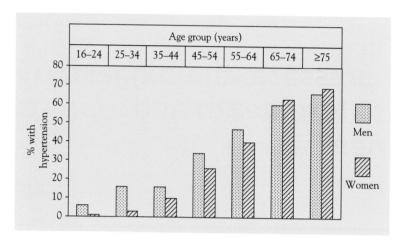

Figure 10.1. *Prevalence of hypertension for men and women in the Health Survey for England 2006.*[2]

lacuna infarcts as a direct effect of the pressure either bursting or damaging small blood vessels in the brain.

Raised blood pressure is the major cause of heart failure, especially in more elderly patients who already have pre-existing coronary artery disease. Raised blood pressure is also an important accelerating factor in aortic aneurysms as well as accelerating the development of renal disease.

Men have, on average, higher blood pressures than women, particularly at younger ages. Figure 10.1 shows the prevalence of hypertension for men and women by age group in the recent Health Survey for England.[2] Hypertension was defined as systolic blood pressure ≥140 mmHg or diastolic ≥90 mmHg (or both), or as being on treatment for raised blood pressure. As shown in Figure 10.1, the prevalence of hypertension is higher in men than in women until the age of 65 years.[2] This also applies to the average blood pressure, which is higher in men than women at younger ages. As the risk of cardiovascular disease starts at a systolic of 115 mmHg, most adult men are at risk from their blood pressure. Therefore, any approach to the damage that blood pressure does in causing strokes, heart attacks, and heart failure must not seek out only those with high blood pressure and treat them where appropriate, but also ensure that measures are taken to reduce population blood pressure. Even a small reduction in population blood pressure will have a major impact on reducing the number of people dying or suffering from strokes, heart attacks, and heart failure.

What puts up blood pressure?

There is now very compelling evidence that dietary salt is the major factor that puts up blood pressure both in men and women[3] and that this effect starts early in childhood.[4,5] There is also good evidence that increasing potassium intake, particularly through the consumption of fruit and vegetables, results in a lower blood pressure.[6] Individuals or societies that have a lower fruit and vegetable consumption are, therefore, likely to have higher blood pressures. Obesity, especially abdominal obesity, is closely associated with raised blood pressure, although people who are obese tend to eat an unhealthy diet with more salt and less fruit and vegetables. Lack of exercise predisposes to high blood pressure and increasing exercise lowers it. Alcohol excess, in particular acutely, puts up blood pressure but this appears to be a fairly transient effect. Modest consumption of alcohol does not seem to have a great effect on blood pressure. It may raise high-density lipoprotein (HDL) cholesterol and may possibly result in a slight reduction in cardiovascular disease. However, alcohol in excess does cause damage both to the heart and the liver, and it can cause immense social damage as well.

Salt

The evidence that salt relates to blood pressure comes from seven different types of study: epidemiological studies,[7] migration studies,[8] intervention studies,[9] treatment studies,[10] animal studies,[11] and genetic studies,[12] as well as studies on cardiovascular

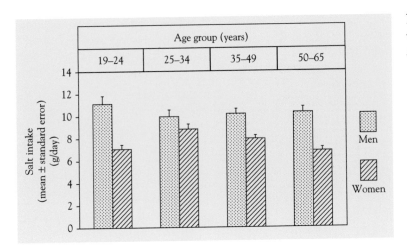

Figure 10.2. *Salt intake as measured by 24-hour urinary sodium in men and women.*[15]

outcome.[13] The average consumption of salt in the UK, as measured by 24-hour urinary sodium, was 10.9 g/day in men, whereas in women, it was only 8.1 g/day according to the National Diet and Nutrition Survey in 2001.[14] A more recent survey in 2005 showed that salt intake has fallen slightly in both men and women, but men still had a much higher salt intake (10.2 g/day) than women (7.7 g/day).[15] The difference in salt intake between men and women exists in all age groups from 16 to 65 years (Fig. 10.2). It would be very interesting to find out whether this sex-based difference in salt intake persists beyond the age of 65 years, as the sex-based difference in the prevalence of hypertension becomes smaller in the elderly. Unfortunately, 24-hour urinary sodium was not measured in those over 65 years of age in this survey.

Based on the different lines of evidence that relates salt intake to blood pressure and cardiovascular disease, it is now recommended both in the UK and worldwide that salt intake needs to be reduced. The current recommended maximum intake for adults is 6 g/day in the UK irrespective of whether the person is male or female.[16] As men have a much higher salt intake than women, in order for men to hit this target, they need to reduce their salt intake to a greater extent (i.e. by an average of 4.2 g/day, from the current intake of 10.2 g/day to the recommended level of 6 g/day), whereas women need to reduce it by only 1.7 g/day (from 7.7 g/day to 6 g/day).

Strategy for reducing salt

In most developed countries approximately 80% of the salt consumed is already present in the food[17] (e.g. in processed, canteen, restaurant, or fast foods). Indeed, on average, only 15% of the salt is added either during the cooking or at the table. Whilst this means that it is extremely difficult for people to reduce their salt intake, it has the major attraction from a public health point of view that, if the food industry can be persuaded to lower gradually the huge amounts of salt that are added to food, salt consumption would fall without the consumers changing the food that they consume. This contrasts with many other public health policies in nutrition where it is necessary to get individual people to change the food that they eat (e.g. by consuming more fruit and vegetables).

Over the past few years, the UK has had an agreed strategy to reduce the amount of salt being added to food by the food industry on a voluntary basis. Most of the food industry is now doing this and the amount of salt added, particularly to processed foods, has already been reduced in the past 2–3 years by 20–30%. Indeed, a recent survey showed that salt intake as measured by 24 hour urinary sodium had already fallen from 9.5 g/day in 2001 to 9.0 g/day in 2005.[15] These reductions have been done without the public noticing any difference in taste, without any technical problems, and without any safety concerns.

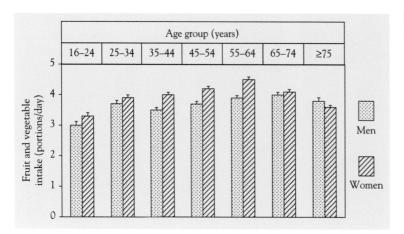

Figure 10.3. *Fruit and vegetable consumption in men and women.*[2]

At the same time, a public campaign drawing attention to the dangers of consuming too much salt has made consumers much more aware of the huge amount of salt that is put into foods and has put further pressure on the food industry to continue to reduce the amount of salt that they add to food. Provided that these cuts are done by small amounts (i.e. 10–20%, the human salt taste receptors cannot distinguish any change in taste)[18] and, very importantly as salt intake falls, the salt taste receptors become much more sensitive to lower concentrations of salt, which means that products with less salt will taste just as salty as they did previously. Indeed, for many people who have reduced their salt intake, high-salt foods then become inedible.

The reductions in salt intake need to start early in childhood.[4] Studies have now shown that, not only does salt intake relate to blood pressure in children,[19] but in controlled trials in which salt intake is reduced, there are falls in blood pressure.[5] These findings are important in view of the fact that blood pressure tracks in children (i.e. the higher the blood pressure during childhood, the higher the blood pressure in adulthood).[20] Therefore, a lower salt diet in children, if continued, may well lessen the subsequent rise in blood pressure with age, which would have major public health implications in terms of preventing the development of hypertension and cardiovascular disease later in life.

Potassium

Epidemiological, animal, and treatment trials have all shown that increasing potassium intake lowers blood pressure.[7,21] The best way of increasing potassium intake is to increase the consumption of fruit and vegetables, which in themselves may have beneficial effects on health, in addition to the potassium that they contain lowering blood pressure.[6,22,23] The recent Health Survey for England showed that men consumed less fruit and vegetables than women in all age groups except that aged 75 years and over (Figure 10.3). On average, men consumed 3.6 portions of fruit and vegetables per day while women consumed 3.9 portions. Only 28% of men consumed the recommended five or more portions per day while 32% of women reached the recommended levels of fruit and vegetable intake.[2] Greater efforts are therefore needed to encourage both men and women to eat more fruit and vegetables.

Importance of identifying and treating high blood pressure

Clinical trials going back to the 1970s have demonstrated the importance of lowering blood pressure when it is elevated.[24] Men should be much more aware of the importance of knowing their blood pressure. Unfortunately, compared with women,

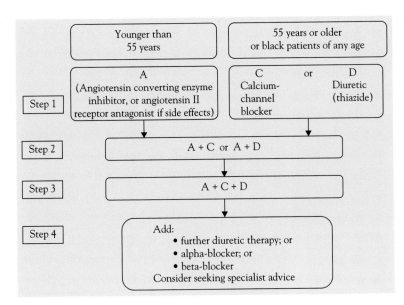

Figure 10.4. *The National Institute for Health and Clinical Excellence and the British Hypertension Society's recommendations for combining blood pressure-lowering drugs.*[25]

men are less likely to have had their blood pressure measured, less likely to go to their doctors, less likely to take action even when they know that their blood pressure is raised, and less likely to take the drugs that they are prescribed.

There is now a range of different blood pressure-lowering drugs available, and by using the right combination – since it is usually necessary to take two or three drugs – blood pressure can be well controlled with the patient feeling well. A simple algorithm produced by the British Hypertension Society and endorsed by the National Institute for Health and Clinical Excellence (NICE) in the UK is an easy way of reminding both health practitioners and patients how their blood pressure should be treated (Fig. 10.4).[25]

Patients need careful explanation of why it is necessary for them to take more than one drug and this relates to the fact that, unlike with cholesterol, when blood pressure is lowered the body tries to put the blood pressure back up by various reflex mechanisms. In order to lower blood pressure, two or three drugs that have different mechanisms are needed to overcome these reflex compensations.

General practitioners are now much more aware, partly through the Quality Outcome Framework, of the importance of identifying people with high blood pressure and getting it controlled. However,

there are still a large number of hypertensive people who have not had their blood pressure controlled to the target of 140/90 mmHg. Indeed, less than 30% have it controlled to the target levels. As a result, very large numbers of strokes and heart attacks are occurring unnecessarily in people with high blood pressure.

Importance of other factors in cardiovascular disease

Saturated fat intake directly affects blood cholesterol levels, and saturated fat intake should be reduced to as low as possible. Most of the fat that we eat is in dairy products, baked products, and meat, particularly processed meat products.

Male-pattern obesity is a particular problem in men and may appear, particularly in Asian men, at quite young ages. Abdominal obesity puts the person at greater risk of cardiovascular disease and high-calorie foods that contain large amounts of fat and sugar, should be avoided. Increasing exercise lowers blood pressure and there is also very good evidence that increasing exercise puts up HDL cholesterol.

Another important point to remember is that men who are very heavy cigarette smokers, because of the peripheral vascular disease that they develop, are much more likely to become impotent at an early age.

Conclusions

Men die before women mainly because of their unhealthy lifestyle and diet and, particularly, they die from cardiovascular disease because of their higher consumption of salt and fat, their lower consumption of fruit and vegetables and, historically, their greater consumption of cigarettes. Men need to be made aware that they are much more likely to develop cardiovascular disease at an earlier age than women and, particularly, to suffer or die from it before the age of 65. A public campaign to make men more aware of the risks they are running and to make them more responsible for their own health would be extremely worthwhile, particularly since it would prevent many men from dying when they are still at a productive age and are often responsible for others (i.e. spouses and children). Most of the diseases from which men die prematurely are almost entirely preventable by a change in lifestyle and diet.

References

1. Lewington S, Clarke R, Qizilbash N, Peto R, Collins R. Age-specific relevance of usual blood pressure to vascular mortality: a meta-analysis of individual data for one million adults in 61 prospective studies. Lancet 2002; 360: 1903–13.
2. Craig R, Mindell J. Health Survey for England, 2006. Volume 1, Cardiovascular disease and risk factors in adults. Available at http://www.ic.nhs.uk/pubs/hse06cvdandriskfactors (accessed on 17 March 2008).
3. He FJ, MacGregor GA. Salt, blood pressure and cardiovascular disease. Curr Opin Cardiol 2007; 22: 298–305.
4. Geleijnse JM, Hofman A, Witteman JC et al. Long-term effects of neonatal sodium restriction on blood pressure. Hypertension 1997; 29: 913–17.
5. He FJ, MacGregor GA. Importance of salt in determining blood pressure in children: meta-analysis of controlled trials. Hypertension 2006; 48: 861–9.
6. Appel LJ, Moore TJ, Obarzanek E et al. A clinical trial of the effects of dietary patterns on blood pressure. DASH Collaborative Research Group. N Engl J Med 1997; 36: 1117–24.
7. Intersalt Cooperative Research Group. Intersalt: an international study of electrolyte excretion and blood pressure. Results for 24 hour urinary sodium and potassium excretion. BMJ 1988; 297: 319–28.
8. Poulter NR, Khaw KT, Hopwood BE et al. The Kenyan Luo migration study: observations on the initiation of a rise in blood pressure. BMJ 1990; 300: 967–72.
9. Forte JG, Miguel JM, Miguel MJ, de Padua F, Rose G. Salt and blood pressure: a community trial. J Hum Hypertens 1989; 3: 179–84.
10. He FJ, MacGregor GA. Effect of modest salt reduction on blood pressure: a meta-analysis of randomized trials. Implications for public health. J Hum Hypertens 2002; 16: 761–70.
11. Denton D, Weisinger R, Mundy NI et al. The effect of increased salt intake on blood pressure of chimpanzees. Nat Med 1995; 1: 1009–16.
12. Lifton RP. Molecular genetics of human blood pressure variation. Science 1996; 272: 676–80.
13. Cook NR, Cutler JA, Obarzanek E et al. Long term effects of dietary sodium reduction on cardiovascular disease outcomes: observational follow-up of the trials of hypertension prevention (TOHP). BMJ 2007; 334: 885.
14. Henderson L, Irving K, Gregory J et al. National Diet and Nutrition Survey: Adults Aged 19 to 64, Volume 3. Norwich, UK: Her Majesty's Stationery Office, 2003: 127–36.
15. Food Standards Agency. Dietary sodium levels surveys. Tuesday 20 March 2007. http://www.food.gov.uk/science/dietarysurveys/urinary (accessed 8 June 2007).
16. Scientific Advisory Committee on Nutrition, Salt and Health. 2003. The Stationery Office. Available at http://www.sacn.gov.uk/pdfs/sacn_salt_final.pdf. Accessed 2005.
17. James WP, Ralph A, Sanchez-Castillo CP. The dominance of salt in manufactured food in the sodium intake of affluent societies. Lancet 1987; 1: 426–9.
18. Girgis S, Neal B, Prescott J et al. A one-quarter reduction in the salt content of bread can be made without detection. Eur J Clin Nutr 2003; 57: 616–20.
19. He FJ, Marrero NM, Macgregor GA. Salt and blood pressure in children and adolescents. J Hum Hypertens 2008; 22: 4–11.
20. Lauer RM, Clarke WR. Childhood risk factors for high adult blood pressure: the Muscatine Study. Pediatrics 1989; 84: 633–41.

21. Whelton PK, He J, Cutler JA et al. Effects of oral potassium on blood pressure. Meta-analysis of randomized controlled clinical trials. JAMA 1997; 277: 1624–32.

22. He FJ, MacGregor GA. Fortnightly review: beneficial effects of potassium. BMJ 2001; 323: 497–501.

23. He FJ, Nowson CA, MacGregor GA. Fruit and vegetable consumption and stroke: meta-analysis of cohort studies. Lancet 2006; 367: 320–6.

24. Anonymous. Effects of treatment on morbidity in hypertension. II. Results in patients with diastolic blood pressure averaging 90 through 114 mm Hg. JAMA 1970; 213: 1143–52.

25. The National Institute for Health and Clinical Excellence (NICE), Hypertension – Management of hypertension in adults in primary care. June 2006. Available at http://www.nice.org.uk/cg034.

CHAPTER 11

Heart failure

John GF Cleland, Alison P Coletta, Klaus KA Witte, Andrew L Clark

Introduction

Heart failure is currently the most common malignant disease in all but the poorest nations. There is no sign that the epidemic is abating. Indeed, improved treatment of hypertension and ischemic heart disease may delay the onset of heart failure but ultimately, by improving survival, increase the prevalence of heart failure.[1] Furthermore, as treatment for heart failure may double life expectancy of patients with this condition, this will increase prevalence further. Overall, heart failure is equally common in men and women[2–7] but important sex-specific differences exist in its pathophysiology and, therefore, presentation and treatment.[6,7] The purpose of this chapter is to describe the causes, consequences and management of heart failure in men and compare these with the situation in women.

Definition of heart failure

Heart failure is a clinical syndrome for which no single specific or sensitive test is entirely satisfactory. The definition proposed originally by the European Society of Cardiology (ESC) in 1995[8] has become widely accepted. This definition requires (a) the presence of appropriate symptoms, (b) objective evidence of important cardiac dysfunction as the likely cause and, (c) when doubt exists about the diagnosis, an improvement in symptoms in response to treatment, particularly diuretics.

The heart failure syndrome is characterized by symptoms such as breathlessness, fatigue and ankle swelling. Simplistically and with some element of truth, these symptoms, in the setting of heart failure, may be generated by a low cardiac output or an inadequate increase on exertion and fluid retention. Symptoms are not very sensitive for serious cardiac disease and have poor specificity.[8] Accordingly, symptoms only alert the clinician to the possibility of cardiac disease and are not robust evidence of its presence. Likewise, absence of symptoms cannot be equated with a lack of serious structural cardiac disease.

A key component of the ESC definition is the demonstration of an important underlying cardiac problem as the likely cause for symptoms.[8] Cardiac dysfunction may result from many different diseases and affect many cardiac structures, most commonly the myocardium, valves, the electrical conducting system or the pericardium. Most studies of heart failure have focused on myocardial disease, particularly when it results in reduced contractility and dilatation of the left ventricle, otherwise known as left ventricular systolic dysfunction (LVSD).

The current definition of heart failure is unsatisfactory for many reasons.[9] As stated above, many patients with serious cardiac disease and failing hearts do not have obvious symptoms or have learnt to live with them and so do not seek help. Symptoms of heart failure are non-specific. Most patients with exertional breathlessness and ankle swelling do not have heart failure. Sorting out which patients with symptoms do have serious heart problems can be a complex and costly process, in terms of financial and human resources. The echocardiogram is ultimately a poor guide to diastolic heart failure (see section on pathophysiology).[10] Moreover, there is no precise cut-off value of ejection fraction or any other measurement of cardiac dysfunction that can be used to define heart failure. Thus, for many patients with a clinical syndrome that looks like heart failure the results of first-line cardiac imaging investigations may be equivocal. More sophisticated techniques such as cine magnetic resonance imaging will reduce such uncertainty considerably but such investigations are expensive and often not available.

More recently, biochemical approaches to detect serious cardiac dysfunction have become available. The most promising group of markers at the moment are the natriuretic peptides, atrial and brain natriuretic peptide (ANP and BNP).[11] Initial data suggest that normal blood concentrations of these peptides reliably exclude serious cardiac disease detected by cardiac imaging, at least in untreated patients. However, many patients have elevated markers but no major cardiac abnormality on imaging. The prognosis of these patients appears to be adverse.[12,13] This raises the question of whether imaging or biochemical tests should now be considered the gold standard for cardiac dysfunction, especially since the blood test could provide a simple, internationally verifiable common standard.

This may lead to a number of different scenarios.

1. Currently, natriuretic peptides are being used to screen patients with symptoms or at risk of serious heart disease, with low values being taken to rule out the diagnosis whilst high values prompt referral for cardiac imaging.[14]
2. However, raised plasma natriuretic peptide concentration could be used to replace cardiac imaging as the gold standard objective measure of cardiac dysfunction. In other words, a patient with elevated blood concentrations of natriuretic peptide should be considered to have serious cardiac disease, even if it is not obvious on conventional imaging, unless there is an obvious alternative reason (such as renal dysfunction).[13]

3. Alternatively, it might be considered that a raised plasma concentration of natriuretic peptide provides complementary information to cardiac imaging. It is clear that echocardiographic evaluation of left ventricular function is operator dependent and only moderately reproducible, especially when disease is only mild or moderate in severity. Discordant results of cardiac imaging and biochemical tests might be used to prompt re-evaluation of both tests.
4. Plasma concentrations of natriuretic peptides could be used to stratify patients into high- and low-risk groups with or without additional information from cardiac imaging. Degree of risk could guide the intensity of therapy and follow-up required. A natural extension of this approach is to use plasma natriuretic peptide concentrations to guide treatment, although this is likely to be a complex process.[15,16]
5. Finally, natriuretic peptides could replace the symptom component of the current ESC definition. Changing the definition of heart failure from 'appropriate symptoms due to significant cardiac dysfunction' to a definition such as 'cardiac dysfunction and activation of compensatory mechanisms, such as natriuretic peptides, above a certain threshold' could lead to earlier and more rigorous diagnosis.

Natriuretic peptides may be used diagnostically in both men and women. However, plasma concentrations increase with normal aging and this rise is greater in women than in men. It is likely that age- and sex-specific cut-off values will be developed for the various tests that are becoming available.

Pathophysiology and etiology

Heart failure should be considered a systemic disease caused by cardiac dysfunction. The fall in cardiac output and/or rise in filling pressures results in activation of a number of different neuroendocrine systems. These hemodynamic and neuroendocrine changes (Fig. 11.1) can then adversely affect myocardial structure and function, vascular and endothelial function, skeletal muscle and the

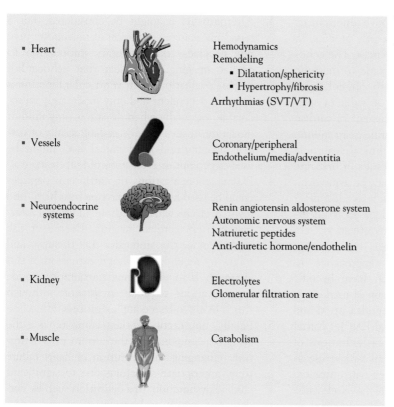

Figure 11.1. *Some pathophysiology of heart failure.*

- Heart
  - Hemodynamics
  - Remodeling
    - Dilatation/sphericity
    - Hypertrophy/fibrosis
  - Arrhythmias (SVT/VT)

- Vessels
  - Coronary/peripheral
  - Endothelium/media/adventitia

- Neuroendocrine systems
  - Renin angiotensin aldosterone system
  - Autonomic nervous system
  - Natriuretic peptides
  - Anti-diuretic hormone/endothelin

- Kidney
  - Electrolytes
  - Glomerular filtration rate

- Muscle
  - Catabolism

Figure 11.2. *Cardiac pathophysiology of heart failure – a simple guide.*

- 'Weak' (Systolic heart failure)
  - Reduced muscle strength and pumping capacity
  - The heart is usually dilated

- 'Stiff' (Diastolic heart failure)
  - The heart pumps adequately but cannot relax to allow proper filling with blood
  - The heart is usually not dilated but the heart muscle is thickened (hypertrophied)

- 'Over-loaded'
  - A narrowed valve or high blood pressure puts excessive load on the heart

- 'Leaking'
  - A heart valve leaks so that much of the blood is pumped backwards rather than forwards.

- 'Confused'
  - Lack of coordination of heart rhythm (atrial fibrillation) or contraction of the different parts of the hearts (dyssynchrony)

function of the kidneys, lungs, liver, pancreas and bone marrow. The causes of heart failure can be simply categorized as shown in Fig. 11.2.

The single most important factor that distinguishes men from women with heart failure (other than their sex) is the prevalence of underlying LVSD. The majority of men with heart failure have global LVSD, the majority of women do not (Fig. 11.3). However, it is not clear that most women have the stiff heart syndrome of diastolic heart failure.[17] Many will have atrial fibrillation as the sole obvious cause whilst others will have impaired long-axis systolic function (i.e. the heart fails to shorten normally although circumferential contraction of the heart is intact). This difference may, in turn, be heavily influenced by the etiology

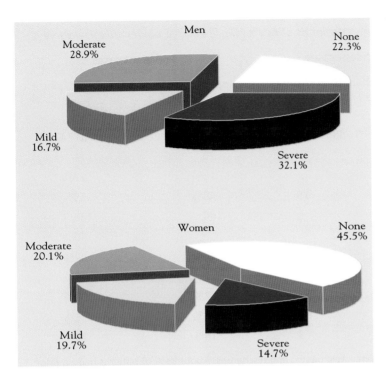

Figure 11.3. *Left ventricular systolic dysfunction in hospital deaths and discharges with suspected heart failure in the EuroHeart Failure Survey (n=6737).*

of the heart failure. Men with heart failure are more likely to have had a myocardial infarction.[5] Women are more likely to be older and more likely to have hypertension as the cause of heart failure.

The development of heart failure is strongly influenced by common comorbidities which are themselves often caused or exacerbated by the presence of heart failure. Heart failure may be exacerbated by anemia, renal dysfunction or atrial fibrillation but may also cause or exacerbate these problems and hence they have become targets for treatment in their own right.[18–20] Other problems, such as gout, may be created by the treatment for heart failure. Pulmonary disease, peripheral and cerebral vascular disease are common in patients with heart failure reflecting the common origins of these conditions.

Common etiologies and co-morbidities of heart failure in men and women in large epidemiological surveys are shown in Table 11.1. The etiology of heart failure differs somewhat from that identified in clinical trials, partly due to selection of patients with LVSD, a selection criterion that also leads to the preferential recruitment of men to these trials (Table 11.2).

Ischemic heart disease is the most common cause of LVSD leading to heart failure, but results in heart failure through very diverse pathophysiological processes.[21–23] Myocardial infarction may result in a full or partial thickness loss of cardiac myocytes and their replacement with scar. On the other hand, sub-lethal coronary occlusion may lead to a chronic loss of myocardial contraction without causing immediate cell death. This phenomenon is known as myocardial hibernation. Hibernating myocardium may not be stable and may induce accelerated death of cardiac myocytes. Less severe coronary occlusion will result in reversible ischemia which may or may not provoke angina. Recurrent ischemia may also lead to prolonged contractile dysfunction which can slowly recover. This phenomenon is called stunning. Clinically, hibernation and stunning are difficult to distinguish. Hibernation, stunning and reversible ischemia are potential key targets for therapy in heart failure although little attention has been paid to these diagnoses so far. How they should be managed is largely anecdotal.

Hypertension may make the single greatest contribution to the development of heart failure

123

Table 11.1. *Common etiologies and co-morbidites of heart failure in large epidemiological surveys*

	Incident cases		Prevalent cases	
	Framingham Heart Study		Improvement	Euroheart failure*
	Men	Women		
N (% women)	N=485		11062 (45%)	10701 (47%)
Age			70	71
Diabetes			18%	27%
Hypertension	76	79	48%	53%
Systolic BP			140	133
Hyperlipidemia				50%**
Atrial fibrillation			22%	42%
Renal dysfunction				17%
Ischemic heart disease	47	27	57%	68%
Dilated cardiomyopathy	NA	NA	6%	6%
Valve disease	2	3	14%	29%

*The Euroheart failure survey included consecutive deaths and discharges. About 35% of patients had no prior history of heart failure. **Percentage of patients with serum cholesterol >5mmol/l. BP, blood pressure; NA, not available.

Table 11.2. *Etiology of heart failure in CHARM (LVSD versus no LVSD) and ATLAS studies*

	CHARM		ATLAS (LVSD)	
	LVSD#	No LVSD	Men	Women
N (% women)	4576 (27%)	3023 (40%)	2516	648
Age	65	67	63	65
Diabetes	28%	28%	19%**	21%**
Hypertension	49%	64%	19%	22%
Systolic BP	128	136	125	129
Hyperlipidemia	41%*	42%*		
Atrial fibrillation	26%	29%	19%	13%
Renal dysfunction				
Ischemic heart disease	65%	56%	68%	52%
Dilated cardiomyopathy	23%	9%	19%	27%
Valve disease			5%	8%

*Percentage of patients receiving lipid-lowering drugs; **, percentage of patients receiving oral hypoglycemic agents and/or insulin; #, data from CHARM–Added[102] and CHARM–Alternative[104] studies combined. LVSD, left ventricular systolic dysfunction; CHARM, candesartan in heart failure assessment of reduction in mortality and morbidity trial; ATLAS, assessment of treatment with lisinopril and survival[159]; BP, blood pressure.

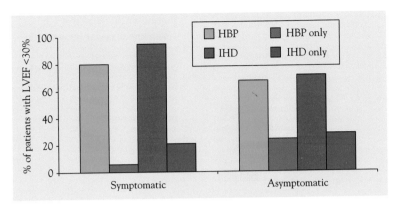

both directly and by inducing coronary disease (Fig. 11.4).[5,24,25] However, hypertension without ischemic heart disease may be more likely to result in heart failure without major impairment of global systolic function.

Presentation

Most patients with heart failure do not present initially with gradually worsening symptoms. Heart failure is diagnosed subsequent to a hospital admission in most cases.[26] In some cases, the development of cardiac dysfunction and of heart failure occurs more or less simultaneously, for instance after a myocardial infarction. In other patients, chronic stable cardiac dysfunction may be precipitated into overt heart failure by an acute event such as an arrhythmia, ischemia, infection, anemia or renal dysfunction. In some patients, it is likely that gradual worsening of heart function eventually reaches a critical threshold that precipitates unheralded severe symptoms without a significant prodrome. The lack of premonitory features may reflect their true absence, patient denial of illness, the attribution of symptoms to another cause (e.g. old age) or to the fact that some people take very little exercise. Acute breathlessness appears to be the most common presentation of heart failure. Only a minority of patients present with progressive symptoms on exertion. Screening high-risk populations by electrocardiography and natriuretic peptides could identify patients at an earlier stage.[14]

Diagnosis of heart failure

Symptoms are a useful alerting mechanism for possible heart failure although perhaps as few as 50% of patients with serious structural heart disease will have overt symptoms (Fig. 11.5).[2,27] A comprehensive approach to diagnosis requires screening of populations at high risk of major cardiac dysfunction (particularly patients with a history of ischemic heart disease). The resources (financial, technological and human skills) available, the cost and the complexity of the test and the efficacy of treatment, will dictate how high the threshold for screening should be set in order for it to be cost effective. Whole (adult) population screening for left ventricular dysfunction has much higher detection rates than for most current cancer screening programs and is much more cost effective, but that is not a justification in itself for such a policy. If a smaller population in which almost all the risks exist can be identified prior to screening tests, then screening is much more efficient. Age, sex and past medical history may indicate which patients may benefit from screening (Figs 11.6 and 11.7).[27] Treatment for asymptomatic LVSD is also much more effective than treatment for other cardiovascular problems, such as hyperlipidemia, for which screening is advocated.

Assuming that the diagnostic pathway begins with symptoms, then two broad approaches to diagnosis can be adopted. The current standard approach is to proceed directly to cardiac imaging (echocardiography) to identify important structural heart disease. Ultimately, such assessments

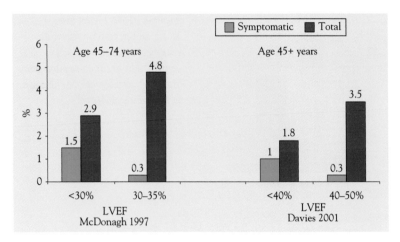

Figure 11.5. *Prevalence of symptomatic and asymptomatic LV systolic dysfunction in two epidemiological studies, according to the severity of left ventricular systolic dysfunction. Adapted from McDonagh et al. Lancet 1997;[27] Davies et al. Lancet 2001.[2]*

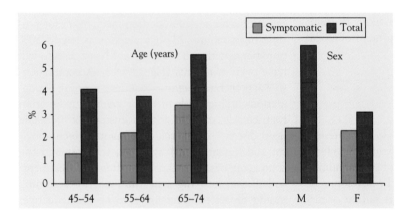

Figure 11.6. *Prevalence of symptomatic and asymptomatic LV systolic dysfunction: effects of age and gender. Adapted from McDonagh et al. Lancet 1997.[27]*

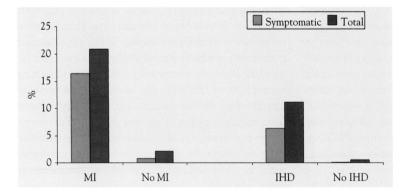

Figure 11.7. *Prevalence of symptomatic and asymptomatic LV systolic dysfunction: according to history of myocardial infarction or ischemic heart disease. Adapted from McDonagh et al. Lancet 1997.[27]*

depend on the quality of the image and the experience of the operator. Considerable room for doubt and error exists in patients who are neither clearly abnormal nor clearly normal. Natriuretic peptides may be a useful cross-check or final arbiter. An alternative approach is to try to screen out patients with a low risk of serious cardiac disease using simple, widely available tests such as the electrocardiogram (ECG) and natriuretic peptides. This approach is very attractive but little practical experience is available. It is not clear whether patients will end up proceeding to echocardiography regardless of the results of screening tests if symptoms persist. The use of natriuretic peptides for diagnosis may be better suited to screening of asymptomatic patients than as a solitary assessment in symptomatic patients. Possible diagnostic algorithms are shown in Figs. 11.8 and 11.9.

Diagnosing the cause of heart failure

Once a diagnosis of heart failure has been made the potential causes, contributory or exacerbating factors and important concomitant diagnoses should be considered.

Some diagnoses will be obvious and others will require further investigation. It is a good policy to first consider how the investigation is going to influence management before requesting it.

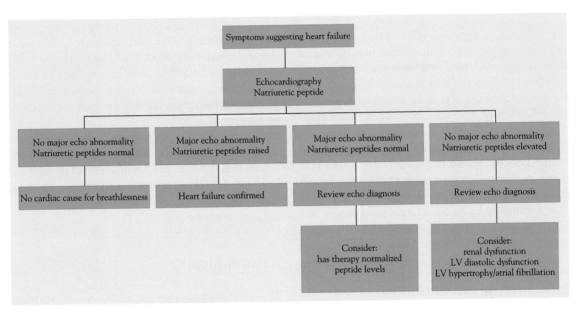

Figure 11.8. *Suggested diagnostic algorithm for symptoms of heart failure.*

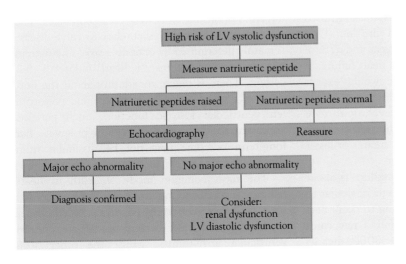

Figure 11.9. *Suggested diagnostic algorithm for patients without heart failure symptoms but at high risk of left ventricular systolic dysfunction.*

- Cardiac imaging test (usually echocardiography)
- ECG
- Chest X-ray
- Full blood count
- Urea and electrolytes/liver function tests
- Natriuretic peptides

Figure 11.10. *Investigations currently recommended by the European Society of Cardiology for all patients with suspected heart failure.*

For instance, in a patient with heart failure and a prior myocardial infarction who is free of angina there is no evidence that revascularization will improve outcome and therefore little reason to ask for an angiogram. There is no evidence as yet that identification of myocardium affected by hibernation, stunning or ischemia should alter therapy.

Routine investigations currently recommended by the ESC are shown in Figure 11.10. Table 11.3 shows problems that commonly contribute chronically to the development of heart failure, factors that commonly cause an acute exacerbation and common concomitant diagnoses that may complicate the management of heart failure.

Incidence, prevalence and lifetime risk

The overall incidence of LVSD is unknown. However, the incidence of hospital-diagnosed myocardial infarction in the United Kingdom (UK) is 1.5–2.0 per 1000 population per year and 37% of such events are expected to lead to heart failure.[1,28] Therefore, in this population we would expect slightly less than one new case of major LVSD per 1000 population per year. However, up to 25% of infarcts do not result in hospitalization and it is not clear whether this group has a greater or lesser likelihood of developing heart failure.

The overall incidence of heart failure is about two per 1000 population per year in men, similar to that observed in women, but tending to occur at a younger age. This equates to about 60 000 new cases in men annually in the UK or about 300 000 men in the USA. This is consistent with the annual incidence of first hospitalization for heart failure reported in Scotland and therefore with the concept that most first presentations are in hospital.

The prevalence of heart failure must be linked to its incidence and prognosis. Assuming that the median survival of heart failure is about 5 years, according to incidence data its prevalence must be about 2%. Again this is very close to estimates of its overall prevalence in men. The prevalence of heart failure increases with age. However, the prevalence of LVSD appears to plateau around 65 years of age (Fig. 11.11). This may reflect poorer survival amongst older patients with LVSD (and therefore under-representation in prevalence data) or may reflect the fact that the etiology of heart failure changes from one driven predominantly by myocardial infarction (in men) to one driven more by hypertension in both sexes. As women have an overall greater life expectancy, there are more women left to develop heart failure in older age groups (Fig. 11.12). The lifetime risk of developing heart failure is about one in five and similar amongst men and women regardless of the age at which assessment begins (Fig. 11.13).

Natural history

The overall prognosis of heart failure is poor, equally bad in men and women and worse than for many cancers (Fig. 11.14). It is clear that patients with myocardial disease resulting in LVSD are largely responsible for this poor outcome. The outcome of heart failure secondary to valve disease is mainly determined by operative risk. The natural history of other forms of heart failure is less certain. There is much uncertainty about the outcome of patients with heart failure and preserved left ventricular systolic function. Such patients appear to have a better short-term prognosis but long-term outcome may not be dissimilar from those with LVSD.

The most common mode of death in heart failure is sudden, which may or may not be preceded by a period of worsening symptoms.[31,32] Probably about 50% of these sudden deaths are due to ventricular arrhythmias, whilst the other 50%

Table 11.3. *Problems which commonly contribute chronically to the development of heart failure, cause acute exacerbations and concomitant diagnoses that complicate treatment*

Problem	Contributes to the development of chronic heart failure (although not the primary cause)	Causes acute exacerbation of heart failure (HF)	Concomitant diagnoses that complicate treatment
Atrial fibrillation (AF)	20–25% will have chronic AF	New onset or uncontrolled AF contributes to about 20% of acute exacerbations of HF	Patients with AF require digoxin in addition to β-blockers for adequate ventricular rate control and warfarin to prevent systemic emboli
Ventricular arrhythmias	Rare	Ventricular arrhythmias are an infrequent cause of acute exacerbation but a common complication of it	Require assessment regarding intensified medical therapy or an ICD (or possibly specific anti-arrhythmic drug therapy)
Pacemakers	5–10% of patients with HF will have a pacemaker	Usually occurs at time of implantation if an acute exacerbation	May cause dyssynchrony and worsening chronic HF requiring upgrade to a cardiac resynchronization device
Angina/myocardial ischemia	Part of the spectrum of ischemic left ventricular dysfunction	Ischemic syndromes contribute to about 25% of acute exacerbations of HF	Angina may require revascularization for relief of symptoms (no evidence of prognostic benefit)
Hypertension	Hypertension is a major risk factor for the development of HF in most patients	Acute exacerbation of heart failure is commonly associated with systemic vasoconstriction and a rise in blood pressure	Most treatments for heart failure reduce arterial pressure
Diabetes	25% of patients will have diabetes – often antedating the onset of HF	Treatment with glitazones may cause fluid retention and acute exacerbation	Requires additional antidiabetic therapy and may cause renal dysfunction
Renal dysfunction	Prevalence depends on definition applied. About 30% will have serum creatinine above upper limit of normal	Worsening renal function is responsible for about 10% of acute exacerbations of HF	Treatment for HF generally causes a deterioration in renal function, especially if BP drops. Requires modification of many drug doses and limits use of spironolactone and ACE inhibitors

(Continued)

Table 11.3. (Continued)

Problem	Contributes to the development of chronic heart failure (although not the primary cause)	Causes acute exacerbation of heart failure (HF)	Concomitant diagnoses that complicate treatment
Anemia	Prevalence depends on definition applied. About 15% will have hemoglobin <11.5g/dl	An occasional cause of acute worsening of HF	May require treatment in its own right
Mitral regurgitation	Affects about 25% of patients	An occasional cause of acute exacerbation	Drug therapy fairly ineffective. Cardiac resynchronization and surgery effective
Aortic valve disease	Affects 5–10% of patients	An occasional cause of acute exacerbation	Drug therapy fairly ineffective. May require surgery
Infection	Rare	Common, usually respiratory or renal. Causes at least 10% of acute deterioration	Septicemia may cause multiorgan failure
Chronic lung disease	Affects about 30% of patients		
Prostatic disease	Common in men	Occasional when acute retention occurs	Acute retention with diuretics. Renal dysfunction
Arthritis	Affects about 10% of patients	Non-steroidal anti-inflammatory drugs may cause fluid retention	Non-steroidal anti-inflammatory drugs (including aspirin) may negate the benefits of ACE inhibitors and cause hyponatremia and renal failure
Pulmonary embolism	Rarely recognized	Recognized in about 3% of cases but may often be occult	Treatment may be inappropriate without correct diagnosis

BP, blood pressure; ACE, angiotensin-converting enzyme; ICD, implantable cardioverter defibrillator.

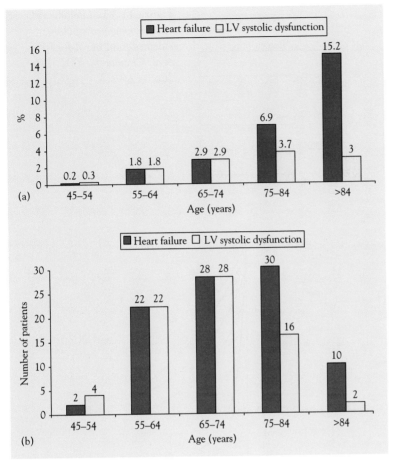

Figure 11.11 (a) Prevalence of LV systolic dysfunction and heart failure. Adapted from McDonagh et al. Lancet 1997,[27] Davies et al. Lancet 2001.[2] (b) Number of people with LV systolic dysfunction and heart failure. Adapted from McDonagh et al. Lancet 1997;[27] Davies et al. Lancet 2001.[2]

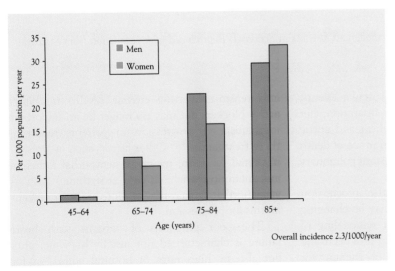

Figure 11.12. Incidence of heart failure in men and women. Adapted from Royal College of General Practitioners. Office of Population Census and Survey, and Department of Health and Social Security. Morbidity Statistics from general practice; fourth national study. 1991–92. London: HMSO, 1995.

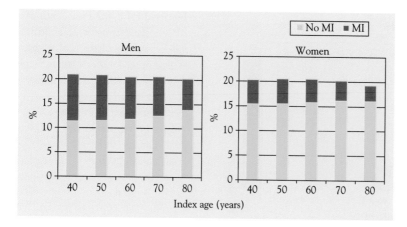

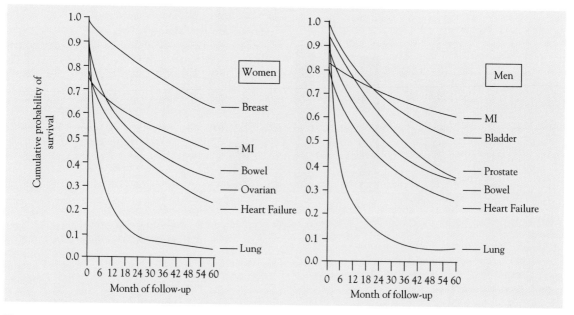

Figure 11.13. *Life time risk of developing heart failure. Adapted from Lloyd-Jones et al. Circulation 2002; 106: 3068–72.[5]*

Figure 11.14. *Prognosis of common malignant diseases in Scotland. Reproduced with permission from Stewart et al. Eur J Heart Fail 2001; 3:315–22.*

are probably due to a variety of vascular events, most commonly acute myocardial infarction, but including stroke, pulmonary embolism and aortic rupture.[31,33] The next most common mode of death is intractable heart failure due to resistant pulmonary edema or cardiogenic shock.

The mechanisms underlying the progression of heart failure are uncertain and may be changing in response to therapy. Structural remodeling of the heart with progressive dilatation and declining function is an important target of therapy for

angiotensin-converting enzyme (ACE) inhibitors and β-blockers but may no longer be an important mechanism of progression in patients receiving these treatments.[34–36] Other factors such as worsening renal function, recurrent myocardial ischemia and infarction, cachexia and arrhythmias such as atrial fibrillation may now be more important mechanisms for progression.

The poor prognosis of patients with heart failure is characterized not just by high mortality but also by high rates of hospital admission for heart failure and other reasons, including chest pain, arrhythmias and stroke.[29,34,35] Admissions are often prolonged and recurrent. Patients with heart failure will spend 5–10% of their remaining life in hospital, with women faring slightly worse than men.[3] Heart failure entails high management costs, much of which are squandered on disorganized care.[37-40]

Many patients with heart failure have severe and persisting symptoms and report anxiety, depression and a poor quality of life.[41,42] Little attention has been paid to how such problems are best managed. It is not clear if there are sex-specific issues here.

Risk stratification

Many factors predict outcome in heart failure but it is unclear which are best since the tests tend to be applied to selected populations (for instance those with systolic dysfunction) that may eliminate the real value of the test. In patients who do have LVSD, natriuretic peptides appear to be one of the best markers and probably superior to grading the severity of ventricular dysfunction. Simple clinical information that suggests an adverse prognosis includes ischemic heart disease as the cause of heart failure, more severe symptoms, lower (systolic) blood pressure, higher diuretic requirements and weight loss.[43] Other biochemical markers such as raised serum creatinine and lower serum sodium also appear to indicate an adverse prognosis. A wide QRS width on the 12-lead ECG, a marker of cardiac dyssynchrony, is also an adverse prognostic sign.[44] These appear to operate similarly in men and women.

Management

This section will focus on the management of heart failure due either to left ventricular systolic or to diastolic heart failure. Patients with heart failure due to other causes, such as valve disease require specialist referral to a cardiologist.

There is little evidence of difference in outcome according to sex in patients with heart failure due to LVSD. However, as LVSD is predominantly a problem affecting men, most of the large clinical trials that have used left ventricular ejection fraction as an entry criterion have recruited mainly men and as a consequence most of the end-points have occurred amongst men. Thus, the apparent sex bias of clinical trials mainly reflects the use of ejection fraction as an entry criterion.

General management

These are mainly opinion based and are well reviewed in the ESC guidelines.[11]

Diet

Patients with heart failure should eat a healthy, well-balanced diet. Those who are somewhat overweight,[45] who have somewhat elevated blood pressure and high blood cholesterol have the best prognosis.[46] So until information that treatment directed at these conditions benefits patients becomes available, healthcare staff should not be excessively concerned about controlling them. It is probably wise to avoid very salty foods in all patients. In patients with advanced heart failure, dietary salt restriction is probably advisable. Alcohol intake should not be excessive. Patients on warfarin should be warned that changes in diet may result in loss of anticoagulant control.

Exercise

Patients should be encouraged to take regular, light exercise, although no more than enough to provoke modest levels of breathlessness.[47] Exercise may have several benefits. Improved cardiovascular fitness will improve exertional capacity, ameliorate muscle wasting and possibly improve prognosis. Exercise, by provoking symptoms, may act as an early warning of deterioration requiring more intensive therapy. There is little evidence to support a benefit from intensive physical training programs.

Travel

Patients are at increased risk of venous thrombosis and changes in diet and climate may affect diuretic and anticoagulant requirements. Issues such as insurance and assistance to avoid long walks at airports should be discussed in advance.

Vaccination

Regular influenza vaccination is recommended although there is little evidence that such practice is safe or effective.

Pharmacological therapy of systolic heart failure

Triple therapy, with ACE inhibitors, β-blockers and aldosterone antagonists, with diuretics to control fluid retention is rapidly becoming the standard treatment for heart failure due to LVSD.[46]

Loop and thiazide diuretics

Diuretics are required for the control of salt and water retention, which may be obvious when peripheral or pulmonary edema develops, or more subtly expressed as exertional breathlessness. They are useful in improving symptoms. The limited data that exist suggest that they reduce hospital admissions and mortality,[48] but they do activate the renin–angiotensin system and probably the sympathetic nervous system which could be deleterious and limit their effectiveness.[49]

'Loop' diuretics act on the Loop of Henle and produce a very potent diuresis over 4–8 hours with a subsequent anti-natriuresis. These are the most widely used diuretics in heart failure, although this is based more on convention than evidence. The vigorous diuresis can cause considerable social inconvenience and may precipitate urinary retention in men with prostatism. With regular treatment the volume and duration of diuresis wane[50] although this also depends on salt and water intake – diuretics tend to be more effective when salt and water excess is present. Loop diuretics are less effective in renal dysfunction and higher doses are needed.

Thiazide diuretics work on the proximal part of the distal convoluted tubule. They are less potent but more long acting and the resultant effect over 24 hours may be similar to loop diuretics. They are more likely to cause hypokalemia and are more diabetogenic than loop diuretics. They may cause less social inconvenience, although diuresis persisting into the night may cause annoying nocturia. They are said to be ineffective in patients with a glomerular filtration rate <30 ml/minute although this is poorly substantiated. Their limited potency means that their use as monotherapy is mainly for patients with milder problems. There are no important sex-specific issues with these agents.

In patients with severe heart failure resistant to loop diuretics, combining loop and thiazide diuretics to induce sequential blockade of the nephron can provoke an extremely marked diuresis.[51] Care must be taken not to cause dehydration and renal dysfunction. This is a useful combination when other options have failed.

Potassium-sparing diuretics

These agents can be divided into aldosterone antagonists and agents working directly on the distal convoluted tubule. Potassium-sparing diuretics can be used to prevent hypokalemia which may provoke arrhythmias. ACE inhibitors and aldosterone antagonists both increase serum potassium and improve patient outcome. Accordingly, the role of potassium-sparing diuretics other than aldosterone antagonists for the management of heart failure has diminished. There are no important sex-specific issues with these agents.

ACE inhibitors (Table 11.4)

ACE inhibitors block the degradation of bradykinin and the formation of angiotensin II, the product of the heightened renin–angiotensin system activity due to heart failure and the diuretics used to treat it. This results in venous and arterial dilatation, a slight fall in arterial pressure and an improvement in renal blood flow. Blockade of these systems also has favorable effects on cardiac and vascular structural remodeling.

ACE inhibitors improve symptoms and retard the progression of ventricular dysfunction and consequently worsening of symptoms.[52–55] Treatment of patients with asymptomatic left ventricular dysfunction, either chronic[53] or occurring soon after a myocardial infarction,[28,56–58] will delay the development of heart failure and reduce mortality,[59,60] predominantly by reducing sudden death.[31] In patients with chronic heart failure, ACE inhibitors will reduce the risk and duration of hospitalization, mainly by reducing the risk of worsening heart failure but also by reducing the risk and duration of recurrent myocardial infarction and other cardiovascular events.[28,34,52,54–66]. ACE inhibitors also increase average life expectancy by 6–36 months depending on the patient's risk profile.[28,34,52,54–66] Reduction in mortality is due to fewer sudden deaths and fewer deaths from worsening heart failure.

Higher doses appear more effective in reducing morbidity.[64,66] Longer-acting agents that can be taken once or twice daily are most convenient for

Table 11.4. *ACE inhibitors (all differences are significant unless otherwise stated)*

Study	Men	Women	Men (%)	Intervention	Outcome	Outcome in men	Outcome in women
(a) *Trials of patients with or at high risk* * *of developing heart failure*							
Meta-analysis(1995)[61]	5399	1587	77%	ACE inhibitors	Mortality Death or HF Hosp	24% reduction 37% reduction	21% reduction 22% reduction
Meta-analysis (2000)[58]	10367	2396	81%	ACE inhibitors	Mortality Death, HF or recurrent MI	21% reduction 29% reduction	15% reduction 21% reduction
CONSENSUS (1998)[59]	178	75	70%	Enalapril	Mortality	31% reduction at 1 year	21% reduction at 1 year[†]
SOLVD-Treatment (1991)[52]	2065	504	80%	Enalapril	Mortality Death or HF Hosp	16% reduction at 3.5 years 26% reduction at 3.5 years	16% reduction at 3.5 years[†] 26% reduction at 3.5 years[†]
SOLVD-Prevention* (1992)[62]	3744	484	89%	Enalapril	Mortality Death or HF	8% reduction (sig) at 3 years 29% reduction at 3 years	8% reduction (sig) at 3 years (ns)[†] 29% reduction at 3 years[†]
SOLVD-Extension (2003)[55]	5817	980	83%	Enalapril	Mortality	10% reduction in mortality over 12 years; 3–4 years treatment increases longevity by 9.4 months over 12 years; similar effect in men and women	10% reduction in mortality over 12 years treatment increases longevity by 9.4 months over 12 years; similar effect in men and women
HOPE* (1992, 2000)[54,62]	6817	2480	73%	Ramipril	MI/CVA/CVS death	22% reduction; similar effects in men and women	22% reduction; similar effects in men and women
(b) *Post-myocardial infarction trials*							
SAVE(1992)[56]	1840	391	82%	Captopril	Mortality	22% reduction 28% reduction	2% reduction[‡] 4% reduction[‡]
AIRE(1993)[57]	1461	525	74%	Ramipril	Mortality	27% reduction; slightly (NS) greater effect in women	27% reduction; slightly (NS) greater effect in women
TRACE (1995)[28], (1999)[63]	1251	498	71%	Trandolapril	Mortality	24% reduction	10% reduction[‡]

(Continued)

135

Table 11.4. (Continued)							
Study	Men	Women	Men (%)	Intervention	Outcome	Outcome in men	Outcome in women
(c) Dose-ranging studies							
ATLAS (1998),[65] (1999),[64] (2001)[34]	2516	648	80%	Lisinopril 5 mg/day versus 35 mg/day	Mortality / Death or Hosp	15% reduction with higher dose / 12% reduction; simililar effect in men and women	5% excess with higher dose (NS)
NETWORK (1998)[66]	976	556	64%	Enalapril 5 mg/day, 10 mg/day or 20 mg/day	Death or worsening HF	No difference between doses†	

*Trials of patients at high risk of developing HF.
†Sex-specific data not reported.
‡Strong trend but not significantly different outcome from that observed in men.
NS, not significant; HF, heart failure; MI, myocardial infarction; CVA, stroke; CVS = cardiovascular; NA, not available; Hosp, hospitalization.

patients but otherwise there appears to be little difference between the efficacy of agents.

Side effects include hypotension (which may be serious with the first dose), renal dysfunction, a persistent dry cough and rarely angio-neurotic edema. Captopril may cause taste disturbances.

Clinical trials suggest that ACE inhibitors may be more effective in men than in women and men appear less prone to side effects such as cough.[61,67]

Adrenergic receptor (β)-blockers (Table 11.5)

The sympathetic nervous system is activated in heart failure and causes vasoconstriction, accelerates adverse remodeling, provokes arrhythmias, may be directly toxic to cardiac myocytes and can stimulate renin–angiotensin system activation and hypokalemia.[68] These effects are mediated by β-1, β-2 and α-1 receptors. Agents that block the β-1 receptor can improve many of the aspects of sympathetic activation, although agents that block a greater array of receptors may be even more effective.[69] Increased sympathetic activity predicts (and is a probable cause of) a worse outcome.[68,70]

β-Blockers do not improve symptoms in the short-term and they may make them worse.[71] In the long term they improve symptoms in many patients and stop them getting worse in many more.[72] Beta-blockers markedly reduce mortality after myocardial infarction, predominantly by reducing sudden death and the risk of recurrent infarction.[73,74] It is likely that they will reduce the risk of asymptomatic left-ventricular dysfunction progressing to heart failure although this is not yet proved. In patients with chronic heart failure, β-blockers will reduce the risk of hospitalization, mainly by reducing the risk of worsening heart failure.[72,75–81] Clinical trials of heart failure have not shown a consistent reduction in non-fatal myocardial infarction or in stroke, perhaps because they preferentially reduce the risk of such events presenting as sudden death.[72,76] Patients who die rapidly will not have time to be diagnosed with a myocardial infarction or stroke. β-Blockers also reduce the overall proportion of time alive spent in hospital.[72,75–81] β-Blockers may increase average life expectancy by 12–24 months,[72,75–82] probably a somewhat larger effect than seen with ACE inhibitors alone. However, the benefits of β-blockade have only been observed in addition to ACE

Table 11.5. β-blockers (all differences are significant unless otherwise stated)

Study	Men	Women	Men (%)	Intervention	Follow-up	Outcome	Outcome in men	Outcome in women
(a) Heart failure								
US Carvedilol trial (1996)[82]	838	256	77%	Carvedilol	7 months	Mortality	59% reduction	77% reduction
CIBIS-II (1999–2001)[75–77]	2132	515	81%	Bisoprolol	16 months	Mortality	30% reduction	54% reduction
MERIT (1999)[78,79,81]	3093	898	77%	Metoprolol	12 months	Mortality Hosp CVS Hosp HF Hosp	Reduced by 39% Reduced by 10% Reduced by 14% Reduced by 18%	Reduced by 8% (NS) Reduced by 19% Reduced by 29% Reduced by 42%
COPERNICUS (2002)[72,80]	1819	470	79%	Carvedilol	10 months	Mortality Death or CVS Hosp Death or HF Hosp	Overall 35% reduction with similar effect in men and women Overall 27% reduction with trend (NS) for less effect in men Overall 31% reduction with trend (NS) for less effect in men	
COMET (2003)[87]	2417	612	80%	Carvedilol vs metoprolol	58 months	Mortality	20% lower risk on carvedilol	3% lower risk on carvedilol*
(b) Post-myocardial infarction								
CAPRICORN (2001)	1440	519	74%	Carvedilol	16 months	Mortality		

*No statistical heterogeneity.
For abbreviations see Table 11.4.

137

Table 11.6. Aldosterone antagonists (all differences significant unless otherwise stated)

Study	Men	Women	Men (%)	Intervention	Follow-up	Outcome	Outcome in men	Outcome in women
RALES (1999)[93]	1217	446	73%	Spironolactone	24 months	Mortality		Overall 30% reduction with similar effect in men and women
EPHESUS (2003)[92]	4714	1918	71%	Eplerenone	16 months	Mortality		Overall 15% reduction with trend (NS) to smaller effect in men
						CVS Death or CVS Hosp		Overall 15% reduction with trend (NS) to greater effect in men

For abbreviations see Table 11.4.

inhibitors, so far. Indeed, there are only limited data to show that β-blockers are effective in the absence of an ACE inhibitor.[83,84]

Little is known about which dose of β-blocker is most effective.[85] There are arguments for the use of low, medium and high doses. Much depends on how well tolerated they are by patients. There also appear to be important differences between β-blockers. Some β-blockers such as bucindolol appear ineffective or harmful.[86] Carvedilol, an agent that blocks β-1, β-2 and α-1 receptors and has antioxidant effects, appears superior to metoprolol, a β-1 selective agent.[87]

Side effects include bradycardia, hypotension, temporary worsening of heart failure and fatigue. β-Blockers are probably not as well tolerated as ACE inhibitors but this partly reflects out-of-date medical training from a time when these agents were considered to be contraindicated in heart failure.[88,89]

Trials of β-blockers suggest that men and women benefit similarly.

Aldosterone antagonists (Table 11.6)

Activation of the renin–angiotensin system and impaired liver function conspire to increase aldosterone levels in heart failure.[90,91] This results, in turn, in renal potassium wasting and hypokalemia which inhibits further increases in aldosterone. Aldosterone is purported to stimulate myocardial and vascular collagen synthesis and therefore have adverse effects on cardiovascular function. ACE inhibitors reduce plasma aldosterone acutely (due to a reduction in angiotensin II) but have little long-term effect, probably reflecting restoration of body potassium levels which had previously held aldosterone secretion in check.

There are few data examining the effects of aldosterone antagonists on symptoms in heart failure, but in patients with right-sided heart failure and persistent edema they are anecdotally very effective. Used in the post-infarction setting,[92] aldosterone antagonists reduce hospital admissions with heart failure and mortality, again predominantly sudden death, indicating that they may have a role for the management of asymptomatic patients. Like ACE inhibitors and β-blockers, aldosterone antagonists reduce hospital admissions, predominantly by reducing heart failure-related and cardiovascular admissions, and increase life expectancy by a substantial amount.[92,93] Aldosterone antagonists seem most effective when added on top of ACE inhibitors and β-blockers.[92,93] There are limited data to show if they are effective without at least one of these other agents also being present. There are no data to indicate whether benefits are dose related but higher doses are more likely to provoke dangerous hyperkalemia.[94]

Side effects of spironolactone include hyperkalemia, renal dysfunction, gynecomastia and testicular atrophy. Selective aldosterone receptor antagonists, such as eplerenone, cause less feminizing side effects than spironolactone.[95]

Trials of aldosterone antagonists suggest that men and women benefit similarly.

Angiotensin-receptor blockers (Table 11.7)

These agents block the effects of angiotensin II and could be used as an alternative or in addition to ACE inhibitors. Studies suggest that they are as effective as ACE inhibitors when used in adequate doses, but given the higher cost of angiotensin receptor blockers (ARBs), ACE inhibitors probably remain the treatment of first choice.[96,97,102–105] Also, the synergy between ACE inhibitors and β-blockers may be greater than any that might exist with angiotensin receptor blockers and β-blockers[96] although there is now conclusive evidence that there is no adverse interaction between ARBs and beta-blockers. A trial comparing high- versus low-dose losartan in patients intolerant of ACE inhibitors is ongoing. For patients who cannot tolerate ACE inhibitors, for example, due to cough or angioneurotic edema, then ARBs may be used as an alternative.[98]

The data so far suggest modest incremental benefits from adding an ARB to an ACE inhibitor (with or without a β-blocker) in terms of symptoms, ventricular function and morbidity.[98–107,160,161] Overall, the addition of an ARB to an ACE inhibitor does not appear to result in a further improvement in mortality.[160,161] Further interpretation and analyses of the benefits of ARBs on symptoms is required before the true value of this treatment combination can be judged.

Effects appear similar in men and women.

Digoxin (Table 11.8)

Digoxin has been used for the treatment of heart failure for over 200 years. It has modest inotropic and diuretic properties, modulates neuroendocrine functions and slows heart rate and atrioventricular conduction.[108–111] Its predominant modern use is for the control of ventricular rate in patients with atrial fibrillation.[36,112,113] β-Blockers or digoxin alone do not appear to control ventricular rate adequately in patients with heart failure but the effects of these agents are synergistic.[113]

In patients in sinus rhythm, digoxin appears to improve symptoms[114] but has no overall effect on mortality when added to an ACE inhibitor.[115] A small reduction in hospitalizations was observed, predominantly due to a reduction in death from worsening heart failure but this was balanced by an increased propensity to sudden death.[115] There are no data investigating the effects of digoxin on symptoms, morbidity or mortality when added on top of β-blockers or aldosterone antagonists. The therapeutic range of digoxin is uncertain. Lower than conventional doses may be effective.[108–111] Higher than conventional doses are associated with side effects such as nausea, vomiting, confusion, arrhythmias and potentially sudden death.[116] Excretion of digoxin is highly dependent on renal function.

The use of digoxin in women in sinus rhythm has been associated with an increase in mortality, perhaps reflecting the use of relatively higher doses in relationship to their renal function. Digoxin[116] did not influence overall mortality in either direction in men.

Other vasodilators

The advent of triple therapy for heart failure has made the existing information in favor of vasodilator therapy – which was never robust – redundant.[117] These trials either excluded women or found no sex-related differences.

Inotropic agents

This class of agent is mainly represented by β-agonists and phosphodiesterase inhibitors. These agents increase intracellular cyclic AMP and cytosolic calcium and have been associated with an increased risk of death when given orally over several months[118] or of adverse effects with

Table 11.7. *Angiotensin receptor blockers (all differences significant unless otherwise stated)*

Study	Men	Women	Men (%)	Intervention	Follow-up	Outcome	Outcome in men	Outcome in women
(a) Heart failure								
ELITE-II (2000)[96]	2185	966	69%	Losartan vs captopril	18 months	Mortality	Overall 13% lower (NS) on captopril vs losartan; similar trend in men and women	
Valsartan (2001)[97–101] (Background ACEi)	4005	1005	80%	Valsartan vs placebo	23 months	Death or worsening HF	Overall 13% lower on valsartan; similar trend in men and women	
CHARM-Added (2003)[102,103] (Background ACEi)	2013	535	79%	Candesartan vs placebo	41 months	CV death or CHF hosp	Overall 15% lower (sig) on candesartan vs placebo; similar trend in men and women	
CHARM – Alternative (2003)[103,104] (ACEi intolerant)	1379	649	68%	Candesartan vs placebo	34 months	CV death or CHF hosp	Overall 23% lower (sig) on candesartan vs placebo; similar trend in men and women	
CHARM – Preserved (2003)[103,105] (normal systolic function)	1814	1209	60%	Candesartan vs placebo	37 months	CV death or CHF hosp	Overall 11% lower (ns) on candesartan vs placebo; similar trend in men and women	
(b) Post-myocardial infarction								
OPTIMAAL (2002)[97]	3902	1575	71%	Losartan vs captopril	32 months	Mortality	Overall 13% lower (NS) on captopril vs losartan; similar trend in men and women	
VALIANT (2003)[106,107]	10133	4570	69%	Valsartan vs Captopril vs Vals + Capto	25 months	Mortality	Similar mortality rates: valsartan 19.9% captopril 19.5% and valsartan plus captopril 19.3%	

For abbreviations see Table 10.4.

Table 11.8. *Miscellaneous (all differences are significant unless otherwise stated)*

Study	Men	Women	Men (%)	Intervention	Follow-up	Outcome	Outcome in men	Outcome in women
Digoxin (2000)[116]	5281	1519	78%	Digoxin	37 months	Mortality	4% reduction (NS)	15% increase (NS)
Digoxin in Patients with Preserved LV Function (2002)[116]	NA	NA	NA	Digoxin	37 months	HF-related death or hosp	14% reduction (NS)	29% reduction (NS)
MADIT-II (2002)[143,145]	1040	192	84%	Defibrillator	20 months	Mortality	Overall 31% reduction with trend (NS) to lesser effect in men	
COMPANION (2003)[116,132,140]	1018	520	67%	Defibrillator with resynchronization	16 months	Mortality	Overall 43% reduction with slight trend (NS) to lesser effect in men	

For abbreviations see Table 11.4.

short-term therapy.[119] Trends to an adverse outcome have also been observed with short-term intravenous therapy with dobutamine and milrinone.[120,162]

The first of a new class of inotropic agent, levosimendan, has recently become available.[121–124] It is a concentration-dependent calcium sensitizer that also has potassium channel-mediated peripheral vasodilator effects. It does not affect intracellular calcium concentrations and sensitizes the myofilaments only during systole so it does not impair diastolic relaxation. It increases cardiac output and reduces filling pressures whilst arterial pressure falls with higher doses. The hemodynamic effectiveness of levosimendan is enhanced in the presence of a β-blocker.[121,122] Compared to placebo or dobutamine, a single infusion lasting 6–24 hours resulted in a substantial reduction in 1-month mortality which persisted out to 6 months. Further trials are underway to confirm these data.

Pharmacological therapy of diastolic heart failure

There are few data with which to guide treatment for diastolic heart failure, although a few observations can be made.

The only substantial randomized controlled trials that included patients with heart failure and preserved left ventricular systolic function were with digoxin[115] (Table 11.8) and candesartan (Table 11.7). Both studies were essentially neutral although showing trends to a reduction in hospitalization but no effect on mortality.[163,164] Admission for heart failure but not the overall risk of hospitalization was reduced by candesartan. Further, substantial trials of ACE inhibitors, angiotensin receptor blockers and β-blockers that will give insights into the efficacy of these agents in patients with heart failure and preserved left ventricular systolic function should report within the next 12–18 months. Only some will focus specifically on diastolic heart failure.[17]

Diuretics should be used to control fluid retention. Digoxin and/or β-blockers may be used to control ventricular rate in patients with atrial fibrillation.[11] Treatment for hypertension, which is common in this population, may include diuretics, β-blockers, ACE inhibitors, aldosterone antagonists and a range of vasodilators. Alpha-blockers cause further activation of the sympathetic nervous system and should be avoided without concomitant β-blocker therapy. The data suggesting benefit with verapamil are weak.

Treatments for ancillary problems

Antithrombotic agents

As much of the morbidity and mortality of heart failure may be related to vascular events it is logical to investigate the safety and utility of antithrombotic agents in this setting.[34,35] Unfortunately, few data exist, as yet, on whether such agents are safe and effective. Aspirin may be ineffective or harmful,[125–129] partly because it may reduce the benefits of ACE inhibitors and partly due to its effects on intrinsic vascular prostaglandin defenses that negate any putative benefit from inhibition of platelet adhesion. Antiplatelet agents that work through other mechanisms, such as dipyridamole or clopidogrel, may be safer and more effective. However, formal anticoagulation with warfarin may be the best method to reduce vascular events. All patients with atrial fibrillation, who are at especial risk of vascular events, should be considered for formal anticoagulation. A large trial comparing aspirin, clopidogrel and warfarin should report soon.[130,131] New anticoagulant agents that are safer and do not require intense monitoring, such as ximelagatran, have also produced some encouraging results.[132,160]

Lipid-lowering therapy

Coronary disease is the commonest cause of heart failure due to left ventricular dysfunction and treatment could make a substantial contribution to slowing progression of heart failure and reducing mortality.[165] However, there are no data to support such a hypothesis as yet and this is reflected by current guidelines on heart failure, which do not support the use of these agents in this setting. Low cholesterol levels predict a worse outcome in patients with heart failure, although this may be because cholesterol levels fall as patients become sicker.[165,166] Statins may also reduce endogenous anti-oxidant defenses such as ubiquinone. On the other hand, statins could reduce coronary events and improve endothelial function and myocardial

perfusion. It is also possible that treatment with statins is futile in patients with heart failure and coronary disease. Patients with heart failure already endure polypharmacy and ineffective or harmful agents should not be allowed to contribute to this burden. A large randomized controlled mortality trial has just begun. Until it reports, there is no justification for prescribing statins routinely in patients with heart failure.[166]

Antiarrhythmic agents

Antiarrhythmic agents, other than β-blockers, amiodarone and possibly dofetilide, are contraindicated in heart failure as they can cause worsening heart failure and increase the risk of sudden death.[32,133] Amiodarone and dofetilide reduce the risk of developing atrial fibrillation and assist cardioversion.[36,112,134,135] Neither agent has been shown to reduce mortality.

Erythropoietin

Patients with heart failure have high levels of erythropoietin but are resistant to its effects, leading to the development of a normochromic normocytic anemia.[19] Plasma volume expansion with hemodilution may also contribute. Anemia is associated with worsening renal function and symptoms and an increase in morbidity and mortality.[137] Treatment with erythropoietin improves exercise capacity.[138] Large trials are underway to investigate the potential therapeutic role of erythropoietin in patients with heart failure.

Devices and surgery

Cardiac resynchronization

Cardiac dyssynchrony is a complex entity comprising one or more of the following: prolonged atrioventricular conduction resulting in atrioventricular dyssynchrony; delayed activation of the left ventricular free wall resulting in dyssynchronous contraction and relaxation of the septum and free wall causing the heart to expend most of its energy deforming its shape rather than ejecting blood; incoordinate activation of the right and left ventricles which reduces the efficiency of both.[44,139] About 25% of patients with advanced heart failure will have a broad QRS width (>120 msec) on their ECG which is a useful (although not perfect) clinical marker for ventricular dyssynchrony.[44,139]

Recent data suggest that atrio-biventricular pacing can correct dyssynchrony and improve symptoms.[44,132,139–142] There is preliminary evidence that resynchronization may also reduce hospitalizations. It is not yet clear if this is associated with a reduction in mortality.

Implantable defibrillators (see Table 11.8)

Sudden death remains the commonest mode of death, despite the ability of ACE inhibitors, β-blockers and aldosterone antagonists to delay such events. Defibrillators can reduce the risk of sudden death by about 50%, implying that defibrillators cannot prevent all arrhythmic deaths or that many sudden deaths are due to another cause, probably vascular events.[132,139,140,143,144] The trials

reporting so far have shown large relative benefits but rather modest absolute benefits from defibrillators, suggesting that patient selection should be improved.[145] Right ventricular or atrio-biventricular pacing back-up is preferred and atrio-right-ventricular pacing should be avoided based on present evidence.[146]

Enhanced external counterpulsation

This non-invasive technique acts in the same way as an intra-aortic balloon pump. A course of 1-hour sessions of counterpulsation (conventionally 35 sessions) has been shown to dramatically reduce severe angina and improve myocardial perfusion.[147,148] Its role for the management of heart failure is now being investigated.[149,150]

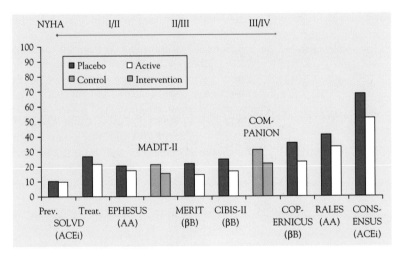

Figure 11.15. *Two-year mortality in contemporary clinical trials. Adapted from: Cleland JGF, Clark AL. JACC 2003.*[46]

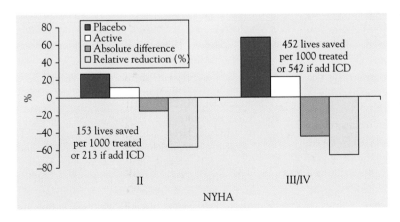

Figure 11.16. *Lives saved over two years per 1000 treated: Effect of triple therapy with ACE inhibitor/beta-blocker/aldosterone antagonist. Adapted from Cleland JGF, Clark AL. JACC 2003.*[46]

Cardiac surgery

A variety of surgical procedures may be considered for patients with heart failure including aneurysmectomy, surgical remodeling of the ventricle, mitral valve repair and coronary artery bypass.[21,151–154] Whether such interventions are beneficial or not is largely anecdotal and depends on skilled judgment. The perceived prognostic benefits of revascularization are more expressions of desperation, ignorance or 'spin' than based on fact.[155] These interventions do not have a role in routine clinical practice at the moment. Trials are underway.[21]

Heart transplantation

There is a diminishing role for conventional heart transplantation procedures as medical therapy improves and the donor supplies decline.[156] Most patients with heart failure are considered too old for transplantation. There are concerns that heart transplantation may have little impact on the prognosis of patients with heart failure unless they are carefully selected.[156] The morbidity associated with repeated biopsy and immunosuppressant therapy is substantial. The development of mechanical assist devices as alternatives to biological transplantation is progressing rapidly.[157] However, for some patients, there is no doubt that heart transplantation is life transforming.

Summary

The understanding and management of heart failure has progressed dramatically over the last 20 years. The 2-year mortality of heart failure due to LVSD has been more than halved (Figs. 11.15 and 11.16).[37,38,46,132] Treating just two patients with moderately severe heart failure will save one life over just 2 years of treatment. Effective, safe treatment requires a highly organized system[37–40,46,132,158] with integrated care between the community, the hospital, the primary care physician and the heart failure specialist (who may or may not be a cardiologist).[46,132] However, we may become victims of our own success because problems are probably being deferred rather than prevented. Understanding and managing patients who appear to have heart failure but who have preserved left ventricular systolic function will be a major challenge.

References

1. Cleland JGF, Khand A, Clark AC. The heart failure epidemic: exactly how big is it? Eur Heart J 2001; 22: 623–6.
2. Davies MK, Hobbs FDR, Davis RC et al. Prevalence of left-ventricular systolic dysfunction and heart failure in the Echocardiographic Heart of England Screening study: a population based study. Lancet 2001; 358: 439–44.
3. Cleland JGF, Gemmel I, Khand A, Boddy A. Is the prognosis of heart failure improving? Eur J Heart Fail 1999; 1: 229–41.
4. Cowie MR, Wood DA, Coats AJS et al. Incidence and aetiology of heart failure. A population based study. Eur Heart J 1999; 20: 421–8.
5. Lloyd-Jones DM, Larson MG, Leip MS et al. Lifetime risk for developing congestive heart failure – The Framingham Heart Study. Circulation 2002; 106: 3068–72.
6. Cleland JGF, Swedberg K, Follath F et al, for the Study Group on Diagnosis of the Working Group on Heart Failure of the European Society of Cardiology. The EuroHeart Failure Survey Programme: survey on the quality of care among patients with heart failure in Europe. Part 1: patient characteristics and diagnosis. Eur Heart J 2003; 24: 422–63.
7. Cleland JGF, Cohen-Solal A, Cosin-Aguilar J et al, for the IMPROVEMENT of Heart Failure Programme Committees and Investigators and the Study Group on Diagnosis of the Working Group on Heart Failure of the European Society of Cardiology. An international survey of the management of heart failure in primary care. The IMPROVEMENT of Heart Failure Programme. Lancet 2002; 360: 1631–9.
8. Cleland JGF, Erdmann E, Ferrari R et al. Task Force on Heart Failure of the European Society of Cardiology. Guidelines for the diagnosis of heart failure. Eur Heart J 1995; 16: 741–51.
9. Cleland JGF. Diagnosis of heart failure. Heart 1998; 79: S10–S16.
10. Vasan RS, Levy D. Defining diastolic heart failure: a call for standardized diagnostic criteria. Circulation 2000; 101: 2118–121.
11. Task Force for the Diagnosis and Treatment of Chronic Heart Failure ESoC, Remme WJ, Swedberg K. Guidelines for the diagnosis and treatment of chronic heart failure. Eur Heart J 2001; 22: 1527–60.
12. McDonagh T, Cunningham AD, Morrison CE et al. Left ventricular dysfunction, natriuretic

peptides and mortality in an urban population. Heart 2002; 86: 21–6.

13. Richards AM, Nicholls MG, Espiner EA et al. B-type natriuretic peptides and ejection fraction for prognosis after myocardial infarction. Circulation 2003; 107: 2786–92.

14. Hobbs FDR, Davis RC, Roalfe AK, Davies MK, Kenkre JE. Reliability of N-terminal pro-brain natriuretic peptide assay in diagnosis of heart failure: cohort study in representative and high risk community populations. BMJ 2002; 324: 1498–500.

15. Troughton RW, Frampton C, Yandle TG et al. Treatment of heart failure guided by plasma aminoterminal brain natriuretic peptide (N-BNP) concentrations. Lancet 2000; 355: 1112–13.

16. Cleland JGF. Commentary on: N-BNP-guided treatment of heart failure resulted in a reduction in total cardiovascular events when compared to usual clinical care by Troughton RW et al. Evidence Based Cardiov Med 2000; 4: 78.

17. Banerjee P, Banerjee T, Khand A, Clark AL, Cleland JGF. Diastolic heart failure – neglected or misdiagnosed? J Am Coll Cardiol 2002; 39: 138–41.

18. Hillege H, Girbes AR, de Kam PJ et al. Renal function, neurohormonal activation and survival inpatients with chronic heart failure. Circulation 2000; 102: 203–10.

19. Silverberg DS, Wexler D, Blum M et al. The use of subcutaneous erythropoietin and intravenous iron for the treatment of the anaemia of severe, resistant congestive heart failure improves cardiac and renal function and functional cardiac class, and markedly reduces hospitalizations. J Am Coll Cardiol 2000; 35: 1737–44.

20. Khand AU, Rankin AC, Kaye GC, Cleland JGF. Systematic review of the management of atrial fibrillation in patients with heart failure. Eur Heart J 2000; 21: 614–32.

21. Cleland JGF, Freemantle N, Ball SG et al. The heart failure revascularization trial (HEART): rationale design and methodology. Eur J Heart Fail 2003; 5: 295–303.

22. Cleland JGF, Pennell DJ, Ray SG et al, on behalf of the CHRISTMAS (carvedilol hibernating reversible ischaemia trial: marker of success) investigators. Myocardial viability as a determinant of the ejection fraction response to carvedilol in patients with heart failure (CHRISTMAS trial): randomised controlled trial. Lancet 2003; 362: 14–21.

23. Cleland JGF, Pennell DJ, Ray S et al. The CHRISTMAS Study Steering Committee and Investigators. The Carvedilol Hibernation Reversible Ischaemia Trial: marker of success (CHRISTMAS). Eur J Heart Fail 1999; 1: 191–6.

24. Levy D, Larson MG, Vasan RS, Kannel WB, Ho KKL. The progression from hypertension to congestive heart failure. JAMA 1996; 275: 1557–62.

25. McDonagh T, Morrison CE, McMurray JJ et al. Global left ventricular systolic dysfunction in north Glasgow. J Am Coll Cardiol 1996; 27(Spec Issue): 106A.

26. Cleland JGF, Clark AL, Caplin JL. Taking heart failure seriously. BMJ 2000; 321: 1095–6.

27. McDonagh TA, Morrison CE, Lawrence A et al. Symptomatic and asymptomatic left-ventricular systolic dysfunction in an urban population. Lancet 1997; 350: 829–33.

28. Kober L, Torp Pedersen C, Carlsen JE et al. A clinical trial of the angiotensin-converting-enzyme inhibitor trandolapril in patients with left ventricular dysfunction after myocardial infarction. New Engl J Med 1995; 333: 1670–6.

29. Brown A, Cleland JGF. Influence of concomitant disease on patterns of hospitalisation in patients with heart failure discharged from Scottish hospitals in 1995. Eur Heart J 1998; 19: 1063–9.

30. Cowie MR, Mosterd A, Wood DA et al. The epidemiology of heart failure. Eur Heart J 1997; 18: 208–23.

31. Cleland JGF, Massie BM, Packer M. Sudden death in heart failure: vascular or electrical? Eur J Heart Fail 1999; 1: 41–5.

32. Cleland JGF, Chattopadhyay S, Khand A, Houghton T, Kaye GC. Prevalence and incidence of arrhythmias and sudden death in heart failure. Heart Fail Rev 2002; 7: 229–42.

33. Uretsky B, Thygesen K, Armstrong PW et al. Acute coronary findings at autopsy in heart failure patients with sudden death: Results from the assessment of treatment with lisinopril and survival study (ATLAS) trial. Circulation 2000; 102: 611–16.

34. Cleland JGF, Thygesen K, Uretsky BF et al. Cardiovascular critical event pathways for the progression of heart failure. A report from the ATLAS study. Eur Heart J 2001; 22: 1601–12.

35. Khand AU, Gemmell I, Rankin AC, Cleland JGF. Clinical events leading to the progression of heart failure: insights from a national database of hospital discharges. Eur Heart J 2001; 22: 153–64.

36. Khand A, Rankin AC, Kaye GC, Cleland JGF. Systematic review of the management of atrial fibrillation in patients with heart failure. Eur Heart J 2000; 21: 614–32.

37. Stewart S, Marley JE, Horowitz JD. Effects of a multidisciplinary, home-based intervention on unplanned readmissions and survival among patients with chronic congestive heart failure: a randomised trial. Lancet 1999; 354: 1077–83.

38. Stewart S, Jenkins A, Buchan S et al. The current cost of heart failure to the National Health Service in the UK. Eur J Heart Fail 2002; 4: 361–71.

39. Stewart S, Blue L, Walker A, Morrison C, McMurray JJ. An economic analysis of specialist heart failure nurse management in the UK: can we afford not to implement it? Eur Heart J 2002; 23: 1369–78.

40. Blue L, Lang E, McMurray JJ et al. Randomised controlled trial of specialist nurse intervention for heart failure. BMJ 2001; 323: 718.

41. Miller AB. Heart failure and depression. Eur J Heart Fail 2002; 4: 402.

42. Cleland JGF, Wang M. Depression and heart failure – not yet a target for therapy? Eur Heart J 1999; 20: 1529–30.

43. Cowburn PJ, Cleland JGF, Coats AJS, Komajda M. Risk stratification in chronic heart failure. Eur Heart J 1998; 19: 696–710.

44. Cleland JGF, Ghosh J, Khan NK et al. Multi-chamber pacing: a perfect solution for cardiac mechanical dyssynchrony? Eur Heart J 2003; 24: 384–90.

45. Davos CH, Doehner W, Rauchhaus M et al. Body mass and survival in patients with chronic heart failure without cachexia: the importance of obesity. J Card Failure 2003; 9: 29–35.

46. Cleland JGF, Clark AL. Delivering the cumulative benefits of triple therapy to improve outcomes in heart failure: too many cooks will spoil the broth. J Am Coll Cardiol 2003; 42: 1234–7.

47. Clark AL, Cleland JGF. Assessing the effect of exercise training in men with heart failure. Eur Heart J 2001; 22: 627–8.

48. Faris R, Flather M, Purcell H et al. Current evidence supporting the role of diuretics in heart failure: a meta analysis of randomised controlled trials. Int J Cardiol 2002; 82: 149–58.

49. Bayliss J, Norell M, Canepa Anson R et al. Untreated heart failure: clinical and neuroen-docrine effects of introducing diuretics. Br Heart J 1987; 57: 17–22.

50. Stewart JH, Edwards KDG. Clinical comparison of frusemide with bendrofluazide, mersalyl, and ethacrynic acid. BMJ 1965; 2: 1277–81.

51. Channer KS, McLean KA, Lawson Mathew P, Richardson M. Combination diuretic treatment in severe heart failure: a randomised controlled trial. Br Heart J 1994; 71: 146–50.

52. The SOLVD investigators. Effect of enalapril on survival in patients with reduced left ventricular ejection fractions and congestive heart failure. New Engl J Med 1991; 325: 293–302.

53. Yusuf S, Nicklas JM, Timmis G et al. Effect of enalapril on mortality and the development of heart failure in asymptomatic patients with reduced left ventricular ejection fractions. New Engl J Med 1992; 327: 685–91.

54. Yusuf S, Sleight P, Pogue J et al. Effects of the angiotensin converting enzyme inhibitor, ramipril, on cardiovascular events in high risk patients. The Heart Outcomes Prevention Evaluation study investigators. New Engl J Med 2000; 342: 145–53.

55. Jong P, Yusuf S, Rousseau MF, Ahn SA, Bangdiwala SI. Effect of enalapril on 12-year survival and life expectancy in patients with left ventricular systolic dysfunction: a follow-up study. Lancet 2003; 361: 1843–8.

56. Pfeffer MA, Braunwald E, Moye LA et al. Effect of captopril on mortality and morbidity in patients with left ventricular dysfunction after myocardial-infarction – results of the survival and ventricular enlargement trial. New Engl J Med 1992; 327: 669–77.

57. Ball SG, Hall AS, Mackintosh AF et al. Effect of ramipril and morbidity of survivors of acute myo-cardial infarction with clinical evidence of heart failure. Lancet 1993; 342: 821–8.

58. Flather MD, Yusuf S, Kober L et al, for the ACE inhibitor Myocardial Infarction Collaborative Group. Long term ACE-inhibitor therapy in patients with heart failure or left ventricular dysfunction: a systematic overview of data from individual patients. Lancet 2000; 355: 1575–81.

59. Swedberg K, Kjekshus J. Effects of enalapril on mortality in severe congestive heart failure: results of the cooperative north Scandinavian enalapril survival trial (CONSENSUS). Am J Cardiol 1988; 62 (Suppl A): 60A–66A.

60. Cohn JN, Johnson G, Ziesche S et al. A comparison of enalapril with hydralazine-isosorbide dinitrate in the treatment of chronic congestive heart failure. New Engl J Med 1991; 325: 303–10.

61. Garg R, Yusuf S. Overview of randomized trials of angiotensin-converting enzyme inhibitors on mortality and morbidity in patients with heart failure. JAMA 1995; 273: 1450–6.

62. Yusuf S, Pepine CJ, Garces C et al. Effect of enalapril on myocardial infarction and unstable angina in patients with low ejection fractions. Lancet 1992; 340: 1173–8.

63. Torp-Pedersen C, Kober L. Effect of ACE inhibitor trandolapril on life expectancy of patients with reduced left ventricular function after acute myocardial infarction. TRACE study group. Lancet 1999; 354: 9–12.

64. Packer M, Poole Wilson PA, Armstrong PW et al, on behalf of the ATLAS investigators. Comparative effects of low and high doses of the angiotensin-converting enzyme inhibitor, lisinopril, on morbidity and mortality in chronic heart failure. Circulation 1999; 100: 2312–18.

65. Cleland JGF, Massie BM, Packer M et al. Health economic benefits of treating patients with heart failure with high dose lisinopril versus low dose lisinopril: The Atlas Study. Circulation 1998 98(Suppl); Abs 698: 1–35.

66. The NETWORK Investigators. Clinical outcome with enalapril in symptomatic chronic heart failure; a dose comparison. Eur Heart J 1998; 19: 481–9.

67. Robinson TD, Celermajer DS, Bye PTP. How to stop ACE inhibitor-induced cough. Lancet 1997; 350: 3–4.

68. Cleland JGF, Bristow M, Erdmann E. Beta-blocking agents in heart failure. Should they be used and how? Eur Heart J 1996; 17: 1629–39.

69. Poole-Wilson PA, Cleland JGF, Hanrath P et al, on behalf of the COMET study investigators. Rationale and design of the carvedilol or metoprolol European trial in patients with chronic heart failure; the COMET trial. Eur J Heart Fail 2002; 4: 321–9.

70. Cohn J, Levine TB, Olivari MT et al. Plasma norepinephrine as a guide to prognosis in patients with chronic congestive heart failure. New Engl J Med 1984; 311: 819–23.

71. MacMahon S, Sharpe N, Doughty R et al. Randomised, placebo-controlled trial of carvedilol in patients with congestive heart failure due to ischaemic heart disease. Lancet 1997; 349: 375–80.

72. Packer M, Fowler MB, Roecker EB et al. Carvedilol prospective randomized cumulative survival COPERNICUS study group. Effect of carvedilol on the morbidity of patients with severe chronic heart failure: results of the carvedilol prospective randomized cumulative survival (COPERNICUS) study. Circulation 2002; 106: 2194–9.

73. Freemantle N, Cleland JGF, Young S, Mason J, Harrison J. Beta blockade after myocardial infarction: systematic review and meta regression analysis. BMJ 1999; 318: 1730–7.

74. Houghton T, Freemantle N, Cleland JGF. Are beta-blockers effective in patients who develop heart failure soon after myocardial infarction? A meta-regression analysis of randomised trials. Eur J Heart Fail 2000; 2: 333–40.

75. Simon T, Mary-Krause M, Funck-Brentano C, Jaillon P, on behalf of the CIBIS II investigators. Sex differences in the prognosis of congestive heart failure. Results from the cardiac insufficiency bisoprolol study (CIBIS-II). Circulation 2001; 103: 375–80.

76. CIBIS-II Investigators and Committee. The cardiac insufficiency bisoprolol study II (CIBIS-II): a randomised trial. Lancet 1999; 353: 9–13.

77. Funck-Brentano C, Lancar R, Hansen S, Hohnloser SHVE. Predictors of medical events and of their competitive interactions in the cardiac insufficiency bisoprolol study 2 (CIBIS-2). Am Heart J 2001; 142: 989–97.

78. Ghali JK, Pina IL, Gottlieb SS, Deedwania PC, Wikstrand JC, The MERIT-HF study group. Metoprolol CR/XL in female patients with heart failure: analysis of the experience in metoprolol extended-release randomized intervention trial in heart failure (MERIT-HF). Circulation 2002; 105: 1585–91.

79. MERIT-HF Study Group. Effect of metoprolol CR/XL in chronic heart failure: metoprolol CR/XL randomised intervention trial in congestive heart failure (MERIT-HF). Lancet 1999; 333: 2001–7.

80. Packer M, Coates AJS, Fowler MD et al. Effect of carvedilol on survival in severe chronic heart failure. N Engl J Med 2001; 344: 1651–8.

81. Hjalmarson A, Goldstein S, Fagerberg B et al. Effects of controlled-release metoprolol on total

mortality, hospitalization, and well-being in patients with heart failure: the metoprolol CR-XL randomized intervention trial in congestive heart failure (MERIT-HF). JAMA 2000; 283: 1295–302.

82. Packer M, Bristow MR, Cohn JN et al, for the US carvedilol study group. The effect of carvedilol on morbidity and mortality in patients with chronic heart failure. New Engl J Med 1996; 334: 1349–55.

83. Remme WJ, CARMEN steering committee and investigators. The carvedilol and ACE-inhibitor remodelling mild heart failure evaluation trial (CARMEN) – rationale and design. Cardiovasc Drugs Ther 2001; 15: 69–77.

84. Coletta A, Louis AA, Clark AL, Nikitin N, Cleland JGF. Clinical trials update from the European Society of Cardiology: CARMEN, EARTH, OPTI-MAAL, ACE, TEN_HMS, MAGIC, RITA-3, SOLVD-X and PATH-CHF. Eur J Heart Fail 2002; 4: 661–6.

85. Bristow MR, Gilbert EM, Abraham WT et al, for the Mocha Investigators. Carvedilol produces dose-related improvements in left ventricular function and survival in subjects with chronic heart failure. Circulation 1996; 94: 2807–16.

86. The beta-blocker evaluation of survival trial investigators. A trial of the beta-blocker bucindolol in patients with advanced chronic heart failure. New Engl J Med 2001; 344: 1659–67.

87. Poole-Wilson PA, Swedberg K, Cleland JGF et al, for the COMET investigators. Comparison of carvedilol and metoprolol on clinical outcomes in patients with chronic heart failure in the Carvedilol or Metoprolol European Trial (COMET): randomised controlled trial. Lancet 2003; 362: 7–13.

88. Cleland JGF, Freemantle N, McGowan J, Clark A. The evidence for beta-blockers equals or surpasses that for ACE inhibitors in heart failure. BMJ 1999; 318: 824–5.

89. Cleland JGF, McGowan J, Cowburn PJ. β-blockers for chronic heart failure: from prejudice to enlightenment. J Cardiovasc Pharm 1998; 32(Suppl 1): S52–S60.

90. Pitt B. 'Escape' of aldosterone production in patients with left ventricular dysfunction treated with an angiotensin converting enzyme inhibitor: implications for therapy. Cardiovasc Drugs Ther 1995; 9: 145–9.

91. Struthers AD. Why does spironalactone improve mortality over and above an ACE inhibitor in

chronic heart failure. Br J Clin Pharmacol 1999; 47: 479–82.

92. Pitt B, Remme W, Zannad F et al, for the Eplerenone Post-acute Myocardial Infarction Heart Failure Efficacy and Survival Study Investigators. Eplerenone, a selective aldosterone blocker, in patients with left ventricular dysfunction after myocardial infarction. N Engl J Med 2003; 348: 1309–21.

93. Pitt B, Zannad F, Remme WJ et al. The effect of spironolactone on morbidity and mortality in patients with severe heart failure. N Engl J Med 1999; 341: 709–17.

94. Effectiveness of spironolactone added to an angiotensin-converting enzyme inhibitor and a loop diuretic for severe chronic congestive heart failure (the randomized aldactone evaluation study (RALES)). Am J Cardiol 1996; 78: 902–7.

95. Pitt B, Williams G, Remme W et al. The EPHESUS trial: eplerenone in patients with heart failure due to systolic dysfunction complicating acute myocardial infarction. Eplerenone post-AMI heart failure efficacy and survival study. Cardiovasc Drugs Ther 2003; 15: 79–87.

96. Pitt B, Poole Wilson PA, Segal R et al, on behalf of the ELITE II investigators. Effect of losartan compared with captopril on mortality in patients with symptomatic heart failure: randomised trial – the losartan heart failure survival study ELITE II. Lancet 2000; 355: 1582–7.

97. Dickstein K, Kjekshus J, and the OPTIMAAL steering committee for the OPTIMAAL study group. Effects of losartan and captopril on mortality and morbidity in high-risk patients after acute myocardial infarction: the OPTIMAAL randomised trial. Lancet 2002; 360: 752–60.

98. Maggioni A, Anand I, Gottlieb SO et al, for the Valsartan Heart Failure Trial Investigators. Effects of valsartan on morbidity and mortality in patients with heart failure not receiving angiotensin converting enzyme inhibitors. J Am Coll Cardiol 2002; 40: 1414–21.

99. Cohn JN, Tognoni G for the Valsartan Heart Failure Trial Investigators. A randomized trial of the angiotensin-receptor blocker valsartan in chronic heart failure. N Engl J Med 2001; 345: 1667–75.

100. Cohn JN, Tognoni G, Glazer RD, Spormann D. Baseline demographics of the Valsartan Heart Failure Trial. Eur J Heart Fail 2000; 2: 439–46.

101. Carson P, Tognoni G, Cohn JN. Effect of valsartan on hospitalization: results from Val-HeFT. J Card Fail 2003; 9: 164–71.

102. McMurray JJV, Ostergren J, Swedberg K et al, for the CHARM investigators and committees. Effects of candesartan in patients with chronic heart failure and reduced left ventricular ejection fraction taking angiotensin-converting enzyme inhibitors: the CHARM-Added trial. Lancet 2003; 362: 767–71.

103. McMurray J, Ostergren J, Pfeffer M et al, on behalf of the CHARM committees and investigators. Clinical features and contemporary management of patients with low and preserved ejection fraction heart failure: baseline characteristics of patients in the candesartan in heart failure – assessment of reduction in mortality and morbidity (CHARM) programme. Eur J Heart Fail 2003; 5: 261–70.

104. Granger CB, McMurray JJV, Yusuf S, for the CHARM investigators and committees. Effects of candesartan in patients with chronic heart failure and reduced ventricular systolic function intolerant to angiotensin converting enzyme inhibitors: the CHARM-Alternative trial. Lancet 2003; 362: 772–6.

105. Yusuf S, Pfeffer MA, Swedberg K, for the CHARM investigators and committees. Effects of candesartan in patients with chronic heart failure and preserved left-ventricular ejection fraction: the CHARM-Preserved trial. Lancet 2003; 362: 777–81.

106. Pfeffer MA, McMurray JJV, Velazquez EJ, for the Valsartan in Acute Myocardial Infarction Trial Investigators. Valsartan, Captopril, or both in myocardial infarction complicated by heart failure, left ventricular systolic dysfunction, or both. New Engl J Med 2003; 349: 1893–906.

107. Velazquez EJ, Pfeffer MA, McMurray JJV, for the VALIANT investigators. Valsartan in acute myocardial infarction (VALIANT) trial: baseline characteristics in context. Eur J Heart Fail 2003; 5: 537–44.

108. Slatton ML, Irani WN, Hall SA et al. Does digoxin provide additional hemodynamic and autonomic benefit at higher doses in patients with mild to moderate heart failure and normal sinus rhythm? J Am Coll Cardiol 1997; 29: 1206–13.

109. Gheorghiade M, Hall VB, Jacobsen G et al. Effects of increasing maintenance dose of digoxin on left ventricular function and neurohormones in patients with chronic heart failure treated with diuretics and angiotensin-converting enzyme inhibitors. Circulation 1995; 92: 1801–7.

110. Krum H, Bigger JTJ, Goldsmith RL et al. Effect of long-term digoxin therapy on autonomic function in patients with chronic heart failure. J Am Coll Cardiol 1995; 25: 289–94.

111. Van Veldhuisen DJ, Brouwer J, Man in 't Veld AJ et al. Progression of mild untreated heart failure during six months follow-up and clinical and neurohumoral effects of ibopamine and digoxin as monotherapy. Am J Cardiol 1995; 75: 796–800.

112. Khand A, Cleland JGF, Deedwania P. Prevention of and medical therapy for atrial arrhythmias in heart failure. Heart Fail Rev 2002; 7: 267–83.

113. Khand AU, Rankin AC, Martin W, Taylor J, Cleland JGF. Digoxin or carvedilol for the treatment of atrial fibrillation in patients with heart failure? Heart 2000; 83(Suppl 1): 30.

114. Packer M, Gheorghiade M, Young JB et al. Withdrawal of digoxin from patients with chronic heart failure treated with angiotensin-converting-enzyme inhibitors. N Engl J Med 1993; 329: 1–7.

115. The Digitalis Investigation Group. The effect of digoxin on mortality and morbidity in patients with heart failure. N Engl J Med 1997; 336: 525–33.

116. Rathore SS, Wang Y, Krumholz HM. Sex-based differences in the effect of digoxin for the treatment of heart failure. N Engl J Med 2002; 347: 1403–11.

117. Cohn JN, Archibald DG, Ziesche S et al. Effect of vasodilator therapy on mortality in chronic congestive heart failure: results of a Veterans Administration Cooperative Study. N Engl J Med 1986; 314: 1547–52.

118. Packer M, Carver JR, Rodeheffer RJ et al. Effect of oral milrinone on mortality in severe chronic heart failure. N Engl J Med 1991; 325: 1468–75.

119. Cuffe M, Califf RM, Adams KF et al. Outcomes of a prospective trial of intravenous milrinone for exacerbations of chronic heart failure (OPTIME-CHF) investigators. JAMA 2002; 287: 1541–7.

120. Thackray S, Eastaugh J, Freemantle N, Cleland JGF. The effectiveness and relative effectiveness of intravenous inotropic drugs acting through adrenergic pathways in patients with heart failure – a meta-regression analysis. Eur J Heart Fail 2002; 4: 515–29.

121. Cleland JGF, McGowan J. Levosimendan: a new era for inodilator therapy for heart failure? Curr Opin Cardiol 2002; 17: 257–65.

122. Follath F, Cleland JGF, Just H et al, for the steering committee and investigators of the LIDO study. Efficacy and safety of intravenous levosimendan compared with dobutamine in severe low-output heart failure (the LIDO study): a randomised double-blind trial. Lancet 2002; 360: 196–202.

123. Moiseyev VS, Poder P, Andrejevs N et al. Safety and efficacy of a novel calcium sensitizer, levosimendan, in patients with left ventricular failure due to an acute myocardial infarction. A randomized, placebo-controlled, double-blind study (RUSSLAN). Eur Heart J 2002; 23: 1422–32.

124. Cleland JGF, Takala A, Apajasalo M, Zethraeus N, Kobelt G. Intravenous levosimendan treatment is cost-effective compared with dobutamine in severe low-output heart failure: an analysis based on the international LIDO trial. Eur J Heart Fail 2003; 5: 101–8.

125. Cleland JGF, Bulpitt CJ, Falk RH et al. Is aspirin safe for patients with heart failure? Br Heart J 1995; 74: 215–19.

126. Cleland JGF. Is aspirin 'The Weakest Link' in cardiovascular prophylaxis. The surprising lack of evidence supporting the use of aspirin for cardiovascular disease. Prog Cardiovasc Dis 2002; 44: 275–92.

127. Cleland JGF. For debate: preventing atherosclerotic events with aspirin. BMJ 2002; 324: 103–5.

128. Cleland JGF. No reduction in cardiovascular risk with NSAIDs – including aspirin? Lancet 2002; 359: 92–3.

129. Cleland JGF. Anticoagulant and antiplatelet therapy in heart failure. Curr Opin Cardiol 1997; 12: 276–87.

130. Jones CG, Cleland JGF. Meeting report – LIDO, HOPE, MOXCON and WASH studies. Eur J Heart Fail 1999; 1: 425–31.

131. The WASH study steering committee and investigators. The WASH study (warfarin/aspirin study in heart failure): rationale, design and methods. Eur J Heart Fail 1999; 1: 95–9.

132. Cleland JGF, Coletta A, Nikitin N, Louis A, Clark AL. Update of clinical trials from the American College of Cardiology 2003. EPHESUS, SPORTIF-III, ASCOT, COMPANION, UK-PACE and T-Wave Alternans. Eur J Heart Fail 2003; 5: 389–94.

133. Amiodarone Trials Meta-analysis investigators. Effect of prophylactic amiodarone on mortality after acute myocardial infarction and in congestive heart failure: meta-analysis of individual data from 6500 patients in randomised trials. Lancet 1997; 350: 1417–24.

134. Pedersen OD, Bagger H, Keller N et al, for the Danish Investigations of Arrhythmia and Mortality on Dofetilide Study Group. Efficacy of dofetilide in the treatment of atrial fibrillation-flutter in patients with reduced left ventricular function: a Danish Investigations of Arrhythmia and Mortality on Dofetilide (DIAMOND) substudy. Circulation 2001; 104: 292–6.

135. Deedwania PC, Singh BN, Ellenbogen K et al, for the Department of Veterans Affairs CHF–STAT investigators. Spontaneous conversion and maintenance of sinus rhythm by amiodarone in patients with heart failure and atrial fibrillation. Circulation 1998; 98: 2574–9.

136. Androne AS, Katz SD, Lund L et al. Hemodilution is common in patients with advanced heart failure. Circulation 2003; 107: 229.

137. Anker SD, Steinborn W. Definition, type, frequency and prognostic impact of anaemia in chronic heart failure. Eur J Heart Fail (Suppl) 2003; 2: 217–20.

138. Mancini DM, Katz SD, Lang CC et al. Effect of erythropoietin on exercise capacity in patients with moderate to severe chronic heart failure. Circulation 2003; 107: 299.

139. Cleland JGF, Thackray S, Goodge L, Kaye GC, Cooklin M. Outcome studies with device therapy in patients with heart failure. J Cardiovasc Electrophysiol 2002; 13: S73–S91.

140. Coletta A, Nikitin N, Clark AL, Cleland JGF. Clinical trials update from the American Heart Association meeting: PROSPER, DIAL home care monitoring trials, immune modulation therapy, COMPANION and anaemia in heart failure. Eur J Heart Fail 2003; 5: 95–9.

141. Young J, Abraham WT, Smith AL et al. Combined cardiac resynchronisation and implantable cardioversion defibrillation in advanced chronic heart failure. The MIRACLE ICD trial. JAMA 2003; 289: 2685–94.

142. Abraham WT, Fisher WG, Smith AL et al, for the MIRACLE Study Group. Cardiac resynchronisation in chronic heart failure. N Engl J Med 2002; 346: 1845–53.

143. Moss AJ, Zareba W, Hall WJ et al, for the Multicenter Automatic Defibrillator Implantation Trial II Investigators. Prophylactic implantation of a defibrillator in patients with myocardial infarction

and reduced ejection fraction. N Engl J Med 2002; 346: 877–83.

144. Moss AJ, Hall WJ, Cannom DS et al. Improved survival with an implanted defibrillator in patients with coronary disease at high risk for ventricular arrhythmia. N Engl J Med 1996; 335: 1933–40.

145. Coletta AP, Thackray S, Nikitin N, Cleland JGF. Clinical trials update: highlights of the scientific sessions of the American College of Cardiology 2002: LIFE, DANAMI 2, MADIT-2, MIRACLE-ICD, OVERTURE, OCTAVE, ENABLE 1&2, CHRISTMAS, AFFIRM, RACE, WIZARD, AZACS, REMATCH, BNP trial and HARD-BALL. Eur J Heart Fail 2002; 4: 381–8.

146. Wilkoff B, Cook JR, Epstein AE et al. Dual chamber and VVI implantable defibrillator trial investigators. Dual-chamber pacing or ventricular backup pacing in patients with an implantable defibrillator: the Dual Chamber and VVI Implantable Defibrillator (DAVID) trial. JAMA 2002; 288: 3115–23.

147. Stys TP, Lawson WE, Hui JCK et al. Effects of enhanced external counterpulsation on stress radionuclide coronary perfusion and exercise capacity in chronic stable angina pectoris. Am J Cardiol 2002; 89: 822–4.

148. Arora RR, Chou TM, Jain D et al. The multicenter study of enhanced external counterpulsation (MUST-EECP): effect of EECP on exercise-induced myocardial ischemia and anginal episodes. J Am Coll Cardiol 1999; 33: 1833–40.

149. Soran O, Fleishman B, DeMarco T et al. Enhanced external counterpulsation in patients with heart failure: a multicenter feasibility study. Congest Heart Fail 2002; 8: 201–3.

150. Lawson WE, Kennard ED, Holubkov R, et al for the IEPR investigators. Benefit and safety of enhanced external counterpulsation in treating coronary artery disease patients with a history of congestive heart failure. Cardiology 2001; 96: 78–84.

151. Smolens IA, Pagani FD, Bolling SF. Mitral valve repair in heart failure. Eur J Heart Fail 2000; 2: 365–71.

152. Izzat MB, Angelini GD. Surgical alternatives to transplantation for treatment of heart failure. Eur J Heart Fail 1999; 1: 47–9.

153. Starling RC, McCarthy PM. Partial left ventriculectomy: sunrise or sunset? Eur J Heart Fail 1999; 1: 313–17.

154. Angelini GD, Pryn S, Mehta D et al. Left-ventricular-volume reduction for end-stage heart failure. Lancet 1997; 350: 489.

155. Cleland JGF, Alamgir F, Nikitin N, Clark A, Norell M. What is the optimal medical management of ischaemic heart failure? Prog Cardiovasc Dis 2001; 43: 433–55.

156. Deng MC, De Meester JM, Smits JM, Heinecke J, Scheld HH. Effect of receiving a heart transplant: analysis of a national cohort entered on to a waiting list, stratified by heart failure severity. Comparative Outcome and Clinical Profiles In Transplantation (COCPIT) Study Group. BMJ 2000; 321: 540–5.

157. Rose EA, Gelijns AC, Moskowitz AJ et al. Long-term mechanical left ventricular assistance for end-stage heart failure. N Engl J Med 2001; 345: 1435–43.

158. Louis AA, Turner T, Baksh A, Cleland JGF. A systematic review of telemonitoring for the management of heart failure. Eur J Heart Fail 2003; 5: 583–90.

159. Cleland JGF, Armstrong P, Horowitz JD et al. Baseline characteristics of patients recruited into the assessment of treatment with lisinopril and survival study. Eur J Heart fail 1999; 1: 73–9.

160. Coletta AP, Cleland JGF, Freemantle N et al. Clinical trials update from the European Society of Cardiology: CHARM, BASEL, EUROPA and ESTEEM. Eur J Heart Fail 2003; 5: 697–704.

161. Cleland JGF, Freemantle N, Kaye G et al. Clinical trials update from the American Heart Association meeting. Q-3 fatty acids and arrhythmia risk in patients with an implantable defibrillator, ACTIV in CHF, VALIANT, The Hanover Autologous-Bone Marrow Transplantation Study, SPORTIF V, ORBIT and PAD and DEFINITE. Eur J Heart Fail 2004; 6: 109–15.

162. Cuffe M, Califf RM, Adams KF et al. Outcomes of a prospective trial of intravenous milrinone for exacerbations of chronic heart failure (OPTIME-CHF) Investigators. JAMA 2002; 287(12): 1541–7.

163. Coletta AP, Cleland JGF, Freemantle N et al. Clinical trials update from the European Society of Cardiology: CHARM, BASEL, EUROPA and ESTEEM. Eur J Heart Fail 2003; 5: 697–704.

164. Cleland JGF, Freemantle N, Kaye G et al. Clinical trials update from the American Heart Association meeting. Q-3 fatty acids and arrhythmia risk in patients with an implantable defibrillator, ACTIV in CHF, VALIANT, The Hanover Autologous

Bone Marrow Transplantation Study, SPORTIF V, ORBIT and PAD and DEFINITE. Eur J Heart Fail 2004; 6: 109–115.

165. Krum H, McMurray JJ. Statins and chronic heart failure: do we need a large-scale outcome trial? J Am Coll Cardiol 2002; 39(10): 1567–73.

166. Cleland JGF, Coletta A, Nikirin N, Louis A, Clark AL. Update of clinical trials from the American College of Cardiology 2003. EPHESUS, SPORTIF-III, ASCOT, COMPANION, UK-PACE and T-Wave Alternans. Eur J Heart Fail 2003; 5(3): 389–94.

CHAPTER 12

Lipids and lipid-modifying therapy

Moira MB Mungall, Allan Gaw

Introduction

The study of cholesterol, one of the principal lipids in our bodies, has probably earned more Nobel prizes than any other aspect of biochemistry. While cholesterol is undoubtedly a fascinating molecule, it is the well-recognized association between the plasma lipid concentrations and the risk of cardiovascular disease that has fuelled medical and scientific interest. In this chapter we look at the evidence that links cholesterol with cardiovascular disease, the pathogenic mechanisms that bring this about, current treatment strategies and future developments in targeting the process of atherosclerosis.

Lipids and cardiovascular disease

During the last quarter of the twentieth century a compelling body of evidence accumulated linking cholesterol with coronary heart disease (CHD). Epidemiological studies such as that of Simons et al,[1] demonstrated that in countries with a high mean blood cholesterol the mortality from CHD was also high. This is illustrated in Fig. 12.1.

In order to quantify this relationship prospective cohort trials were undertaken. These showed that the relation between cholesterol and CHD risk was graded and continuous and there was probably no threshold cholesterol level that could be considered completely safe.[2,3] There were initial concerns regarding the potential risks of lowering cholesterol as the MR FIT (Multiple Risk Factor Intervention Trial) study exhibited a J-shaped relationship between blood cholesterol and total mortality with death rates appearing to rise at cholesterol levels below 4 mmol/l, as illustrated in Fig. 12.2. However, these fears have proved to be unfounded as studies examining specific causes of mortality such as cancer, hemorrhagic stroke and suicide demonstrated no causal relation with low cholesterol.[4-6] But the most compelling evidence for the safety of lipid lowering comes from the recent large-scale clinical trials of the statin drugs which will be considered later.

These studies identified total cholesterol as a risk factor and since 60–70% of plasma cholesterol is transported in the form of low density lipoprotein (LDL) the effects of total cholesterol reflect the effects of LDL cholesterol. However, the contribution of the other lipid subfractions to CHD risk is increasingly being recognized.

HDL cholesterol

There is considerable evidence to support an inverse relationship between plasma high density lipoprotein (HDL) and CHD risk.[7,8] The importance of HDL as a risk factor is related to LDL levels, and the ratio of total cholesterol to HDL cholesterol is a better predictor of CHD risk than either of the variables alone. A ratio of 5 or less appears to be desirable.

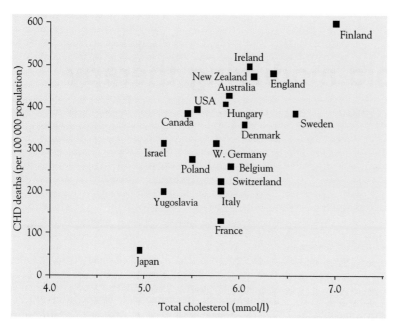

Figure 12.1. *Relationship between coronary heart disease (CHD) mortality and total serum cholesterol worldwide. (Adapted from LA Simons et al. Am J Cardiol 1986; 57: G5-10.[1])*

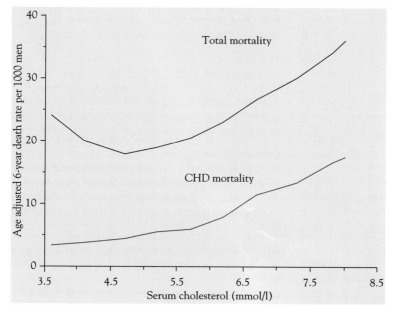

Figure 12.2. *Relationship between coronary heart disease (CHD) and total mortality according to serum total cholesterol. (Adapted from MJ Martin et al. Lancet 1986; 2: 933-6.[3])*

Triglyceride

Plasma triglyceride has been shown to be an independent risk factor for CHD in men in studies such as the Copenhagen Male Study.[9] However, in patients hypertriglyceridemia frequently coexists with low HDL and a particularly atherogenic type of LDL called small, dense LDL. This combination is termed the atherogenic lipoprotein profile (ALP),[8] which confers increased CHD risk. Assman and Schulte quantified this by noting that the combination of plasma triglyceride >2.3 mmol/l; total cholesterol/HDL cholesterol ratio >5; and HDL <1.0 mmol/l for men is a predictor of particularly high CHD risk.[8]

The importance of 'metabolic' or 'insulin resistance' syndrome as a risk factor for both CHD and type 2 diabetes has recently been recognized. The Adult Treatment Panel (ATP) III of the National Cholesterol Education Program[10] recently proposed a definition for metabolic syndrome incorporating thresholds for five easily measured variables linked to insulin resistance: triglyceride, HDL cholesterol, waist circumference, fasting plasma glucose concentration and blood pressure. A patient exhibiting three or more abnormalities is considered to be suffering from metabolic syndrome.

Lipids and lipoprotein biochemistry

Although studies have attempted to isolate the role of different lipoproteins and quantify their independent risk, it is clear that they are closely interrelated and they act synergistically to increase CHD risk. These interrelations may be understood by examining the metabolic pathways in which lipids are involved.[11] All lipids are, by definition, insoluble in water so in order to facilitate transport through the aqueous medium of the plasma, cholesterol is packaged into lipoproteins. These are multi-molecular complexes with a hydrophobic lipid core surrounded by a shell of molecules with water and lipid soluble faces.

There are a number of different lipoproteins which interact at different points along the pathway that transports cholesterol, from its origins as either an endogenously produced molecule or a dietary component, to one of its many target tissues. Cholesterol is required throughout the body as it is an integral component of all animal cell membranes as well as being a starting block in steroid hormone and bile acid biosynthesis. The different lipoproteins and their functions are summarized in Table 12.1.

Lipoprotein metabolism may be thought of as two interconnected cycles centered on the liver. Two important enzymes are involved: lipoprotein lipase (LPL) acts on chylomicrons and very low density lipoprotein (VLDL) and releases free fatty acids and glycerol into the tissues; while lecithin-cholesterol acyl transferase (LCAT) forms cholesteryl esters from free cholesterol and fatty acids. The LDL receptor is another key element present on cell surfaces that binds lipoproteins containing the protein components apolipoprotein (Apo) B and E. This receptor internalizes the lipoproteins within the cell where they are broken down. The number and activity of the receptors largely dictate the level of circulating LDL.

Dietary fats are dealt with via the exogenous lipid cycle, which involves lipid absorption via the small intestine and their incorporation into chylomicrons. These large particles are secreted into the lymphatics and reach the bloodstream via the thoracic duct. Within the circulation LPL gradually depletes triglyceride from the chylomicron, producing deflated remnant particles that are removed by the liver.

Usually about 25–30% of the body's cholesterol is from dietary sources, while the remainder is

Table 12.1. *The principal plasma lipoproteins*

Lipoprotein	Function
Chylomicron	Largest lipoprotein. Synthesized by gut after fatty meal. Main carrier of dietary lipid. Rapid clearance, undetectable after 12-hour fast
Very low density lipoprotein (VLDL)	Similar in structure to chylomicrons but smaller. Synthesized in liver. Main carrier of endogenously produced triglyceride
Low density lipoprotein (LDL)	Generated from VLDL in the circulation. Main carrier of cholesterol, accounting for 60–70% of plasma cholesterol
High density lipoprotein (HDL)	Smallest but most numerous. Protective function. Returns cholesterol to liver for excretion from peripheral tissues. Carries 20–30% of plasma cholesterol

synthesized mainly by the liver and metabolized via the endogenous lipid pathway. VLDL particles are produced which then undergo the same form of delipidation as chylomicrons. This occurs in a stepwise fashion producing intermediate density lipoprotein (IDL) then LDL. At this stage LDL may be removed from the circulation through the action of the LDL receptor or by other scavenger routes, such as those involved in the creation of atherosclerotic plaques.

HDL particles originate in the liver and the gut. They act as cholesteryl ester shuttles, removing the sterol from the peripheral tissues and returning it to the liver. This process is known as reverse cholesterol transport and is thought to be antiatherogenic.

Atherogenesis

Atherosclerosis, the pathological process that results in CHD, has been defined as a focal, inflammatory, fibro-proliferative response to multiple forms of endothelial injury.[12] The first lesions that may be recognized as truly atherosclerotic are called fatty streaks (Fig. 12.3a). They occur when monocytes/macrophages adhere to an injured endothelial surface and begin to invade the subendothelial space. By ingesting lipoproteins these cells become lipid-filled foam cells, which localize within the intima. They may be the precursor of larger atherosclerotic plaques but may also be an entirely reversible phenomenon.[13] The oxidation of LDL particles facilitates uptake into macrophages and there is no regulatory mechanism within these scavenger cells to limit lipid accumulation.[14]

Progression of a fatty streak to a larger more complex lesion is believed to occur through two key processes. First the foam cells begin to die and break down in the center of the fatty streak. Release of their cytoplasmic contents leads to the presence of extracellular lipids and the secretion of growth factors as part of the inflammatory response (Fig. 12.3b).

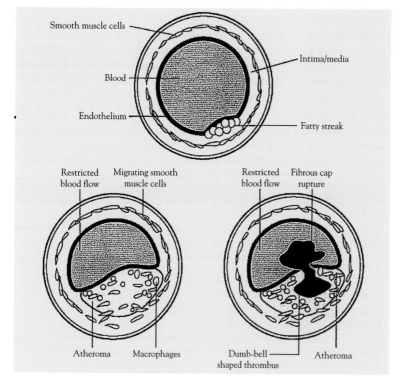

Figure 12.3. *Pathogenesis of atherosclerosis.*

Vascular smooth muscle cell migration and proliferation then follows, resulting in an increase in cell numbers and the laying down of collagenous matrix. This increases the bulk of the plaque, which may now protrude into the artery lumen and is referred to as a raised fibrolipid or advanced plaque.

The integrity of the coronary blood flow may be compromised by the size of the atherosclerotic plaque, but more importantly by its tendency to fissure and rupture. The final pathway to a major clinical event, such as an acute myocardial infarction, is thought to involve rupture or fissuring of the plaque's fibrous cap, hemorrhage into the plaque, or thrombosis on its surface.[15] Figure 12.3c shows a ruptured plaque through which a large dumb-bell-shaped thrombus has formed.

The concept of therapeutic intervention to produce reversal or regression of atherosclerotic lesions originated more than 50 years ago when anecdotal reports of post-mortem examinations on individuals who had suffered great weight losses prior to their death, claimed that the extent of plaque development in the aorta and coronary arteries was much less than expected.

That regression is possible clinically has since been proved in randomized controlled clinical studies using lipid-lowering therapy. In the Familial Atherosclerosis Treatment Study,[16] middle-aged men who had moderately elevated LDL, a family history and angiographic evidence of CHD, had reduced frequency of progression of coronary lesions, increased frequency of regression and reduced incidence of CHD events if prescribed lipid-lowering therapy.

Dietary modification of lipids

Recognition of the role of cholesterol in CHD has led to attempts to optimize lipid profiles and improve patient outcome. Dietary modification has been regarded as the first line of attack in this respect since the publication of studies such as the Seven Countries Study,[17] which showed that CHD is inversely related to the ratio of polyunsaturated to saturated fats in the diet.

Recent work suggests that dietary modification may have an effect independent of any apparent effect on the plasma cholesterol concentration. In the Lyon Diet Heart Study[18] postmyocardial infarction patients were randomized to regular or Mediterranean-style diets and after a mean follow-up of 27 months there was a 73% reduction in cardiovascular death and non-fatal myocardial infarction in the group following the Mediterranean diet. This occurred despite unaltered lipid profiles.

For some clinicians, the introduction of effective lipid-lowering drugs has superseded dietary advice in the management of patients at risk of CHD. However, studies indicate that as an adjunct to drug treatment, a diet rich in mono-unsaturated fatty acids, antioxidant vitamins and fiber, while low in saturated fat, provides an additional reduction of coronary risk independent of cholesterol levels and other traditional cardiovascular risk factors.[19]

Pharmacological modification of lipids

The earliest drug intervention trials took place in the 1970s using the best available lipid-lowering drugs in the pre-statin era. The two most important trials, which were of a randomized, double-blind and placebo-controlled design, are discussed below. These were followed by a series of important studies using statins (see later).

Lipid Research Clinics Coronary Primary Prevention Study

This study involved 3806 middle-aged men with primary hypercholesterolemia[20] who were followed for an average of 7.4 years. Those treated with the bile acid sequestrant drug, cholestyramine, showed on average, an 8.5% reduction in total cholesterol, a 12.6% reduction in LDL cholesterol, a 3% rise in HDL cholesterol and a 4.5% rise in triglyceride, over the placebo-treated control group. The drug-induced lipid changes were associated with a 24% fall in definite CHD deaths and a 19% fall in nonfatal MI. These findings provided the impetus for other groups to investigate the efficacy of other lipid-lowering agents.

The Helsinki Heart Study

The next major study confirmed the clinical efficacy of one of the fibrates, gemfibrozil. The Helsinki Heart Study[21] was conducted in a group of over 4000 middle-aged men (40–55 years) with primary dyslipidemia (non-HDL cholesterol >5.2 mmol/l). Gemfibrozil therapy was associated with reductions in triglyceride of 35%, in LDL cholesterol of 11%, and an increase in HDL cholesterol of 11% and the 5-year reduction in CHD risk of the treatment group was 34% (P<0.02).

Statin Trials

The introduction of the 3-hydroxy-3-methyl glutaryl coenzyme A (HMG-CoA) reductase inhibitors, or statins, was arguably the most effective development in the prevention of cardiovascular disease.[22] These drugs lower total cholesterol, LDL cholesterol, and triglyceride, while raising HDL and have been extensively studied in a series of large-scale, randomized, placebo-controlled, double-blind trials covering a wide variety of patient groups (Table 12.2).

Scandinavian Simvastatin Survival Study (4S)

This secondary prevention study, reported in 1994, included men and women aged between 35 and 70 years who had a history of angina or myocardial infarction.[23] Subjects with cholesterol levels between 5.5 and 8.0 mmol/l and triglycerides of <2.5 mmol/l were given either simvastatin, 20–40 mg, or placebo, and reviewed over a 5-year period.

In addition to beneficial changes in their lipid profiles the simvastatin-treated group exhibited a 30% reduction in the primary endpoint of total mortality and a 34% reduction in the secondary endpoint which was major coronary events. Moreover the trial demonstrated that simvastatin had an excellent safety record putting to rest the suggestion that lowering cholesterol leads to increased mortality from non-cardiovascular causes. A recent update on 4S reported that statin treatment in patients with CHD for up to 8 years was safe and yielded continued survival benefit.[24]

The results of the trial may be summarized by considering the implications for practice. If 100 middle-aged CHD patients were prescribed

Table 12.2. *Major studies of prevention of coronary heart disease with statins*

Clinical trial	Drug used	No. of subjects	Relative reduction in fatal or non-fatal MI (%)
Scandinavian Simvastatin Survival Study (4S)	Simvastatin	4444	34
West of Scotland Coronary Prevention Study (WOSCOPS)	Pravastatin	6595	31
Cholesterol and Recurrent Events (CARE) Study	Pravastatin	4159	24
Air Force/Texas Coronary Prevention Study(AF/TEXCAPS)	Lovastatin	6605	37*
Long Term Intervention with Pravastatin in Ischaemic Disease (LIPID)	Pravastatin	9014	23
Heart Protection Study (HPS)	Simvastatin	20 536	24**
Anglo-Scandinavian Cardiac Outcomes Trial – Lipid Lowering Arm (ASCOT-LLA)	Atorvastatin	10 305	36

*Expanded endpoint of combined unstable angina, fatal and non-fatal MI and sudden cardiac death.
**Major vascular events.
MI, myocardial infarction.

simvastatin for 6 years then four of the expected nine deaths would be avoided; seven of the 21 expected myocardial infarctions would be prevented; and six out of 19 revascularization procedures would be unnecessary.

West of Scotland Coronary Prevention Study (WOSCOPS)

This study published in 1995 was a primary prevention study that included only men and the active treatment was pravastatin 40 mg.[25] A total of 6595 men, aged between 45 and 64 years with LDL cholesterol levels of 4.5–6.0 mmol/l, were recruited. Subjects were required to have no history of myocardial infarction, however, they were eligible for inclusion if they had stable angina provided they had not been hospitalized over the past 12 months. The subjects were followed up over a 5-year period. The primary endpoint was combined CHD death and non-fatal myocardial infarction, which was significantly reduced by 31%. Deaths from any cause were also reduced in the pravastatin group by 22%, and as with 4S, there was no excess of non-cardiac deaths.

Extrapolating the WOSCOPS data into practice reveals that treating 1000 middle-aged men who are hypercholesterolemic but otherwise healthy with pravastatin for 5 years, will avoid 14 coronary angiograms; eight revascularization procedures; 20 non-fatal myocardial infarctions; seven cardiovascular deaths; and two deaths from other causes.

Cholesterol and Recurrent Events (CARE)

This was a secondary prevention trial published in 1996[26] whose objective was to evaluate the effects of pravastatin (40 mg) therapy on post-myocardial infarction patients who did not have elevated total plasma cholesterol concentrations. Subjects received standard post-myocardial infarction treatments including aspirin, β-blockers and percutaneous transluminal coronary angioplasty (PTCA) and coronary artery bypass grafts (CABG).

In total, 4159 subjects aged 21–75 years who were 3–20 months post-myocardial infarction were randomized and followed-up for an average of 5 years. The pravastatin treated group demonstrated a 24% reduction in fatal or non-fatal myocardial

infarction. Analysis of the secondary endpoints of the study showed a 31% reduction in stroke; 26% reduction in CABG and 22% reduction in PTCA for the active treatment group.

These results may be summarized by considering the effects of treating 1000 post-myocardial infarction patients, whose total cholesterol levels are less than 6.2 mmol/l (240 mg/dl) for 5 years. In this scenario we would prevent 150 cardiovascular events and 51 patients would be spared from having at least one such event. For patients >60 years the corresponding figures would be 207 cardiovascular events and 71 patients.

Air Force/Texas Coronary Atherosclerosis Prevention Study (AF/TEXCAPS)

This study randomized 6605 subjects (85% men) who had no clinical evidence of atherosclerotic cardiovascular disease to either placebo or lovastatin.[27] Baseline lipid levels were not elevated, average total plasma cholesterol level was 5.7 mmol/l (220 mg/dl) and average LDL cholesterol was 3.9 mmol/l (150 mg/dl). However, lovastatin was titrated up to 40 mg/day in order to achieve a target LDL cholesterol goal of less than 2.8 mmol/l (110 mg/dl). Five years of therapy lowered total cholesterol by 18% and LDL cholesterol by 25%. Triglyceride levels were reduced by 25% and HDL cholesterol was raised by 6%.

These lipid changes did not result in significant reductions in CHD/death or total mortality, however, they did have a significant impact in preventing coronary occlusive events as the combined primary endpoint of the trial (unstable angina, fatal and non-fatal myocardial infarction or sudden cardiac death) was reduced by 37%.

Long Term Intervention with Pravastatin in Ischaemic Disease Study (LIPID)

Like 4S and CARE, the LIPID Study was concerned with secondary prevention, however it recruited substantial numbers of patients with unstable angina and these individuals benefited in terms of event avoidance as much as recruits with a history of myocardial infarction. A total of 9014 subjects (83% male) drawn from 87 centers in Australia and New Zealand and with an average total cholesterol level of 5.65 mmol/l (218 mg/dl) were randomized to pravastatin (40 mg/day) or placebo and followed for an average of 6 years.[28] All-cause mortality was reduced by 22% while CHD death fell by 24%. The number of strokes was also reduced by 19%.

Pravastatin Pooling Project Study (PPP)

The PPP was a prospectively planned study, designed to evaluate the consistency of the treatment effect of pravastatin at 40 mg/day. It combined the clinical outcomes of WOSCOPS, CARE and LIPID, providing a combined patient population of approximately 20 000 patients who were followed for 5 or more years, yielding approximately 100 000 patient-years experience.

The results of the PPP subgroup analyses clearly demonstrate the significant clinical benefits achieved in a broad spectrum of patients using pravastatin.[29] Furthermore, mortality data confirm the highly significant reductions in total mortality and CHD mortality.[30] Equally important, the PPP investigators confirmed that pravastatin was not associated with any increase in non-cardiovascular mortality.

Heart Protection Study (HPS)

The HPS is a large trial designed to examine the effects of simvastatin and antioxidant vitamins in high-risk subjects.[31] Over 20 000 subjects were recruited into the HPS across a wide age range, all with a total cholesterol >3.5 mmol/l. In addition all subjects were either 'secondary' prevention candidates with a history of CHD, stroke or other vascular disease, or were at high risk because of a history of hypertension or diabetes. The study was designed in a 2×2 factorial format, comparing simvastatin 40 mg with antioxidants and placebo, singly or in combination. The mean follow-up was 5.5 years.

The main findings of the statin arm of HPS were total mortality fell by 13%, cardiovascular death by 17%, fatal and non-fatal stroke by 25% and all major vascular events by 24%. The results of this study demonstrated the benefits of statin therapy across a wide range of subjects with low as well as high cholesterol values. However, the antioxidant vitamin arm of the HPS showed no benefit at all in the prevention of vascular events or all-cause mortality.

Anglo-Scandinavian Cardiac Outcomes Trial – Lipid Lowering Arm (ASCOT-LLA)

The Anglo-Scandinavian Cardiac Outcomes Trial set out to examine hypertensive patients (treated and untreated) who had at least three cardiovascular risk factors.[32] More than 19 000 patients were recruited to receive one of two antihypertensive therapies for a period of 5 years. The lipid-lowering arm consisted of 10 305 patients, with cholesterol levels up to 6.5 mmol/l (250 mg/dl) who were randomized to receive either atorvastatin 10 mg/day or placebo. After a mean follow-up period of 3.3 years the data and safety monitoring committee recommended the early termination of the lipid-lowering arm because there had been a 36% reduction in fatal CHD and non-fatal myocardial infarction in the atorvastatin treated group. Other major cardiovascular events were also significantly reduced: fatal and non-fatal strokes fell by 27%; fatal CHD and non-fatal myocardial infarction (excluding silent) were reduced by 38%; total cardiovascular and total coronary events were down by 21% and 29%, respectively.

Current guidelines and future therapies

There now exists a wealth of clinical trial data covering men over a wide age range. This has been translated into various guidelines for the management of patients who either already manifest, or are at risk of developing CHD.[10,33] These depend upon an assessment of overall CHD risk and take into account the presence of multiple risk factors. Individually these risk factors may represent only minor deviations from the optimum, but in combination they are thought to confer a much greater risk than a single risk factor.

Increasingly it is being recognized that statins are not merely lipid-modifying drugs,[34] but rather they are viewed as drugs that promote vascular health, and which reduce cardiovascular events in patients at risk almost irrespective of their baseline lipid values.

More potent statins such as rosuvastatin are being developed and introduced on to the market[35] and alternative approaches to optimizing lipid management are being attempted by combining statins with other lipid-lowering drugs such as fibrates and niacin.[36] There have been some safety concerns about increased levels of adverse events with these combinations but studies suggest that this will be a promising area.[37,38] Completely novel therapies are also being developed including cholesterol absorption inhibitors such as ezetimibe,[39] which is being advocated as an adjunct to statins.[40]

References

1. Simons LA. Interrelations of lipids and lipoproteins with coronary artery disease mortality in 19 countries. Am J Cardiol 1986; 57: G5–10.
2. Stamler J, Wentworth D, Neaton JD for the MRFIT Research Group. Is relationship between serum cholesterol and risk of premature death from coronary heart disease continuous and graded? Findings in 356 222 primary screenees of the Multiple Risk Factor Intervention Trial (MRFIT). JAMA 1986; 256: 2823–8.
3. Martin MJ, Hulley SB, Browner WS et al. Serum cholesterol, blood pressure and mortality: implications from a cohort of 361 662 men. Lancet 1986; 2: 933–6.
4. Katan MB. Effects of cholesterol lowering on the risk for cancer and other non-cardiovascular diseases. In: Atherosclerosis VII 1986; 657–61.
5. Iso H, Jacobs DR, Wentworth D et al. Serum cholesterol levels and six year mortality from stroke in 350 977 men screening for the Multiple Risk Factor Intervention Trial. N Engl J Med 1989; 320: 904–10.
6. Davey Smith G, Pekkanen J. Should there be a moratorium on the use of cholesterol lowering drugs? BMJ 1992; 304: 431–4.
7. Pocock SJ, Shaper AG, Phillips AN. Concentrations of high density lipoprotein cholesterol, triglycerides and total cholesterol in ischemic heart disease. BMJ 1989; 298: 998–1002.
8. Assman G, Schulte H. Relation of high density lipoprotein cholesterol and triglyceride to incidence of atherosclerosis coronary artery disease (the PROCAM experience). Am J Cardiol 1992; 70: 733–7.
9. Jeppesen J, Hein HO, Suadicani P, Gyntelberg F. Triglyceride concentration in ischemic heart disease: an eight-year follow-up in the Copenhagen Male Study. Circulation 1998; 97: 1029–36.
10. Executive summary of the third report of the National Cholesterol Education Program (NCEP) expert panel on detection, evaluation and treatment of high blood cholesterol in adults (Adults Treatment Panel III). JAMA 2001; 285: 2486–97.
11. Gaw A, Shepherd J. Cholesterol and lipoproteins. In: Lindsay GM, Gaw A (eds). Coronary Heart Disease Prevention: A Handbook for the Healthcare Team. Edinburgh: Churchill Livingstone, 1997.
12. Ross R. The pathogenesis of atherosclerosis: a perspective for the 1990s. Nature 1993; 362: 801–9.
13. Freedman D, Newman WP, Tracy RE et al. Black–white differences in aortic fatty streaks in adolescence and early adulthood: the Bogalusa Heart Study. Circulation 1989; 77: 856–64.
14. Steinberg D, Parthasarathy S, Carew TE, Khoo JC, Witztum JL. Beyond cholesterol: modifications of low density lipoprotein that increase its atherogenicity. N Engl J Med 1989; 320: 915–24.
15. Davies MJ, Thomas AC. Plaque Assuring – the cause of acute myocardial infarction, sudden death, and crescendo angina. Br Heart J 1985; 53: 363–73.
16. Brown G, Albers JJ, Fisher LD et al. Regression of coronary artery disease as a result of intensive lipid-lowering in men with high levels of apolipoprotein B. N Engl J Med 1990; 323: 1289–98.
17. Keys A. Seven countries: A Multivariate Analysis of Death and Coronary Heart Disease. Cambridge, Massachusetts: Harvard University Press, 1980.
18. de Lorgeril M, Salen P, Martin J-L et al. Mediterranean diet, traditional risk factors, and the rate of cardiovascular complications after myocardial infarction: final report of the Lyon Diet Heart Study. Circulation 1999; 99: 779–85.
19. Pitsavos C, Panagiotakos DB, Chryohoou C et al. The effect of Mediterranean diet on the risk of the development of acute coronary syndromes in hyper-cholesterolemic people: a case-control study (CARDIO2000). Coron Artery Dis 2002; 13: 295–300.
20. Lipid Research Clinics Program. The Lipid Research Clinics Coronary Primary Prevention Trial results. I. Reduction in incidence of coronary heart disease. JAMA 1984; 251: 351–64.
21. Frick MH, Elo O, Haapa K et al. Helsinki Heart Study: primary-prevention trial with gemfibrozil in middle-aged men with dyslipidemia. N Engl J Med 1987; 317: 1237–45.
22. Roberts WC. The underused miracle: the statin drugs are to atherosclerosis what penicillin was to infectious diseases. Am J Cardiol 1996; 78: 377–8.

23. Scandinavian Simvastatin Survival Study Group. Randomised trial of cholesterol lowering in 4444 patients with coronary heart disease: The Scandinavian Simvastatin Survival Study (4S). Lancet 1994; 344: 1383–9.

24. Pedersen TR, Wilhelmsen L, Faergeman O et al. Follow-up study of patients randomized in the Scandinavian Simvastatin Survival Study (4S) of cholesterol lowering. Am J Cardiol 2000; 86: 257–62.

25. Shepherd J, Cobbe SM, Ford I et al. Prevention of coronary heart disease with pravastatin in men with hypercholesterolaemia. N Engl J Med 1995; 333: 1301–7.

26. Sacks FM, Pfeffer MA, Moye LA et al for the Cholesterol and Recurrent Events Trial Investigators. The effect of pravastatin on coronary events after myocardial infarction in patients with average cholesterol levels. N Engl J Med 1996; 335: 1001–9.

27. Downs JR, Clearfield M, Weis S et al. Primary prevention of acute coronary events with lovastatin in men and women with average cholesterol levels: results of AFCAPS/TEXCAPS Research Group. JAMA 1998; 279: 1615–22.

28. Long-term Intervention with Pravastatin in Ischaemic Disease (LIPID) Study Group. Prevention of cardiovascular events and death with pravastatin in patients with coronary heart disease and a broad range of initial cholesterol levels. N Engl J Med 1998; 339: 1349–57.

29. Sacks FM, Tonkin AM, Shepherd J et al. Effect of pravastatin on coronary disease events in subgroups defined by coronary risk factors: the Prospective Pravastatin Pooling Project. Circulation 2000; 102: 1893–900.

30. Simes J, Furberg CD, Braunwald E et al. Effects of pravastatin on mortality in patients with and without coronary disease across a broad range of cholesterol levels. Eur Heart J 2002; 23: 207–15.

31. Heart Protection Study Collaborative Group. MRC/BHF Heart Protection Study of cholesterol lowering with simvastatin in 20 536 high-risk individuals: a randomized placebo-controlled trial. Lancet 2002; 360: 7–22.

32. Sever PS, Dahlof B, Poulter NR et al. Prevention of coronary and stroke events with atorvastatin in hypertensive patients who have average or lower-than-average cholesterol concentrations, in the Anglo-Scandinavian Cardiac Outcomes Trial – Lipid Lowering Arm (ASCOT-LLA): a multicentre randomized controlled trial. Lancet 2003; 361: 1149–58.

33. Wood DA, De Backer G, Faergeman O et al. Prevention of coronary heart disease in clinical practice. Recommendation of the second joint task force of the European Society of Cardiology, European Atherosclerosis Society and European Society of Hypertension. Eur Heart J 1998; 19: 1434–503.

34. Vaughan CJ, Murphy MB, Buckley BM. Statins do more than just lower cholesterol. Lancet 1997; 348: 1079–82.

35. Olsson AG, Pears J, McKellar J, Mizan J, Raza A. Effect of rosuvastatin on low-density lipoprotein cholesterol in patients with hypercholesterolemia. Am J Cardiol 2001; 88: 504–8.

36. Ballantyne CM. Treating mixed dyslipidemias: why and how. Clin Cardiol 2001; 24 (Suppl II): II-6–II-9.

37. Pauciullo P, Borgnino C, Paoletti R, Mariani M, Mancini M. Efficacy and safety of a combination of fluvastatin and bezafibrate in patients with mixed hyperlipidaemia (FACT study). Atherosclerosis 2000; 150: 429–36.

38. Kashyap ML, Evans R, Simmons PD, Kohler RM, McGovern ME. New combination niacin/statin formulation shows pronounced effects on major lipoproteins and is well tolerated. J Am Coll Cardiol 2000; 35(Suppl A): 326.

39. Leitersdorf E. Selective cholesterol absorption inhibition: a novel strategy in lipid-lowering management. Int J Clin Pract 2002; 56: 116–19.

40. Kosoglou T, Meyer I, Veltri EP et al. Pharmacodynamic interaction between the new selective cholesterol absorption inhibitor ezetimibe and simvastatin. Br J Clin Pharmacol 2002; 54: 309–19.

CHAPTER 13

Erectile dysfunction: cardiovascular risk and the primary care clinician

Louis Kuritzky, Martin Miner

Introduction

The recognition that erectile dysfunction (ED) has a strong association with vascular disease, and particularly endothelial dysfunction, is relatively new. In the not too distant past, in the textbook *Impotence*[1] less than 0.3% of the book – a single page in this 320 page text – focused upon the relationship between cardiovascular disease and ED (see Fig. 13.1). Indeed, discussion about the vasculature in ED at that point in time gave special attention to rare disorders such as vascular dysplasia or flow-limiting stenotic lesions, some of which might be surgically remediable, but remain to this date in the category of 'investigational'.

The discovery of the place of nitric oxide and the critical role of the endothelium in vascular health were critical to the evolution of both pathophysiologic and therapeutic growth in the field of sexual medicine. One of the authors of this chapter (LK) had the privilege of being in the audience at the New York meeting of the American Society of Hypertension in the early 1990s where one of the discoverers of endothelial-derived relaxing factor (EDRF), shortly afterwards identified as nitric oxide, humbly described his serendipitous insight that an intact endothelium was necessary for vasorelaxation and appropriate responses to vascular stimuli. This same man accepted, in 1998, a Nobel Prize for his discovery. In 1992, the journal *Science* published a cover story about nitric oxide, calling it 'Molecule of the Year,'[2] anticipated by an article earlier that same year by Jacob Rajfer, a urologist at the University of California, Los Angeles, who published the first article asserting that it is indeed nitric oxide that mediates erections, based on his studies in rabbits.[3]

Since the discovery of the role of nitric oxide, the evidence relating ED to vascular disease has become essentially incontrovertible. Primary care clinicians are the healthcare providers of first contact for most patients with vascular disease in all tissue compartments, so whether patients manifest their vascular dysfunction as stroke, transient ischemic attack (TIA), myocardial infarction (MI), angina, ED, or intermittent claudication, the likelihood is that a primary care clinician (PCC) will be involved in their care. Similarly, since the recognized risk factors that lead to vascular disease are also managed primarily by PCCs in the ambulatory setting, care of patients with ED, vascular disease, and those with risk factors for vasculopathy will ultimately require appropriate intervention in the primary care setting.

Epidemiology of erectile dysfunction and cardiovascular disease

Probably the most oft-cited epidemiologic survey of sexual function in American men is the Massachusetts Male Aging Study (MMAS).[4] If we acknowledge that this study appropriately identifies the prevalence of ED in the USA, then as many as

50% or more of men over the age of 40 have some degree of ED, the majority of which is attributable to underlying vasculopathy (see Fig. 13.2). The MMAS study demonstrated that erectile dysfunction is an age-dependent disorder: 'between the ages of 40 and 70 years the probability of complete impotence tripled from 5.1% to 15%, moderate impotence

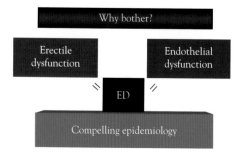

Figure 13.1. *ED, by happy coincidence, stands for both erectile dysfunction and endothelial dysfunction. Since endothelial dysfunction is indeed the most common etiology of erectile dysfunction, and merits close scrutiny of cardiovascular risk-factor burden, recognition of the dual meaning of 'ED' is important. Were either erectile dysfunction or endothelial dysfunction uncommon, energies to identify them might be ill spent; however, both share a dramatically compelling epidemiologic presence in midlife men worldwide.*

doubled from 17% to 34% while the probability of minimal impotence remained constant at 17%.' By age 70, only 32% were free of ED (Fig. 13.3). Finally, in this population, cigarette smoking increased the probability of total ED in men with treated heart disease or hypertension (HTN). It similarly increased ED probability for men on cardiac, anti-hypertensive, or vasodilator medications. Men treated for diabetes mellitus, heart disease, and HTN had significantly higher probabilities for ED than the sample as a whole. ED prevalence varied inversely with high-density lipoprotein in this population.

Since 2004, the diagnosis of diabetes has been recognized as a coronary heart disease risk equivalent, placing a diabetic patient at equal (or greater) risk of subsequent MI than a person who has already sustained an MI. In concrete terms, for an adult diabetic the likelihood of an MI within the next 10 years is greater than 20%.[5] Accordingly, in the diabetic population, there is a 'shift to the left' in ED prevalence, such that even by age 30 years, as many as 15% of diabetic men suffer impotence.[6] (see Table 13.1).

In a landmark 2005 publication, Thompson et al. confirmed what had been long believed: that ED is a sentinel marker of and risk factor for future cardiovascular events.[7] Their data originated in men aged 55 years and older (n = 18 882) participating in the Prostate Cancer Prevention Trial. Amongst the

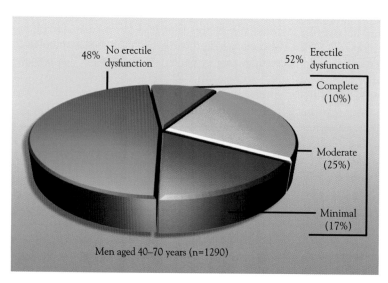

Figure 13.2. *The Massachusetts Male Aging Study (MMAS) is one of the most important studies of the epidemiology of erectile dysfunction in American men. Based on a population of almost 1300 men aged 40 and above, fully 52% acknowledged some degree of erectile dysfunction. Adapted from reference 4.*

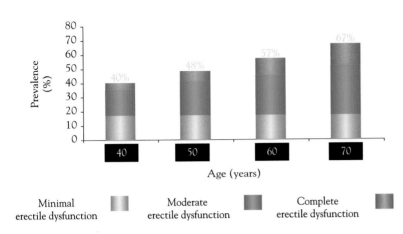

Minimal erectile dysfunction Moderate erectile dysfunction Complete erectile dysfunction

Figure 13.3. *According to the Massachusetts Male Aging Study, as many as 40% of men even as young as age 40 to 50 have some degree of ED. Over time, the frequency of ED increases; of concern, it is the degree of moderate to complete ED that increases most (as opposed to minimal ED). Adapted from reference 4.*

Table 13.1. *Diabetes mellitus induces endothelial dysfunction at a macrovascular and microvascular level, as well as neuropathic changes. Accordingly, the prevalence of ED in diabetes is age-related, but may appear more prominently in younger persons that those without diabetes. Adapted from reference 1*

Impotence and diabetes mellitus

Age-dependent

Age (years)	Frequency
20–29	9%
30–34	15%
60–64	55%

men receiving placebo (n > 9000), 47% had ED at study baseline. Both placebo and treated groups were followed for the development of ED and cardiovascular end-points every 3 months for the 9-year duration of the study. Attesting to the strong age-related epidemiology of ED, after 5 years, 57% of the 4300 men without ED at study entry reported incident ED. The adjusted hazard ratio for new cardiovascular events during study follow-up (1994–2003) in these men was 1.25. For men with either incident or prevalent ED, the hazard ratio was 1.45. Thus, men with ED are at risk for developing cardiac events over the next 10 years, with ED being as strong a risk factor as current smoking

or premature family history of cardiac disease. In this population, the relationship between incident ED (the first report of ED of any grade) and CVD was comparable to that of current smoking, family history of MI, or hyperlipidemia.

Seftel et al.[8] quantified the prevalence of diagnosed HTN, hyperlipidemia, diabetes, and depression in men with ED using a nationally representative managed care claims database that covered 51 health plans with 28 million lives from 1995 to 2002. Based on 272 325 identified patients with ED, population and age-specific prevalence rates were calculated. Crude population prevalence rates in this study population were 41.6% for HTN, 42.4% for hyperlipidemia, 20.2% for diabetes, and 11.1% for depression. Of 87 163 patients with ED, 68% had one or more of the comorbidities of HTN, hyperlipidemia, diabetes, or depression. This evidence supports the concept that ED can be viewed as a marker for these concurrent comorbidities[8] (see also Table 13.2).

In accordance with the concept that ED is a predictor of cardiovascular risk, Min et al.[10] studied 221 men referred for stress myocardial perfusion single-photon emission computed tomography (MPS), an imaging method commonly used to diagnose and stratify CVD risk. They found that 55% of the patients had ED, and that these men exhibited more severe coronary heart disease ($p < 0.001$) and left ventricular dysfunction ($p = 0.01$) than those without ED. These data suggest that ED is an independent predictor of more severe coronary artery disease.

Table 13.2. *Because erectile dysfunction and endothelial dysfunction are inextricably linked, recognition of the relationship between hyperlipidemia and ED would be anticipated. There is a linear relationship between increases in cholesterol and ED. Similarly, HDL increases are associated with a lesser relative risk for ED. Adapted from reference 9*

ED correlates with hyperlipidemia

- Prospective study examined relationship between total cholesterol and erectile dysfunction in 71 subjects

- Every mmol/L of increase in total cholesterol associated with 1.32 (95% CI, 1.04–1.68) times relative risk (RR)* of erectile dysfunction (i.e. 32% increase in risk for erectile dysfunction)

- Every mmol/L of increase in HDL-C associated with 0.38 times RR of erectile dysfunction (i.e. 62% decrease in risk for erectile dysfunction)

- Results support cause–effect relation between high level of total cholesterol, low level of HDL-C and erectile dysfunction

*Relative risk is, within specified period, probability of developing an outcome if risk factor present, divided by probability of developing outcome if risk factor absent.

Further data support the ED–cardiovascular paradigm. A sample of nearly 4000 Canadian men aged 40–88 years reported on erectile function as measured by the International Index of Erectile Function (IIEF) score.[11] The presence of CVD or diabetes increased the probability of ED. Among those patients without established CVD or diabetes, the calculated 10-year Framingham score and fasting glucose level were independently associated with ED (Fig. 13.4).

Subsequent to the analysis by Thompson et al.[7] and lending further support to the idea of ED as a precursor of CVD, Montorsi et al.[13] investigated 285 patients with coronary artery disease. Nearly all patients who developed symptoms had experienced ED symptoms first, on average 3 years beforehand.

More recent data added greater depth to our epidemiologic knowledge of ED and its related disorders in the USA. The National Health and Nutrition Examination Survey (NHANES) conducted surveys and examinations of 11 039 adults over a 2-year period. The prevalence of ED increased dramatically with advanced age; 77.5% of men aged 75 years and older were affected. In addition, there were several modifiable risk factors that were independently associated with ED, including diabetes mellitus (OR, 2.69), obesity (OR, 1.60), current smoking (OR, 1.74), and hypertension (OR, 1.56).[14]

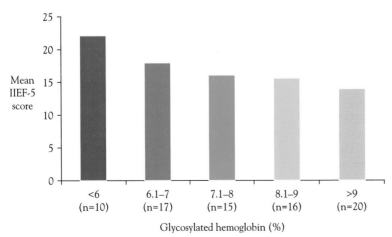

Figure 13.4. *The association of erectile dysfunction, as measured by the IIEF score, and degree of control of diabetes is linear and consistent. Unfortunately, there are little data to suggest that improvements in glycemic control reverse this association. Adapted from reference 12.*

Table 13.3. *Any disorder that is linked with development of vasculopathy may be anticipated to increase likelihood of ED. Medication, lifestyle factors and disease states that lead to endothelial dysfunction and vascular disease are all strong risk factors for ED. HCTZ, hydrochlorthiazide. Adapted from reference 4*

Major risk factors for ED

- Chronic diseases
  - Hypertension
  - Diabetes
  - Depression
  - Cardiovascular disease
- Medications
  - HCTZ
  - β-blockers
- Lifestyle
  - Stress
  - Alcohol abuse
  - Smoking

Based upon the above considerations, Kuritzky (2004) suggested that 'the man with ED ... should be considered a vasculopath until proven otherwise'. Accordingly, men with ED merit a thorough investigation of cardiovascular risk factors. Subsequently, in support of this concept the Second Princeton Consensus Conference on Sexual Dysfunction and Cardiac Risk recommended screening men with ED for vascular disease and abnormal metabolic parameters, including glucose, lipids, and blood pressure. It stressed that men with ED and no cardiac disease should be considered at risk for CVD until proven otherwise.[15] A summary of risk factors for ED is presented in Table 13.3.

Ultimately, some clinicians will prefer formal risk stratification for men with ED. The Princeton Consensus Conference document provides guidance in this regard.[15]

Intervention by risk factor modification

Esposito et al.[16] determined the effect of weight loss and increased physical activity on erectile and endothelial function in obese men. They conducted a randomized, single-blind trial of 110 obese men aged 35–55 years without diabetes, HTN, or hyperlipidemia, who had ED. The study was conducted from October 2000 to October 2003 at a university hospital in Italy. The intervention group received detailed advice about how to achieve a loss of 10% or more in their total body weight by reducing caloric intake and increasing their level of physical activity. Men in the control group (n = 55) were given general information about healthy food choices and exercise.

After 2 years, body mass index decreased more in the intervention group (from a mean of 36.9 g/m^2 to 31.2 g/m^2) than in the control group (from 36.4 g/m^2 to 35.7 g/m^2) ($p < 0.001$). The mean level of physical activity increased more in the intervention group than in the control group. The mean IIEF score improved in the intervention group (from 13.9 to 17, $p < 0.001$), but remained stable in the control group. In multivariate analyses, changes in body mass index ($p = 0.02$) and physical activity ($p = 0.02$) were independently associated with changes in IIEF score. The investigators concluded that lifestyle changes were associated with improvement in sexual function in about one-third of obese men with ED.

If these clinical associations are valid, then one could argue that there should be mechanistic data supporting these concepts. Eaton et al.[17] evaluated the association between the degree of ED and levels of atherosclerotic biomarkers in a cross-sectional study of 988 US male health professionals between the ages 46 and 81 years who were participating as part of an ongoing epidemiologic study, which included atherosclerotic biomarkers measured from blood collected in 1994–1995. Men with poor to very poor erectile function had 2.1 times the odds of having an elevated total cholesterol:high-density lipoprotein ratio ($p = 0.02$) compared with men with good and very good erectile funtion after multivariate adjustment.

167

Addressing cardiovascular risk issues in men with erectile dysfunction

Four pertinent clinical questions follow from the above epidemiologic and pathophysiologic considerations:

1. When men (or their partners) inform the clinician that ED is an issue, what is appropriate to suggest as far as scrutiny of cardiovascular risk factors?
2. Because ED may reflect underlying vascular disease, which symptoms of vasculopathy should be sought (e.g. angina, intermittent claudication, transient ischemic attacks)?
3. Should men with ED be screened for CVD by more advanced techniques, such as exercise treadmill testing?
4. What advice should be given to men with ED with regard to engaging in sexual activity? More directly, considering the fact that men with ED have a disproportionate incidence of underlying cardiovascular atherosclerosis, is it safe for them to engage in sexual activity?

What cardiovascular risk factor screening is appropriate for men with erectile dysfunction?

Traditional risk factors for ED are the same as those for cardiovascular disease: hypertension, dyslipidemia, diabetes, cigarette smoking, obesity, and sedentary lifestyle. Although a multitude of other 'minor' risk factors have been identified (e.g. fibrinogen, Lp(a), C-reactive protein), there is insufficient evidence for any of these to be regarded yet as an important modifiable risk factor. Given that there has been some evidence that risk factor modification may benefit sexual function in men with existing ED, the authors recommend the following goals to optimize sexual function (as well as general health) in men with ED:

- low-density lipoprotein <100 mg/dL;
- triglycerides <150 mg/dL;
- high-density lipoprotein >45 mg/dL;
- blood pressure <140/90 mmHg;

- glycosylated hemoglobin <7.0%;
- body mass index <26 kg/m^2;
- vigorous physical activity (i.e. 4 METS) to an average of 30 minutes daily; and
- abstinence from cigarette smoking.

Based upon these goals, it is appropriate to screen men for fasting lipid levels, blood pressure, glycosylated hemoglobin, and fasting or postprandial glucose levels. Recommendations about treatment interventions to address each of these components is beyond the scope of this chapter.

What symptoms of vaculopathy should be sought?

We now recognize that ED is more often than not a symptom of vasculopathy. The three other tissue compartments most often symptomatic for vascular disease are the heart, the central nervous system, and the peripheral circulation. Most commonly, symptomatic coronary ischemia manifests as chest pain, but sometimes exertional fatigue or dyspnea may be anginal equivalents. Clinical inquiry should include not only episodes of chest pain, but any changes in physical activities that have occurred (i.e. restrictions of activity) secondary to physical symptoms. Patients who have given up golf or tennis because of activity-related 'fatigue' may be actually suffering coronary ischemia.

Should men with erectile dysfunction be screened for cardiovascular disease with advanced screening techniques?

If we must rely on the available evidence base, the simplest and most direct answer to this question is 'no'. There is no evidence that investigation of any asymptomatic population by exercise testing improves outcomes. If we were to invite any population of 70-year-old men to be exercise tested, there would be a very substantial number who would be found to have coronary disease, and a similarly impressive number who would have coronary disease that would be viewed as appropriate for surgical intervention. The reason we don't screen elderly men is because we do not have data that show that screening of asymptomatic men improves outcomes. We know that screening produces harm in several ways:

- Patients have to undergo the inconvenience of the test
- Patients may have to shoulder the expense of the test
- Treadmill testing has resulted in death (albeit rarely)
- Some patients will be referred for cardiologic consultation and undergo interventions which are costly and have important morbidity and mortality
- Referral for testing implies that the patient is at risk for an MI, adding to 'imagined disease burden'
- Findings on a treadmill may alter a person's insurability
- Findings from a treadmill may alter a person's long-term self-perception as either healthy or unhealthy.

To counterbalance these known harms, we can hope that treadmill testing will have some benefits:

- It may underscore for our patients that those with ED have a greater than average CVD risk
- It may identify hitherto silent but clinically important coronary vascular lesions that would be interventionally remediable
- It may save the lives of people who might otherwise go on to have their first (and last) MI.

To reiterate: the harms of exercise treadmill testing are certain and established; the benefits are not.

Casting even greater doubt on the value of exercise testing is the recently published COURAGE trial.[18] In this randomized trial (n = 2287) of people who had symptomatic coronary artery disease (a higher risk group than those with asymptomatic coronary artery disease, the group we seek insight about), the authors sought to discern whether interventional management is superior to simply managing risk factors (e.g. by management of lipid levels, blood pressure, and glucose levels) for reducing cardiovascular events. The primary outcome was death from any cause and non-fatal MI during a mean follow-up of 4.6 years. There was actually a trend towards more coronary events in the intervention group than in the medically managed group. These data have reinforced the propriety of managing even stable symptomatic angina with medical risk factor modification, rather than intervention. Certainly, in the lower risk group of asymptomatic patients with ED and no chest pain, there is even less rationale for surgical intervention, and hence no evidence-based rationale for exercise testing.

If, then, the potential value of treadmill testing lies in discovery of potentially surgical coronary vascular lesions, the preponderance of current evidence suggests that the best course of action is simply vigorous modification of cardiovascular risk factors.

Is it safe for men with erectile dysfunction to engage in sexual activity?

Vigorous sexual activity typically requires a workload of approximately 3–5 METS.[19] Hence, the American College of Cardiology guidelines suggest that risk of coitus-induced ischemia is low in men who can exercise to an equivalent to a treadmill exercise of 5–6 METS.[20] Men do not generally require treadmill testing to discern their level of fitness for intercourse, because men who regularly engage in vigorous physical activity without evidence of coronary ischemia are at very low likelihood of coitus-induced cardiac events.[6] Because treadmill testing is expensive, inconvenient, and may lead to the above-mentioned harms, it is preferred that a clinical assessment be done instead. If a man can climb two flights of stairs without chest pain or dyspnea, it is likely that his cardiac reserve is sufficient for intercourse.[21] Another simple clinical decision rule is that if a patient can walk 1 mile within 15 minutes (the equivalent of 4 METS) without symptoms, he has done his own 'free living treadmill', and his risk of cardiovascular misadventure from sexual activity is minimal.[6]

Treatment-associated cardiovascular risks

Shortly after the advent of highly effective oral agents to treat ED (sildenafil, tadalafil, and vardenafil), reports surfaced of MI occurring in men using these phosphodiesterase type 5 (PDE-5) inhibitors. Subsequently, population data have been reassuring that, if anything, MI occurs less frequently in men who use PDE-5 inhibitors than their age-matched counterparts in the general population. That this should occur should not be surprising, given that PDE-5 inhibitors were originally investigated as anti-anginal agents.[22]

The contraindication for co-administration of nitrates with PDE-5 inhibitors remains absolute. Clinical data have shown that co-administration of nitrates with PDE-5 inhibitors can produce dramatic and precipitous declines in blood pressure, resulting in MI. Unfortunately, some clinicians have interpreted this restriction in two ways that merit addressing further:

- they consider this essentially to preclude *ever* using PDE-5 inhibitors for anyone who has used or does use nitrates; and
- they consider the use of a PDE-5 inhibitor as a 'nitrate disservice', because someone who has taken a PDE-5 inhibitor and then gets an episode of myocardial ischemia cannot receive the 'therapeutic benefit' of nitrates.

Let us address both of these issues. First, although coadministration of nitrates with PDE-5 inhibitors is an appropriate absolute contraindication, there are many persons who use nitrates intermittently (as opposed to daily). There is no reason that a well-informed patient who has nitrates on hand to treat angina cannot use a PDE-5 inhibitor, and be warned that he must not take a nitrate as treatment for his chest pain. Such advice should not be undertaken lightly. Indeed, most clinicians find it simpler to tell patients who have nitrates in their therapeutic regimen with any schedule of administration that they may not use PDE-5 inhibitors. Alternatively, there are some persons who have nitrates in their regimen that may be supplanted with other agents, or eliminated with better alternative pharmacotherapy: perhaps a patient with angina can improve anginal control by adding a calcium-channel blocker to his beta-blocker regimen, obviating the need for nitrates.

Next, the duration of time following a PDE-5 inhibitor after which it is considered safe to employ a nitrate has been established: 48 hours for tadalafil, and 24 hours for either sildenafil or vardenafil.

Finally, we must recognize that although nitrates are highly effective, well-targeted treatments to reduce chest pain, their use has not been shown to alter outcomes for people with chest pain or ischemia. According to the reference text Clinical Evidence: 'During the thrombolytic era, two large randomized controlled trials compared nitrates given acutely versus placebo in 58050 and 17817 people with acute MI ... Neither trial found a significant improvement in survival.'[23] In other words, in the event a patient has taken a PDE-5 inhibitor and does sustain an MI, another analgesic intervention is appropriate, but inability to use nitrates does not alter outcomes.

Conclusions

In middle-aged and more mature men, ED most commonly reflects vasculopathy that is not compartmentalized to the penis. If a man has endothelial dysfunction in the corpora cavernosa of his penis, it is likely that vascular disease exists elsewhere, and his risk for cardiovascular morbidity and mortality is predictably higher. When the clinician sees a patient with ED, or his partner, the authors suggest that information be shared, that a man with ED should be considered a vasculopath until proven otherwise. Rather than being necessarily frightening news, this message should be delivered with the encouraging principle that the presence of the ED may have given us the earliest possible time of discovery of important vascular dysfunction, meriting scrutiny for cardiovascular risk factors, and vigorous application of risk factor reduction.

References

1. Bennett AH, ed. Impotence. Philadelphia: WB Saunders, 1994.
2. Koshland DE. The molecule of the year. Science 1992; 258: 1861–5.

3. Rajfer J, Aronson WJ, Bush PA, Dorey FJ, Ignaro IJ. Nitric oxide as a mediator of relaxation of the corpus cavernosum in response to nonadrenergic, noncholinergic neurotransmission. N Engl J Med 1992; 326: 90–4.

4. Feldman HA, Goldstein I, Hatzichristou DG, Krane RJ, McKinlay JG. Impotence and its medical and psychosocial correlates: results of the Massachusetts Male Aging Study. J Urol 1994; 151: 54–61.

5. Grundy SM, Cleeman JI, Merz CNB et al. Coordinating Committee of the National Cholesterol Education Program. Implications of recent clinical trials for the National Cholesterol Program Adult Treatment Panel III Guidelines. Circulation 2004; 110: 227–39.

6. Kuritzky L. Primary care issues in the management of erectile dysfunction. In: Seftel AD, Padma-Nathan H, McMahon CG, Giuliano F, Althof SE, eds. Male and Female Sexual Dysfunction. Edinburgh Mosby, 2004: 229–33.

7. Thompson IM, Tangen CM, Goodman PJ et al. Erectile dysfunction and subsequent cardiovascular disease. JAMA 2005; 294: 2996–3002.

8. Seftel AD, Sun P, Swindle R. The prevalence of hypertension, hyperlipidemia, diabetes mellitus and depression in men with erectile dysfunction. J Urol 2004; 171: 2341–5.

9. Wei M, Macera CA, Davis DR et al. Total cholesterol and high density lipoprotein cholesterol as important predictors of erectile dysfunction. Am I Epidemiol 1994; 140: 930–7.

10. Min JK, Williams KA, Okwuosa TM et al. Prediction of coronary heart disease by erectile dysfunction in men referred for nuclear stress testing. Arch Intern Med 2006; 166: 201–6.

11. Grover SA, Lowensteyn I, Kaouache M et al. The prevalence of erectile dysfunction in the primary care setting. Arch Intern Med 2006; 166: 213–19.

12. Romeo JH, Seftel AD, Madhan ZT, Aron DC. Sexual function in men with diabetes type 2: association with glycemic control. J Urol 2000; 163: 788–91.

13. Montorsi P, Ravagnani PM, Galli S et al. Association between erectile dysfunction and coronary artery disease. Role of coronary clinical presentation and extent of coronary vessels involvement: the COBRA trial. Eur Heart J 2006; 27: 2632–9.

14. Saigal CS, Wessels H, Pace J et al. Predictors and prevalence of erectile dysfunction in a racially diverse population. Arch Intern Med 2006; 166: 207–12.

15. Kostis JB, Jackson G, Rosen R et al. Sexual dysfunction and cardiac risk (the Second Princeton Consensus Conference). Am J Cardiol 2005; 96: 313–21.

16. Esposito K, Giugliano F, Di Palo C et al. Effect of lifestyle changes on erectile dysfunction in obese men: a randomized controlled trial. JAMA 2004; 291: 2978–84.

17. Eaton CB, Liu YL, Mittleman MA et al. A retrospective study of the relationship between biomarkers of atherosclerosis and erectile dysfunction in 988 men. Int J Impot Res 2007; 19: 218–25.

18. Boden WE, O'Rourke RA, Teo KK et al. Optimal medical therapy with or without PCI for stable coronary disease. N Engl J Med 2007; 356: 1503–16.

19. Arruda-Olson AM, Mahoney DW, Nehra A. Cardiovascular effects of sildenafil during exercise in men with known or probably coronary artery disease. JAMA 2002; 287: 719–25.

20. Cheitlin MD, Hutter AM Jr, Brindis RG et al. Use of sildenafil in patients with cardiovascular disease. Circulation 1999; 99: 168–77.

21. Mobley DF, Baum NH. What you need to know before prescribing Viagra. Hosp Med 1999: 20–6.

22. Katzenstein L. Viagra: The Remarkable Story of the Discovery and Launch. New York: Medical Information Press, 2001.

23. Barton S, ed. Clinical Evidence. London: BMJ Publishing, 2001.

Sexual health and men

CHAPTER 14

Risk factors in men with erectile dysfunction

Hemant Solomon

Introduction

Erectile dysfunction (ED) is one of the most distressing conditions a man can experience. It is defined by the National Institutes of Health as 'the inability to achieve and maintain an erection sufficient to permit satisfactory sexual intercourse'.[1] It has a significant adverse impact on quality of life, reducing self-esteem, compromising wellbeing, and limiting interpersonal relationships.[2] In 1995, studies estimated ED to affect over 152 million men worldwide,[3] with a projected 322 million men being affected by 2025. The potential increase in the prevalence of ED, the social stigma attached to it, and its strong association with cardiovascular disease have prompted a significant amount of research. The breadth of this investigation ranges from elucidating pathophysiological mechanisms at the cellular level to, more recently, identifying a prognostic significance of ED at the population level. This chapter discusses the risk factors associated with the occurrence of vascular ED, and proposes the novel concept that vascular ED represents a systemic cardiovascular condition with an unfavorable cardiovascular prognosis.

Background studies

In 1994, the Massachusettes Male Aging Study (MMAS), a large population-based random sample of 1290 'healthy' men provided the first dataset on the prevalence of ED, along with its physiological and psychological correlates.[4] Surprisingly, 52% of all men aged 40–70 years experienced some degree of ED. This landmark study provided the impetus for investigators throughout the world to evaluate the prevalence and clinical correlates of ED in other continents (Table 14.1). In Brazil, of 1286 men aged 18–70 years, 46.2% reported having ED,[5] whilst in France 39% reported ED.[6] Among 1240 Australian men aged over 18 years, ED was reported in 39.4%,[7] and in Thailand, 37.5% of 1250 men aged 40–70 years admitted to having ED.[8] All of these studies demonstrated that the severity and frequency of ED increased with age. Among Brazilian men, complete ED increased from 1% in those under 40 years old to 11% in those over 70 years old (Fig. 14.1). In Australian men aged 50–69 years old, complete ED was present in 15.7%, increasing to 47.0% in those over 70 years old.[7] The MMAS found that ED affected as many as 70% in those approaching 70 years of age.

The erectile response declines with age owing to a failure of both cellular and molecular processes. In a healthy young male, penile erection is mediated by a neurovascular event.[9] On sexual stimulation, an increase in parasympathetic activity causes the release of neurotransmitters from the cavernous nerve terminals and of relaxing factors from the endothelial cells in the penis (Fig. 14.2). This results in smooth muscle relaxation in the arteries and arterioles supplying the erectile tissue and a several-fold increase in blood flow to the penis.

Table 14.1. *Prevalence rates of erectile dysfunction in various areas of the world.*

	Year	Men (n)	Age (years)	Prevalence (%)
Thailand[8]	2000	1250	40–70	37.5
Brazil[5]	2001	1286	18–70+	46.2
France[6]	1997	>1200	18–70	39.0
Australia[7]	2000	1240	18–91	39.4
New York State[75]	2000	1650	50–76	46.3

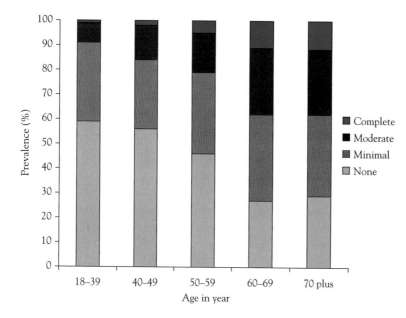

Figure 14.1. *Prevalence and severity of erectile dysfunction by age.*[5]

The smooth muscle relaxation is brought about by the release of nitric oxide (NO) from both the endothelial cells and neural tissue supplying the corpora cavernosa. NO activates a soluble guanylyl cyclase, which raises the intracellular concentration of cyclic guanosine monophosphate (cGMP), which in turn activates a specific protein kinase, ultimately blocking calcium influx by inhibition of calcium channels. This causes a drop in cytosolic calcium concentrations and results in relaxation of smooth muscle, vasodilatation, an increase in penile blood flow, and a subsequent erection.

Aging is associated with a decreased availability of NO in the endothelium of the penis. Haas et al. have studied the differences in this neurovascular event in the young (6-month-old) and the older

(2.5–3.5-year-old) rabbit *in vitro*.[10] They compared the ability of rabbit cavernosal smooth muscle to relax in an organ bath in response to acetylcholine (Ach), an endothelium-dependent vasodilator and sodium nitroprusside (SNP), an NO donor. They also examined the endothelial integrity using immunohistochemical techniques. The endothelium was equally well preserved in both age groups, thereby excluding any anatomical deficit in the older animals. Ach-mediated relaxation of penile corporal tissue was significantly attenuated from a maximum of 68.4% in young rabbits to 39.0% in older rabbits, but no difference was seen in cavernosal relaxation to SNP between young and older rabbits. Impaired relaxation of the older rabbit cavernosal smooth muscle was due to a defect in Ach-induced NO

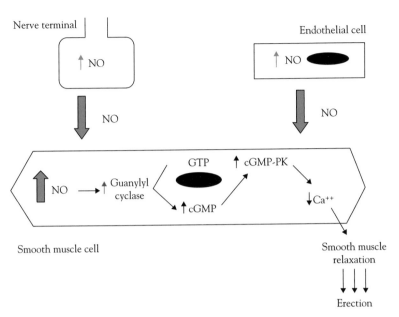

Figure 14.2. *Mechanisms involved in smooth muscle cell relaxation in the corpus carvenosum. GTP, guanosine triphosphate; cGMP, cyclic guanosine monophosphate; cGMP-PK, cGMP-dependent protein kinase; NO, nitric oxide; CA²⁺, calcium.*

production and not in NO *activity*. The authors concluded that ED in the aging rabbit cavernosum is not related to anatomical disturbances, but to endothelial dysfunction through an impaired ability to produce NO, although the response to NO was well preserved. Thus, the correlation between ED and aging is not simply due to a degenerative aging process *per se*. The endothelium plays a significant role in penile erection and, in fact, those conditions that cause endothelial dysfunction (and hence ED) happen to be more prevalent in the elderly and are therefore accountable for this relationship.

Endothelial dysfunction

The endothelium is an active paracrine, autocrine, and endocrine organ that is instrumental in maintaining vascular tone and homeostasis through its fine balance of vasodilators and vasoconstrictors. A relative reduction in the bioavailability of the potent vasodilator NO shifts the balance towards a state of impaired endothelium-dependent vasodilatation (Fig. 14.3), which represents the functional characteristic of endothelial dysfunction. In addition, dysfunction of the endothelium comprises a proinflammatory, proliferative, and procoagulatory

milieu that favors all stages of atherosclerosis. Thus, endothelial function reflects the likelihood of a person to develop atherosclerosis, and in fact some studies have shown that the presence of endothelial dysfunction is associated with an increased propensity to developing adverse cardiovascular events.[11,12]

Erectile function relies on the integrity of the smooth muscle cells in the walls of the cavernosal arterioles and the trabeculae of cavernous sinuses in the penis. NO, released by endothelial cells, is the principal chemical mediator responsible for smooth muscle cell relaxation in the penile tissue, resulting in vasodilatation and engorgement of blood within the penis (see Fig. 14.2). Therefore, erectile function depends on an intact endothelium, and endothelial dysfunction within the penile tissue may result in vascular ED. However, endothelial dysfunction is not necessarily limited to a single arterial bed. It is usually a diffuse systemic process, affecting multiple peripheral vascular beds, including both conduit arteries and small resistance vessels in the extremities.[13] Measurements of endothelial function in the forearm, using venous occlusion plethysmography, demonstrated that brachial artery endothelial dysfunction was associated with an increased incidence of cardiovascular (CV) events

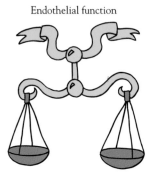

Endothelial function

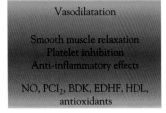

Vasodilatation

Smooth muscle relaxation
Platelet inhibition
Anti-inflammatory effects

NO, PCI$_2$, BDK, EDHF, HDL,
antioxidants

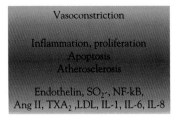

Vasoconstriction

Inflammation, proliferation
Apoptosis
Atherosclerosis

Endothelin, SO$_2$-, NF-kB,
Ang II, TXA$_2$,LDL, IL-1, IL-6, IL-8

Figure 14.3. *Endothelial balance of vasodilators and vasocontrictors. NO, nitric oxide; PCI$_2$, prostacyclin, BDK, bradykinin; EDHF, endothelium-derived hyperpolarizing factor; HDL, high-density lipoprotein; SO$_2$, sulfur dioxide; NF-kB, nuclear factor kB; Ang II, angiotensin II; TXA$_2$, thromboxane A$_2$; LDL, low-density lipoprotein, IL, interleukin.*

in other organs, including myocardial infarction and the need for coronary angioplasty in the heart, and ischemic stroke in the brain.[14]

Recently, studies have shown that ED is also associated with systemic endothelial dysfunction, implying that ED is not simply a manifestation of a localized disorder within the urogenital system, but a clinical surrogate of a diffuse systemic process.[15] Men with CV risk factors and ED have significantly impaired brachial artery flow-mediated dilatation compared with men with CV risk factors without ED (3.2% vs 6.0%, $p < 0.001$). Furthermore, endothelial function in men with vascular ED without CV risk factors is significantly reduced (1.3 vs 2.4%, $p = 0.014$) compared with potent men.[16] The latter study is the first to demonstrate that impotent men, even without significant CV risk factors, have peripheral endothelial dysfunction, suggesting that ED alone could be a manifestation of endothelial dysfunction.

We recently looked at the association of ED and endothelial dysfunction in the coronary circulation.[17] We studied coronary endothelial function in a group of 60 men with normal coronary angiograms (no evidence of significant obstructive coronary disease) and assessed their erectile function score.[18] In addition, we measured systemic levels of asymmetric

dimethylarginine (ADMA), a competitive inhibitor of NO and a serum marker for systemic endothelial dysfunction.[19] Men with coronary endothelial dysfunction had significant impairment of erectile function ($p = 0.008$) and significantly higher levels of ADMA (0.5 ± 0.06 ng/mL vs 0.45 ± 0.07 ng/mL, $p = 0.017$). Additionally, significant correlations were found between both the severity of ED and coronary endothelial dysfunction ($p < 0.001$) and the severity of ED and elevated ADMA levels ($p = 0.001$). This was the first study to identify a significant relationship between ED and coronary endothelial dysfunction in men with normal coronary angiograms.

Together, these studies substantiate the hypothesis that ED is not a condition localized to the penis but is a clinical manifestation of the unfavorable vascular milieu that gives rise to the systemic condition of endothelial dysfunction. The relationship between ED with systemic endothelial dysfunction may initially appear rather inconsequential, but further analysis is concerning. Endothelial dysfunction is not a benign phenomenon. In a study assessing brachial artery flow-mediated dilatation among 225 hypertensive patients, there were 29 major adverse cardiovascular events at an average of 31.5 months follow-up. Events included myocardial infarction, angina, coronary revascularization procedures, stroke, transient cerebral ischemic attack, and aortoiliac occlusive disease. Event rate was highest amongst the group with endothelial dysfunction, with a relative risk of 2.84 (95% CI, 1.25–3.48; $p = 0.0049$).[11]

Patients with coronary endothelial dysfunction are also at a significant risk. Among 157 patients with mildly diseased coronary arteries who had undergone coronary endothelial evaluation, 14% of patients with severe coronary endothelial dysfunction had 10 cardiac events at 28 months follow-up ($p < 0.05$ vs control group), including myocardial infarction, coronary revascularization, and cardiac death.[20]

Since endothelial dysfunction is associated with a poor cardiac prognosis and ED is a manifestation of endothelial dysfunction, then the prognosis for ED should also be guarded. Although no long-term randomized prospective study has been performed to establish that ED has a poor cardiac prognosis, its proven association with endothelial dysfunction and atherosclerosis must encourage healthcare workers to interpret ED as having an unfavorable CV outcome.

Atherosclerosis

The association between atherosclerosis and ED has been established for decades. In the 1920s, Leriche described the well-known syndrome of ED, buttock claudication, and aorto-iliac atherosclerosis.[21] Behr-Roussel et al. studied the mechanisms implicated in atherosclerosis-induced ED.[22] They assessed erectile responses *in vivo* from young adult, adult, and age-matched, cholesterol-fed, atherosclerotic rabbits. In addition, they studied endothelium-dependent and -independent relaxations of corporal strips *in vitro* from the three groups of animals. Measurement of intima–media (I/M) ratio on iliac arteries from the atherosclerotic rabbits determined those with moderate or severe atherosclerotic lesions. The electrically stimulated erectile responses were reduced in the adult rabbits compared with the young adult rabbits (51.6% vs 57.5%); they were similar in the adult rabbits and the rabbits with moderate atherosclerosis (48.1%), but drastically impaired ($p < 0.05$)

in the rabbits with severe atherosclerosis (34.8%). Corporal endothelium-dependent and -independent relaxations were similar in the young adult and the adult rabbits (maximum relaxation to acetylcholine: 51.3% vs 56.1%) but decreased in the atherosclerotic rabbits (37.1%, $p < 0.001$).

Although the erectile response is diminished both with age and atherosclerosis, atherosclerosis causes more severe ED. These studies corroborate the results of previous human clinical studies demonstrating the association of ED and atherosclerosis. In the MMAS the probability of ED increased to as much as 56% in patients with established cardiac disease. The suggestion that atherosclerosis is associated with ED is also supported by a meta-analysis of four studies involving 1476 men with heart disease, myocardial infarction, or vascular surgery. Incidences of ED ranged from 39% to 64% in each patient group.[23] Furthermore, the severity of ED has been linked to the severity of coronary atherosclerosis. Men with one-vessel disease have more erections ($p < 0.04$) and firmer erections ($p < 0.001$) with fewer difficulties in achieving an erection ($p < 0.007$) than men with two- or three-vessel disease.[24]

Vascular ED is now considered as a clinical surrogate for the co-existence of occult CV disease. In 1999, Pritzker reviewed the results of CV stress testing, risk profile analysis, and angiography in 50 men with ED of presumed vascular origin aged between 40 and 60 years, all of whom were asymptomatic from cardiovascular disease.[25] Multiple CV risk factors were present in 80% of men, and graded exercise testing was electrically positive in 28 of the 50 men. Coronary angiography was performed in 20 men. Left main stem or severe three-vessel disease was found in 6 men, moderate two-vessel disease was identified in 7 men, and significant single vessel in a further 7 men (Fig. 14.4). In a Korean study, 97 men complaining of ED were given repeated pharmacological tests with $10\,\mu g$ of prostaglandin E_1 to try to induce the erectile state.[26] They were divided according to the results of the pharmacological tests as responders (n = 46) or non-responders (n = 51). Men from both groups underwent exercise treadmill testing as a screening method for ischemic heart disease. Ischemic ST segment changes on the exercise test were seen only

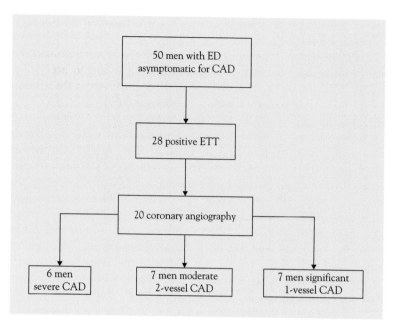

Figure 14.4. *The penile stress test: a window to the hearts of man?*[25] *ED, erectile dysfunction; CAD, coronary artery disease; ETT, exercise treadmill test.*

in non-responders (15.7%, $p = 0.006$). Thus, men with ED who do not respond to pharmacotherapy have more severe ED *and* are at a greater risk of occult coronary artery disease than those who respond. A study by Kawanishi et al. also supports this concept.[27] Among 52 men complaining of ED, 24.1% were diagnosed with ischemic heart disease (IHD) on the basis of a positive stress test or coronary angiography. The mean peak systolic velocity (PSV) in the penile cavernous artery in patients with IHD was 22.0 cm/s compared with a PSV of 35 cm/s in patients without IHD ($p < 0.01$). Furthermore, only 3.7% of patients in whom PSV values exceeded 35 cm/s had IHD whereas 41.9% of men with a PSV less than 35 cm/s had IHD ($p < 0.01$). The investigators concluded that in men with ED, the incidence of asymptomatic IHD was high and that men who had low PSV values (representing more severe form of ED) should undergo screening for IHD.

Over the past decade the co-existence of ED with cardiovascular disease has become increasingly established. Of concern is that the treatment of ED without prior thorough CV assessment has triggered cardiac events and resulted in significant morbidity or even mortality in some cases.[28] We have found that 30% of men presenting to a urologist with ED

were at such high risk of significant cardiovascular disease that ED therapy was deferred until further CV evaluation and treatment could establish them as low cardiac risk.[29] Most recent data suggest that ED may precede and hence predict the development of coronary artery disease. Of 300 men who presented with an acute coronary syndrome, ED was present in 49%.[30] Of this group, ED symptoms preceded a diagnosis of coronary artery disease in 67% (99 of 147 men) by a mean time interval of 38 months. Among 4247 men in the Prostate Cancer Prevention Trial who were potent at study entry, 57% reported ED after 5 years.[31] Incident ED was associated with a hazard ratio of 1.25 (95% CI 1.02–1.53, $p = 0.04$) for subsequent CV events during study follow up. For men with either incident or prevalent ED, the hazard ratio was 1.45 (95% CI 1.25–1.69, $p < 0.01$) for subsequent CV events. Similarly, in the COBRA study, amongst men who had stable coronary artery disease and ED, almost all of them (93%) had their ED symptoms preceding their coronary artery disease diagnosis.[32]

The risk factors for coronary artery disease and ED are identical and it has been only 20 years since the presence of ED has been closely linked to arterial risk factors.[33] Thus, men with CV risk factors such as hyperlipidemia, diabetes mellitus, hypertension, and a history of smoking are at an increased risk of developing ED. Paradoxically, however, some medications that are used to control these risk factors may worsen or even precipitate ED. The role by which each of these individual risk factors produces ED is examined separately below. In addition, how the medications that control these risk factors may exacerbate ED is also presented.

Diabetes mellitus

Diabetes mellitus is a well-known cause of ED. Data from the MMAS identified a 28% probability of complete ED among diabetics versus a 9% probability among non-diabetics. This increased probability has been associated with the duration of the disease and the paucity of glycemic control. The incidence of ED is 1.6-fold higher in men with a history of diabetes of at least 11 year's duration compared with men who have had diabetes for 5 years or less.[34] Patients also have a 1.7-fold increased incidence if the glycosylated hemoglobin is greater than 9% compared with a level of 7.5% or less. This prolonged hyperglycemic state appears to have a deleterious effect on both the endothelium and the nerve fibers supplying the smooth muscle cells,

which together prevent vasodilatation of the penile microvasculature (Fig. 14.5).

Diabetes appears to affect the endothelium both by anatomical changes as well as a reduction in endothelial function. Diabetic rats had a reduced cavernosal smooth muscle cell content of 9.83% compared to controls, which had a cavernosal smooth muscle cell content of 15.28% ($p = 0.0001$).[35] Cavernosal endothelial cell content is also reduced in the diabetic group (4.01%) compared with the control group (6.93%, $p < 0.0001$). Human studies have shown deterioration in endothelial function in diabetic men with ED.[36] Endothelial function was compared between diabetic impotent men and diabetic potent men by measuring mean reduction in blood pressure after an intravenous infusion of the NO precursor L-arginine. The blood pressure response in men with ED was significantly impaired ($+0.3$ mmHg vs -4.5 mmHg in potent men, $p < 0.05$), suggesting endothelial dysfunction as the mechanism for their ED. This study also assessed the degree of peripheral and autonomic neurological impairment in both groups of men. Quantitative sensory testing (QST) using vibratory, thermal, and pain sensory thresholds was performed to assess the peripheral nervous system. QST was pathological in 40% of impotent diabetic men but in only 15% of potent diabetic men ($p > 0.05$). Autonomic nerve

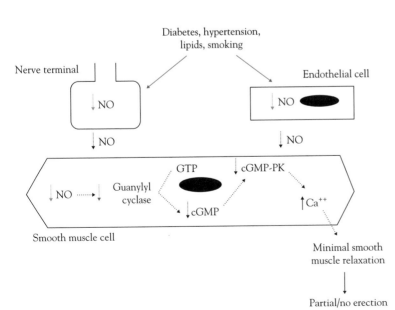

Figure 14.5. *The mechanism of risk factors in causing erectile dysfunction. GTP, guanosine triphosphate; cGMP, cyclic guanosine monophosphate; cGMP-PK, cGMP-dependent protein kinase; NO, nitric oxide; CA^{2+}, calcium.*

function tests were impaired in 70% of impotent men compared with only 30% of potent men ($p = 0.02$). Other studies have also shown a reduction in both autonomic and peripheral nerve function in diabetic men with ED.[37,38]

The relative contribution of endothelial and neurological dysfunction in the etiology of diabetic-induced ED remains unclear, but, nonetheless, the final common pathway for both mechanisms terminates in reduced vascular flow. A long duration of the diabetic state and poor hyperglycemic control significantly impair erectile function through mechanisms involving neural and endothelial cells. This reduced vascular flow in the penile tissues causes ED, probably in a similar manner to the reduction in coronary blood flow that is commonly seen in these poorly controlled diabetic patients.

Hypertension

Hypertension is often cited as a risk factor for ED. The MMAS found that hypertensive patients only had an 8.5% risk of acquiring ED, but more recent data suggest that the prevalence of ED in hypertensive men may in fact be as high as 68.3%, with 45.2% of hypertensive men having severe ED.[39] Animal studies addressing the cellular effects of hypertension on penile tissue provide significant insight. Changes in cavernous tissue from spontaneously hypertensive rats were compared with normotensive Wistar–Kyoto rats over 8 months.[40] The spontaneously hypertensive rats had a higher proliferative score in cavernous smooth muscle (2.7 vs 1.1, $p < 0.001$) and in vascular smooth muscle (2.7 vs 1.0, $p < 0.001$), and a higher cavernous tissue fibrosis score (2.8 vs 0.1, $p < 0.001$) compared with normotensive rats. An increase in surrounding connective tissue at the epineurium and endoneurium in the cavernous tissue was also found in the spontaneously hypertensive rats. The degree of proliferation and fibrosis in the penile tissue positively correlated to systolic blood pressure in the spontaneously hypertensive rats, indicating that a higher systolic blood pressure was associated with worsening morphological change. The focal alterations were not found in age-matched normotensive controls. Interestingly, these morphological changes

might be responsible for the functional impairment in erectile tissue that was found in the same species by Behr-Roussel in a more recent study.[41] In vivo electrical stimulation of the cavernous nerve demonstrated a reduction in the frequency-dependent erectile response in the spontaneously hypertensive rats compared with normotensive animals. In vitro endothelium-dependent relaxations of corporal strips to ACh were significantly impaired in the spontaneously hypertensive rats, suggesting a defect in endothelium dependent reactivity associated with ED in the spontaneously hypertensive rats.

The question inevitably arises as to whether the ED is caused by penile atherosclerosis resulting from arterial hypertension or whether it is a result of antihypertensive therapy used to lower blood pressure. Bansal reviewed various studies comparing the onset of ED in hypertensive men after the initiation of either antihypertensive medication or placebo.[42] In one study he found no difference in the incidence of ED in the active drug arm compared with the placebo arm. However, in a second study he found a 3.39-fold increase in the incidence of ED after active treatment was initiated. Jensen et al. found that 44% of hypertensive men with ED attributed their ED to antihypertensive therapy.[43] Although many studies report an increased incidence of ED after initiation of drug therapy, they often fail to identify a specific drug class with the onset of ED. Burchardt et al. could not establish any relationship between drug class and ED, in spite of the high prevalence of ED among hypertensive men in their study.[39]

Therefore, although hypertensive men may have a tendency towards experiencing ED as a result of the penile morphological changes that occur from the persistently elevated arterial pressure, the effect of these anatomical alterations may not become apparent until the addition of antihypertensive therapy. Precise control of blood pressure from the outset, thereby minimizing smooth muscle cell proliferation and fibrosis, may be the best method of preventing ED. Sexual performance should be discussed frequently with male hypertensive patients, especially when antihypertensive medication is initiated. Careful consideration must be made when selecting antihypertensive medications, especially with regard to their propensity to produce ED, so that subsequent patient non-compliance is avoided (see the section on medications, below).

Cigarette smoking

The original MMAS demonstrated that the effect of smoking was not directly associated with ED but that, when combined with other risk factors, it augmented the likelihood of ED. In subjects with heart disease, the probability of ED was 56.1% amongst smokers compared with 21% for non-smokers. Hypertensive men had a probability of ED of 20% if they smoked compared with 8.5% if they did not. Between 1995 and 1997, Feldman et al. re-interviewed a cohort of men for the presence of ED, who during the original MMAS study (1987–1989) were healthy at baseline and taking no medications.[44] Cigarette smoking at baseline almost doubled the likelihood of moderate or complete ED at follow-up (24% vs 14%, adjusted for age and covariates, $p=0.01$). A cross-sectional survey of 4462 US army veterans demonstrated that, after controlling for multiple cofounders, cigarette smoking was associated with an almost two-fold increase in ED prevalence.[45]

Cigarette smoking has been objectively demonstrated to cause a reduction in erectile response in humans. Among 314 smokers, penile rigidity during nocturnal erection inversely correlated with the number of cigarettes smoked per day.[45] Men who smoked more than 40 cigarettes a day had the fewest minutes of nocturnal tumescence and they detumesced fastest. Penile microcirculatory blood flow was measured among 26 impotent smokers at 1 day and 4 weeks abstention from smoking and finally 10 minutes after smoking one cigarette following the 4-week abstention period. Penile blood flow improved considerably after 4 weeks of abstention from smoking but was significantly lower 10 minutes after smoking one cigarette compared with after 1 day without smoking.[46]

The effect of cigarette smoking at the penile molecular level remains to be fully elucidated. One study did show that cigarette smoke inhibited penile prostacyclin (PGI_2) synthesis in rats and therefore potentially reduced the vasodilatation produced by PGI_2.[47] A second study, however, revealed conflicting results. The effects on erectile function of 8 weeks' chronic exposure to cigarette smoke in rats was studied. Although hypertension developed and penile neuronal NO synthase expression was decreased, no impairment of erection was noted.[48] Nicotine has been documented to enhance platelet aggregation to endothelial cells and to induce vasospasm.[49] Therefore, smoking-induced ED may be mediated through the production of microthrombi within the penile vasculature, which subsequently reduces penile blood flow rather than causing endothelial dysfunction.

Although further research needs to be focused on smoking and its mechanistic role in inducing ED, there exists abundant evidence to support healthcare initiatives aimed at eliminating cigarette smoking altogether.

Dyslipidemia

The association between ED and hypercholesterolemia has been documented in a group of apparently healthy men complaining of ED. More than 60% of men had abnormal cholesterol levels and over 90% of these men showed evidence of penile arterial disease on Doppler ultrasound testing.[50] In fact, the risk of ED appears to increase with the level of serum cholesterol. Amongst a cohort of 71 men, for every 1 mmol/L increase in total cholesterol, there was a 1.32-fold increase in the risk of ED.[51]

ED appears to be associated not only with the severity of dyslipidemia but also with the type of dyslipidemia. Among the lipid fractions, low-density lipoprotein (LDL) is known to be the greatest determinant for the development of atherosclerosis, whilst high-density lipoprotein (HDL) protects against it. A marked increase in LDL fraction has been reported in men with ED compared with potent men.[52] In addition, the MMAS reported a 0% probability of complete ED in men with HDL values more than 90 mg/dL, but a 16.1% probability if the HDL values dropped to below 30 mg/dL (1 mg/dL=0.02586 mmol/L). The dyslipidemic state appears to produce an anatomical as well as a functional disruption in cavernosal tissue. Anatomical alterations were found in cavernous tissue biopsies taken from rabbits that were fed on a cholesterol-enriched diet for 3 months.[53] Ultramorphological examination of a normal cholesterol diet group showed normal smooth muscle cell architecture. The high cholesterol diet group showed significant smooth muscle cell degeneration with loss of intercellular contacts, suggesting that impaired lipid metabolism causes cavernous smooth muscle cell degeneration.

Functional studies have produced consistent results with regard to the effects of hypercholesterolemia on corpora cavernosal tissue. Rabbits with diet-induced severe hypercholesterolemia demonstrated a reduction in endothelium-dependent relaxation in penile tissue, which was partially reversed by the supplementation of L-arginine, an NO precursor.[54] The hypercholesterolemic state increased the production of superoxide radicals in rabbit cavernosal tissue, leading to functional impairment of cavernous smooth muscle relaxation in response to endothelium-mediated stimuli.[55] Similar hypercholesterolemic rabbits also had atheroma in cavernosal sinusoids, and both endothelium-dependent and endothelium-independent relaxation of isolated cavernosal strips were impaired.[56]

Triglycerides have a less significant association with atherosclerosis compared with LDL-cholesterol, and studies considering the effects of triglycerides on cavernosal smooth muscle relaxation or contractile responses are rare. One study did demonstrate a significant impairment of rabbit cavernous smooth muscle contraction in response to norepinephrine, but no significant alteration of the relaxation response to endothelium-dependent and endothelium-independent vasodilators was noted.[55] This group also found no increase in the prevalence of ED in men with abnormally high triglyceride levels compared with control patients. Hence it appears that triglycerides may not have as significant a role to play in the development of ED as does elevated LDL-cholesterol.

There is no doubt that there is an association between lipid disorders and ED, and in particular, the person with high LDL and low HDL levels appears to be at significant risk. Attempts to increase the HDL–LDL ratio may prevent erectile function from deteriorating, and dietary supplementation with L-arginine may be an appropriate step towards

preventing ED. It would be interesting to see the results of further studies aimed at reversing dyslipidemia-induced ED based on this approach.

Medications

Although ED can be produced by many of the risk factors known to cause atherosclerosis, initiation of pharmacological measures to control these vascular risk factors may in fact worsen or even precipitate ED. Clearly, this unwanted side effect may limit adherence to proven medical therapy and hence interfere with the potential advantages to be gained by these therapeutic approaches. The precise mechanisms by which medications are able to produce ED are not well understood. Their differing mechanisms of action and vast side-effect profiles make it almost impossible to identify why one particular drug should cause ED in one person but not in others. Nonetheless, the following section attempts to address some of the current hypotheses and supporting evidence for proposed mechanisms by which cardiovascular drugs might produce ED, and to provide the reader with a more thorough understanding of the complexity of this subject.

Statins
Statin therapy routinely recommended for cardiovascular disease has been associated with differing effects on erectile function. Case reports and small randomized control studies of statin therapy and erectile function have been published. Men with ED for at least 6 months, secondary to an elevated LDL (mean LDL 173 mg/dL) as their only risk factor, were given titrated doses of atorvastatin for 4 months until LDL reached <120 mg/dL.[57] Erectile function and RigiScan measurements (a measure of penile rigidity) significantly improved after atorvastatin treatment (mean LDL, 98 mg/dL). Herrman et al. demonstrated that in men with ED unresponsive to oral sildenafil 100 mg, atorvastatin not only decreased LDL cholesterol from 135 mg/dL to 78 mg/dL (43% reduction, $p=0.012$), but also significantly improved erectile function in response to sildenafil ($p=0.036$).[58] This improved response to sildenafil is thought to be due to an atorvastatin-mediated increase in the bioavailability of NO, as

shown by *in vitro* studies performed on rat aortic rings.[59]

Not all statins have shown such promising results. Simvastatin was found to cause impotence in five men with coronary artery disease after its initiation, but within 1 week of its discontinuation, sexual function was restored.[60] The Australian Adverse Drug Reactions Committee reported 42 cases of ED associated with simvastatin.[61] In this study, 50% of men with previously normal erectile function experienced some degree of impotence after the addition of statin therapy. However, the casual association of statin therapy with ED has been questioned. The ability of statins to induce ED is surprising since these drugs have been shown to improve endothelial function in other parts of the vasculature.[62,63] One possible mechanism postulated is that some statins, such as simvastatin, are more lipophilic than other statins and may be more likely to produce ED through actions on the central nervous system or to induce a neuropathy in the penile nerves.

β-blockers

Like statins, β-blockers have produced varying reports regarding their effects on erectile function. In the large Medical Research Council (MRC) Trial, effects of propranolol and placebo on sexual function were compared over 23 582 patient-years.[64] The incidence of withdrawal from randomized treatment was 5.48 per 1000 patient-years in the propanolol group vs 0.89 per 1000 patient-years in the placebo group ($p < 0.001$). In a randomized, double-blind, cross-over trial comparing valsartan with carvedilol, carvedilol consistently decreased frequency of sexual activity, in contrast to valsartan, which was found to increase sexual activity.[65]

Both carvedilol and propranolol are non-selective β-blockers and decrease sexual function in men. The more selective β-blockers, however, have shown mixed effects. In the TOHMS trial, a study comparing the effects of five differing classes of antihypertensives on erectile function. Acebutalol had a similar effect to placebo on erectile function, whilst diuretic therapy produced a significant worsening.[66]

However, in the TAIM study,[67] 878 overweight hypertensive patients were randomized to

chlorthalidone 25 mg orally daily, atenolol 50 mg orally daily, or placebo. Although chlorthalidone was associated with the greatest incidence of ED (28%), atenolol also produced worsening of erectile function in 11% of subjects, whereas the placebo group was not as severely affected (3%). Some studies argue that the ED effect of atenolol may be purely psychological.[68]

Ninety-six hypertensive patients without ED were given atenolol 50 mg orally daily and randomized into one of three groups: group A was blinded to the identity of the drug, group B knew the name of the drug only, and group C knew the name of the drug and that it had a possible side effect of ED. Surprisingly, the incidence of ED was 3.1% in group A, 15.6% in group B, and 31.2% in group C ($p < 0.01$). All patients reporting ED were then randomized to either sildenafil 50 mg orally or placebo in a cross-over study. Both sildenafil and placebo were equally effective at reversing the ED. The authors conclude that the occurrence of organic ED whilst taking β-blockers is much lower than thought and that knowledge about side effects may influence their propensity to occur.

Angiotensin-1 receptor blockers

Angiotensin-1 receptor blockers (ARBs) are the only class of antihypertensive drugs that have consistently shown a favorable effect on erectile function. Hypertensive men all with ED at baseline on monotherapy for hypertension discontinued their blood pressure medication and switched to a 12-week trial of losartan 50 mg orally daily.[69] Losartan improved sexual satisfaction from 7.3% to 58.5% ($p = 0.01$), and only 11.8% reported any ED at the end of the study. In the previously reported cross-over study comparing the effects of valsartan with carvedilol on sexual activity,[65] valsartan tended to increase sexual activity whereas carvedilol was associated with a significant reduction ($p < 0.01$). In an open-label, prospective study,[70] 75% of 3502 hypertensive patients were found to have ED at baseline. After 6 months of switching antihypertensive therapy to valsartan 80–160 mg/day, valsartan decreased the prevalence of ED to 53% ($p < 0.0001$).

Angiotensin-1 receptors (AT_1R) are found throughout the vasculature, particularly in smooth muscle and endothelial cells. Preferential activation of these receptors over the angiotensin-2 receptors (AT$_2$R) by angiotensin II produces vasoconstriction, cell proliferation, sodium resorption, aldosterone, and inflammatory mediator release, all of which have a tendency to produce endothelial dysfunction (Fig. 14.6). Blockade of AT$_1$R with ARBs produces a relative rise in bradykinin levels, and preferential

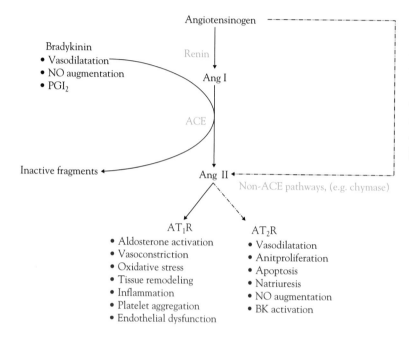

Figure 14.6. *The renin–angiotensin pathway, activating angiotensin-1 receptors (AT$_1$R) more than angiotensin-2 receptors (AT$_2$R). ACE, angiotensin-converting enzyme; Ang I, angiotensin I; Ang II, angiotensin II; BK, bradykinin; PGI$_2$, prostacyclin; NO, nitric oxide.*

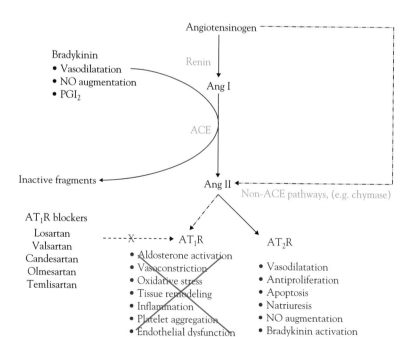

Figure 14.7. *The renin–angiotensin pathway: blockade of angiotensin-1 receptors (AT$_1$R) producing preferential activation of angiotension-2 receptors (AT$_2$R). ACE, angiotensin converting enzyme; Ang I, angiotensin I; Ang II, angiotensin II; BK, bradykinin; PGI$_2$, prostacyclin; NO, nitric oxide.*

angiotensin II-mediated activation of the AT_2R, which in turn causes NO augmentation, bradykinin release, and vasodilatation (Fig. 14.7). Bradykinin is known to activate NO and PGI_2, both of which have a favorable effect on the endothelium, producing vasodilatation. ARBs have been shown to improve endothelial function both in animal and human studies,[71,72] and since ED is already known to be associated with endothelial dysfunction, it is not surprising that these drugs also improve erectile function.

Other antihypertensive drugs

Diuretics, in particular the thiazide class, appear to be considered a risk factor for the development of ED. After 2 years of treatment for hypertension with bendrofluazide 5 mg orally twice daily, ED prevalence was 22.6% compared with 10.1% after placebo treatment ($p<0.001$).[64] In the TOMHS trial,[66] chlorthalidone 15 mg/day was the only class of five different antihypertensive drugs to produce a statistically elevated incidence of ED compared with the placebo group after 24 months' treatment ($p=0.025$). Adverse effects of thiazide diuretics on sexual function have been reported by several groups,[67,73] although no concise explanation for this adverse effect has been put forward. Some authors suggest that chronically hypertensive patients are more prone to experiencing side effects related to acute lowering of blood pressure. A reduction in blood flow to the penile artery as a consequence of diuretic therapy may account for the ED side effect. However, this is purely speculation and the precise mechanisms by which these agents cause ED remain to be ascertained.

Few data from small studies are available with respect to calcium-channel blockers and angiotensin-converting enzyme inhibitors and sexual function. The available information suggests that there is no overall negative effect on sexual function caused by these two classes of drugs.

Conclusion

ED is common and its prevalence is increasing. It is associated with a number of cardiovascular risk factors that affect the endothelium, producing both anatomical and functional alterations of NO activity, leading to impairment of erectile function. Vascular ED must be recognized as a systemic condition, and is often the hallmark for undiagnosed cardiovascular disease. Increasing data suggest that ED pertains a poorer long-term prognosis. Thus, the cardiovascular risks of the individual patient must be addressed as part of the treatment plan for ED.

Some medications used to treat CV risk factors can paradoxically cause ED. The side-effect profile of these drugs invariably results in a reduction in treatment compliance and thereby increased vascular risk.[74] Patients need to be warned about this potential side effect when initiating any of these drugs so that compliance can be maintained by offering alternative therapy, if required. Provided that cardiovascular risk factors are well controlled and that patients are counseled with regard to CV disease, the treatment of ED and its risk factors can be successfully and safely accomplished.

References

1. NIH Consensus Development Panel on Impotence. Impotence. JAMA 1993; 270: 83–90.
2. Krane RJ, Goldstein I, Saenz de Tejada I. Impotence. N Engl J Med 1989; 321: 1648–59.
3. Ayta IA, McKinlay JB, Krane RJ. The likely worldwide increase in erectile dysfunction between 1995 and 2025 and some possible policy consequences. BJU Int 1999; 84: 50–6.
4. Feldman HA, Goldstein I, Hatzichristou DG, Krane RJ, McKinlay JB. Impotence and its medical and psychosocial correlates: results of the Massachusetts Male Aging Study. J Urol 1994; 151: 54–61.
5. Moreira ED Jr, Abdo CH, Torres EB, Lobo CF, Fittipaldi JA. Prevalence and correlates of erectile dysfunction: results of the Brazilian study of sexual behavior. Urology 2001; 58: 583–8.
6. Virag R, Beck-Ardilly L. Nosology, epidemiology, clinical quantification of erectile dysfunctions. Rev Med Interne 1997; 1(18 Suppl): 10s–13s.
7. Chew KK, Earle CM, Stuckey BG, Jamrozik K, Keogh EJ. Erectile dysfunction in general medicine practice: prevalence and clinical correlates. Int J Impot Res 2000; 12: 41–5.
8. Thai Erectile Dysfunction Epidemiologic Study Group (TEDES). An epidemiologic study of erectile

dysfunction in Thailand (Part 1: Prevalence). J Med Assoc Thai 2000; 83: 872–9.

9. Lue TF. Erectile dysfunction. N Engl J Med 2000; 342: 1802–13.

10. Haas CA, Seftel AD, Razmjouei K et al. Erectile dysfunction in aging: upregulation of endothelial nitric oxide synthase. Urology 1998; 51: 516–22.

11. Perticone F, Ceravolo R, Pujia A et al. Prognostic significance of endothelial dysfunction in hypertensive patients. Circulation 2001; 104: 191–6.

12. Halcox JP, Schenke WH, Zalos G et al. Prognostic value of coronary vascular endothelial dysfunction. Circulation 2002; 106: 653–8.

13. Anderson TJ, Gerhard MD, Meredith IT et al. Systemic nature of endothelial dysfunction in atherosclerosis. Am J Cardiol 1995; 75: 71B–4B.

14. Heitzer T, Schlinzig T, Krohn K, Meinertz T, Munzel T. Endothelial dysfunction, oxidative stress, and risk of cardiovascular events in patients with coronary artery disease. Circulation 2001; 104: 2673–8.

15. Yavuzgil O, Altay B, Zoghi M et al. Endothelial function in patients with vasculogenic erectile dysfunction. Int J Cardiol 2005; 103: 19–26.

16. Kaiser DR, Billups K, Mason C et al. Impaired brachial artery endothelium-dependent and -independent vasodilation in men with erectile dysfunction and no other clinical cardiovascular disease. J Am Coll Cardiol 2004; 43: 179–84.

17. Elesber AA, Solomon H, Lennon RJ et al. Coronary endothelial dysfunction is associated with erectile dysfunction and elevated asymmetric dimethylarginine in patients with early atherosclerosis. Eur Heart J 2006; 27: 824–31.

18. Rosen RC, Riley A, Wagner G et al. The International Index of Erectile Function (IIEF): a multidimensional scale for assessment of erectile dysfunction. Urology 1997; 49: 822–30.

19. Kielstein JT, Impraim B, Simmel S et al. Cardiovascular effects of systemic nitric oxide synthase inhibition with asymmetrical dimethylarginine in humans. Circulation 2004; 109: 172–7.

20. Suwaidi JA, Hamasaki S, Higano ST et al. Long-term follow-up of patients with mild coronary artery disease and endothelial dysfunction. Circulation 2000; 101: 948–54.

21. Leriche R. Des obliterations artérielles hautes comme cause d'une insuffisance circulatoire des membres inférieurs. Bull Soc Chirurigie 1923; 49: 1404.

22. Behr-Roussel D, Bernabe J, Compagnie S et al. Distinct mechanisms implicated in atherosclerosis-induced erectile dysfunction in rabbits. Atherosclerosis 2002; 162: 355–62.

23. Bortolotti A, Parazzini F, Colli E, Landoni M. The epidemiology of erectile dysfunction and its risk factors. Int J Androl 1997; 20: 323–34.

24. Greenstein A, Chen J, Miller H et al. Does severity of ischemic coronary disease correlate with erectile function? Int J Impot Res 1997; 9: 123–6.

25. Pritzker M. The penile stress test: a window to the hearts of man? Circulation 2000; 100: P3751.

26. Kim SW, Paick J, Park DW, Chae I, Oh B. Potential predictors of asymptomatic ischemic heart disease in patients with vasculogenic erectile dysfunction. Urology 2001; 58: 441–5.

27. Kawanishi Y, Lee KS, Kimura K et al. Screening of ischemic heart disease with cavernous artery blood flow in erectile dysfunctional patients. Int J Impot Res 2001; 13: 100–3.

28. Solomon H, Man J, Gill J, Jackson G. Viagra on the internet: unsafe sexual practice. Int J Clin Pract 2002; 56: 403–4.

29. Solomon H, Man J, Wierzbicki AS, O'Brien T, Jackson G. The value of routine cardiovascular assessment in patients with erectile dysfunction. Circulation 2002; 106: 749.

30. Montorsi F, Briganti A, Salonia A et al. Erectile dysfunction prevalence, time of onset and association with risk factors in 300 consecutive patients with acute chest pain and angiographically documented coronary artery disease. Eur Urol 2003; 44: 360–4; discussion 364–5.

31. Thompson IM, Tangen CM, Goodman PJ et al. Erectile dysfunction and subsequent cardiovascular disease. JAMA 2005; 294: 2996–3002.

32. Montorsi P, Ravagnani PM, Galli S et al. Association between erectile dysfunction and coronary artery disease. Role of coronary clinical presentation and extent of coronary vessels involvement: the COBRA trial. Eur Heart J 2006; 27: 2632–9.

33. Virag R, Bouilly P, Frydman D. Is impotence an arterial disorder? A study of arterial risk factors in 440 impotent men. Lancet 1985; 1: 181–4.

34. Fedele D, Coscelli C, Cucinotta D et al. Incidence of erectile dysfunction in Italian men with diabetes. J Urol 2001; 166: 1368–71.

35. Burchardt T, Burchardt M, Karden J et al. Reduction of endothelial and smooth muscle density in the corpora cavernosa of the streptozotocin induced diabetic rat. J Urol 2000; 164: 1807–11.

36. De Angelis L, Marfella MA, Siniscalchi M et al. Erectile and endothelial dysfunction in type II diabetes: a possible link. Diabetologia 2001; 44: 1155–60.

37. Wellmer A, Sharief MK, Knowles CH et al. Quantitative sensory and autonomic testing in male

diabetic patients with erectile dysfunction. BJU Int 1999; 83: 66–70.

38. Bemelmans BL, Meuleman EJ, Doesburg WH, Notermans SL, Debruyne FM. Erectile dysfunction in diabetic men: the neurological factor revisited. J Urol 1994; 151: 884–9.

39. Burchardt M, Burchardt T, Baer L et al. Hypertension is associated with severe erectile dysfunction. J Urol 2000; 164: 1188–91.

40. Toblli JE, Stella I, Inserra F et al. Morphological changes in cavernous tissue in spontaneously hypertensive rats. Am J Hypertens 2000; 13: 686–92.

41. Behr-Roussel D, Chamiot-Clerc P, Bernabe J et al. Erectile dysfunction in spontaneously hypertensive rats: pathophysiological mechanisms. Am J Physiol Regul Integr Comp Physiol 2003; 284: R682–8.

42. Bansal S. Sexual dysfunction in hypertensive men. A critical review of the literature. Hypertension 1988; 12: 1–10.

43. Jensen J, Lendorf A, Stimpel H et al. The prevalence and etiology of impotence in 101 male hypertensive outpatients. Am J Hypertens 1999; 12: 271–5.

44. Feldman HA, Johannes CB, Derby CA et al. Erectile dysfunction and coronary risk factors: prospective results from the Massachusetts Male Aging Study. Prev Med 2000; 30: 328–38.

45. Mannino DM, Klevens RM, Flanders WD. Cigarette smoking: an independent risk factor for impotence? Am J Epidemiol 1994; 140: 1003–8.

46. Ledda ABG. Evaluation of penile microcirculation. In: Ledda ABG, ed. Vascular Andrology. Heidelberg, Germany: Springer-Verlag, 1996: 29–36.

47. Jeremy JY, Mikhailidis DP, Thompson CS, Dandona P. The effect of cigarette smoke and diabetes mellitus on muscarinic stimulation of prostacyclin synthesis by the rat penis. Diabetes Res 1986; 3: 467–9.

48. Xie Y, Garban H, Ng C, Rajfer J, Gonzalez-Cadavid NF. Effect of long-term passive smoking on erectile function and penile nitric oxide synthase in the rat. J Urol 1997; 157: 1121–6.

49. Jeremy JY, Mikhailidis DP. Vascular and platelet eicosanoids, smoking and atherosclerosis. Adv Exp Med Biol 1990; 273: 135–46.

50. Billups K, Friedrich S. Assessment of fasting lipid panels and Doppler ultrasound testing in men presenting with erectile dysfunction and no other problems. Program and abstracts of the American Urological Association 95th Annual Meeting; Atlanta, Georgia; April 29–May 4, 2000. Abstract 655.

51. Wei M, Macera CA, Davis DR et al. Total cholesterol and high density lipoprotein cholesterol as important predictors of erectile dysfunction. Am J Epidemiol 1994; 140: 930–7.

52. Juenemann KP, Rohr G, Siegsmund M, Alken P. Does lipid metabolism influence the pathogenesis of vascular impotence. Int J Impot Res 1990; 2: 33.

53. Junemann KP, Aufenanger J, Konrad T et al. The effect of impaired lipid metabolism on the smooth muscle cells of rabbits. Urol Res 1991; 19: 271–5.

54. Azadzoi KM, Goldstein I, Siroky MB et al. Mechanisms of ischemia-induced cavernosal smooth muscle relaxation impairment in a rabbit model of vasculogenic erectile dysfunction. J Urol 1998; 160: 2216–22.

55. Kim SC. Hyperlipidemia and erectile dysfunction. Asian J Androl 2000; 2: 161–6.

56. Kim JH, Klyachkin ML, Svendsen E et al. Experimental hypercholesterolemia in rabbits induces cavernosal atherosclerosis with endothelial and smooth muscle cell dysfunction. J Urol 1994; 151: 198–205.

57. Saltzman EA, Guay AT, Jacobson J. Improvement in erectile function in men with organic erectile dysfunction by correction of elevated cholesterol levels: a clinical observation. J Urol 2004; 172: 255–8.

58. Herrmann HC, Levine LA, Macaluso J Jr et al. Can atorvastatin improve the response to sildenafil in men with erectile dysfunction not initially responsive to sildenafil? Hypothesis and pilot trial results. J Sex Med 2006; 3: 303–8.

59. Castro MM, Rizzi E, Rascado RR et al. Atorvastatin enhances sildenafil-induced vasodilation through nitric oxide-mediated mechanisms. Eur J Pharmacol 2004; 498: 189–94.

60. Jackson G. Simvastatin and impotence. BMJ 1997; 315: 31.

61. Boyd IW. Comment: HMG-CoA reductase inhibitor-induced impotence. Ann Pharmacother 1996; 30: 1199.

62. Pedersen TR, Faergeman O. Simvastatin seems unlikely to cause impotence. BMJ 1999; 318: 192.

63. O'Driscoll G, Green D, Taylor RR. Simvastatin, an HMG-coenzyme A reductase inhibitor, improves endothelial function within 1 month. Circulation 1997; 95: 1126–31.

64. Adverse reactions to bendrofluazide and propranolol for the treatment of mild hypertension. Report of Medical Research Council working party on mild to moderate hypertension. Lancet 1981; 2: 539–43.

65. Fogari R, Zoppi A, Poletti L et al. Sexual activity in hypertensive men treated with valsartan or carvedilol: a crossover study. Am J Hypertens 2001; 14: 27–31.

66. Grimm RH, Jr, Grandits GA, Prineas RJ et al. Long-term effects on sexual function of five antihypertensive drugs and nutritional hygienic treatment in hypertensive men and women. Treatment of Mild Hypertension Study (TOMHS). Hypertension 1997; 29: 8–14.

67. Wassertheil-Smoller S, Blaufox MD, Oberman A et al. Effect of antihypertensives on sexual function and quality of life: the TAIM Study. Ann Intern Med 1991; 114: 613–20.

68. Silvestri A, Galetta P, Cerquetani E et al. Report of erectile dysfunction after therapy with beta-blockers is related to patient knowledge of side effects and is reversed by placebo. Eur Heart J 2003; 24: 1928–32.

69. Llisterri JL, Lozano Vidal JV et al. Sexual dysfunction in hypertensive patients treated with losartan. Am J Med Sci 2001; 321: 336–41.

70. Dusing R. Effect of the angiotensin II antagonist valsartan on sexual function in hypertensive men. Blood Press Suppl 2003; 2: 29–34.

71. Sierra C, de la Sierra A. Antihypertensive, cardiovascular, and pleiotropic effects of angiotensin-receptor blockers. Curr Opin Nephrol Hypertens 2005; 14: 435–41.

72. De Gennaro Colonna V, Fioretti S, Rigamonti A et al. Angiotensin II type 1 receptor antagonism improves endothelial vasodilator function in L-NAME-induced hypertensive rats by a kinin-dependent mechanism. J Hypertens 2006; 24: 95–102.

73. Chang SW, Fine R, Siegel D et al. The impact of diuretic therapy on reported sexual function. Arch Intern Med 1991; 151: 2402–8.

74. Brock G, Lue TF. Drug induced male sexual dysfunction. An update. Drug Saf 1993; 8: 414–26.

75. Ansong KS, Lewis C, Jenkins P, Bell J. Epidemiology of erectile dysfunction: a community-based study in rural New York State. Ann Epidemiol 2000; 10: 293–6.

CHAPTER 15

Evaluation and treatment of male infertility

Joseph Dall'Era, Craig S Niederberger, Randall B Meacham

Introduction

Infertility is defined by the World Health Organization (WHO) as the inability to conceive after 1 year of intercourse without the use of birth control. Based on this criterion, approximately one in seven couples experience infertility. Male factor infertility has been shown to play a role in up to 50% of couples unable to conceive. Ongoing advances in the management of this disorder have led to improved treatment options. Ideally, evaluation and treatment of the infertile male will allow the development of an effective therapeutic plan, while minimizing overall cost. This chapter reviews the work-up for male factor infertility, and the evidence-based treatment options available.

History and physical examination

The general history should begin with details of prior pregnancies in the patient or his partner, coital habits, female partner fertility history, and duration of attempted conception. Approximately 5% of couples report sexual behavior that is counterproductive to conception. A detailed medical history should be included to identify any systemic illnesses (diabetes, cancer, history of sexually transmitted diseases) or possible genetic causes. A surgical history focused on pelvic trauma, prior hernia repair, and bladder, prostate, or scrotal surgery should also be elicited in the history. It is important to enquire about a childhood history of cryptorchidism, orchidopexy, torsion, and timing of puberty, since many patients do not relate pediatric history to problems with fertility. Finally, a thorough medication and social history (including occupational exposures) can often identify possible etiologies of infertility.

A systematic physical examination should begin with observations of overall body habitus and hair distribution. Gynecomastia or abnormal hair distribution may indicate incomplete virilization or etiologies warranting a more thorough hormonal evaluation. An examination of the phallus, looking for chordee, hypospadias, and other lesions is aimed at ruling out structural impediments to effective sperm delivery. Next, the scrotal contents should be examined to evaluate the size, position, and consistency of the testes, as well as the presence and characteristics of the vas deferens (looking for vasal agenesis), spermatic cord (looking for clinically significant varicocele), and epididymis (looking for induration, which may indicate obstruction). Finally, a digital rectal examination should be performed to evaluate the prostate, seminal vesicles, and anal sphincter tone, since findings may indicate infection, obstruction, or a neurological disorder.

Laboratory examinations

Semen analysis

The semen analysis is a critical component of the initial laboratory investigation. An analysis of the ejaculate volume, sperm count, sperm morphology, and sperm motility provides information regarding the chances for normal conception but are generally poor in predicting those chances unless the patient is severely oligospermic or azoospermic.

Proper collection is required to validate the results of the semen analysis. The current recommendations are for two or three semen collections (each performed after 2–5 days of abstinence) over the course of several weeks. This has been shown to minimize intraindividual variation, most notably seen in sperm concentration.[1] The ejaculated semen should be collected in the physician's office in a clean container, free of lubricants or contaminants. If a specimen is collected at home, the patient should transport the container to the laboratory within 45 minutes of collection.

Table 15.1 lists the WHO reference values for an adequate semen sample.[2] These values correspond only to the likelihood of conception, and should not be used to evaluate a patient for advanced reproductive techniques. Though the nuances of the semen analysis are beyond the scope of this chapter, special attention should be paid to the patient with azoospermia because of its impact on further evaluation.

Azoospermia is found in 10–15% of infertile men,[3] and is differentiated from oligospermia by centrifugation of the semen sample and analysis of the pellet. Any sperm in the pellet excludes the diagnosis of azoospermia. A patient with confirmed azoospermia should be evaluated for obstruction or testicular failure. A physical examination must be performed to confirm the presence of each vas deferens, since congenital bilateral absence of the vas deferens (CBAVD) precludes the possibility of surgical reconstruction. Moreover, CBAVD is found to be associated with an 80% risk of mutation in the cystic fibrosis transmembrane conductance regulator (CFTR) gene.[4] Thus, a genetic assessment and appropriate genetic counseling is mandated in these patients and their female partners prior to sperm retrieval for advanced reproductive techniques.

Endocrine evaluation

Figure 15.1 illustrates the hypothalamic–pituitary–testis axis involving gonadotropin-releasing hormone (GnRH), luteinizing hormone (LH), and follicle stimulating hormone (FSH). An understanding of this control mechanism for spermatogenesis and the production of testosterone is critical for the correct interpretation of hormonal assays. The hypothalamus secretes GnRH in a pulsatile fashion

Table 15.1. *Reference values for semen analysis from the World Health Organization (1999)*

Volume	2 ml or greater
Sperm concentration	20 × 10⁶ or greater sperm/ml
Total sperm no.	40 × 10⁶ or greater
Sperm morphology	15% or greater
Sperm viability	75% or greater viable sperm
WBCs	<1 million/ml

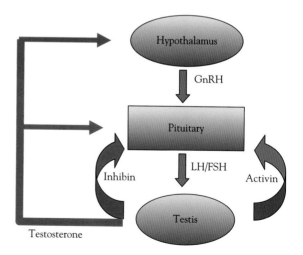

Figure 15.1. *Diagram of the hypothalamic–pituitary–testis axis. GnRH, gonadotropin releasing hormone; LH, luteinizing hormone; FSH, follicle stimulating hormone.*

into the portal system, which leads to the pituitary gland. The anterior pituitary in turn secretes LH and FSH which diffuse into the bloodstream and act at the level of the testes. LH stimulates Leydig cells to secrete testosterone, and FSH acts on the Sertoli cells to stimulate spermatogenesis. Negative feedback occurs via testosterone at the levels of the hypothalamus and pituitary to regulate testosterone and sperm production. Additional feedback to the pituitary is supported by Sertoli cell production of inhibin and activin, suppressing and stimulating FSH production, respectively.

In the present era, it is unclear what the endocrine evaluation should entail or on whom it should be performed. Sigman and Jarow noted a hormonal etiology for male infertility in 3% of patients, but the assessment for hypoandrogenism used in the study is not currently in common use.[5] At present, we recommend a morning testosterone assay for all patients, and an FSH for men with azoospermia.[6] Patients with erectile dysfunction or decreased libido are particularly likely to have hypoandrogenism.[7,8] Computational techniques may allow a more accurate prediction of which patients have a significant endocrine abnormality based on sperm count, testis volume, and percentage of motile sperm.[9] If the testosterone level is found to be low in the initial screen, LH and prolactin levels should be determined to characterize further the hormonal etiology.

Genetic evaluation

A genetic etiology may be found in up to 12% of infertile men who have azoospermia or severe oligospermia, but the incidence according to geographic region is highly variable.[10] According to guidelines from the American Urological Association and the American Society for Reproductive Medicine, genetic screening should be considered in infertile men presenting with sperm counts of less than 5 million/mL or non-obstructive azoospermia who are considering advanced reproductive techniques. Patients with at least one absent vas deferens or a family history suggestive of other infertility-associated syndromes should be offered genetic screening.

Genetic screening for male infertility may include a karyotype analysis, Y chromosome microdeletion

analysis, and gene mutation analysis for specific genes associated with infertility. A karyotype analysis identifies patients with ultrastructural DNA changes or supranumerary chromosomes, such as those seen in Klinefelter's syndrome. Y chromosome microdeletions represent the most common molecular abnormality found in infertile men.[11] Three loci on the long arm of the Y chromosome involved in spermatogenesis, designated azoospermia factor (AZF)a, AZFb, and AZFc, are the most common sites of microdeletions found. Further, it has been shown that longer segments of microdeletion confer a poorer rate of sperm retrieval for in vitro fertilization (IVF).[12] Finally, specific gene mutation analyses are used to identify several clinically relevant genetic abnormalities among the many genes involved in sexual development. The most commonly detected are mutations in the CFTR, androgen receptor, insulin like factor-3, and leucine rich repeat containing G protein coupled receptor 8 genes.[13]

Klinefelter's syndrome (47, XXY) occurs in 0.1–0.2% of all newborn males and is found in 10% of infertile men with azoospermia.[13,14] Primary testicular failure is among the phenotypic abnormalities found in patients with Klinefelter's syndrome and is characterized by increased gonadotropins and small, firm testicles. Historically, hypogonadism was treated with testosterone replacement, but the reproductive outlook remained poor until the advent of newer advanced reproductive techniques. Currently, men with Klinefelter's syndrome may achieve reproductive success with intracytoplasmic sperm injection (ICSI).[13]

Treatment

The treatment of male infertility begins with the identification of a medically or surgically correctable etiology. Surgically treatable causes of male factor infertility discussed here include varicocele, ductal obstruction, and certain congenital anomalies. In addition, medical causes such as hormonal abnormalities and certain immunological conditions will be included. Other key issues in the decision algorithm include maternal age and overall cost. In cases of advanced maternal age, one must consider that conception may not occur for up to a year after treatment of the male factor. These patients, therefore, may be counseled to pursue immediate advanced reproductive techniques rather than surgical treatment. The cost of treatment is another important consideration, since the majority of infertility treatments and advanced reproductive techniques are not covered by health insurance.[15] Overall, when considering the cost of advanced reproductive techniques, the expense generated by correcting the male infertility factor is often more cost-effective.[8]

Varicocele

A varicocele is a dilatation and tortuosity of the spermatic veins within the pampiniform plexus. This condition is found in 19% of healthy young men and up to 40% of men presenting with infertility.[8,16] The mechanism behind the harmful effect on spermatogenesis and testicular volume remains unknown, but is likely to be due to a combination of increased testicular temperature, reflux of adrenal and renal metabolites from the renal vein, hypoxia, and decreased testicular blood flow. Only varicoceles identified by palpation or those that are visible are clinically significant. A non-palpable varicocele that is demonstrated only on radiographic assessment such as ultrasonography is highly unlikely to contribute to male reproductive dysfunction.

The most common abnormalities seen on semen analysis in men with varicoceles are decreased sperm motility and concentration. After surgical repair, improvements in sperm motility are most common, though increased sperm concentrations may be noted as well. The indication for surgical correction in adolescents remains controversial, but most agree that a clinically detected varicocele with ipsilateral testicular hypotrophy should be repaired for potential preservation of fertility.[16] A recent study has shown significantly decreased sperm motility and concentration in adolescents with a varicocele and 10% volume discrepancy between testicles.[17] Adolescents in this group should at least undergo routine semen analysis to ensure stability of sperm parameters. Relative indications for varicocele repair in adolescents include grade 3 varicocele without testicular hypotrophy, palpable varicocele in a solitary testis, or an abnormal semen analysis in an

otherwise normally developed adolescent. In adult, infertile men, on the other hand, varicocelectomy is recommended for those with at least one abnormal semen parameter on semen analysis and a palpable varicocele. Studies have shown improved pregnancy rates and a decreased need for advanced reproductive techniques in this population of men.[18,19]

Several options are available for the surgical correction of varicocele, including open or laparoscopic repair and the use of radiographically injected sclerotic or embolic agents. The main objective of any operation is to ligate the spermatic veins while preserving the testicular artery. An inguinal or subinguinal approach, with or without the use of an operating microscope, is the most common approach. Complication and recurrence rates are minimized with the use of microsurgical techniques by preserving lymphatics and the testicular artery. Percutaneous embolization and sclerotherapy techniques are currently in practice at many institutions, and are associated with relatively good success rates with somewhat decreased postoperative discomfort.

Reversal of vasectomy

Predictors of success following vasectomy reversal are important to the discussion of this option, especially in those couples with advanced maternal age. A time interval less than 8 years from vasectomy to reversal and the intraoperative finding of motile sperm in the vas are the best predictors of success following vasectomy reversal.[20] If no sperm are noted in the fluid emerging from the testicular limb of the vas and the fluid is thick and opaque, obstruction of the epididymis may be present, necessitating an epididymovasostomy.[21]

Success rates vary depending on the time interval from vasectomy to reversal. In a study of 1247 patients undergoing vasectomy reversal, the rates of return of sperm to the semen and pregnancy were 97% and 76%, respectively, if the obstructive interval was less than 3 years, 88% and 53% if 3–8 years, 79% and 44% if 9–14 years, and 71% and 30% if longer than 15 years.[22]

Ejaculatory duct obstruction

Ejaculatory duct obstruction may be diagnosed in up to 5% of men presenting with infertility and is most commonly caused by congenital anomalies of the Wolffian and Müllerian ducts, trauma, or inflammation.[23,24] Complete obstruction should be suspected in patients with low ejaculate volume (<1.0 mL), azoospermia, a normal endocrine panel, and absent sperm in a post-ejaculate urinalysis. Fructose, normally secreted by the seminal vesicles, is absent or decreased in the semen of men with ejaculatory duct obstruction and can be assessed as part of the semen analysis. Partial ejaculatory duct obstruction may present with less dramatic abnormalities in the semen analysis. If suspected, a transrectal ultrasound to evaluate for dilated seminal vesicles or ejaculatory duct cysts can add diagnostic information.

The primary surgical treatment for ejaculatory duct obstruction is transurethral resection of the ejaculatory ducts. The verumontanum is resected until the opening of the dilated ejaculatory duct is seen. Care is taken to avoid the bladder neck and external urethral sphincter, and additional incisions may be made using an endoscopic knife to unroof occluding cysts. Some have proposed the use of a balloon dilating device to open the ejaculatory ducts after a resection.[25] Post-operative urine reflux into dilated ducts following resection may lead to recurrent epididymitis, and all patients should be warned of this potential complication prior to proceeding. Overall success rates with this technique have been reported at 60% for improvement in seminal fluid and 20% pregnancy rate.[23,26]

Hypospadias

Hypospadias can be an anatomic cause of infertility in some men because it impairs normal deposition of semen in the vagina. Although correction is often performed in childhood, patients may present in adulthood. Surgical correction can restore fertility, but intrauterine insemination is an alternative solution for affected couples. These patients should also be evaluated for a hormonal abnormality since this may be present in a small subset of these patients.[27]

Peyronie's disease

Peyronie's disease is an acquired curvature of the penis resulting from abnormal plaque formation within the cavernosal tissue. The etiology of this plaque formation is unknown, and is often not related to penile trauma. An inability to penetrate the vagina or penile pain may become a factor in male fertility. Surgical correction can be performed with a plication procedure or the use of a graft. However, intrauterine insemination may also be a viable alternative among affected couples.

Advanced reproductive techniques

Among the most dramatic advances in the management of male factor infertility have been in the development of advanced reproductive techniques. These techniques include IVF, ICSI, intrauterine insemination (IUI), and various forms of microsurgical sperm acquisition. A complete description of advanced reproductive techniques is beyond the scope of this chapter, but the most commonly employed techniques are described.

IUI is the most frequently used advanced reproductive techniques worldwide and has been shown to yield a three-fold increase in the probability of conception among couples with persistent infertility.[28] The technique involves the use of a small catheter to inject sperm into the uterus, thus bypassing the cervix. This technique may be especially helpful to couples in whom the male infertility factor is identified to be anatomic in nature, such as severe hypospadias, erectile dysfunction, or ejaculatory dysfunction. Other indications include female factors such as painful intercourse or anatomic abnormalities. The technique of ovarian hyperstimulation is often combined with IUI; however, this has not been shown to have an added benefit in couples with a low sperm count (<10 million motile sperm).[28]

IVF has become a mainstay of infertility treatment when other therapies are unsuccessful.[29] The combination with ICSI has provided pregnancies in couples previously considered 'infertile', and it is more commonly employed in younger women.[15] The greatest hurdle to this technology is the logistical and financial strain placed on couples. The woman must undergo hormone injections, and frequent ultrasound examination, and she may require more than one IVF cycle. The cost of IVF is roughly US$10 000–US$20 000, and even higher when

ICSI is employed.[15] Data from the Society for Assisted Reproductive Technology (SART) and the US Centers for Disease Control and Prevention (CDC), regarding 94 242 IVF cycles initiated in 2004, indicate that 36 760 live births resulted from these cycles, with a pregnancy rate and live birth rate of 34% and 28%, respectively, per cycle.[30] For couples with severe male factor infertility, the use of ICSI has improved the success rates of IVF to levels similar to those achieved among couples with normal male fertility status.[29]

The techniques of microsurgical sperm retrieval have developed in parallel with the increasing utilization of ICSI. Patients previously thought to have no hope of fertility, such as those with Klinefelter's syndrome, have been helped to achieve paternity.[31] In patients with obstructive azoospermia, sperm can be retrieved with techniques such as microsurgical epididymal sperm aspiration and percutaneous sperm aspiration. In men with non-obstructive azoospermia or primary testicular failure, testicular biopsy is required to retrieve sperm from seminiferous tissue for subsequent use in advanced reproductive techniques. Ramasamy and Schlegel described a microsurgical technique that may obtain sperm from men with non-obstructive azoospermia in cases where multiple biopsies are negative.[32] Pretreatment with clomiphene citrate may improve the chances of obtaining sperm surgically in men with spermatogenic dysfunction.[33]

Non-surgical causes of male infertility and their treatments

Specific medical therapies are available for several recognized etiologies of male infertility, and empiric therapies are available for cases of idiopathic infertility. For cases of hypogonadotrophic hypogonadism, such as in Kallman's syndrome, treatment is aimed at gonadotropin replacement. This is accomplished with human chorionic gonadotropin as an LH analog, human menopausal gonadotropin as an LH and FSH analog, or purified FSH. A more cumbersome and expensive alternative is pulsatile GnRH, which can closely mimic normal physiology.[34] Hypothyroidism has been recognized as a cause of male infertility, and thyroid replacement

may restore fertility in these individuals.[35] Androgen excess, most commonly from exogenous testosterone or anabolic steroid abuse, can be corrected with withdrawal of the agent.[36]

Occasionally, prolactin excess is found as an etiology in cases of male infertility. Magnetic resonance imaging of the brain should be employed to rule out pituitary tumor in such patients. In cases of idiopathic hyperprolactinemia, dopaminergic agonists such as bromocriptine and cabergoline may be used to normalize prolactin levels.[35] Estrogen excess secondary to morbid obesity or liver dysfunction may be identified as an etiology of male infertility, and treatment is aimed at correcting the underlying cause.

Men with idiopathic infertility may undergo non-specific medical therapy in an effort to improve semen parameters. Clomiphene citrate, a synthetic antiestrogen, has been used in many cases of idiopathic infertility to increase production of testosterone and gonadotropins. Success in stimulating the production of testosterone has been demonstrated, though increased pregnancy rates have not been shown.[34] Recent data, however, suggest there may be a role for clomiphene citrate in augmenting spermatogenesis prior to testis biopsy.[33]

Conclusion

Male factor infertility is often a treatable condition when the etiology is correctly identified. A thorough history and physical examination can often elucidate the abnormality and allow for goal-directed therapy. Recent developments in advanced reproductive techniques may allow couples with severe, intractable male factor infertility to achieve conception.

References

1. Carlsen E, Petersen JH, Anderson AM, Skakkebaek NE. Effects of ejaculatory frequency and season on variations in semen quality. Fertil Steril 2004; 82: 358–66.
2. World Health Organization. WHO Laboratory Manual for the Examination of Human Semen and

Sperm–Cervical Mucus Interaction. New York: Cambridge University Press, 1999.

3. Jarow JP, Espeland MA, Lipshultz LI. Evaluation of the azoospermic patient. J Urol 1989; 142: 62–5.

4. Ratbi I, Legendre M, Niel F et al. Detection of cystic fibrosis transmembrane conductance regulator (CFTR) gene rearrangements enriches the mutation spectrum in congenital bilateral absence of the vas deferens and impacts on genetic counselling. Hum Reprod 2007; 22: 1285–91.

5. Sigman M, Jarow JP. Endocrine evaluation of infertile men. Urol 1997; 50: 659–64.

6. Schoor RA, Elhanbly S, Niederberger CS, Ross LS. The role of testicular biopsy in the modern management of male infertility. J Urol 2002; 167: 197–200.

7. Sharlip ID, Jarow JP, Belker AM et al. Best practice policies for male infertility. Fertil Steril 2002; 77: 873–82.

8. Shefi S, Turek PJ. Definition and current evaluation of subfertile men. Int Braz J Urol 2006; 32: 385–97.

9. Powell CR, Desai RA, Makhlouf AA et al. Computational models for detection of endocrinopathy in subfertile males. Int J Impot Res 2008; 20: 79–84. Epub 2007 Aug 23.

10. De Braekeleer M, Dao TN. Cytogenetic studies in male infertility: a review. Hum Reprod 1991; 6: 245–50.

11. Foresta C, Moro E, Ferlin A. Y chromosome microdeletions and alterations of spermatogenesis. Endocr Rev 2001; 22: 226–329.

12. Hopps CV, Mielnik A, Goldstein M et al. Detection of sperm in men with Y chromosome microdeletions of the AZFa, AZFb and AZFc regions. Hum Reprod 2003; 18: 1660–5.

13. Ferlin A, Raicu F, Gatta V et al. Male infertility: role of genetic background. Reprod Biomed Online 2007; 14: 734–45.

14. Foresta C, Garolla A, Bartoloni L, Bettella A, Ferlin A. Genetic abnormalities among severely oligospermic men who are candidates for intracytoplasmic sperm injection. J Clin Endocr Metab 2005; 90: 152–6.

15. Meacham RB, Joyce GF, Wise M, Kparker A, Niederberger C (Urologic Diseases in America Project). Male infertility. J Urol 2007; 177: 2058–66.

16. Cayan S, Woodhouse CRJ. The treatment of adolescents presenting with a varicocele. BJU Int 2007; 100: 744–7.

17. Diamond DA, Zurakowski D, Bauer SB et al. Relationship of varicocele grade and testicular hypotrophy to semen parameters in adolescents. J Urol 2007; 178: 1584–8.

18. Marmar JL, Agarwal A, Prabakaran S et al. Reassessing the value of varicocelectomy as a treatment for male subfertility with a new meta-analysis. Fertil Steril 2007; 88: 639–48.

19. Cayan S, Erdemir F, Ozbey I et al. Can varicocelectomy significantly change the way couples use assisted reproductive technologies. J Urol 2002; 167: 1749–52.

20. Yang G, Walsh TJ, Shefi S, Turek PJ. The kinetics of the return of motile sperm to the ejaculate after vasectomy reversal. J Urol 2007; 177: 2272–6.

21. The Practice Committee of the American Society for Reproductive Medicine. Vasectomy reversal. Fertil Steril 2006; 86: S268–71.

22. Belker AM, Thomas AJ Jr, Fuchs EF, Konnak JW, Sharlip ID. Results of 1,469 microsurgical vasectomy reversals by the Vasovasostomy Study Group. J Urol 1991; 145: 505–11.

23. Pryor JP, Hendry WF. Ejaculatory duct obstruction in subfertile males: analysis of 87 patients. Fertil Steril 1991; 56: 725–30.

24. Jarow JP. Transrectal ultrasonography in the diagnosis and management of ejaculatory duct obstruction. J Androl 1996; 17: 467–72.

25. Schlegel PN. Is assisted reproduction the optimal treatment for varicocele-associated male infertility? A cost-effectiveness analysis. Urol 1997; 49: 83–90.

26. Meacham RB, Hellerstein DK, Lipshultz LI. Evaluation and treatment of ejaculatory duct obstruction in the infertile male. Fertil Steril 1993; 59: 393–7.

27. Rey RA, Codner E, Iniguez G et al. Low risk of impaired testicular Sertoli and Leydig cell functions in boys with isolated hypospadias. J Clin Endocr Metab 2005; 90: 6035–40.

28. Cantineau AEP, Cohlen BJ, Heineman MJ. Ovarian stimulation protocols (anti-oestrogens, gonadotropins with and without GnRH agonists/antagonists) for intrauterine insemination (IUI) in women with subfertility. Cochrane Database Syst Rev 2007; 2: CD 005356.

29. Goldberg JM, Falcone T, Attaran M. In vitro fertilization update. Clev Clin J Med 2007; 74: 329–38.

30. Wright VC, Chang J, Jeng G et al. Centers for Disease Control and Prevention. Assisted Reproductive Technology Surveillance – United States, 2004. MMWR Surveill Summ 2007; 56: 1–22. Erratum in: MMWR Morb Mortal Wkly Rep 2007; 56: 658.

31. Schoor RA, Elhanbly S, Niederberger CS, Ross LS. The role of testicular biopsy in the modern

management of male infertility. J Urol 2002; 167: 197–200.

32. Ramasamy R, Schlegel PN. Microdissection testicular sperm extraction: effect of prior biopsy on success of sperm retrieval. J Urol 2007; 177: 1447–9.

33. Hussein A, Ozgok Y, Ross L, Niederberger C. Clomiphene administration for cases of nonobstructive asoospermia: a multicenter study. J Androl 2005; 26: 787–91.

34. Schiff JD, Ramirez ML, Bar-Chama NB. Medical and surgical management of male infertility. Endocr Metab Clin North Am 2007; 36: 313–31.

35. Siddiq FM, Sigman M. A new look at the medical management of infertility. Urol Clin North Am 2002; 29: 949–63.

36. Nudell DM, Monoski MM, Lipshultz LI. Common medications and drugs: how they affect male fertility. Urol Clin North Am 2002; 29: 965–73.

CHAPTER 16

Effects of testosterone replacement therapy on the prostate in the aging male

Michael G Kirby, Melanie E Cunningham, Frances Bunn

Introduction

There is an increasing interest in the use of testosterone replacement therapy (TRT) for late-onset hypogonadism (LOH). Mean testosterone values can decline by as much as 50% between the ages of 25 and 75.[1] This results in 20% of men being androgen-deficient by the age of 60, increasing to 40% by the age of 80 (Fig. 16.1).[2] Clinically, this can lead to symptoms, including fatigue, depression, impaired memory, poor concentration, and loss of muscle mass and sexual vigor.[3] TRT has been found to be of use in decreasing the severity of these symptoms;[4] however, there remain considerable concerns regarding the potential long-term effect of such treatment, particularly on the prostate. Concerns about TRT on the prostate stem from knowledge that medical or surgical castration in prostate cancer patients can lead to delayed disease progression, at least initially. Therefore, it has been suggested that increasing testosterone could lead to an over-expression of prostate cancer or other prostate-related diseases such as benign prostate hyperplasia (BPH) and associated lower urinary tract symptoms (LUTS).

This chapter aims to provide a brief outline of the rationale for TRT in the aging male, to address the concerns regarding effects of TRT on the prostate, and to give a brief description of the recommendations for the pre- and post-treatment assessment of prostate safety.

Clinical rationale for TRT in the aging male

The term 'male climacteric' was first coined by Werner in 1939.[5] Hellers and Myers in 1944 described a symptom complex, reversed by testosterone replacement but not by placebo, seen in men suffering from an age-associated decline in testosterone concentrations. The symptoms described in the male climacteric syndrome were depression, nervousness, flushes and sweats, decreased libido, erectile dysfunction, fatigue, and poor concentration and memory.[6]

Since then, this group of symptoms has been referred to as the 'male menopause', or 'andropause'. Yet this comparison to the female menopause is incorrect in that there is no discontinuity in the reproductive lives of men and the decline in testosterone levels is not absolute or inevitable. Recently, other terms such as androgen deficiency in the aging male (ADAM), the viropause, and LOH have come into being. The reduction in testosterone in the aging male is though to be due to a decrease in hypothalamic–pituitary function or a depletion of Leydig cell mass, or both. Although most men will experience a gradual and progressive decline in serum testosterone levels of about 1% per year after the age of 30,[7] inter-individual variability is significant and some men will have larger reductions than others. As such, not all men will become clinically hypogonadal or express symptoms of hypogonadism.

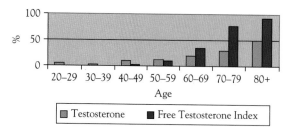

Figure 16.1. *Hypogonadism in the aging male. From Harman et al., 2001.*[2]

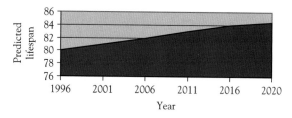

Figure 16.2. *Predicted lifespan for men, 1996–2020. From Morales and Lunenfeld, 2002.*[8]

For example, testosterone levels can be influenced by past and concurrent illnesses, heredity, lifestyle, or medication. Hypogonadism has been defined as 'a biochemical syndrome associated with advancing aging and characterized by a deficiency in serum androgen levels with or without a decreased genomic sensitivity to androgens. It may result in significant alterations in the quality of life and adversely affect the function of multiple organ systems.'[8] As the average lifespan of men continues to increase, the potential for age-related hypogonadism can be expected to increase (Fig. 16.2).[9] However, people are generally hoping to enjoy their extended lifespan and do not wish to be limited by poor strength and function, poor memory or depression, or sexual dysfunction. Therefore, it is important to consider the most effective way to treat men with clinically significant LOH.

TRT has been found useful in improving body composition, strength and functional ability, erythrocytosis, cognitive function, sexual function and enjoyment, cardiovascular risk factors (cholesterol, glycemic and insulin status, fat mass, and thrombotic profile), and vasodilatation of the coronary arteries.[10–14]

Yet despite this, few men receive treatment, possibly due to the controversy surrounding risks associated with hormone treatments.[15] The main area of debate surrounds the potential effect of testosterone treatment on rates of prostate cancer and, to a lesser extent, its effects upon the progression of BPH. This debate has been compounded by recent reports demonstrating a link between hormone replacement therapy in women and an increased risk of breast cancer.[16,17] In addition,

knowledge that androgen deprivation can slow the development of prostate cancer and improve other prostate-related symptoms such as BPH-induced LUTS has led to concern regarding the use of long-term TRT in the aging male.

Effects of testosterone on BPH

BPH is the most prevalent disorder of the prostate, affecting 43% of men over their lifetime.[18] BPH requires the presence of androgens to develop, and it regresses with androgen-deprivation therapy.[19] Testosterone is converted by 5-alpha reductase to dihydrotestosterone (DHT), the latter exhibiting a five- to 10-fold greater potency within the prostate. Although plasma androgen levels decline with age, intraprostatic levels of DHT have not been shown to do so and remain relatively constant. Indeed, prostate volume continues to increase with age despite falls in circulating testosterone levels. By inhibiting the effect of DHT on prostatic cellular processes, inhibitors of the enzyme 5-alpha reductase have been shown to reduce prostate volume in men with BPH by almost 30%. Interestingly, some studies have shown that androgen deficiency is associated with smaller prostate volumes and circulating prostate-specific antigen (PSA) levels,[20–24] indicating that significantly low circulating testosterone levels may result in diminished intraprostatic androgen concentrations. The use of TRT in hypogonadal men has been shown in some studies to restore prostate volumes and PSA concentrations, but not to levels beyond those seen in eugonadal men of the same age.[22–25]

One long-term study showed that PSA levels do not continue to increase after 6 months of TRT.[25] A recent study using planimetric prostate ultrasound lent support to hypogonadism being associated with lower PSA levels and prostate volumes; however, when such men were given long-term TRT, prostate volumes did not increase to those of age-matched eugonadal controls, whereas PSA levels did.[26] Androgen use and abuse in eugonadal men, with physiological and supraphysiological doses of androgens, have also not been associated with an increase in PSA levels and prostate volume.[27,28] Prostatic responses to increasing serum androgen levels in terms of cellular proliferation and PSA secretion therefore appear to reach a threshold, supporting a view that intraprostatic mechanisms ultimately control such factors.

With regard to symptoms associated with BPH, TRT has not been shown to exacerbate LUTS; however, data are limited.[25,29–32] A recent study using a testosterone gel preparation in 123 evaluable hypogonadal men over a period of 42 months failed to shown a worsening of LUTS as measured using the International Prostate Symptom Score or urinary flow rates.[25,33]

Effects of testosterone replacement on PSA and prostate cancer risk

The possibility that testosterone may initiate prostate cancer is a major concern and has been a subject of great debate. It has long been recognized that once a cancer is present, testosterone can stimulate its development, and therefore TRT is contraindicated in men with evidence of prostate cancer.

There appears to be no compelling evidence that testosterone has a causative role in prostrate carcinogenesis, and the association between circulating androgen levels and prostatic carcinoma has been the subject of several reviews and papers.[33–36] Slater and Oliver[37] concluded that the link between testosterone and development of prostate cancer was weak and that there are many other factors (including genetic predisposition, diet, infection, and environment) that have an impact on the gland at different stages of life.

A review of 10 prospective epidemiological studies found no evidence that serum levels of endogenous sex hormones were associated with a risk of developing prostate cancer.[38] Three studies published after this review found that higher levels of serum testosterone were indeed associated with a reduced risk of prostate cancer.[39–41] In a recently published large prospective cohort study, high levels of testosterone and adrenal androgens were significantly associated with a reduced risk of aggressive prostate cancer but not of non-aggressive prostate cancer.[42] Conversely, others have reported that low testosterone levels have been associated with aggressive cancer.[43]

A recent review concluded that to date there is no evidence from studies of TRT in hypogonadal men or from prescription event monitoring that testosterone usage is associated with an increased risk of developing prostate cancer above that in a healthy age-matched population.[36] There have been few randomized controlled studies of TRT in hypogonadal men despite the availability of testosterone for the past 70 years. Data from uncontrolled and controlled trials along with a lack of signal from prescription event monitoring would suggest that there is no appreciable risk of inducing prostate cancer with testosterone treatment.[36] A definitive answer, however, is lacking, and it has been estimated that a placebo-controlled trial involving 6000 older men treated for an average of 5 years would be required to detect a statistical difference with adequate power.[44] At present no plans exist to conduct such a study and therefore the answer to whether TRT causes prostate cancer will continue to elude us.

Monitoring before and after TRT

Guidelines exist for the diagnosis and management of LOH; those from the International Society for the Study of the Aging Male have been utilized in the production of the tripartite recommendations of the International Society of Andrology, the International Society for the Study of the Aging Male, and the European Association of Urology.[45,46] US guidelines also exist, having been produced by the American Association of Clinical

Table 16.1. *Study reports of increases in BPH, LUTS, PSA or prostate cancer*

Study	Methods	Outcome	Testosterone dose and route		Results
Bakhashi et al. (2000)[50]	Double-blind RCT Length of follow-up: 8 weeks	Rehabilitation in ill older males	Testosterone enanthate 100 mg IM vs placebo	15 males (T=9, C=6) Age range: 65–90 Mean age: T, 78.3±5.6; C, 75.7±5.3	PSA/cancer incidence: N/S changes (i.e elevation in PSA >4.5 ng/dl or symptoms of obstructive uropathy)
Carani et al. (1990)	Double-blind RCT Length of follow-up: 6 months	Erectile dysfunction	Dehydroepian drosterone 50 mg daily vs placebo	40 males (T=20, C=20) Mean age: 56.5 (41–69)	PSA/cancer incidence: N/S changes Sexual function: significant effects in improved erectile function, intercourse satisfaction, sexual desire and overall satisfaction ($p<0.001$) and orgasmic function ($p<0.01$)
Cherrier et al. (2001)[51]	Double-blind RCT Length of follow-up: 6 weeks	Spatial and verbal memory	Testosterone enanthate 100 mg IM vs placebo	28 entered the trial, 25 completed follow-up Mean age: T, 65; C, 70	PSA: levels significantly increased at week 4 compared with baseline, ($F_{[2,21]}=5.54$). Returned to normal at follow-up
English et al. (2000)[52]	Double-blind RCT Length of follow-up: 14 weeks	Angina thresholds	Testosterone patch (two 2.5 mg patches daily) vs placebo	53 entered (mean age 62), 46 completed follow-up (T=22, C=24)	PSA/cancer incidence: N/S changes
Gerstenbluth et al. (2002)[53]	Retrospective analysis Length of follow-up (mean): 30.2 months	PSA in hypogonadal men receiving TRT	Testosterone IM injection every 2–4 weeks	54 men aged 42–76 (mean 60.4)	PSA: 6 men required prostate biopsy because of raised PSA >4.0 ng/ml; 1 developed prostate cancer; result N/S increase in risk of prostate cancer

Study	Design	Objective	Intervention	Participants	Results
Hajjar et al. (1997)[29]	Retrospective analysis Length of follow-up: 2 years	Body composition and sexual function	Testosterone enanthate or testosterone cypionate 200 mg IM vs no intervention	72 male participants (T=45 entered, 26 completed follow-up; C=27 entered, 23 completed follow-up) Mean age: T=69.9±1.9, C=71.8±1.7 years	PSA/cancer incidence: N/S changes 14 participants (31.1%) in the treatment group withdrew from testosterone treatment within the 2 years Reasons for withdrawal: no improvement: 5; gynecomastia: 1; reaction at injection site: 1; sleep apnea: 1; inconvenience: 1; concern about side effects: 2; loss to follow-up: 3
Holmang et al. (1993)[54]	Double-blind RCT Length of follow-up: 8 months	Effect of testosterone on prostate volume and PSA	Testosterone undecanoate 160 mg vs placebo	25 males (T=11, C=8) Age range 40–65, median 52	PSA/cancer incidence: N/S changes
Jin et al. (2001)[26]	Pair-matched clinical trial	Effect of androgen replacement on prostate zonal volumes	Testosterone implants (n = 27), ester injections (n = 24), other treatment (n = 3), no treatment (n=17)	71 men aged 18–78 (mean 40±2), compared with age-matched healthy pairs	PSA: concentrations were significantly lower among men with untreated androgen deficiency. PSA concentrations in treated androgen deficiency were higher than those with untreated androgen deficiency ($p=0.078$), but similar to that of age-matched controls ($p=0.35$) BPH: N/S changes
Kenny et al. (2001)[55]	RCT Length of follow-up: 1 year	Assess bone and muscle mass	Transdermal testosterone patches (two 2.5 mg patches) vs placebo patches	76 hypogonadal men aged 65–87 (mean 76 ±4) were randomized; 44 men completed the trial	PSA/ cancer incidence: N/S changes ($p=0.09$) BPH: N/S changes IPSS: N/S changes

(Continued)

Table 16.1. *(Continued)*

Study	Methods	Outcome	Testosterone dose and route		Results
Márin et al. (1993)[30]	Double-blind RCT Length of follow-up: 9 months	Effects on abdominal obesity	Group 1; Testogel 5g; group 2: Andractim 5g; group 3: placebo gel	31 men aged 40 or above (mean 57.7±2.1) Numbers per treatment arm not recorded	PSA/ cancer incidence: N/S changes LUTS: N/S changes BPH: N/S changes
McNicholas et al. (2003)[56]	RCT Length of follow-up: 60 days	Body composition and sexual function	Testim patch 50 mg/day, Testim patch 100 mg/day, or Andropatch two 2.5 mg patches/day	208 men Mean age 57.9 years Testim 50: 68 participants, Testim 100 mg: 72 participants; Andropatch: 68 participants	Sexual function: all three groups improved in relation to sexual motivation, desire, and performance Men receiving Testim 100 mg had twice the incidence of spontaneous erections than at baseline Testim was significantly better than Andropatch at 30 days ($p \leq 0.05$) PSA/cancer incidence: N/S changes
Park et al. (2003)[57]	Placebo-controlled clinical trial, single-blinded Length of follow-up: 3 months	Quality of life, including sexual function as primary outcome	Testosterone undecanoate (Andriol) 80 mg orally, twice daily	39 men entered, 35 completed Age not documented NB: 7 men had primary hypogonadism and 26 had secondary hypogonadism T=33, C=6	N/S changes The overall improvement in sexual function from baseline was 43.9% better in the group treated with testosterone ($p=<0.05$)
Pope et al. (2003)[31]	RCT Length of follow-up: 8 weeks	Depressive symptoms	1% testosterone gel vs placebo gel	22 men aged 30–65 (mean T, 48.9, mean C, 49.5) T=12 (10 completed follow-up), C=10 (9 completed follow-up)	PSA/cancer incidence: N/S changes LUTS: 1 withdrawal because of LUTS, otherwise N/S BPH: N/S changes

Study	Design	Purpose	Intervention	Participants	PSA/ cancer incidence
Rhoden and Morgentaler (2003)[58]	Retrospective analysis. Length of follow-up: 1 year	PIN (to see if PIN-positive patients are at higher risk of prostate cancer)	Testosterone enanthate IM vs patch	75 men aged 42–77 (mean 59.6±9.0)	PSA/ cancer incidence: N/S changes
Sih et al. (1997)[59]	RCT. Length of follow-up: 1 year	12 month trial of TRT	Testosterone cypionate (200 mg) IM every 14–17 days for 12 months or placebo	32 men aged 51–79 (mean 65±1.2) T=17, C=15	PSA did not change significantly compared with controls over the study period. Baseline PSA: T, 1.0±0.2; C, 1.5±0.4. Completion PSA: T, 1.9±0.3; C, 2.0±0.4. No changes were detected on DRE
Swerloff and Wang (2003)[60]	Randomized, multi-center, parallel study. Length of follow-up: 3 years (This is an initial conclusions paper, not a full report)	TRT	Androgel 5g/day, 7.5g/day, vs 10g/day	163 men were randomized, 122 were evaluated. Two age groups were evaluated: 19–57 (mean 47.5) and 60–67 (mean 63)	PSA: significant increase in PSA levels at 36 months from baseline measurements (0.37 ng/ml); 7 participants had rises above 5.5 ng/dl (in 2, this was transient). 1 stopped testosterone treatment and PSA normalized; 1 was found to have prostatitis, which was treated and PSA resolved; 2 developed prostate cancer; and 1 developed PBH – all found through rises in PSA. Sexual function: treatment group reported improved sexual desire, enjoyment, percentage total erections, and self-assessed satisfaction with erections
Snyder et al. (1999)[61]	Double-blind RCT. Length of follow-up: 36 months	Effects of TRT on bone mineral density in men over 65	Testogel patch 6mg vs placebo gel patch	108 men randomized, 96 completed. Mean age 73 T=54, C=54	16 participants in the treatment arm and 11 in the placebo arm had clinically significant prostate events. PSA: T=10 transient rises, C=6 transient rises, 1 prostate cancer. There were significant changes in PSA in the testosterone-treated group ($p<0.001$)

(Continued)

Table 16.1. *(Continued)*

Study	Methods	Outcome	Testosterone dose and route		Results
Tan and Pu (2003)[62]	Clinical pilot study	Effects of testosterone on Alzheimer's disease	Testosterone 200 mg IM every 2 weeks	10 men Mean age: 72.4 (range: 68–80) T=5, C=5	PSA: N/S changes (*p*=0.07) Sexual function: 1 patient withdrawn because of hypersexual behavior
Tenover (1992)[63]	Randomized cross-over trial Length of follow-up: 6 months	Effects of testosterone on the aging male	Testosterone enanthate IM vs placebo	13 men aged 57–76 (mean 67.5±1.5) T=7, C=6	PSA levels increased significantly in the treatment group from 2.1±0.4 to 2.7±0.5 ng/ml (*p*=0.01) Testosterone supplementation resulted in a significant decrease in urinary excretion of hydroxyproline (*p*=0.001): baseline, 151±10; placebo, 142±13; treatment, 108±8 BPH: N/S changes

BPH, benign prostatic hyperplasia; LUTS, lower urinary tract symptoms; PSA, prostate-specific antigen; RCT, randomized controlled trial; TRT, testosterone replacement therapy; PIN, prostate intraepithelial neoplasia; IM, intramuscular; T, treatment group; C, control group; N/S, not significant; DRE, digital rectal examination.

Endocrinologists.[47] Both sets of guidelines stress the importance of a biochemical diagnosis as well as a symptomatic complaint, and both discuss contra-indications to treatment and the assessment and monitoring of patients before and after the start of treatment. Of importance is the issue of excluding prostate cancer prior to therapy and monitoring of prostate status thereafter. Using conventional screening tools, exclusion of the presence of cancer is never absolute but investigation by digital rectal examination (DRE) and PSA level analysis are considered essential. Using conventional PSA cut-off values may be inadequate, since not only can prostate cancer be present in a proportion of men with PSA levels below 4 ng/ml, but also men with LOH frequently have lower PSA levels than healthy age-matched controls, thereby begging the question of whether cut-off values should be reduced in such men before treatment or further investigation for prostate cancer is contemplated. In one study of 77 hypogonadal men with a mean age of 58 years, PSA values of 4 ng/mL or less, and non-suspicious DRE, 14% had prostate cancer on prostate biopsy prior to planned treatment with testosterone. This figure rose to 29% when data for men over 60 were analyzed. Gleason scores for all cancers were 6 or 7. The authors suggest that findings on DRE and PSA levels are insensitive indicators of prostate cancer in men with low total or free testosterone levels.[48] Owing to these problems with PSA testing, some routinely perform transrectal ultrasound (TRUS)-guided prostate biopsy on men with LOH prior to initiating TRT.[49] This practice is questionable, owing to the substantial overall negative biopsy rate; it is, however, imperative that, if doubt exists as to the presence or not of malignancy, further opinion should be sought and further investigation should be undertaken. Other measures may be considered prior to treatment, such as taking into consideration the pre-treatment ratio of free-to-total PSA, or the assessment of PSA density if prostate volume has been recorded through TRUS. Prostate safety needs to be evaluated after initiation of TRT through DRE and PSA testing every 3 months during the first year of treatment and yearly thereafter. TRUS-guided biopsies of

the prostate are indicated only if the DRE or serum PSA levels are abnormal.[46]

Summary

There is currently no significant evidence to indicate that testosterone replacement should be withheld on the grounds that it increases the risk of LUTS or BPH, causes a significant rise in PSA value, or induces prostate cancer. The findings of studies in this area are summarized in Table 16.1. However, within this rubric there is the acknowledgement that further long-term research is required to consolidate current evidence and draw informed conclusions. Such information is not forthcoming and no proposed studies are in planning to help answer the question.

Any patient considering testosterone therapy should be counseled as to the possible association between testosterone and prostate cancer but that definitive evidence is lacking. When patients are treated with testosterone and regularly reviewed, there is an opportunity to detect important prostate cancer at an early stage when it is potentially curable.

References

1. Matsumoto AM. Fundamental aspects of hypogonadism in the aging male. Rev Urol 2003; 5(Suppl 1): S3–S10.
2. Harman SM, Metter EJ, Tobin JD et al. Longitudinal effects of aging on serum and free testosterone levels in healthy men: Baltimore Longitudinal Study of Aging. J Clin Endocrinol Metab 2001; 86: 724–31.
3. Heaton JPW. Hormone treatments and preventative strategies in the aging male: whom and when to treat? Rev Urol 2003; 5(Suppl 1): S16–21.
4. Gooren L. Testosterone supplementation: why and for whom? Aging Male 2003; 6: 184–99.
5. Werner AA. The male climacteric. JAMA 1939; 112: 1441–3.
6. Heller CG, Myers GB. The male climacteric, its symptomatology, diagnosis and treatment. JAMA 1944; 126: 472–7.

7. Gray A, Feldman HA, McKinlay JB et al. Age, disease and changing sex hormone levels in middle-aged men: results of the Massachusetts Male Aging Study. J Clin Endocrinol Metab 1991; 73: 1016–25.

8. Morales A, Lunenfeld B. Investigation, treatment and monitoring of late-onset hypogonadism in males. Official recommendations of the International Society for the Study of the Aging Male. Aging Male 2002; 5: 74–86.

9. Department of Health. National Statistics: Life Expectancy. London: Department of Health, 7 May 2004. [http://www.statistics.gov.uk/cci/nugget.asp?id=881]

10. Webb CM, McNeill JG, Hayward CS et al. Effects of testosterone on coronary vasomotor regulation in men with coronary artery disease. Circulation 1999; 19: 1690–6.

11. Mårin P, Holmang S, Jonsson L et al. The effects of testosterone treatment on body composition and metabolism in middle-aged obese men. Int J Obes Relat Metab Disord 1992; 16: 991–7.

12. Wang C, Swedloff RS, Iranmanesh A et al. Transdermal testosterone gel improves sexual function, mood, muscle strength and body composition parameters in hypogonadal men. J Clin Endocrinol Metab 2000; 85: 2839.

13. Boyanov MA, Boneva Z, Christov VG. Testosterone supplementation in men with type 2 diabetes, visceral obesity and partial androgen deficiency. Aging Male 2003; 6: 1.

14. Mårin P. Testosterone and regional fat distribution. Obes Res 1995; 3(Suppl 4): 609S–12S.

15. Skin Patch Replaces Testosterone. FDA Updates. Rockville, MD: Food and Drug Administration, 1996. [http://www.fda.gov/fdac/departs/196_upd.html]

16. Rossouwe JE, Anderson GL, Prentice RL et al. Risks and benefits of estrogen plus progestin in healthy postmenopausal women: principal results from the Women's Health Initiative randomised controlled trial. JAMA 2002; 288: 321–33.

17. Manson JE, Hsai J, Johnson KC et al. Estrogen plus progestin and the rise of coronary heart disease. N Engl J Med 2003; 349: 523–34.

18. Kirby SR, Kirby MG. Benign and malignant diseases of the prostate. In: Kirby RS, Carson CC, Kirby MG, Farah RN, eds. Men's Health, 2nd edn. London: Taylor and Francis, 2004; 287.

19. Huggins C, Stevens RE, Hodges CV. Studies on prostatic cancer II. The effects of castration on advanced carcinoma of the prostate gland. Arch Surg 1941; 43: 209–23.

20. Canale D, Andreini F, Mais V et al. Ultrasound monitoring of testis and prostate maturation in hypogonadotropic hypogonadic males during gonadotropin-releasing hormone treatment. Fertil Steril 1990; 53: 537–40.

21. Sasagawa I, Nakada T, Kazama T et al. Volume change of the prostate and seminal vesicles in male hypogonadism after androgen therapy. Int Urol Nephrol 1990; 22: 279–84.

22. Behre HM, Bohmeyer J, Nieschlag E. Prostate volume in testosterone-treated and untreated hypogonadal men in comparison to age-matched normal controls. Clin Endocrinol 1994; 40: 341–9.

23. Meikle AW, Stephenson RA, Lewis CM, Middleton RG. Effects of age and sex hormones on transition and peripheral zone volumes of prostate and benign prostatic hyperplasia in twins. J Clin Endocrinol Metab 1997; 82: 571–5.

24. Ozata M, Bulur M, Beyhan Z et al. Effects of gonadotropin and testosterone treatments on prostate volume and serum prostate-specific antigen levels in male hypogonadism. Endocr J 1997; 44: 719–24.

25. Wang C, Cunningham G, Dobs A et al. Long-term testosterone gel (Androgel) treatment maintains beneficial effects on sexual function and mood, lean and fat mass, and bone mineral density in hypogonadal men. J Clin Endocrinol Metab 2004; 89: 2085–98.

26. Jin B, Conway AJ, Handelsman DJ. Effects of androgen deficiency and replacement on prostate zonal volumes. Clin Endocrinol 2001; 54: 437–45.

27. Cooper CS, Perry PJ, Sparks AE et al. Effect of exogenous testosterone on prostate volume, serum and semen prostate specific antigen levels in healthy young men. J Urol 1998; 159: 441–3.

28. Jin B, Turner L, Walters WAW, Handelsman DJ. Androgen or estrogen effects on the human prostate. J Clin Endocrinol Metab 1996; 81: 4290–5.

29. Hajjar RR, Kaiser FE, Morley JE. Outcomes of long-term testosterone replacement in older hypogonadal males: a retrospective analysis. J Endocrinol Metab1997; 82: 3793–6.

30. Mårin, P, Holmang, S, Gustafsson C et al. Androgen treatment of abdominally obese men. Obes Res 1993; 1: 245–51.

31. Pope HG Jr, Cohane GH, Siegel AJ, Hudson JI. Testosterone gel for men with refractory depression: a randomized controlled trial. Am J Psychiatry 2003; 160:105–11.

32. Snyder PJ, Peachey H, Berlin JA et al. Effects of testosterone replacement on bone mineral density

in men over 65 years of age. J Clin Endocrinol Metab 2005; 84: 1966–72.

33. Carter HB, Pearson JD, Metter EJ et al. Longitudinal evaluation of serum androgen levels in men with and without prostate cancer. Prostate 1995; 27: 25–31.

34. Heikkila R, Aho K, Heliovaara M et al. Serum testosterone and sex hormone binding globulin concentrations and the risk of prostate carcinoma: a longitudinal study. Cancer 1999; 86: 312–15.

35. Hsing AW. Hormones and prostate cancer: what's next? Epidemiol Rev 2001; 23: 42–58.

36. Gould DC, Kirby RS. Testosterone replacement threapy for late onset hypogonadism: what is the risk of inducing prostate cancer? Prostate Cancer Prostatic Dis 2006; 9: 14–18.

37. Slater S, Oliver RT. Testosterone: its role in development of prostate cancer and potential risk from use as hormone replacement therapy. Drugs Aging 2000; 17: 431–9.

38. Eaton NE, Reeves GK, Appleby PN et al. Endrogenous sex hormones and prostate cancer: a quantitative review of prospective studies. Br J Cancer 1999; 80: 930–4.

39. Chen C, Weiss NS, Stanczyk FZ et al. Endogenous sex hormones and prostate cancer risk: a case-control study nested within the Carotene and Retinol Efficacy Trial. Cancer Epidemiol Biomarkers Prev 2003; 12: 1410–16.

40. Platz EA, Leitzmann MF, Rifai N et al. Sex steroid hormones and the androgen receptor gene CAG repeat and subsequent risk of prostate cancer in the prostate-specific antigen era. Cancer Epidemiol Biomarkers Prev 2005; 14: 1262–9.

41. Stattin P, Lumme S, Tenkanen L et al. High levels of circulating testosterone are not associated with increased prostate cancer risk: a pooled prospective study. Int J Cancer 2004; 108: 418–24.

42. Severi G, Morris HA, MacInnis RJ et al. Circulating steroid hormones and the risk of prostate cancer. Cancer Epidemiol Biomarkers Prev 2006; 15: 86–91.

43. Hoffman MA, DeWolf WC, Morgentaler A. Is low serum free testosterone a marker for high grade prostate cancer? J Urol 2000; 163: 824–7.

44. Bhasin S, Singh AB, Mac RP et al. Managing the risks of prostate disease during testosterone replacement therapy in older men: recommendations for a standardized monitoring plan. J Androl 2003; 24: 299–311.

45. Morales A, Lunenfeld B. Investigation, treatment and monitoring of late-onset hypogonadism. Aging Male 2002; 5: 74–86.

46. Nieschlag E, Swerdloff R, Behre HM et al. Investigation, treatment and monitoring of late-onset hypogonadism in males: ISA, ISSAM and EAU recommendations. Int J Androl 2005; 28: 125–7.

47. American Association of Clinical Endocrinologists. American Association of Clinical Endocrinologists medical guidelines for clinical practice for the evaluation and treatment of hypogonadism in adult male patients – 2002 update. Endocr Pract 2002; 8: 440–56.

48. Morgentaler A, Bruning CO III, DeWolf WC. Occult prostate cancer in men with low serum testosterone levels. JAMA 1996; 276: 1904–6.

49. Rhoden El, Morgentaler A. Risks of testosterone-replacement therapy and recommendations for monitoring. N Engl J Med 2004; 350: 482–92.

50. Bakhashi V, Elliot M, Gentili A et al. Testosterone improves rehabilitation outcomes in ill older men. J Amer Ger Soc 2000; 48: 550–3.

51. Cherrier MM, Asthana S, Plymate S et al. Testosterone supplementation improves spatial and verbal memory in healthy older men. Neurology 2001; 57: 80–8.

52. English KM, Steeds RP, Jones HT et al. Low-dose transdermal testosterone therapy improves angina threshold in men with chronic stable angina: a randomized, double-blind, placebo-controlled study. Circulation 2000; 102: 1906–11.

53. Gerstenbluth RE, Maniam PN, Corty EW, Seftel AD. Prostate-specific antigen changes in hypogonadal men treated with testosterone replacement. J Androl 2002; 23: 922–6.

54. Holmang S, Mårin P, Lindstedt G, Hedelin H. Effects of long-term oral testosterone undecanoate treatment on prostate volume and serum prostate-specific antigen concentration in eugonadal middle-aged men. Prostate 1993; 23: 99–106.

55. Kenny AM, Prestwood KM, Gruman CA et al. Effects of transdermal testosterone on bone and muscle in older men with low bioavailable testosterone levels. J Gerontol A Biol Sci Med Sci 2001; 56: M266–72.

56. McNicholas TA, Dean JD, Mulder H et al. A novel testosterone gel formulation normalizes androgen levels in hypogonadal men, with improvements in body composition and sexual function. BJU Int 2003; 91: 69–74.

57. Park NC, Yan BQ, Chung JM, Lee KM. Oral testosterone undecanoate (Andriol®) supplement therapy improves the quality of life for men with

testosterone deficiency. Aging Male 2003; 6: 86–93.

58. Rhoden EL, Morgentaler A. Testosterone replacement therapy in hypogonadal men at high risk for prostate cancer: results of 1 year of treatment in men with prostatic intraepithelial neoplasia. J Urol 2003; 170: 2348–51.

59. Sih R, Morley JE, Kaiser FE et al. Testosterone replacement in older hypogonadal men: a 12 month randomised controlled trial. J Clin Endocrinol Metab 1997; 82: 1661–7.

60. Swerloff RS, Wang C. Three year follow-up of androgen treatment in hypogonadal men: preliminary report with testosterone gel. Aging Male 2003; 6: 207–11.

61. Snyder PJ, Peachey H, Hannoush P et al. Effects of testosterone treatment on bone mineral density in men over 65 years of age. J Clin Endocrinol Metab 1999; 84: 1966–72.

62. Tan RS, Pu SJ. A pilot study on the effects of testosterone in hypogonadal aging male patients with Alzheimers disease. Aging Male 2003; 6: 13–7.

63. Tenover JS. Effects of testosterone supplementation in the aging male. J Clin Endocrinol Metab 1992; 75: 1092–8.

CHAPTER 17

Novel approaches to male contraception

RA Anderson

Introduction

The development of a range of effective methods of contraception is an essential element of reproductive health. Female-dependent methods have been the subject of considerable scientific advance as a result of advances in steroid chemistry in the past half century and the development of effective and autonomous contraception, but there has been an emerging emphasis that men should be more involved in family planning.[1] The supremacy of modern, female methods in the developed world obscures the fact that one-third of all couples worldwide rely on a male-dependent method of contraception, mostly the condom or withdrawal, methods that have been used for millennia with only minimal development in recent years. While the development of new effective methods of male contraception has been identified as a high priority by international organizations, including the World Health Organization (WHO),[2,3] and there are both hormonal and non-hormonal methods in advanced clinical trials, the limited involvement of the pharmaceutical industry in this research suggests caution in prophesying the availability of new products in the near future.

Developments in existing methods

Condoms are very widely used by men at some point in their lives, with past usage at up to 90%, higher than any other method in a survey across different cultures.[4] Estimates of the pregnancy rate with condom usage vary greatly according to the population studied. With near-perfect use, pregnancy rates as low as 3% have been reported, although national data probably more closely reflecting typical use show a rate of 14% in the first year.[5] There have also been large increases in the use of condoms over the past 2 decades, associated with increased awareness of HIV and public information campaigns.[6,7] Recent UK data indicate that the proportion of family planning clinic attenders using condoms rose from 6% to 35% over the years 1975 to 2000–2001. Condoms also reduce the risk of sexually transmitted disease, although good-quality data are lacking for many diseases.[8] However, the results of meta-analysis of 12 studies of the potential protective effect of condom usage on HIV transmission that were regarded as sufficiently informative clearly shows a reduction in risk of infection with condom usage of approximately 87%.[9]

The use of new materials for the manufacture of condoms shows advantages in some but not all respects. The polyurethane condom may give better sensitivity than latex but it has slippage and breakage rates up to five times higher.[10] In a randomized trial, two-thirds of both male and female participants preferred one of the synthetic condoms.[11] No information is available regarding protection from sexually transmitted diseases, and there are only limited data on protection from pregnancy.[10]

Some 40–60 million couples in the world depend on vasectomy as their method of contraception;[12] in the UK nearly 30% of couples over 35 years old use vasectomy as their contraceptive method, compared with approximately 20% using female sterilization.[13] Assessment of efficacy is complicated by the marked decline in fertility of older women. Case series by individual surgeons report failure rates of 0–2%, probably an underestimate caused by under-reporting, and there are no prospective studies equivalent to those for female sterilization.[14]

Novel potential approaches to contraception

The male reproductive system offers a number of potential targets for new contraceptives (Fig. 17.1).

However in contrast to the female, millions of mature gametes are produced daily in a continuous process. Spermatogenesis takes approximately 75 days and involves reduction of the chromosome number from 46 to the haploid number of 23 and enormous modification of the round spermatogonium into the elongated, motile spermatozoon. Meiosis occurs only in the gonad in the adult and its careful regulation is indicated by the precisely ordered arrangement of specific stages of development with the Sertoli cell population, each of which can support only a limited number of germ cells. Hence, it should be potentially possible to interfere specifically with key processes unique to the testis – the non-hormonal approach.

One problem with the non-hormonal approach is limited knowledge as to the molecular details of the regulation of spermatogenesis and spermiogenesis

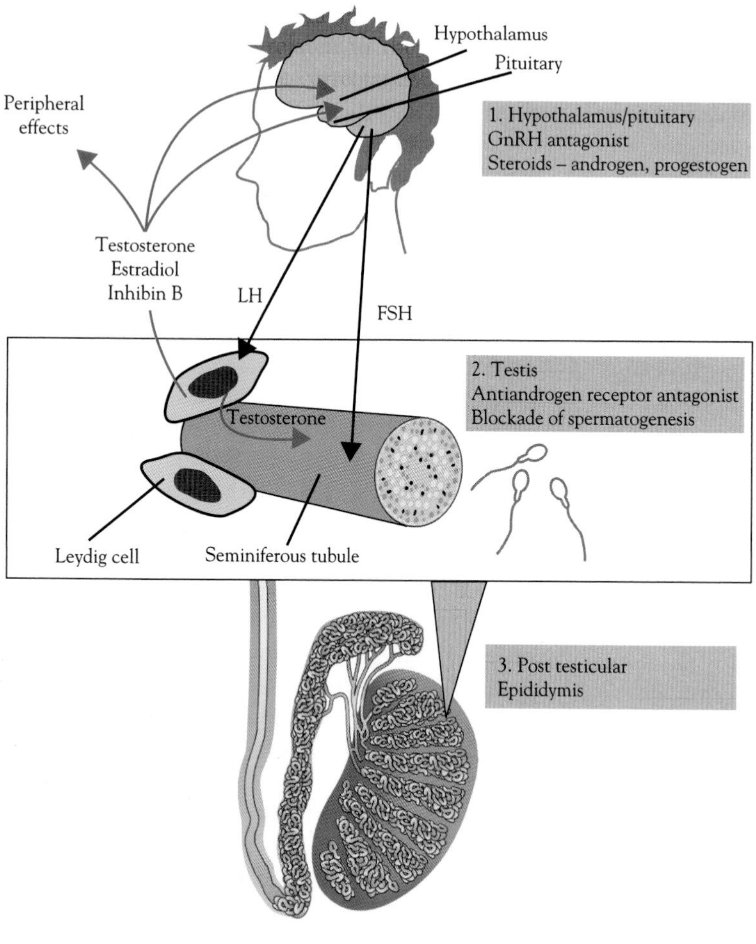

Figure 17.1. *Novel approaches to male contraception.*

(the release of spermatozoa from the Sertoli cells) in the testis and sperm maturation in the epididymis. Thus potential contraceptives have at times been identified serendipitously and when problems (such as with toxicity) are identified, rational approaches to address them can be difficult. One example of how this might be addressed comes from the compound adjudin, which has for many years been know to interfere with adhesion between Sertoli cells and developing germ cells and which results in reversible infertility in animal models.[15] However, cell adhesion in other organs is also affected, resulting in toxicity. This has been strikingly reduced by linking adjudin to a variant of FSH. This allows a much lower dose to be administered, removing the toxicity, while the testicular targeting conferred by the FSH enhances its anti-spermatogenic potency.

An alternative approach is exemplified by the recent identification of a cation channel specific for sperm motility specifically expressed on the sperm tail. Targeted disruption reduced sperm motility and abolished their ability to penetrate the zona pellucida and fertilize the egg but had no other apparent effect.[16] These approaches are some way from clinical investigation.

The non-hormonal methods in clinical trials are not based on targeting the testis, but on preventing sperm getting into the ejaculate. Some of these are effectively a reversible vasectomy with a removable barrier introduced into the vas lumen. A recent randomized trial compared a urethane intravas device (IVD) versus no-scalpel vasectomy in nearly 300 men in China. The IVD was slightly less effective and took a little longer to insert, but postoperative recovery was quicker and satisfaction was scored higher.[17] Long-term failure rates remain to be established. Pressure within the proximal vas is lower than following vasectomy because the IVD acts as a filter rather than a complete plug, which may account for the reduction in complications. More subtly, the RISUG method (reversible inhibition of sperm under guidance) involves injection of a steric acid anhydride compound into the vas.[18] This does not result in luminal obstruction, but destroys the sperm as they pass by damaging the cell membrane. Reversibility can be achieved by injection of a solvent. There are limited clinical data as to its efficacy and duration of action, and reversibility

has thus far only been demonstrated in non-human primates, but the method looks promising at present.

Hormonal contraception

The most widely studied approach, with recent European phase II clinical trials, is the hormonal one. It has been known for over 75 years that normal testicular function is dependent on pituitary gonadotrophins, the secretion of which is stimulated by gonadotrophin hormone-releasing hormone (GnRH) from the hypothalamus and regulated by the negative feedback activity of testosterone and inhibin B secreted by the testis. Luteinizing hormone acts on the Leydig cells to stimulate testosterone production, and follicle stimulating hormone acts on the Sertoli cells to support spermatogenesis. Suppression of both is required for adequate inhibition of spermatogenesis, indicating the importance of testosterone in supporting normal spermatogenesis. As a result of this, hormonal contraceptive regimens also induce suppression of testicular steroidogenesis, requiring co-administration of androgen to prevent the symptoms and consequences of hypogonadism.

Suppression of gonadotrophin secretion can be achieved by over-riding the physiological negative feedback control mechanisms at the hypothalamus and pituitary gland by administration of exogenous steroids, more directly by administration of a GnRH analog to block the effect of GnRH on the pituitary, or by a combination of such agents (see Fig. 17.1). The requirement for androgen to provide replacement for the secondary hypogonadism will also provide a physiological feedback signal at the hypothalamus preventing increased GnRH secretion, which may increase the effectiveness of a co-administered GnRH analog. The major issues are the need for rapid, consistent yet reversible suppression of spermatogenesis to a level that will give adequate contraceptive efficacy, potential adverse effects of administered steroids or other agents, and the need for appropriately acceptable drug formulations. Conversely there is the potential for non-contraceptive health benefits as well as risks from such alterations in the hormonal milieu, as with the female combined contraceptive pill.

Establishment of contraceptive efficacy

The principle of hormonal contraception for men was established over 60 years ago when it was shown that men became azoospermic when injected every day with testosterone propionate.[19–21] The subsequent development of longer-acting testosterone injections allowed a more systematic approach but it rapidly became apparent that azoospermia was not achieved in all men. It thus became important to explore the degree of spermatogenic suppression necessary for contraceptive protection since induced oligozoospermia may carry a very different risk of pregnancy from that observed in sub-fertile men. This was investigated in two large international studies sponsored by WHO. The regimen investigated was testosterone enanthate (TE) 200 mg intramuscularly weekly, and subjects used no other contraceptive for 12 months once their sperm concentration had fallen below the set threshold. In the first study,[22] the threshold was azoospermia and 137 men (70%) entered the efficacy phase. Only one pregnancy resulted, demonstrating that hormonal male contraception could really work. This large study, however, also illustrated the variable degree of suppression of spermatogenesis achieved, with only two-thirds of men achieving azoospermia within 6 months of TE treatment.

This relatively low proportion allowed the investigation of the contraceptive efficacy of induced oligozoospermia in a second study,[23,24] with the threshold for entering the efficacy phase set at 3 million sperm/mL. Inadequate suppression of spermatogenesis to preclude entry to the efficacy phase occurred in only 8 (2.2%) of the total of 357 men who completed the suppression phase. Four pregnancies occurred during the nearly 50 person-years of exposure in the oligozoospermic (0.1–3.0 million sperm/mL) group with none in 230 years of exposure in the azoospermic group. These data gave a pregnancy rate of 1.4 per 100 years exposure (95% CI 0.4–3.7) overall and of 8.1 (95% CI 2.2–20.7) in the oligozoospermic group alone. These landmark studies clearly demonstrate the contraceptive efficacy of hormonally induced azoospermia. While induced oligozoospermia also appears to offer contraceptive efficacy similar to other male methods, i.e. condoms, the number of pregnancies involved was very small and thus the confidence intervals are wide.

The precise degree of suppression required remains uncertain, although there is a consensus among researchers in the field that the goal is a sperm concentration of <1 million/mL in all men.[25] It is likely that the final decision will be whether a particular regimen can be marketed with an acknowledged failure rate because of its otherwise attractive attributes, as with all other methods of contraception. The degree of contraceptive risk that is acceptable will vary according to a couple's needs, both over time and between individual couples. Awareness of differences in contraceptive reliability are an accepted part of the current decision-making process with current methods and may indicate possible markets for several hormonal male methods differing in their reliability and method of administration.

Refinement of the method

The WHO studies described above utilized a high dose of testosterone, administered weekly. It is important to recognize that this regimen was never intended to be developed as a practical method, but was used to demonstrate that the hormonal approach could deliver acceptable contraceptive efficacy. Subsequent studies, mostly involving much smaller groups of men, have subsequently investigated a range of testosterone preparations and a wider range of progestogens covering the range from oral, transdermal, injectable, and implant-based regimens. Table 17.1 lists the main testosterone preparations investigated in this context, and Table 17.2 lists recently investigated progestogens. That so many variations have been investigated illustrates the point that none shows a clear overall advantage at present, although there have been few studies comparing different progestogens with a constant testosterone regimen. In addition, the small size of many studies, often with 8–20 men per group, limits their power to demonstrate statistically significant differences in the degree of spermatogenic suppression between the regimens tested.[26] The apparently high efficacy of certain regimens, with which all or nearly all men have become azoospermic, may not be confirmed in larger, adequately powered studies.

Table 17.1. *Currently available androgens for male contraception*

Androgen preparation	Administration interval	Characteristics
Testosterone enanthate	1–2 weeks	Poor pharmacokinetics
Testosterone undecanoate (injectable)	Up to 3 months	Much longer duration of action
Testosterone implants (pellets)	3–4 months	Near-zero order release, but minor insertion procedure, risk of expulsion
Testosterone patches (transdermal)	Daily	Low efficacy in contraceptive studies
Testosterone gel (transdermal)	Daily	Untested in this context
17α-methyl-19-nortestosterone acetate implants	6 months or more	Long duration, tissue selectivity, theoretical prostate-sparing

Table 17.2. *Progestogens currently investigated as potential components of a hormonal male contraceptive regimen*

Progestogen	Formulations	Special notes
Medroxyprogesterone acetate	Oral or injection	Low androgenicity, tissue accumulation
Levonorgestrel	Oral or implant	Significant metabolic effects, e.g. lipoproteins
Cyproterone acetate	Oral	Antiandrogenic activity
Desogestrel, etonogestrel	Oral or implant	Implant formulations allow dose-sparing
Norethisterone enanthate	Injection	Complex metabolism, including estrogenicity

The central component of a hormonal male contraceptive is the testosterone preparation. Despite this, the testosterone component remains one of the major problems. Up until very recently available testosterone esters had a short duration of action, needing to be injected at 1–2-week intervals for contraceptive use. This is clearly unacceptable. A much longer acting ester, testosterone buciclate, was developed by WHO and the National Institutes for Health, and initial studies were promising[27] but further development did not proceed. Injectable formulations of testosterone undecanoate have now been developed both in China and in Europe, and the product marketed by Schering is now licensed in the UK with an injection interval of approximately 12 weeks for replacement in hypogonadal men.

These have both been used at 4-week intervals alone or with a progestogen, and the Chinese preparation has been used in large contraceptive efficacy studies.[28] This preparation has also been used in a recent commercially backed study in Europe (yet to be published). This collaboration between Organon and Schering was hoped to be a major step forward towards the commercialization of the development of hormonal male contraception, but both companies have subsequently announced withdrawal from this field. This is a major blow to hopes for a hormonal product in the medium term.

Transdermal testosterone preparations, including patches and gels, are available and may seem more user-friendly (see Table 17.1). As their main value is in maintaining physiological testosterone concentrations, data so far on their potential in contraception have been related to them as components of a combination preparation,[29–31] in which the degree of spermatogenic suppression achieved has been surprisingly low. This may in part reflect poor compliance, because the transdermal patches currently available are irritant to the skin,[32] and early data suggest that testosterone gels are likely to be substantially more effective.[33]

Testosterone pellets are also available in some countries, and have been investigated as a component of a male contraceptive in the UK and Australia. They require a minor surgical procedure for insertion, and there is a low (<10%) extrusion rate. Despite these drawbacks they are very well tolerated and indeed preferred by some hypogonadal men because of the relatively constant testosterone concentrations achieved, compared with the large swings from supraphysiological to subphysiological over 2–3 weeks with injectable preparations.[34] As a contraceptive, the excellent pharmacokinetics are also advantageous, and my group has used them in our own studies, in which they are administered at 12-week intervals.[35,36] A contraceptive efficacy study investigating their potential in combination with depot medroxyprogesterone acetate (DMPA) in Australia showed very promising results.[37] While their disadvantages prevent their use outside a research environment, they remain a valuable prototype of a preparation with zero order testosterone release characteristics.

Synthetic androgens

An alternative approach is the use of a synthetic androgen. 17α-alkylated androgens cause occasional hepatotoxicity and are not used clinically; however, 7α-methyl-19-nortestosterone (MENT), which was first described in the 1960s, has become the subject of considerable interest because of its differential metabolism compared with testosterone. It is 10-fold more potent than testosterone at effects mediated directly by the androgen receptor without intermediate metabolism, such as on muscle mass and at suppressing gonadotrophin secretion, but it is resistant to metabolism by the enzyme 5α-reductase.[38] This enzyme normally converts testosterone to the more potent dihydrotestosterone, thus acting as a tissue-specific amplifier of androgen action. This is particularly important in the prostate. Resistance to this enzyme will thus confer relative sparing of the prostate gland, while maintaining androgen action at other tissues.

The other major pathway of testosterone metabolism is aromatization to estradiol, the importance of which is demonstrated by the phenotype of people with mutations of either the estrogen receptor[39] or the aromatase enzyme.[40] One striking feature in these people is marked osteoporosis. MENT is subject to aromatization,[41] and thus might be expected to support the effects of androgen in bone. It is rapidly cleared from the circulation, and it is therefore formulated as the acetate in silastic implants. Transdermal application is also possible, particularly in view of its high potency. While the prostate-sparing effect of MENT has been confirmed in animal models,[42,43] only limited clinical data on the prostate and bone are available.[44] The combination of MENT and progestogen implants offers the possibility for long-acting contraception.[45]

There is also considerable interest in the development of non-steroidal molecules that have selectivity and specificity for the androgen receptor.[46] The further modification of these selective androgen-receptor modulators (SARMs) may lead to them displaying agonist, antagonist, or partial effects. Not only may this be of great benefit in the area of male hormonal contraception but it may also have more widespread clinical applications in the treatment of hypogonadism, androgen-dependent malignancy, and sarcopenia and in the development of replacement therapy in aging men.

Progestogen–testosterone combinations

Progestogens are as potent suppressors of gonadotrophin secretion in men as in women. Progesterone itself inhibits spermatogenesis,[47] and a wide range of synthetic progestogens and preparations have been investigated (see Table 17.2). Their main value is that, by the nature of their effect on gonadotrophin suppression, a much lower dose of testosterone is required. This dose can in fact be reduced to low-physiological levels,[35] although most studies have used mildly supraphysiological doses. The combination of a progestogen with testosterone has the advantage of the availability of a wide range of drugs and preparations and is currently at the most advanced stage of development, although at present no one combination is clearly 'better' than others.[26]

Initial studies used DMPA.[48–50] The combination with testosterone is highly effective, and a study investigating the contraceptive efficacy of testosterone pellets with DMPA (i.e. a dual-depot regimen), gave encouraging results.[37] One feature of DMPA is that it accumulates in adipose tissue, resulting in sometimes prolonged effects in women, which may be a complication for long-term studies involving repeated administration.

Some of the most striking data derive from studies using the potent oral progestogen cyproterone acetate (CPA). These studies, although involving small numbers of men, suggested that the combination of CPA in doses of 25–100 mg/day with 100 mg TE per week resulted in the rapid onset of azoospermia in all subjects.[51,52] The antiandrogenic effect of CPA appeared to be reflected in a dose-dependent fall in hemoglobin concentration and in hematocrit and also in body weight, despite the mildly supraphysiological dose of testosterone. The antiandrogenic activity may enhance the efficacy of this regimen by antagonizing the supportive effect of the low but continuing rate of testicular testosterone synthesis on spermatogenesis despite gonadotrophin suppression.

Levonorgestrel and desogestrel have the potential advantages of availability in both oral and implant preparations. Both levonorgestrel and desogestrel result in dose-dependent suppression of spermatogenesis when administered with testosterone.[35,53,54] Preliminary studies using both steroid components as implants have been carried out with promising results.[31,55] The significantly higher doses required in men than in women reflect the need for much more complete suppression of gonadotrophin secretion. Implant formulations have the advantage of reducing compliance problems, but men may prefer an oral formulation,[4] perhaps reflecting the synonymy of contraception with 'the pill' in Western society.

An alternative approach might be to combine the testosterone and progestogen as injections. This would be a possibility with DMPA, and also with norethisterone acetate, widely used around the world as a depot contraceptive administered every 8 weeks. Given its widespread use in women, it has been relatively little studied in men although the available data are very promising[56] and it may be the combination for future investigation by WHO.

Testosterone with gonadotrop in-releasing hormone analogs

The secretion of LH and FSH from the pituitary are under the stimulatory control of GnRH, thus the most direct approach to the suppression of gonadotrophin secretion is the blockade of the effect of GnRH. The GnRH analogs, which have been available for many years and are effective suppressors of gonadal function in a wide range of clinical conditions such as prostate and breast cancer, endometriosis, and in vitro fertilization, have agonist activity causing secondary receptor down-regulation. As part of a male contraceptive regimen the degree of gonadotrophin and spermatogenic suppression was, however, incomplete.[57] The development of GnRH antagonists has been complicated by their short duration of action, their expense, and their histamine-like side effects, but early results were encouraging.[58,59] More recent studies have investigated the concept of using the antagonist with testosterone for a suppression phase, with administration of testosterone alone for maintenance of suppression.[60] GnRH antagonists are now becoming clinically available, and it is likely that further studies will provide clearer evidence as to whether or not they have real advantages over the progestogens.[61]

Side effects of hormonal male contraception

The administration of high doses of testosterone has predictable effects, particularly on the skin and on lipoprotein metabolism.[62] Effects on the prostate gland may be more difficult to detect in short-term studies,[63] but are of concern for the widespread introduction of this method. The use of testosterone in strictly physiological replacement doses in a combination regimen may prevent many of these effects, but some may be induced by a progestogen component. This appears to be the case with weight gain and changes in lipoprotein metabolism. The real consequences of these changes will not be apparent until post-marketing surveillance data are available, but meanwhile the objective of many studies is to derive a 'metabolically neutral' regimen. There is conversely the possibility of reproductive or non-reproductive benefits, analogous to the benefits of the female contraceptive pill. These may arise, for example, from the use of synthetic androgens with selective metabolism at different tissues, such as the prostate, as discussed above.

The potential market

The question of whether there is a market for hormonal male contraception is a subject of considerable uncertainty although there are grounds for cautious optimism. The past 50 years have seen the provision of contraception change from male-based methods – the condom and withdrawal – to relatively 'high-tech' methods for women. These are predominantly hormone-based, and represent the application of advances in steroid chemistry dating back to the 1950s. There has thus been, within a single reproductive lifetime, a complete change in accompanying attitudes to contraception. While hormonal male methods of contraception are still under development, the speed and degree of the sea-change in contraception we have seen suggests that attitudes to contraception may not be firmly entrenched in our society, but rather reflect the convenience and safety of currently available methods. There is also considerable use of male contraceptives at the moment despite the drawbacks of currently available methods: condoms and vasectomy provide contraception for approximately 35%

of couples in the UK, and withdrawal is used by more men than the number of women who use the intrauterine device.[64] Moreover, there is an increasing awareness that men should share, to a greater extent, responsibility for contraception.[65] This is strongly supported by recent surveys of attitudes of men and women to the use of novel hormonal male methods.[4,66] Despite large differences between current and past experience of different contraceptive methods there was significant support for a male hormonal method and 44–83% of men surveyed would use a male pill if it was available (Fig. 17.2). In a parallel survey, women were asked what they thought about the use of a male hormonal method.[66] More than 70% of women in Shanghai and Edinburgh and of white women in South Africa stated that they would consider using a hormonal male method (Fig. 17.3). Remarkably, only 2% of women said they wouldn't trust their partner to take a 'male pill'. It is interesting that the acceptability was lowest among both men and women in Hong Kong, where condoms are the commonest current method; thus, widespread use of one male method does not predict that different approaches would also show high acceptability.

Conclusion

Of the range of potential targets for the development of novel male contraceptive agents, the hormonal approach is closest to fruition, although

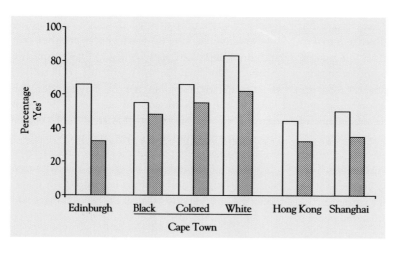

Figure 17.2. *The percentage of men in different cities who would definitely or probably use an oral (open columns) or injectable (shaded columns) male hormonal contraceptive (n=1829). Data from Martin et al.[4]*

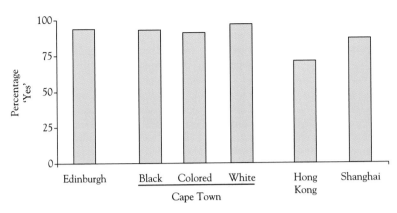

Figure 17.3. *The percentage of women in different cities who would definitely or probably use a hormonal male contraceptive, n=1781. Data from Glasier et al.*[66]

the withdrawal of pharmaceutical company involvement is a concern. One major difficulty is the limited range of androgen preparations: it is likely that the rapidly increasing interest in androgen supplementation of the aging male will provide a further spur to development in this field. This may at last give men the opportunity for fuller involvement in family planning, and reveal quite how far they wish to go to take up an equal share in this responsibility.

References

1. International Conference on Population and Development. Programme of Action. New York: United Nations, 1994.
2. United Nations Population Fund (UNFPA). Report of the International Conference on Population and Development. New York: United Nations Annual Conference 171/13, 1994.
3. World Health Organization. World Health Day 1998 Fact Sheets: prevent unwanted pregnancy. Geneva: World Health Organization, 1998.
4. Martin CW, Anderson RA, Cheng L et al. Potential impact of hormonal male contraception: cross-cultural implications for development of novel preparations. Hum Reprod 2000; 15: 637–45.
5. Fu H, Darroch JE, Haas T, Ranjit N. Contraceptive failure rates: new estimates from the 1995 National Survey of Family Growth. Fam Plan Perspect 1999; 31: 56–63.
6. Bankole A, Darroch JE, Singh S. Determinants of trends in condom use in the United States, 1988–1995. Fam Plan Perspect 1999; 31: 264–71.
7. Catania JA, Canchola J, Binson D et al. National trends in condom use among at-risk heterosexuals in the United States. J Acquir Immune Defic Syndr 2001; 27: 176–82.
8. Workshop summary. Scientific evidence on condom effectiveness for sexually transmitted disease (STD) prevention. Washington, DC: National Institute of Allergy and Infectious Diseases, National Institutes of Health, Department of Health and Human Services, 2001.
9. Davis KR, Weller SC. The effectiveness of condoms in reducing heterosexual transmission of HIV. Fam Plan Perspect 1999; 31: 272–9.
10. Gallo MF, Grimes DA, Schulz KF. Nonlatex vs. latex male condoms for contraception: a systematic review of randomized controlled trials. Contraception 2003; 68: 319–26.
11. Frezieres RG, Walsh TL. Acceptability evaluation of a natural rubber latex, a polyurethane, and a new non-latex condom. Contraception 2000; 61: 369–77.
12. Schlegel PN, Goldstein M. Vasectomy. In: Sharpe D, Haseltine FP, eds. Contraception. New York: Springer-Verlag, 1993: 181–91.
13. Oddens BJ, Visser AP, Vemer HM, Everaerd WT, Lehert P. Contraceptive use and attitudes in Great Britain. Contraception 1994; 49: 73–86.
14. Peterson H, Xia Z, Hughes J et al. The risk of pregnancy after tubal sterilization: findings from the US Collaborative Review of Sterilization. Am J Obstet Gynecol 1996; 174: 1161–70.
15. Akama TO, Nakagawa H, Sugihara K et al. Germ cell survival through carbohydrate-mediated interaction with Sertoli cells. Science 2002; 295: 124–7.
16. Ren D, Navarro B, Perez G et al. A sperm ion channel required for sperm motility and male fertility. Nature 2001; 413: 603–9.

17. Song L, Gu Y, Lu W, Liang X, Chen Z. A phase II randomized controlled trial of a novel male contraception, an intra-vas device. Int J Androl 2006; 29: 489–95.

18. Chaudhury K, Bhattacharyya AK, Guha SK. Studies on the membrane integrity of human sperm treated with a new injectable male contraceptive. Hum Reprod 2004; 19: 1826–30.

19. McCullagh EP, McGurl FJ. Further observations on the clinical use of testosterone propionate. J Urol 1939; 42: 1265–7.

20. Heckel NJ. Production of oligospermia in a man by the use of testosterone propionate. Proc Soc Exp Biol Med 1939; 40: 658–9.

21. Reddy PR, Rao JM. Reversible antifertility action of testosterone propionate in human males. Contraception 1972; 5: 295–301.

22. World Health Organization Task Force on Methods for the Regulation of Male Fertility. Contraceptive efficacy of testosterone-induced azoospermia in normal men. Lancet 1990; 336: 955–9.

23. World Health Organization Task Force on Methods for the Regulation of Male Fertility. Rates of testosterone-induced suppression to severe oligozoospermia or azoospermia in two multinational clinical studies. Int J Androl 1995; 18: 157–65.

24. World Health Organization Task Force on Methods for the Regulation of Male Fertilty. Contraceptive efficacy of testosterone-induced azoospermia and oligozoospermia in normal men. Fertil Steril 1996; 65: 821–9.

25. Aaltonen P, Amory JK, Anderson RA et al. 10th Summit Meeting consensus: recommendations for regulatory approval for hormonal male contraception. J Androl 2007; 28: 362–3.

26. Grimes DA, Lopez LM, Gallo MF et al. Steroid hormones for contraception in men. Cochrane Database Syst Rev 2007: CD004316.

27. Behre HM, Nieschlag E. Testosterone buciclate (20-Aet-1) in hypogonadal men: pharmacokinetics and pharmacodynamics of the new long-acting androgen ester. J Clin Endocrinol Metab 1992; 75: 1204–10.

28. Gu YQ, Wang XH, Xu D et al. A multicenter contraceptive efficacy study of injectable testosterone undecanoate in healthy Chinese men. J Clin Endocrinol Metab 2003; 88: 562–8.

29. Büchter D, von Eckardstein S, von Eckardstein A et al. Clinical trial of transdermal testosterone and oral levonorgestrel for male contraception. J Clin Endocrinol Metab 1999; 84: 1244–9.

30. Hair WM, Kitteridge K, O'Connor DB, Wu FCW. A novel male contraceptive pill-patch combination: oral desogestrel and transdermal testosterone in the suppression of spermatogenesis in normal men. J Clin Endocrinol Metab 2001; 86: 5201–9.

31. Gonzalo IT, Swerdloff RS, Nelson AL et al. Levonorgestrel implants (Norplant II) for male contraception clinical trials: combination with transdermal and injectable testosterone. J Clin Endocrinol Metab 2002; 87: 3562–72.

32. Jordan WP, Jr. Allergy and topical irritation associated with transdermal testosterone administration: a comparison of scrotal and nonscrotal transdermal systems. Am J Contact Dermatol 1997; 8: 108–13.

33. Page ST, Amory JK, Anawalt BD et al. Testosterone gel combined with depomedroxyprogesterone acetate is an effective male hormonal contraceptive regimen and is not enhanced by the addition of a GnRH antagonist. J Clin Endocrinol Metab 2006; 91: 4374–80.

34. Handelsman DJ, Mackey MA, Howe C, Turner L, Conway AJ. An analysis of testosterone implants for androgen replacement therapy. Clin Endocrinol 1997; 47: 311–16.

35. Kinniburgh D, Zhu H, Cheng L, Kicman AT, Baird DT, Anderson RA. Oral desogestrel with testosterone pellets induces consistent suppression of spermatogenesis to azoospermia in both Caucasian and Chinese men. Hum Reprod 2002; 17: 1490–501.

36. Anderson RA, Kinniburgh D, Baird DT. Suppression of spermatogenesis by etonogestrel implants with depot testosterone: potential for long-acting male contraception. J Clin Endocrinol Metab 2002; 87: 3640–9.

37. Turner L, Conway AJ, Jimenez M et al. Contraceptive efficacy of a depot progestin and androgen combination in men. J Clin Endocrinol Metab 2003; 88: 4659–67.

38. Sundaram K, Kumar N, Bardin CW. 7a-methyl-nortestosterone (MENT): the optimal androgen for male contraception. Ann Med 1993; 25: 199–205.

39. Smith EP, Boyd J, Frank GR et al. Estrogen resistance caused by a mutation in the estrogen-receptor gene in a man. N Engl J Med 1994; 331: 1056–61.

40. Morishima A, Grumbach MM, Simpson ER, Fisher C, Qin K. Aromatase deficiency in male and female siblings caused by a novel mutation and the physiological role of estrogens. J Clin Endocrinol Metab 1995; 80: 3689–98.

41. LaMorte A, Kumar N, Bardin CW, Sundaram K. Aromatization of 7α-methyl-19-nortestosterone by human placental microsomes *in vitro*. J Steroid Biochem Mol Biol 1994; 48: 297–304.

42. Kumar N, Didolkar AK, Monder C, Bardin CW, Sundaram K. The biological activity of 7α-methyl-19-nortestosterone is not amplified in male reproductive tract as is that of testosterone. Endocrinology 1992; 130: 3677–83.

43. Cummings DE, Kumar N, Bardin CW, Sundaram K, Bremner WJ. Prostate-sparing effects in primates of the potent androgen 7α-methyl-19-nortestosterone: a potential alternative to testosterone for androgen replacement and male contraception. J Clin Endocrinol Metab 1998; 83: 4212–19.

44. Anderson RA, Wallace AM, Sattar N, Kumar N, Sundaram K. Evidence for tissue selectivity of the synthetic androgen 7α-methyl-19-nortestosterone in hypogonadal men. J Clin Endocrinol Metab 2003; 88: 2784–893.

45. Walton MJ, Kumar N, Baird DT, Ludlow H, Anderson RA. 7α-methyl-19-nortestosterone (MENT) vs testosterone in combination with etonogestrel implants for spermatogenic suppression in normal men. J Androl 2007; 28: 679–88.

46. Omwancha J, Brown TR. Selective androgen receptor modulators: in pursuit of tissue-selective androgens. Curr Opin Investig Drugs 2006; 7: 873–1.

47. Heller CG, Laidlaw WM, Harvey HT, Nelson WO. Effects of progestational compounds on the reproductive processes of the human male. Ann N Y Acad Sci 1958; 71: 649–5.

48. Frick J. Control of spermatogenesis in men by combined administration of progestin and androgen. Contraception 1973; 8: 191–206.

49. Coutinho EM, Melo JF. Successful inhibition of spermatogenesis in man without loss of libido: a potential new approach to male contraception. Contraception 1973; 8: 207–17.

50. Johansson EDB, Nygren K-G. Depression of plasma testosterone levels in men with norethindrone. Contraception 1973; 8: 219–26.

51. Meriggiola MC, Bremner WJ, Paulsen CA et al. A combined regimen of cyproterone acetate and testosterone enanthate as a potentially highly effective male contraceptive. J Clin Endocrinol Metab 1996; 81: 3018–23.

52. Meriggiola MC, Bremner WJ, Costantino A, Di Cintio G, Flamigni C. Low dose of cyproterone acetate and testosterone enanthate for contraception in men. Hum Reprod 1998; 13: 1225–9.

53. Anawalt BD, Bebb RA, Bremner WJ, Matsumoto AM. A lower dosage levonorgestrel and testosterone combination effectively suppresses spermatogenesis and circulating gonadotropin levels with fewer metabolic effects than higher dosage combinations. J Androl 1999; 20: 407–14.

54. Anderson RA, van der Spuy ZM, Dada OA et al. Investigation of hormonal male contraception in African men: suppression of spermatogenesis by oral desogestrel with depot testosterone. Hum Reprod 2002; 17: 2869–77.

55. Brady BM, Walton M, Hollow N, Kicman AT, Baird DT, Anderson RA. Depot testosterone with etonogestrel implants result in induction of azoospermia in all men for long-term contraception. Hum Reprod 2004; 11: 2658–67.

56. Kamischke A, Venherm S, Plöger D, von Eckardstein S, Nieschlag E. Intramuscular testosterone undecanoate with norethisterone enanthate in a clinical trial for male contraception. J Clin Endocrinol Metab 2001; 86: 303–9.

57. Behre HM, Nashan D, Hubert W, Nieschlag E. Depot gonadotrophin-releasing hormone agonist blunts the androgen-induced suppression of spermatogenesis in a clinical trial of male contraception. J Clin Endocrinol Metab 1992; 74: 84–90.

58. Pavlou SN, Brewer K, Farley MG et al. Combined administration of a gonadotropin-releasing hormone antagonist and testosterone in men induces reversible azoospermia without loss of libido. J Clin Endocrinol Metab 1991; 73: 1360–9.

59. Tom L, Bhasin S, Salameh W et al. Induction of azoospermia in normal men with combined Nal-Glu gonadotrophin releasing hormone antagonist and testosterone enanthate. J Clin Endocrinol Metab 1992; 75: 476–83.

60. Swerdloff RS, Bagatell CJ, Wang C et al. Suppression of spermatogenesis in man induced by Nal-Glu gonadotrophin releasing hormone antagonist and testosterone enanthate (TE) is maintained by TE alone. J Clin Endocrinol Metab 1998; 83: 3527–33.

61. Matthiesson KL, Amory JK, Berger R et al. Novel male hormonal contraceptive combinations: the hormonal and spermatogenic effects of testosterone and levonorgestrel combined with a 5{alpha}-reductase inhibitor or gonadotropin-releasing hormone antagonist. J Clin Endocrinol Metab 2005; 90: 91–7.

62. Wu FCW, Farley TMM, Peregoudov A, Waites GMH, WHO Task Force on Methods for the Regulation of Male Fertility. Effects of testosterone enanthate in normal men: experience from a

multicenter contraceptive efficacy study. Fertil Steril 1996; 65: 626–36.

63. Wallace EM, Pye SD, Wild SR, Wu FCW. Prostatic specific antigen and prostate gland size in men receiving exogenous testosterone for male contraception. J Androl 1993; 16: 35–40.

64. Wellings K, Field J, Johnson AM, Wadsworth J. Sexual Behaviour, in Britain. The National Survey of Sexual Attitudes and Lifestyles. London: Penguin Books, 1994.

65. Ringheim K. Whither methods for men? Emerging gender issues in contraception. Reprod Health Matters 1996; 7: 79–89.

66. Glasier A, Anakwe R, Everington D et al. Would women trust their partners to use a male pill? Hum Reprod 2000; 15: 646–9.

CHAPTER 18

Peyronie's disease: history and medical therapy

J Slade Hubbard, Culley C Carson III

Introduction and history

Peyronie's disease (PD), also known as induratio penis plastica, is a disorder characterized by plaque formation in the tunica albuginea (TA) of the penis. The disease is named after Francois Gigot de la Peyronie (1678–1747), a Frenchman who served as royal surgeon to King Louis XV and who made significant contributions to intestinal surgical techniques. de la Peyronie was also instrumental in effecting the transition of surgery from a trade into a professional guild in France.[1,2] de la Peyronie described PD in a treatise on ejaculatory dysfunction in 1743, reporting on a patient with 'rosary beads' of scar tissue extending along the dorsum of the penis that was associated with upward penile curvature during erection.[3] de la Peyronie suggested that the best treatment was bathing in the baths of Barèges in southern France. He was not, however, the first to describe the condition that bears his name. In 1561, Fallopius and Vesalius corresponded about a patient with Peyronie's disease, and several earlier references exist, though the vague descriptions make it less clear if these truly refer to the same clinical entity.[1]

Clinical characteristics and epidemiology

PD involves the formation of fibrotic plaques in the TA. Plaques are typically unifocal (78–84% of cases)

and located on the dorsum of the penis, though they may be located in any region of the TA.[4] In one series, dorsal (46%), lateral (29%), and ventral (9%) curvature were the most common abnormalities, with the rest being indeterminate.[5] Scar tissue plaques cause curvature with erection, with the curvature directed toward the site of the plaque. The plaques can also cause penile shortening and other deformities, such as 'hourglass' and 'swanneck' deformities. Penile deformity may develop in an acute manner, in which case patients report development of deformity essentially overnight, while others have a more insidious onset over weeks to months.[5]

The extent of curvature can make sexual intercourse challenging from a mechanical standpoint, and can cause discomfort for a patient and the patient's partner. Curvature can exceed 90°; in one cohort approximately 20% of patients had curvature greater than 60°.[5] In addition, many patients have pain during the early, acute phase of the disease, often associated with penile tumescence or intercourse (or both), though some have pain while flaccid. This pain is believed to be due to active inflammation; biopsy of 12 painful plaques found inflammatory infiltrates in two-thirds of the cases.[4] In most cases pain resolves with time, and pain resolution reflects stabilization of the disease. The acute inflammatory phase typically lasts between 6 and 18 months.[6] The subsequent chronic phase is characterized by little pain, stable penile deformity, and stable plaque size.

Erectile dysfunction (ED) is reported by 20–40% of PD patients, with either generalized lack of tumescence or with flaccidity distal to the plaque.[7,8] PD also affects quality of life, with 77% of afflicted men reporting psychological effects and two-thirds of those reporting frequent concern over the condition.[9,10] Spontaneous disease regression has been noted in 5–40% of cases, with one large series finding a rate of 13%.[2,6,7,10]

PD predominantly affects middle-aged and older men, with prevalence between 0.38 and 3.7% of 40- to 70-year-old men.[6] However, age at diagnosis can vary widely, with reported cases ranging from 18 to 80 years of age.[4,5] The true prevalence may be higher than currently thought, owing to patients' hesitancy in reporting this sensitive condition.[11] This is supported by an autopsy series of 100 men without history of PD, which found pathologic derangements like those seen in PD in 23%.[12] The lowest prevalence of large series, which is probably an underestimate, was a prevalence of 0.38% noted in a retrospective review of medical records of residents of Rochester, Minnesota, between 1950 and 1984.[13] The prevalence of PD noted in contemporary prostate cancer screening populations has been 3.7 to 8.9%.[6,9] The prostate cancer screening model has the potential advantage that patients are not presenting with any particular urologic complaint and diagnosis is defined by a physician's palpating a plaque on examination.[9] A large German study, which assessed for the presence of PD with a questionnaire about the presence of a palpable plaque, found a prevalence of 3.2%.[14] Another point to consider is that approximately 10% of men with ED have PD.[15]

Histological characteristics

The TA is a connective tissue structure composed of inner circular and outer longitudinal layers encompassing the corpora cavernosa.[16] Normal TA is composed of collagen bundles undulating among elastic fibers in an irregular, latticed pattern.[17] The TA of PD plaques is characterized by dysregulated extracellular matrix, with excessive amounts of collagen in a disorganized pattern, loss and fragmentation of elastic fibers, and fibrin deposition.[17,18]

Plaques contain an increased ratio of type III to type I collagen, and collagen fibers are tightly packed with loss of normal intervening ground substance.[19] In addition to decreased elastic fiber density in plaques compared to controls, PD patients with ED have fewer elastic fibers compared with those with PD and normal erections.[19,20] Additionally, plaque-adjacent 'normal' TA has been found to contain excess type III collagen and decreased elastin, indicating that the pathologic disease process is not solely limited to the clinically evident plaque.[20,21]

Peyronie's plaques usually contain an increased density of fibroblasts. Also, myofibroblasts, which produce tractional forces in wound organization and which are normally cleared by apoptosis after wound healing, can persist in plaques.[22,23] A perivascular lymphocytic and plasmacytic infiltrate is noted in some plaques, either within the tunica itself or in surrounding tissues.[18] This inflammatory infiltrate is characteristic of lesions of short duration, suggesting that inflammation is an early, inciting event in pathogenesis. Chronic lesions typically have little inflammation, though inflammatory infiltrates have been noted in chronic plaques.[24–26] Calcification and ectopic ossification have been noted in up to one-third of plaques, typically in those of longer duration.[18,25,27] Also, the connective tissue derangements can extend beyond the TA into the corporal tissue.[18,21,25]

The abnormal extracellular matrix makes plaques inflexible compared with surrounding normal TA. Collagen has great tensile strength, but poor compliance, while elastin can stretch to up to 150% of its length.[16] Thus, with erection, plaques do not expand like normal TA, and so cause curvature or deformity by tethering the TA.[27] Additionally, the abnormal mechanical properties of tunical plaques could contribute to dysfunction of erectile hemodynamics – for instance, with derangement of the normal compression of subtunical venules during tumescence leading to veno-occlusive incompetence or venous leakage.[28]

Etiology

Since the earliest descriptions of PD, authors have speculated about its cause. The Byzantine historian Zonar chronicled the case of Emperor Heraclius, who developed penile deformity causing him to 'urinate into his face', an affliction thought to be punishment for an incestuous relationship with his niece.[1,2] In the 19th and early 20th century, PD was purported to be due to penetrative trauma from having sex with a non-enthusiastic or bored partner. Indeed, it was believed that intercourse with a facilitating partner could reverse the condition. Infections such as syphilis and gonorrhea have been cited as causative, and medical conditions such as gout and diabetes have been implicated. It has even been suggested that the disease reflects an evolutionary regressive phenomenon since some other mammals, such as canines and some primates, have an osseous penis.[1]

It has become clear, however, that most cases are idiopathic and not associated with other disease states, and the cause of PD remains unclear. The current leading theory is that blunt trauma to the TA during intercourse causes micro-hemorrhage, fibrin extravasation, cellular infiltration, and inflammatory response, inducing deposition of abnormal extracellular matrix.[27,29] The inflammatory response may be a self-perpetuating process, with accumulated cytokines and reactive oxygen species inducing more cellular infiltration, which subsequently leads to further cytokine production.[27,30]

It is also believed that PD patients might have a genetic predisposition to abnormal wound healing or be affected by autoimmune, connective tissue, or vasculogenic aberrations.[31] Reasons for this theory include a family history of PD in 2–4% of patients and an association with Dupuytren's contracture in 20% of patients. Dupuytren's contracture, or aponeurotic palmar fibrosis, is a heritable, autosomal-dominant disease with a population prevalence of 4–6%.[31–33] Identical twins have been reported to have Peyronie's disease. Also, in a study of patients with Paget's disease of bone, a condition characterized by abnormal bone turnover, 14–31% of the patients had PD and 23% had Dupuytren's contracture.[32] Studies of human leukocyte antigen linkage have found PD to be associated with the HLA-B7 and HLA-B27 antigens, though results vary and the largest study to date found no association between PD and HLA antigens.[6,34,35] Immunologic studies in PD patients have found at least one abnormal immunologic test in 76%, altered

cell-mediated immunity in 49%, and markers of autoimmunity in 38%.[36] PD patients have also been found to have elevated levels of anti-elastin antibodies, further suggesting autoimmune mechanisms.[37]

Age is a clear risk factor, with prevalence rates in one large survey of 1.5% in men aged 30–39 years, increasing to 6.5% in men older than 70 years.[14] It is speculated that older men may be more susceptible to tunical injury, owing to their having less rigid erections that are more likely to buckle during intercourse. Genital trauma has also been reported as a cause of PD, with a three-fold increased risk of PD in patients with prior genital or perineal trauma in one study.[33,38] An association has also been reported with invasive penile procedures (i.e. cystoscopy).[33] However, a review of 193 patients with surgically corrected penile fracture and 150 with a history of taqaandan (the cultural habit of forceful bending of the erect penis to achieve detumescence) found only one case of PD.[39] This finding brings to question the role of trauma or suggests that trauma only in association with predisposing factors (e.g. autoimmunity) results in PD. Association with hypertension, diabetes, and other risk factors for systemic vascular disease have been found in some studies, but not in others.[5,9,40] While infection has been speculated as a cause of PD, a sensitive molecular analysis found no evidence of bacteria in plaques.[41]

Transforming growth factor (TGF)-beta is believed to play a causative role in fibrotic diseases and is implicated as being central in the pathogenesis of PD. TGF-beta is elevated in the TA of patients with PD.[6] Injection of cytomodulin, a synthetic peptide similar to TGF-beta, into rodent penile tissue produces an intense fibrotic reaction in the TA.[42] TGF-beta promotes expression of other fibrotic cytokines, such as connective tissue growth factor and monocyte chemoattractant protein 1.[42] Several other fibrotic genes are over-expressed in plaques, including basic fibroblast growth factor.[43,44] An interesting theory regarding pathogenesis involves the observation that plasminogen activator inhibitor type-1, an inhibitor of both fibrin and collagen degradation, is over-expressed in plaques.[29] The inciting traumatic event in PD is theorized to cause extravasation of fibrin into the TA, and some believe this extravasated fibrin is the primary trigger to plaque development. Support for this includes the detection of fibrin in plaques that are many years old and the induction of plaque-like histologic changes by injection of fibrin into the TA of rodents.[29] Osteoblast-stimulating factor-1 is also increased in plaques, potentially explaining the high incidence of calcification in Peyronie's plaques.[27] At the same time, genes that are involved in tissue remodeling have been found to be down-regulated in plaques.[44]

Cell cycle dysregulation may play a role in PD. Aberrant p53 function has been found in association with PD, with increased levels of the protein gene product in plaque fibroblasts compared with normal fibroblasts. This promotes cellular proliferation, allowing damaged cells to continue inappropriately through the cell cycle.[42,43] Chromosomal instability, including microsatellite alterations and loss of heterozygosity, has been associated with PD and Dupuytren's contracture.[6,42]

The cause of ED in patients with PD is also controversial. While penile deformity, pain, and psychologic factors may be the cause of ED in some patients, it has been shown that penile vascular derangements are etiologic in 61–88% of Peyronie's patients with ED.[15] The TA plays a key role in the veno-occlusive mechanism of erection, and loss of its normal mechanical properties could contribute to malfunction of the erectile mechanism.[1,45] However, data are conflicting and some believe ED associated with PD is due to venous leak and others think arterial insufficiency is to blame.[46] Veno-occlusive dysfunction has been found in 30–86% of PD patients with ED, while arterial dysfunction has been demonstrated in 44–52%.[8,15] A study using color Doppler ultrasonography to evaluate vascular function in PD patients with and without ED suggested that arterial insufficiency, either alone or in combination with venous dysfunction, was the most important factor in the ED of PD.[15] Another study using ultrasonography compared patients with PD and those with a presenting complaint of ED alone. There was no difference in rates of veno-occlusive dysfunction between PD patients with associated ED and the group with ED alone.[46] Interestingly, patients with ED alone had significantly higher rates of normal vascular function (24%) than those with PD and ED (4%).[46]

Conversely, Lopez and Jarow, in a similar study, found that venous leakage was significantly higher in patients with PD and ED (59%) than in those with ED alone (16%).[8,46] Given that both veno-occlusive and arterial dysfunction are common, determining the exact etiologic factor for ED in every case can be difficult. Moreover, the baseline incidence of ED and the presence of vascular disease risk factors in the age group affected by PD further clouds a clear etiologic theory.

Diagnosis

Diagnosis is based on history and palpating a plaque in the TA. Most plaques are easily palpable, typically being larger than 1.5 cm^2. Presenting symptoms, duration of symptoms, and stability of the lesion should be assessed. Patients should be questioned about potentially associated conditions such as Dupuytren's contracture, Lederhosen disease, family history, diabetes, Paget's disease of bone, systemic vascular disease, and prior genitourinary trauma or instrumentation. A patient should be asked about erectile function, with attention paid to characteristics of dysfunction – poor tumescence distal to the plaque, generalized lack of tumescence, physical inability for intromission due to the degree of curvature, anxiety, and psychological impact. Questioning the partner if possible, or asking about the partner's experience, is also important since dyspareunia experienced by the partner may be relevant. Though it is somewhat imprecise, plaque size should be measured.

Numerous imaging modalities have been used to characterize plaques, including ultrasonography, X-ray in mammography technique, computed tomography (CT), and magnetic resonance imaging (MRI). High-frequency ultrasonography is the only modality that reliably identifies plaque calcification and thickness of the TA.[47] Ultrasound also provides reliable plaque size and is used by some to follow treatment effects.[31] Color Doppler duplex ultrasonography can also be used to evaluate penile vascular function. MRI with gadolinium visualizes inflammation and may provide a method for monitoring plaque inflammation. However, inflammation is associated with pain, and history can provide the basic information garnered from MRI. Thus use of this costly imaging modality cannot be justified on a routine basis.[31,47]

A practical protocol is to limit imaging to the evaluation of ED associated with PD via penile color Doppler ultrasonography after induction of erection with an intracavernosal injectible vasoactive agent. This is the most cost-effective method to evaluate the vascular erectile mechanism in these patients.[15] Evaluation of erectile function is important when planning operative intervention, since patients with preserved erectile function will be candidates for straightening procedures alone, while those with deranged function will probably require prosthesis implantation. Patients are injected with a vasoactive agent (e.g. alprostadil 10–20 μg) and asked to self-stimulate in private, without ejaculation, for 5–10 minutes to obtain penile tumescence equal to or better than obtained at home. Ultrasound is then used to inspect for sufficient arterial flow and for venous leakage. Peak systolic velocity reflects arterial inflow (normal is >35 cm/second), and color Doppler ultrasonography has a sensitivity of 100% and a specificity of 95% for diagnosis of arterial insufficiency compared with pudendal arteriography.[15] Dynamic infusion cavernosometry and cavernosography are gold standards for detecting veno-occlusive dysfunction, with cavernosography in PD typically demonstrating a focal area of venous leakage in the region of the plaque.[15,48] End-diastolic velocity and related measures (e.g. resistive index) derived from ultrasonography provide information about veno-occlusive dysfunction. An end-diastolic velocity >5 cm/second has a sensitivity of 90% and a specificity of 56% for detecting venous leakage compared with cavernosography. Also, a resistive index <75% by ultrasonography is associated with venous leak in 95% of patients compared with cavernosography.[15] Documenting the degree of curvature during erection with photographs allows for future comparison and patient counseling as treatment is undertaken.

Treatment

Owing to lack of a definitive pathogenesis for PD, therapies are often directed at symptoms or speculated mechanisms. The phenomenon of spontaneous disease resolution and the divergent natural history of PD put a premium on double-blind, placebo-controlled trials and mandate caution when interpreting studies.[2] Unfortunately, placebo-controlled trials are lacking, providing little clarity as to the effectiveness of most therapies. Non-surgical management is appropriate during the early phase of the disease with progressive, unstable plaques or painful erections. Such clinical management is usually recommended for at least the first 12 months. However, if a patient presents with a longer-duration plaque with significant symptoms, conservative management is likely to be ineffective.[6] Since symptoms will not resolve spontaneously in the great majority of patients, clinical therapies are usually undertaken. Here, therapies that are currently clinically relevant are reviewed.

Oral therapy

Numerous drugs have been used to treat PD, often with only tangential rationale. Oral therapies have included mineral water, sulfur, mercury, milk, iodides, disodium phosphate, acetyl-l-carnitine, estrogen, procarbazine, vitamin E, para-aminobenzoic acid, tamoxifen, colchicine, and others.[1,49,50] Oral therapy, as opposed to local, intra-plaque drug delivery, is favored by some because of pathologic findings suggesting a generalized derangement of the TA, not simply limited to the plaque.[20,51] One unanswered question regarding oral therapy is what the bioavailability of systemically delivered drug is at the level of the TA.[52] Oral therapy is appropriate in the acute disease phase, though once stable, non-painful deformity is established, oral treatment is likely to have limited benefit.[53]

Vitamin E has been used to treat PD since the 1940s because of its antioxidant properties. Typical dosing is 400 mg twice daily. Non-controlled studies have found improvements in pain in 82–100% of patients, decreased plaque size in 20–91%, and improved deformity in 33–78%.[53–56] However, in a questionnaire survey, Gelbard and colleagues found no differences in changes in disease parameters between patients treated with vitamin E and those who received no treatment.[10] Additionally, a controlled study by Pryor and colleagues found that pain improved in only 35% and that deformity improved in only 10%, and there was minimal decrease in plaque size, findings comparable to those seen in controls.[50,53,57] With the available data, the effect of vitamin E on PD, if any, remains unclear. However, owing to its low cost and lack of side effects, vitamin E continues to be widely used, either alone or with other therapies.[58] Current controversy regarding the cardiovascular effects of vitamin E further add to the controversy of the use of vitamin E in the treatment of PD.

Potassium para-aminobenzoate has anti-inflammatory and anti-fibrotic properties.[59] *In vitro*, para-aminobenzoate inhibits secretion of glycosaminoglycans and mucopolysacharides by fibroblasts. It has been used clinically to treat inflammatory, fibrotic disorders such as scleroderma, dermatomyositis, and pulmonary fibrosis, and it was first used in PD in 1959.[50,52,53] Typical dosing is 12 g per day, usually in three or four divided doses. Uncontrolled studies have noted improvements in pain in 44–100%, in plaque size in 11–100%, and in angulation in 58–82%.[53,60,61] A placebo-controlled, double-blind study of 41 patients found trends toward symptomatic improvement in the treatment group, but there were no statistically significant differences.[62] Weidner and colleagues conducted a prospective, randomized, placebo-controlled trial of para-aminobenzoate (3 g powder four times/day for 12 months) in 75 patients with onset of disease less than 12 months earlier, non-calcified plaques, and no prior treatment. Therapeutic response was defined as regression in plaque-size or reduction in penile curvature of at least 30%, or both. Overall response rates were 74% and 50% for the intervention and placebo arms, respectively. Plaque size decreased significantly in the para-aminobenzoate arm compared with the placebo arm, while there were no differences in improvement in pain or erectile function between the two groups. A protective effect on the development of new or worsening penile curvature was observed, with degree of curvature remaining stable in the treatment arm, while it worsened in 33% of the placebo arm. In fact, none of 13 patients with a straight penis at presentation developed curvature on para-aminobenzoate, while 6 of 8 developed curvature on placebo.[52] Factors limiting the use of para-aminobenzoate include high cost, frequent dosing, and potential

for severe gastrointestinal symptoms.[53] In the study by Weidner et al., 13.7% of patients in the treatment arm and 7.7% in the placebo arm dropped out because of side effects; however, the percentage of patients who dropped out because of gastrointestinal side effects was the same in the two groups. The authors also speculated that the high rate of non-compliance (16%) in their study was related to patients' dislike of powder-form drug, frequent dosing, amount of drug consumed, and poor taste of the drug.[52]

Colchicine binds cellular microtubules, with resulting anti-mitotic, anti-fibrotic, and anti-inflammatory effects.[53] It interferes with intracellular collagen synthesis by fibroblasts and promotes collagenase activity.[51,53,63] It has also been shown to inhibit proliferation of plaque-derived fibroblasts in cell culture.[64] Pathologic clinical case studies of colchicine treatment in other fibromatoses (desmoid tumor and Dupuytren's contracture) have found decreases in abnormal intracellular collagen fibrils and myofibrils.[65] Colchicine's anti-inflammatory actions are related to its inhibitory effects on leukocyte motility and phagocytic activity, secretion of inflammatory cytokines, and on the lipooxygenase pathway.[51] An *in vivo* rodent study evaluated colchicine's effect in inhibiting plaque-like derangements after injection of TGF-beta into the TA. Colchicine-treated rats exhibited less tunical collagen deposition, less elastic fiber fragmentation, a more normal extracellular architecture, and significant down-regulation of TGF-beta expression. Treatment effects were markedly more impressive when treatment was initiated immediately versus 6 weeks after TGF-β injection.[66]

Colchicine was first used to treat PD in a pilot study in 1994. Non-controlled studies have found improved pain in 71–95% of patients, decreased plaque size in 47–50%, and improved deformity in 30–55%.[51,53,67,68] Interestingly, one study found that response was improved in patients with short duration of disease (<6 months), no ED, and degree of curvature <30°.[51] Dosing has varied among studies. Patients are started at a low dose, 0.6–1.2 mg daily for 1 week, and then the dose is gradually increased according to patient tolerance up to a maximum of around 2.4 mg daily (given in divided, twice-daily dosing). Treatment has typically been for 3–6 months.

Controlled studies of colchicine have produced conflicting results. Prieto Castro and colleagues, in a single-blinded study of early PD (duration <6 months, no ED, curvature <30°, pain present), randomized 45 patients to vitamin E (600 mg/day) with colchicine (1 mg every 12 hours) versus ibuprofen (400 mg/day) for 6 months. They found statistically significant objective improvements in plaque size and curvature in the vitamin E–colchicine group compared to the ibuprofen group. Pain improved in 91% of the colchicine–vitamin E group compared with 68% of the ibuprofen group, although the differences were not statistically significant.[58] Safarinejad performed a randomized, double-blind, placebo-controlled trial of colchicine (0.5–2.5 mg/day for 4 months), with 78 patients completing the study. He found no differences compared with placebo in pain resolution, decrease in deformity, or decrease in plaque size. The average disease duration was longer in the Safarinejad study than in the other study (e.g. disease duration <6 months was an inclusion criteria in the study by Prieto Castro et al.). However, subgroup analyses found no differences between drug and placebo when evaluated by severity of disease or disease duration (<1 year versus ≥1 year).[69] Another consideration regarding the use of colchicine is that side effects, often gastrointestinal upset or diarrhea, are not uncommon, and this is the rationale for dosage escalation schemes. One series reported gastrointestinal side effects in 33% of patients, with 17% discontinuing therapy.[67] In contrast, the study by Prieto Castro and colleagues found that 16% of colchicine-treated patients experienced diarrhea, which resolved after temporary dose reduction, and none of the patients dropped out of the study.[58] Hematologic derangements (e.g. bone marrow suppression) can occur, and complete blood count monitoring is prudent while patients are on treatment.[51] Colchicine does have the benefit of being relatively inexpensive.

Tamoxifen, an anti-estrogen, has been studied because of its suppressive effects on TGF-beta production by fibroblasts in vitro.[70] An uncontrolled study found that patients treated with tamoxifen had good clinical response, with greatest improvements noted in patients with disease duration of less than 4 months. Additionally, in a subset of patients with pre-treatment tunical biopsy, 75% of patients with inflammatory infiltrates showed clinical improvement with treatment, compared with none without evidence of inflammation.[70] However, a subsequent randomized, placebo-controlled trial of tamoxifen (20 mg twice daily for 3 months) found no differences in pain resolution or in changes in plaque size or curvature as determined subjectively and objectively between tamoxifen and placebo.[71] A criticism of this subsequent study is that disease duration was longer (with a mean of 20 months) compared with the initial study (with a mean of 8 months).[50] Interestingly, the significance of the placebo effect in PD was clearly demonstrated in this study, with subjective improvements in pain (75%), curvature (42%), and plaque size (25%) in placebo-treated patients.[71] Side effects have been noted in up to 25% of patients, and include decreased libido, facial flushing, reduced ejaculate volume, and gastrointestinal upset.[49,70] Given the lack of supportive data and the potential for side effects, tamoxifen is not recommended for routine use at this time.

Research is suggesting a role for the nitric oxide (NO)–cGMP system in PD pathogenesis. Inducible NO synthase (iNOS) and NO synthesis are upregulated in plaques. Specific inhibition of iNOS in the TGF-beta rat model of PD worsens fibrosis, suggesting that NO production by iNOS may have an anti-fibrotic role in Peyronie's plaques.[22] An in vitro study of human and rodent TA and derived cell cultures and an in vivo rodent study by Valente and colleagues have found that stimulation of the NO–cGMP system might indeed counteract the fibrosis typical of PD. Most interesting was the finding that rats fed substances in their drinking water that stimulate this system, including the phosphodiesterase inhibitor sildenafil, had 80–95% reduction in both plaque size and the collagen-to-fibroblast ratio compared with controls, as well as increased fibroblast apoptosis in the TA.[22] In a follow-up study, this group performed gene transfer of iNOS into rodent TGF-beta-induced PD-like plaques, with resulting decrease in plaque size, decreased expression of pro-fibrotic mediators (e.g. TGF-beta), and increased levels of factors that oppose oxidative damage.[72] This preliminary research awaits clinical evaluation before further conclusions can be drawn.

Local drug therapy (intralesional and iontophoresis)

As with oral therapies, numerous agents have been used for intralesional therapy of PD.[69] Intralesional therapy has the theoretical concern of disrupting tissue planes, causing additional scarring, and making subsequent surgery more difficult. This clinically has been noted with intralesional corticosteroid therapy, making, for instance, dissection of the neurovascular bundles from the TA quite difficult.[73]

Use of verapamil, a calcium-channel blocker, is based on its ability to modulate extracellular matrix metabolism. In vitro study has shown that exocytosis of extracellular matrix molecules is dependent on intracellular calcium ions.[74,75] Verapamil alters fibroblast function, resulting in decreased collagen and extracellular matrix synthesis and secretion. Verapamil also increases extracellular collagenase activity, with a 20-fold increase noted in one in vitro study.[74,76,77] In vitro study has found that verapamil inhibits the proliferation of plaque-derived fibroblasts and modulates the effects of inflammatory and fibrotic cytokines.[64,74,78] It was noted that the concentration of verapamil needed to induce these effects on in vitro fibroblasts was more than 500 times therapeutic serum ranges seen with the use of verapamil for medical conditions such as hypertension, indicating the need to deliver the drug directly into plaques and other fibrotic lesions.[74,79] Animal studies have found improved wound healing with verapamil, and, in humans, direct injection of verapamil has resulted in improved scar size.[77,80]

Multiple non-controlled series have found improvements in objective and subjective parameters of PD with intralesional verapamil treatment.[74,81–85] An Italian study of 39 men found that pain was improved in 91%, plaque size did not change, and curvature improved in 50% with disease duration less than 1 year. However, curvature improved in only 10% of those with disease longer than 1 year.[86] Levine and colleagues reported the largest series to date, a non-controlled, prospective study

of 156 men. In their series, 60% had an objective decrease in curvature while mean plaque volume was 4.2 cm^3 before and 2.7 cm^3 after treatment. Subjective improvements were noted in curvature in 62%, girth in 83%, rigidity distal to the plaque in 80%, sexual function in 71%, and pain in 84%. There were no differences in response to verapamil based on disease duration or severity, and with mean follow-up of 2.5 years no patient who had improvement in penile deformity has reported recurrence of deformity.[82] A small, controlled study of intralesional verapamil versus saline injections (n=14) found that penile curvature improved in 29% of the verapamil-treated patients while there was no improvement in the controls, but this difference was not statistically significant. Plaque volume decreased in 57% of the treatment group vs 28% of the control group, while subjective ED improved in 43% of the verapamil group vs none of the controls.[77] A controlled study of peri-lesional, subcutaneous injection of verapamil found no advantage of verapamil over placebo, indicating the need to deliver the drug into the lesion.[74,87]

Intralesional verapamil has minor side effects. Many men have mild ecchymosis at the injection site. In the series by Levine et al., only 6 of 156 patients (4%) reported any side effects; 3 patients experienced pain at the injection site lasting longer than 1 day but less than 7 days, and 3 patients had transient nausea or lightheadedness without hypotension or dysrhythmia.[74] Levine and colleagues noted that, in their experience, the use of intralesional verapamil has not made subsequent corrective surgery more difficult. In fact, they use verapamil in men for whom they are planning surgical intervention if those men continue to have active, unstable disease or deformity >90°. They find that this hastens stabilization of the plaque; they wait to perform surgery until the deformity is stable for at least 6 months.[74]

A standard regimen for intralesional verapamil is to use 10 mg of verapamil diluted to 10 ml total volume with saline or a local anesthetic agent. After induction of penile block, the verapamil solution is distributed throughout the plaque by passing a 25 gauge needle in and out of the plaque numerous times. Skin is punctured only once and the needle is directed into different regions of the plaque without drawing the needle out of the skin. The needle should typically be inserted in the dorsolateral or lateral region of the penis, depending on the plaque location, to avoid injury to the dorsal penile neurovascular bed.[74,77] Injections are delivered at 2-week intervals for a total of 12 treatments. Injections more frequently than every 2 weeks have been found to induce an increased inflammatory response.[74]

Other modes of verapamil delivery have been tried. Dermal application of verapamil to the penis resulted in a low level of systemic verapamil, but no drug was identified in TA tissue samples.[88] Electromotive transdermal delivery (iontophoresis) of verapamil into plaques has also been used. This method has the benefit of being non-invasive and pain-free and without tissue trauma from injections. Moreover, it is argued that iontophoresis may provide a more homogeneous drug delivery to the plaque.[89] A study of this method found detectable verapamil in 72% of TA specimens, though drug concentration varied widely. The exact implication of this in the clinical setting remains unclear.[90] Both uncontrolled and placebo-controlled studies of electromotive delivery of verapamil combined with dexamethasone have provided positive results.[89,91–94] An example of one dosing regimen is verapamil 5mg (with corticosteroid and with or without lidocaine) delivered via a 2.4mA electric current applied for 20 minutes with four sessions per week for 6 weeks.[92] This regimen is intensive, and 24% of patients withdrew before completing the full course of therapy. Others use a less frequent treatment regimen.[89] Unfortunately, these studies all combine verapamil with corticosteroid and sometimes with lidocaine, making the determination of each drug's independent effect impossible. Based on the purported biologic mechanism of verapamil, however, electromotive delivery should have similar effects as injection of the drug. The effect of electromotively delivered corticosteroid is unclear. Supportive evidence for corticosteroid injections in PD includes uncontrolled case series, while a placebo-controlled study found no benefit.[92,95,96] Another issue is whether corticosteroid delivered by iontophoresis produces sclerosis, which

can hinder future surgery, as has been noted with corticosteroid injection therapy.[73]

Interferons are a group of naturally occurring proteins with numerous biologic properties, including immunomodulatory, anti-tumorigenic, growth-regulating, and cellular differentiation effects, which form the rationale for their use in PD.[97] *In vitro* study of plaque-derived fibroblasts has shown that interferon-alpha-2b inhibits fibroblast proliferation and collagen synthesis and increases collagenase synthesis.[97,98] Moreover, interferon-alpha-2b has been used successfully in the treatment of keloid scars and in scleroderma.[97] Uncontrolled studies have demonstrated mixed results, with some showing marked improvements and others finding no benefit.[99–107] There is also concern about systemic toxicity with the use of interferon, which can produce flu-like side-effects. In one series, such symptoms (fatigue, myalgia, fever >38°C) occurred after only 2% of injections and resolved within 24 hours, while in a different study 74 of 90 injections produced fever >38°C, side effects were significant, and 8 days of work were lost.[101,103] To date, there are no randomized, placebo-controlled trials published on the use of interferon in PD; as such, conclusions regarding its effectiveness are not possible. Given its side-effect profile and high cost, its use should remain limited until further supportive data are available.[50] In a single-blind placebo-controlled trial of interferon 2b, Hellstrom and colleagues report statistically significant improvement in penile curvature, plaque size and density, and penile pain.[108]

Intralesional collagenase has been investigated as a treatment option. Case series and a randomized, placebo-controlled, double-blind study reported positive results with collagenase.[109,110] However, the controlled study provides little detail regarding the clinical improvements and notes that the absolute change in deformity was small.[109] Additionally, treatment with collagenase induced a humoral immune response, with elevated IgG in 88% of treated patients and elevated IgE in 1 of the 44 patients. The authors speculate that future intralesional treatment with collagenase would not be significantly inhibited by preformed IgG antibody, owing to the relative avascular nature of TA, though they do note that the potential for severe allergic reaction exists with IgE antibody sensitization.[111] Given these concerns and the relative lack of significant, supportive data, collagenase is not a current standard therapy. Other drugs, such as orgotein and parathyroid hormone, that have been used for intralesional delivery currently lack sufficient data to draw conclusions regarding effectiveness or to support their usage.[112–115]

Extracorporeal shock-wave therapy and other forms of energy delivery

Modes of energy delivery that have been used to treat PD include radiation, ultrasound, laser therapy, extracorporeal shock-wave therapy (ESWT), and diathermy.[69] ESWT delivers directed ultrasound energy to the plaque. The exact mechanistic rationale for a beneficial effect is unclear. It is interesting that the presumed pathogenesis of PD is trauma to the TA, and that this therapeutic intervention itself is traumatic.[116] Side effects are usually minor and include local pain, bruising, and urethral bleeding with macroscopic hematuria (7% in one large series).[116] No serious side effect has been reported in any study, though there is the theoretical concern for urethral stricture given the occurrence of urethral trauma.[116] Uncontrolled studies of ESWT have provided conflicting results. Results of various studies include decreased plaque size in 0–58%, reduced curvature in 0–74%, decreased pain in 56–100%, and improved sexual function in 12–75%.[116–124] The study most resembling a placebo-controlled study was one in which patients who had previously failed oral therapy were treated with EWST and compared with age-matched patients without previous therapy, who were given oral placebo drug. While the study design makes interpretation of the results unclear, it found no difference in decrease in pain, subjective improvement, or improvement in sexual function. Curvature showed a greater decrease in the ESWT group compared with the placebo group, though this was not statistically significant.[125] An exploratory meta-analysis of outcomes from 17 study groups found no clear effect on plaque size or penile deformity, though it did suggest that ESWT might promote faster resolution of pain compared with the natural course of the disease and that it may also promote improved

sexual function.[126] It has been theorized that the mechanism behind pain relief with ESWT is direct disturbance of pain receptors or hyperstimulation-induced analgesia.[116] However, the natural history of PD is that of pain relief with time for most patients, bringing into question whether the treatment of pain alone should be a primary treatment goal.[116] At a minimum, further study with appropriately conducted, placebo-controlled trials is needed before generalized implementation of this expensive technology can be recommended.

Radiation therapy has also been used to treat PD. Randomized, placebo-controlled studies are lacking and results of non-controlled studies are inconclusive, though most have found a reduction in pain.[38,43,127–132] One large retrospective, non-controlled review of 106 patients treated with radiation therapy found that at an average of 9 years after therapy, 69% with pain prior to radiation therapy reported improved pain, 29% reported decreased curvature, and 13% with pre-intervention ED had improved erections.[38] However, 54% of patients reported not having erections rigid enough for sexual intercourse; this compares with a pre-treatment rate of ED of 18%.[38] Causes for this decrease in erectile function are unclear, but could be related to increased patient age (mean of 9 years between the two assessments), effects of PD itself, as well as possible damaging effects on the neurovascular erectile mechanism by irradiation. Cases have been reported of extensive corporal fibrosis after penile irradiation.[133] Interestingly, an *in vitro* study of plaque-derived fibroblasts found that irradiation significantly increased the expression of pro-fibrotic cytokines.[133]

Treatment of ED in men with PD

Treatment of ED associated with PD can be challenging.[134] In one series of 56 men with PD and complete loss of erectile function, 51 were unresponsive to intracavernosal prostaglandin E1.[8] In another group of patients with less severe baseline ED, 36 of 38 experienced good response to intracavernous injection therapy (papaverine plus phentolamine plus prostaglandin E1).[135] Levine and colleagues evaluated the use of sildenafil in a retrospective review of patients with PD and ED characterized by having lack of rigidity sufficient for vaginal penetration and maintenance throughout sexual intercourse.[81] Of responders, 71% were satisfied or very satisfied with the effect of sildenafil, 10% were neutral, and 19% were dissatisfied or very dissatisfied.[81] In a subgroup analysis, 90% of their patients with venous leakage were satisfied with sildenafil, while only 52% with arterial insufficiency were satisfied. This suggests that patients with more severe arterial dysfunction and those with comorbid vascular risk factors, such as diabetes or hypertension, may respond more poorly to the phosphodiesterase inhibitors. However, given that this class of drugs is generally safe and an effective, first-line therapy for ED, it is still practical to perform a trial of therapy, even if there is evidence of arterial or vascular disease.[81] Vacuum erection devices are another option for patients although the constriction ring has been implicated in the etiology of PD.[136]

Surgery

Given the potential for spontaneous regression, conservative management is appropriate in the acute stage of PD. Surgery should be performed only after an interval of 6–12 months of stable disease. This strategy helps to ensure that the surgical correction is not endangered by continued disease progression.[2] Surgery should be reserved for those with severe deformities causing significant sexual dysfunction. Ultimately, approximately 10% of PD patients will require surgery, a percentage that reflects surgical intervention for straightening alone as well as those who require operations for ED.[8] Options for penile straightening include plication of the TA at a point contralateral to the plaque. This is an option for patients with less severe curvature (<60°), though it has the intrinsic problem of producing penile shortening. Of note, while penile shortening is an intrinsic component of the disease process itself, many patients do not appreciate this at the time of presentation. It is worthwhile to point out the fact that shortening has already occurred before patients undergo surgery.[4] Plaque incision and excision with grafting are other options; these methods are often used for high-grade curvature and in those where loss of penile length would be

problematic. These methods still produce penile shortening, but less so than simple contralateral plication techniques.

In patients with concomitant ED, conservative measures such as oral or injectible vasoactive agents are first-line therapy. If these are unsuccessful, penile prosthesis implantation is often performed, with straightening of the penis performed either by modeling the penis over an inflated prosthesis or by plaque incision or excision with grafting.[2,137]

Summary and practical disease management

PD appears to be more prevalent than previously thought, and its prevalence is likely to increase as our population ages and more men seek treatment for ED. The disease remains enigmatic and incurable, with only limited evidence and speculation as to its pathogenesis. Many medical treatment options have been tried, and conclusions regarding the various therapies are limited given the paucity of randomized, controlled clinical trials. Moreover, the natural history of the disease contributes to the difficulty in interpreting the effectiveness of therapeutic interventions.

A practical treatment algorithm is to manage the patient initially and during the acute phase of the disease expectantly. If the patient is relatively asymptomatic, clinical follow-up may be all that is necessary, at least initially. If the patient has progressive or symptomatic disease, clinical therapy is indicated. Choosing between the different treatment options will depend on the physician's clinical experience and interpretation of the available data and on the patient's comfort with different forms of therapy. Treatment of concomitant ED will be with either oral or injectible erection-promoting agents or a vacuum erection device. Surgical intervention for penile straightening should be reserved for those with severe penile deformity that precludes sexual intercourse, and penile prosthesis implantation is used in impotent patients who fail clinical therapy. Surgical intervention should be performed only after the disease has stabilized for 6–12 months.

References

1. Dunsmuir WD, Kirby RS. Francois de LaPeyronie (1678–1747): the man and the disease he described. Br J Urol 1996; 78: 613–22.

2. Hauck EW, Weidner W. Francois de la Peyronie and the disease named after him. Lancet 2001; 357: 2049–51.

3. De la Peyronie F. Sur quelques obstacles quis'opposent à l'éjaculation naturelle de la semence. Mem Acad Roy Chir 1743; 1: 423–34.

4. Pryor JD, Ralph DJ. Clinical presentations of Peyronie's disease. Int J Impot Res 2002; 12: 414–17.

5. Kadioglu A, Tefekli A, Erol B et al. A retrospective review of 307 men with Peyronie's disease. J Urol 2002; 168: 1075–9.

6. Rodríguez Tolrà J, Franco Miranda E, Prats Puig JM et al. Treatment with the Newbit technique in patients with Peyronie's disease. Int J Impot Res 2003; 15(Suppl 7): S36–40.

7. Hellstrom WJG. History, epidemiology, and clinical presentation of Peyronie's disease. Int J Impot Res 2003; 15(Suppl 5): S91–2.

8. Weidner W, Schroeder-Printzen I, Weiske WH et al. Sexual dysfunction in Peyronie's disease: an analysis of 222 patients without previous local plaque therapy. J Urol 1997; 157: 325–8.

9. Mulhall JP, Creech SD, Boorjian SA et al. Subjective and objective analysis of the prevalence of Peyronie's disease in a population of men presenting for prostate cancer screening. J Urol 2004; 171: 2350–3.

10. Gelbard MK, Dorey F, James K. The natural history of Peyronie's disease. J Urol 1990; 144:1376–9.

11. Sommer F, Schwarzer U, Wassmer G et al. Epidemiology of Peyronie's disease. Int J Impot Res 2002; 14: 379–83.

12. Smith BH. Subclinical Peyronie's disease. Am J Clin Pathol 1969; 52: 385–90.

13. Lindsay MB, Schain DM, Grambsch P et al. The incidence of Peyronie's disease in Rochester, Minnesota, 1950 through 1984. J Urol 1991; 146: 1007–9.

14. Schwarzer U, Sommer F, Klotz T et al. The prevalence of Peyronie's disease: results of a large survey. BJU Int 2001; 88: 727–30.

15. Kadioglu A, Tefekli A, Erol H et al. Color Doppler ultrasound assessment of penile vascular system in men with Peyronie's disease. Int J Impot Res 2000; 12: 263–7.

16. Moreland RB, Nehra A. Pathophysiology of Peyronie's disease. Int J Impot Res 2002; 14: 406–10.

17. Brock G, Hsu G, Nunes L et al. The anatomy of the tunic albuginea in the normal penis and Peyronie's disease. J Urol 1997; 157: 276–81.

18. Davis CJ Jr. The microscopic pathology of Peyronie's disease. J Urol 1997; 157: 282–4.

19. Akkus E, Carrier S, Baba K et al. Structural alterations in the tunica albuginea of the penis: impact of Peyronie's disease, ageing and impotence. Br J Urol 1997; 79: 47–53.

20. Iacono B, Barra S, De Rosa G et al. Microstructural disorders of tunica albuginea in patients affected by Peyronie's disease with or without erection dysfunction. J Urol 1993; 150: 1806–9.

21. Somers KD, Sismour EN, Wright GL et al. Isolation and characterization of collagen in Peyronie's disease. J Urol 1989; 141: 629–31.

22. Valente EGA, Vernet D, Ferrini MG et al. L-Arginine and phosphodiesterase (PDE) inhibitors counteract fibrosis in Peyronie's fibrotic plaque and related fibroblast cultures. Nitric Oxide 2003; 9: 229–44.

23. Hirano D, Takimoto Y, Yamamoto T et al. Electron microscopic study of the penile plaques and adjacent corpora cavernosa in Peyronie's disease. Int J Urol 1997; 4: 274–8.

24. Vande Berg JS, Devine CJ, Horton CE et al. Peyronie's disease: an electron microscopic study. J Urol 1981; 126: 333–6.

25. Smith BH. Peyronie's disease. Am J Clin Pathol 1966; 45: 670–8.

26. Bystrom J, Rubio C. Induratio penis plastica (Peyronie's disease). Scand J Urol Nephrol 1976; 10: 12–20.

27. Lue TF. Peyronie's disease: an anatomically-based hypothesis and beyond. Int J Impot Res 2002; 14: 411–13.

28. Hellstrom WJG, Bivalacqua TJ. Peyronie's disease: etiology, medical, and surgical therapy. J Androl 2000; 21: 347–54.

29. Davila HH, Magee TR, Zuniga FI et al. Peyronie's disease associated with increase in plasminogen activator inhibitor in fibrotic plaque. Urology 2005; 65: 645–8.

30. Sikka SC, Hellstrom WJG. Role of oxidative stress and antioxidants in Peyronie's disease. Int J Impot Res 2002; 14: 353–60.

31. Fornara P, Gerbershagen HP. Ultrasound in patients affected with Peyronie's disease. World J Urol 2004; 22: 365–7.

32. Lyles KW, Gold DT, Newton RA et al. Peyronie's disease is associated with Paget's disease of bone. J Bone Miner Res 1997; 12: 929–34.

33. Patrizia Carrieri M, Serraino D, Palmiotto F et al. A case-control study on risk factors for Peyronie's disease. J Clin Epidemiol 1998; 51: 511–15.

34. Leffell MS, Devine CJ Jr, Horton CE et al. Non-association of Peyronie's disease with HLA B7 cross-reactive antigens. J Urol 1982; 127: 1223–4.

35. Hauck EW, Hauptmann A, Weidner W et al. Prospective analysis of HLA classes I and II antigen frequency in patients with Peyronie's disease. J Urol 2003; 170: 1443–6.

36. Schiavino D, Sasso F, Nucera E et al. Immunologic findings in Peyronie's disease: a controlled study. Urology 1997; 50: 764–8.

37. Stewart S, Malto M, Sandberg L et al. Increased serum levels of anti-elastin antibodies in patients with Peyronie's disease. J Urol 1994; 152: 105–6.

38. Incrocci L, Hop WCJ, Slob AK. Current sexual functioning in 106 patients with Peyronie's disease treated with radiotherapy 9 years earlier. Urology 2000; 56: 1030–4.

39. Zargooshi J. Trauma as the cause of Peyronie's disease: penile fracture as a model of trauma. J Urol 2004; 172: 186–8.

40. Usta MF, Bivalacqua TJ, Jabren GW et al. Relationship between the severity of penile curvature and the presence of comorbidities in men with Peyronie's disease. J Urol 2004; 171: 775–9.

41. Hauck EW, Domann E, Hauptmann A et al. Prospective analysis of 16S rDNA as a highly sensitive marker for bacterial presence in Peyronie's disease plaques. J Urol 2003; 170: 2053–6.

42. Smith CJ, McMahon C, Shabsigh R. Peyronie's disease: the epidemiology, aetiology and clinical evaluation of deformity. BJU Int 2005; 95: 729–32.

43. Mulhall JP, Branch J, Lubrano T et al. Radiation increases fibrogenic cytokine expression by Peyronie's disease fibroblasts. J Urol 2003; 170: 281–4.

44. Magee TR, Qian A, Rajfer J et al. Gene expression in the Peyronie's disease plaque. Urol 2002; 59: 451–7.

45. Bertolotto M, de Stefani S, Martinoli C et al. Color Doppler appearance of penile cavernosal–spongiosal communications in patients with severe Peyronie's disease. Eur Radiol 2002; 12: 2525–31.

46. Usta MF, Bivalacqua, Tokatli Z et al. Stratification of penile vascular pathologies in patients with Peyronie's disease and in men with erectile dysfunction according to age: a comparative study. J Urol 2004; 172: 259–62.

47. Andresen R, Wegner HE, Miller K et al. Imaging modalities in Peyronie's disease. An intrapersonal comparison of ultrasound sonography, X-ray in mammography technique, computer tomography, and nuclear magnetic resonance in 20 patients. Eur Urol 1998; 34: 123–34.

48. Hakim LS. Peyronie's disease: an update. The role of diagnostics. Int J Impot Res 2002; 14: 321–3.

49. Biagiotti G, Cavallini G. Acetyl-l-carnitine vs tamoxifen in the oral therapy of Peyronie's disease: a preliminary report. BJU Int 2001; 88: 63–7.

50. Ralph DJ, Minhas S. The management of Peyronie's disease. BJU Int 2004; 93: 208–15.

51. Kadioglu A, Tefekli A, Koksal T et al. Treatment of Peyronie's disease with oral colchicine: long-term results and predictive parameters of successful outcome. Int J Impot Res 2000; 12: 169–75.

52. Weidner W, Hauck EW, Schnitker J. Potassium paraaminobenzoate (POTABA™) in the treatment of Peyronie's disease: a prospective, placebo-controlled, randomized study. Eur Urol 2005; 47: 530–6.

53. Mynderse LA, Monga M. Oral therapy for Peyronie's disease. Int J Impot Res 2002; 14: 340–4.

54. Scott WW, Scardino PL. A new concept in the treatment of Peyronie's disease. South Med J 1948; 41: 173–7.

55. Chesney J. Peyronie's disease. Br J Urol 1975; 47: 209–18.

56. Scardino PL, Scott WW. The use of tocopherols in the treatment of Peyronie's disease. Ann N Y Acad Sci 1949; 52: 390–401.

57. Pryor JP, Farell CF. Controlled clinical trial of vitamin E in Peyronie's disease. Prog Reprod Biol 1983; 9: 47–60.

58. Prieto Castro RM, Lave Vallejo ME, Regueiro Lopez JC et al. Combined treatment with vitamin E and colchicine in the early stages of Peyronie's disease. BJU Int 2003; 91: 522–4.

59. Sagone AL, Husney RM, Davis WB. Biotransformation of para-aminobenzioc acid and salicylic acid by PMN. Free Radic Biol Med 1993; 14: 27–35.

60. Carson CC. Potassium para-aminobenzoate for the treatment of Peyronie's disease: is it effective? Tech Urol 1997; 3: 135–9.

61. Hasche-Klunder R. Treatment of Peyronie's disease with para-aminobenzoacidic potassium (POTOBA). Urologe A 1978; 17: 224–7.

62. Shah PJR, Green NA, Adib RS et al. A multi-centre double-blind controlled clinical trial of potassium para-amino-benzoate (POTABA) in Peyronie's disease. Prog Reprod Biol 1983; 9: 47–60.

63. Ehrlich HP, Bornstein P. Microtubules in trans-cellular movement of procollagen. Nat New Biol 1972; 238: 257–60.

64. Anderson MS, Shankey TV, Lubrano T et al. Inhibition of Peyronie's plaque fibroblast prolifera-tion by biologic agents. Int J Impot Res 2000; 12(Suppl 3): S25–31.

65. Dominguez-Malagon HR, Alfeiran-Ruiz A, Chavarria-Xicotencatl P et al. Clinical and cellular effects of colchicine in fibromatosis. Cancer 1992; 69: 2478–83.

66. El-Sakka AI, Bakircioglu ME, Bhatnagar RS et al. The effects of colchicine on a Peyronie's-like condition in an animal model. J Urol 1999; 161: 1980–3.

67. Akkus E, Carrier S, Rehman, J et al. Is colchicine effective in Peyronie's disease? A pilot study. Urology 1994; 44: 291–5.

68. Alonso JJ, Amaya J, Vega P et al. Results of the use of colchicine in the treatment of the tunica albuginea fibrosis. J Androl 2001; 22(Suppl): 139.

69. Safarinejad MR. Therapeutic effects of colchicine in the management of Peyronie's disease: a ran-domized double-blind, placebo-controlled study. Int J Impot Res 2004; 16: 238–43.

70. Ralph DJ, Brooks MD, Bottazzo GF et al. The treatment of Peyronie's disease with tamoxifen. Br J Urol 1992; 70: 648–51.

71. Teloken C, Rhoden EL, Grazziotin TM et al. Tamoxifen versus placebo in the treatment of Peyronie's disease. J Urol 199; 162: 2003–5.

72. Davila HH, Magee TR, Vernet D et al. Gene trans-fer of inducible nitric oxide synthase complemen-tary DNA regresses the fibrotic plaque in an animal model of Peyronie's disease. Biol Reprod 2004; 71: 1568–77.

73. Gelbard MK, Hayden B. Expanding contractures of the tunica albuginea due to Peyronie's disease with temporalis fascia free grafts. J Urol 1991; 145: 772–6.

74. Levine LA, Estrada CR. Intralesional verapamil for the treatment of Peyronie's disease: a review. Int J Impot Res 2002; 14: 324–8.

75. Kelly RB. Pathways of protein secretion in eukaryotes. Science 1985; 230: 25–32.

76. Aggeler J, Frisch SM, Werb Z. Changes in cell shape correlate with collagenase gene expression in rabbit synovial fibroblasts. J Cell Biol 1984; 98: 1662–71.

77. Rehman J, Benet A, Melman A. Use of intra-lesional verapamil to dissolve Peyronie's disease plaque: a long-term single-blind study. Urology 1998; 51: 620–6.

78. Rodler S, Roth M, Nauck M et al. Ca(2+)-channel blockers modulate the expression of interleukin-6 and interleukin-8 genes in human vascular smooth muscle cells. J Mol Cell Cardiol 1995; 27: 2295–302.

79. Lee RC, Ping JA. Calcium antagonists retard extracellular matrix production in connective tissue equivalent. J Surg Res 1990; 49: 463–6.

80. Lee RC, Doong H, Jellema AF. The response of burn scars to intralesional verapamil. Report of five cases. Arch Surg 1994; 129: 107–11.

81. Levine, LA. Treatment of Peyronie's disease with intralesional verapamil injection. J Urol 1997; 158: 1395–9.

82. Levine LA, Goldman KE, Greenfield JM. Experi-ence with intraplaque injection of verapamil for Peyronie's disease. J Urol 2002; 168: 621–6.

83. Lasser A, Vandenberg TL, Vincent MJ et al. Intraplaque verapamil injection for treatment of Peyronie's disease. J La State Med Soc 1998; 150: 431–4.

84. Mirone V, Imbimbo C, Palmieri A et al. A new biopsy technique to investigate Peyronie's disease associated histologic alterations: results with two different forms of therapy. Eur Urol 2002; 42: 239–44.

85. Levine LA, Estrada CR, Storm DW et al. Peyronie disease in younger men: characteristics and treatment results. J Androl 2003; 24: 27–32.

86. Arena F, Peracchia G, Di Stefano C et al. Clinical effects of verapamil in the treatment in Peyronie's disease. Acta Biomed 1995; 66: 269–72.

87. Teloken C, Vaccaro F, Da Ros C et al. Objective evaluation of non-surgical approach for Peyronie's disease. J Urol 1996; 155: 633A, abstract 1290.

88. Martin DJ, Badwan K, Parker M et al. Transdermal application of verapamil gel to the penile shaft fails to infiltrate the tunica albuginea. J Urol 2002; 168: 2483–5.

89. Riedl CR, Plas E, Engelhardt P et al. Iontophoresis for treatment of Peyronie's disease. J Urol 2000; 163: 95–9.

90. Levine AL, Estrada CR, Shou Wilson et al. Tunica albuginea tissue analysis after electromotive drug administration. J Urol 2003; 169: 1775–8.

91. Di Stasi SM, Giannantoni G, Capelli G et al. Transdermal electromotive administration of verapamil and dexamethasone for Peyronie's disease. BJU Int 2003; 91: 825–9.

92. Di Stasi SM, Giannantoni A, Stephen RL et al. A prospective, randomized study using transdermal electromotive administration of verapamil and dexamethasone for Peyronie's disease. J Urol 2004; 171: 1605–8.

93. Treffiletti S, Annoscia S, Montefiore F et al. Iontophoresis in the conservative treatment of Peyronie's disease: preliminary experience. Arch Ital Urol Androl 1997; 69: 323–7.

94. Montorsi F, Salonia A, Guazzoni G et al. Transdermal electromotive multi-drug administration for Peyronie's disease: preliminary results. J Androl 2000; 21: 85–90.

95. Winter CC, Khanna R. Peyronie's disease: results with dermo-jet injection of dexamethasone. J Urol 1975; 114: 898–900.

96. Cipollone G, Nicolai M, Mastroprimiano G et al. Betamethasone versus placebo in Peyronie's disease. Arch Ital Urol Androl 1998; 70: 165–8.

97. Lacy GL, Adams DM, Hellstrom WJG. Intralesional interferon-alpha-2b for the treatment of Peyronie's disease. Int J Impot Res 2002; 14: 336–9.

98. Duncan MR, Berman B, Nseyo UO. Regulation of the proliferation and biosynthetic activities of cultured human Peyronie's disease fibroblasts by interferons-alpha, -beta, and -gamma. Scand J Urol Nephrol 1991; 25: 89–94.

99. Astorga R, Cantero O, Contreras D et al. Intralesional recombinant interferon alpha-2b in Peyronie's disease. Arch Esp Urol 2000; 53: 665–71.

100. Ahuja S, Bivalacqua TJ, Case J et al. A pilot study demonstrating clinical benefit from intralesional interferon alpha 2B in the treatment of Peyronie's disease. J Androl 1999; 20: 444–8.

101. Brake M, Loertzer H, Horsch R et al. Treatment of Peyronie's disease with local interferon-α 2b. BJU Int 2001; 87: 654–7.

102. Wegner HE, Andresen R, Knipsel HH et al. Treatment of Peyronie's disease with local interferon-alpha 2b. Eur Urol 1995; 28: 236–40.

103. Wegner HE, Andresen R, Knispel HH et al. Local interferon-alpha 2b is not an effective treatment in early-stage Peyronie's disease. Eur Urol 1997; 32: 190–3.

104. Judge IS, Wisniewski ZS. Intralesional interferon in the treatment of Peyronie's disease: a pilot study. Br J Urol 1997; 79: 40–2.

105. Dang G, Matern R, Bivalacqua TJ et al. Intralesional interferon-alpha-2B injections for the treatment of Peyronie's disease. South Med J 2004; 97: 42–6.

106. Polat O, Gul O, Ozbey I et al. Peyronie's disease: intralesional treatment with interferon alpha-2A and evaluation of the results by magnetic resonance imaging. Int Urol Nephrol 1997; 29: 465–71.

107. Novak TE, Bryan W, Templeton L et al. Combined intralesional interferon alpha 2B and oral vitamin E in the treatment of Peyronie's disease. J La State Med Soc 2001; 153: 358–63.

108. Hellstrom WJ, Kendirci M, Matern R et al. Single-blind, multicenter, placebo controlled, parallel study to assess the safety and efficacy of intralesional interferon alpha-2B for minimally invasive treatment for Peyronie's disease. J Urol 2006; 176: 394–8.

109. Gelbard MK, James K, Riach P et al. Collagenase versus placebo in the treatment of Peyronie's disease: a double-blind study. J Urol 1993; 149: 56–8.

110. Gelbard MK, Lindner JA, Kaufman JJ. The use of collagenase in the treatment of Peyronie's disease. J Urol 1985; 134: 280–3.

111. Hamilton RG, Mintz GR, Gelbard MK. Humoral immune responses in Peyronie's disease patients receiving clostridial collagenase therapy. J Urol 1986; 135: 641–7.

112. Morales A, Bruce AW. The treatment of Peyronie's disease with parathyroid hormone. J Urol 1975; 114: 901–2.

113. Perez Espejo L, Campoy Martinez P, Perez Perez M et al. Iontophoresis in Peyronie's disease. Our experience. Arch Esp Urol 2003; 56: 1133–7.

114. Wagenknecht LV. Differential therapies in various stages of penile induration. Arch Esp Urol 1996; 49: 285–92.

115. Gustafson H, Johansson B, Edsmyr F. Peyronie's disease: experience of local treatment with orgotein. Eur Urol 1981; 7: 346–8.

116. Hauck EW, Hauptmann A, Bschleipfer T et al. Questionable efficacy of extracorporeal shock wave therapy for Peyronie's disease: results of a prospective approach. J Urol 2004; 171: 296–9.

117. Lebret T, Loison G, Herve J et al. Extracorporeal shock wave therapy in the treatment of Peyronie's disease: experience with standard lithotriptor (Siemens-Multiline). Urology 2002; 59: 657–61.

118. Michel MS, Ptaschnyk T, Musial A et al. Objective and subjective changes in patients with Peyronie's disease after management with shockwave therapy. J Endourol 2003; 17: 41–4.

119. Skolarikos A, Alargof E, Rigas A et al. Shockwave therapy as first-line therapy for Peyronie's disease: a prospective study. J Endourol 2005; 19: 11–14.

120. Strebel RT, Suter S, Sautter T et al. Extracorporeal shockwave therapy for Peyronie's disease does not correct penile deformity. Int J Impot Res 2004; 16: 448–51.

121. Manikandan R, Islam W, Srinivasan V et al. Evaluation of extracorporeal shock wave therapy in Peyronie's disease. Urology 2002; 60: 795–800.

122. Kiyota H, Ohishi Y, Asano K et al. Extracorporeal shock wave treatment for Peyronie's disease using EDAP LT-02; preliminary results. Int J Urol 2002; 9: 110–13.

123. Colombo F, Nicola M. Peyronie's disease: ultrasonographic follow-up of ESWT. Arch Ital Urol Androl 2000; 72: 388–91.

124. Husain J, Lynn NNK, Jones DK et al. Extracorporeal shock wave therapy in the management of Peyronie's disease: initial experience. BJU Int 2000; 86: 466–8.

125. Hauck EW, Altinkilic BM, Ludwig M et al. Extracorporal shock wave therapy in the treatment of Peyronie's disease. First results of a case-controlled approach. Eur Urol 2000; 38 (6): 663–9.

126. Hauck EW, Mueller UO, Bschleipfer T et al. Extracorporeal shock wave therapy for Peyronie's disease: exploratory meta-analysis of clinical trials. J Urol 2004; 171: 740–5.

127. Rodrigues CR, Njo KH, Karim ABMF. Results of radiotherapy and vitamin E in the treatment of Peyronie's disease. Int J Radiat Oncol Biol Phys 1995; 31: 571–6.

128. Incrocci L, Wijnmaalen A, Slob AK et al. Low-dose radiotherapy in 179 patients with Peyronie's disease: treatment outcome and current sexual functioning. Int J Radiat Oncol Biol Phys 2000; 47: 1353–6.

129. Carson CC, Coughlin PW. Radiation therapy for Peyronie's disease: is there a place? J Urol 1985; 134: 684–6.

130. Weisser GW, Schmidt B, Hubener KH et al. Radiation treatment of plastic induration of the penis. Strahlenther Onkol 1987; 163: 23–8.

131. Kammerer R. Radiotherapy of induratio penis plastica. Z Urol Nephrol 1988; 81: 323–8.

132. Koren H, Alth G, Schenk GM et al. Induratio penis plastica: effectivity of low-dose radiotherapy at different clinical stages. Urol Res 1996; 24: 245–8.

133. Hall SJ, Basile G, Bertero EB et al. Extensive corporeal fibrosis after penile irradiation. J Urol 1995; 153: 372–7.

134. Krane RJ. The treatment of loss of penile rigidity associated with Peyronie's disease. Scand J Urol Nephrol Suppl 1996; 179: 147–50.

135. Culha M, Mutlu N, Acar O et al. Patient–partner satisfaction with intracavernous medication supported with oral agents in selected cases of Peyronie's disease. Int Urol Nephrol 1999; 31(2): 257–62.

136. Ganem JP, Lucey DT, Janosko EO, Carson CC. Unusual complications of the vacuum erectile device. Urol 1998; 51: 627–31.

137. Wilson SK, Delk JR. A new treatment for Peyronie's disease: modeling the penis over an inflatable penile prosthesis. J Urol 1994; 152: 1121–3.

CHAPTER 19

Hypospadias: uncovering a common problem

Hitendra RH Patel, Christopher RJ Woodhouse

Introduction

Hypospadias is the abnormal development of the anterior urethra in which the external urethral opening can be located on the ventrum of the penis anywhere between the proximal glans penis (Fig. 19.1) and the scrotum or perineum. The penis is more likely to have associated ventral shortening and curvature (chordee) with more proximal urethral defects.

Galen first documented hypospadias during AD 200, with the only treatment being amputation of the distal penis to external urethral opening. Hypospadias repair has come a long way since this time, with many different repairs being described in the medical literature. Clinical outcomes have improved over the past century with modern sutures, dressings, instruments and antibiotics. This has led to more cases being done as a single-stage repair and earlier in life (usually by the age of 2 years; Fig. 19.2).

Epidemiology

Hypospadias occurs in approximately 1 in 300 live male births, but appears to be rising. One reason for this may be increased reporting, however this cannot explain a doubling in incidence over the past two decades.[1] The incidence is higher in whites than in blacks, and it is more common in males of Jewish and Italian descent.

Etiology

Genetic, endocrine and environmental agents have all been blamed for the development of hypospadias. A genetic predisposition has been suggested by the eight-fold increase in incidence of hypospadias among monozygotic twins compared to singletons.

This finding may be related to the demand by two fetuses for human chorionic gonadotrophins (hCGs) produced by the single placenta resulting in an inadequate supply during critical periods of urethral development. A familial trend has been noted with hypospadias. Eight per cent of fathers of affected boys have hypospadias, while 14% of brothers are affected. This suggests the inheritance pattern is polygenic. Baskin suggested epithelial–mesenchymal interactions (local effect) may play a key role after showing that disruption of the FGF10 gene, coding for fibroblast growth factor 10 was associated with hypospadias.[2]

A decrease in available androgen or an inability to use available androgen appropriately may result in hypospadias. Aaronson et al showed that 66% of boys with mild hypospadias and 40% with severe hypospadias had a defect in testicular testosterone biosynthesis.[3] Mutations in the 5-α reductase enzyme, which converts testosterone to the more potent dihydrotestosterone (DHT) have been associated with hypospadias. Silver et al. found that nearly 10% of boys with isolated hypospadias had at least

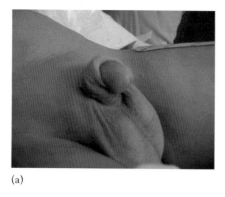

(a)

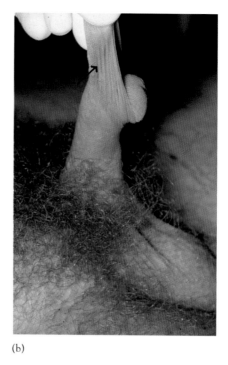

(b)

Figure 19.1. *(a) Preoperative glandular hypospadias in a 1 year old. (b) Preoperative adult hypospadias demonstrating the underdevelopment of the ventral prepuce, with an apparent overgrowth of the dorsal prepuce (arrow).*

one allele affected with a 5-α reductase mutation.[4] Although androgen receptor deficits have been shown to result in hypospadias, this is thought to be a relatively infrequent occurrence and other factors are more commonly implicated.

Males conceived by in vitro fertilization (IVF) had a five times increased risk of hypospadias compared to a control group.[5] This may reflect maternal exposure to progesterone, which is commonly administered in IVF protocols. Progesterone is a substrate for 5-α reductase and can competitively inhibit the conversion of testosterone to DHT. Other factors that contribute to infertility, such as underlying endocrinopathies or fetal endocrine abnormalities may also play a role.[3,6]

The disruption of endocrine pathways by environmental agents is an interesting hypothesis to explain the increased incidence of hypospadias. Estrogens have been implicated in abnormal penile development in many animal models. Environmental substances with significant estrogenic activity are ubiquitous in industrialized society and are ingested as pesticides on fruits and vegetables, endogenous plant estrogens, milk from lactating pregnant dairy cows, from plastic linings in metal cans, and in pharmaceuticals. Hadziselimovic described an increase in estradiol concentration in placental basal syncytiotrophoblasts of boys with undescended testes compared to a control population.[7] Undescended testes and hypospadias have been associated, but increased estradiol concentration has not been implicated in hypospadias. This may support the association of hypospadias with increasing parity, increasing maternal age and low birth weight noted in some studies in relation to lifelong exposure to environmental factors which have a cumulative effect. Aarskog, in a retrospective study, showed that maternal progestin intake may be associated with hypospadias, however,[8] this has been difficult to prove or refute.

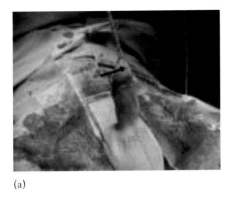

(a)

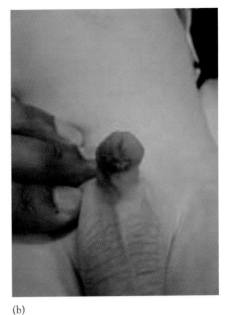

(b)

Figure 19.2. *(a) Immediate postoperative pediatric hypospadias repair in one stage. Note the closure of the ventral defect, with a catheter clearly demonstrating the external neomeatus in the correct position (arrow). (b) Three months after surgery the cosmetic result is close to normal.*

Pathophysiology

Urethral development occurs between 8 and 20 weeks of gestation. The external genital structures develop a masculine phenotype primarily under the influence of testosterone. As the phallus elongates, the open urethral groove extends from the base to the corona. The classic theory is that the urethral folds coalesce in the midline from base to tip, forming a tubularized penile urethra and median scrotal raphe. The anterior or glanular urethra develops in a proximal direction, with canalization of an ectodermal core (programmed cell death or apoptosis) forming at the tip of the glans penis. This joins with the proximal urethra at the corona. The potential weakness in this last step may explain the higher incidence of subcoronal hypospadias.

The circumferential development of the prepuce is obstructed by the failure of urethral folds to fuse, forming the hooded prepuce noted in hypospadias. The exception to this is the megameatus intact prepuce, which appears as suggested by its name.

Chordee (ventral curvature) of the penis is often associated with more severe forms of hypospadias. It occurs by differential growth between the dorsal corporal bodies and the ventral urethral tissues (Fig. 19.3).

The location of the abnormal urethral meatus classifies the hypospadias.[9] The location is anterior (glanular and subcoronal) in 50% of cases, middle (distal penile, midshaft and proximal penile) in 20%, and posterior (penoscrotal, scrotal and perineal) in 30%, with the subcoronal position being the most common overall.

Associated problems

Undescended testes and inguinal hernias are the most common anomalies associated with hypospadias. A review of over 1000 patients with hypospadias found the incidence of undescended testes and inguinal hernias at 9% each.[10] As the severity of hypospadias increased, the incidence of undescended testes and inguinal hernias was >30% and ~20%, respectively.

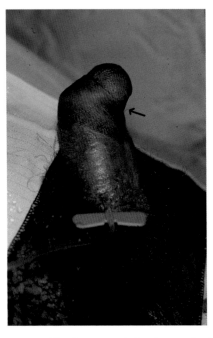

Figure 19.3. *Chordee or penile bending is clearly demonstrated by an artificial erection*

Combined hypospadias and undescended testis are suggestive of intersex disorders found in 30% of cases.[11] The more proximal the location of the meatus the higher the association with intersex states. If bilateral non-palpable gonads are present the occurrence rises to 50%, whereas a unilaterally palpable gonad is associated with a lower intersex occurrence at 15%.

Surgical treatment

Surgical correction aims to return the penis to a normal anatomical and functional state. Various surgical options include chordee repair (straightening the penis), urethroplasty (moving the external urethral meatus to the tip of the penis), glanuloplasty (reformation of the flattened glans into a more natural conical shape), giving cosmetically and functionally acceptable penile skin coverage, and creating a normal-appearing scrotum. The aim should be to enable the patient to have sexual intercourse, void standing and appear normal.

Timing

Before 1980, hypospadias repair was performed after the age of 3 years because the penis is bigger and the operation easier. However, genital surgery at this age can be associated with significant psychological morbidity, including aberrant behavior, guilt and gender identity confusion.

Currently, most surgeons repair hypospadias when the child is aged 6–18 months. This is thought to be associated with an improved emotional and psychological result although evidence is sparse. In addition, some surgeons ask parents to apply DHT cream to stimulate tissue growth and quality at the time of repair, and thus decrease risk of complications. A 5-week course of hCG reduced the difficulty of repair in more proximal hypospadias.[12]

Types of repair

There are many types of repair. Describing each is not the aim of the present chapter. More important are the basic principles. The penis is degloved and examined with and without an erection, to assess for skin tethering and chordee. The latter may be repaired by excising fibrous tethered tissue or by plicating the opposite side to the chordee on the dorsal tunics of the corporal bodies. This will lead to shortening of the penis. Severe chordee requires application of grafts on the ventral corporal bodies (autologous tissues – tunica vaginalis or dermal grafts) to avoid excessive penile shortening. The urethral plate is a good base for the urethroplasty and is only divided if the chordee is particularly severe.

A variety of methods exist to lengthen the urethra (primary tubularization, local pedicled skin flaps, tissue grafting techniques, or meatal advancement). Salvage repairs use buccal mucosal grafts because no local tissue is useful. It has been used successfully. Urethral stents are generally used for bladder drainage while healing occurs over a 5–7-day period.

Complications of surgery

Immediate complications

Postoperative bleeding may occur, but is countered by leaving a pressure dressing on for 5–7 days. Infection now is rare as techniques, materials and antibiotics have improved.

Long-term complications

Fistula
Urethrocutaneous fistula formation generally occurs in less than 10% for most one-stage repairs but increases up to 40% in complex salvage procedures. Decreasing this by a second layer closure of the neourethra has become a standard technique, avoiding overlap of suture lines.[13–15] The basic principles of fistula repair hold (remove non-viable or infected tissue, tension-free repair, dry wound, non-crossing suture lines).

Meatal/urethral stenosis
Meatal stenosis is usually due to the fashioning at surgery. It manifests late as a fine urinary stream and straining to void. Urethral strictures occur more commonly in proximal hypospadias repair. When minor, simple dilatation may suffice. When extensive, however, they require excision with reanastomosis, or patching with a graft or pedicled skin flap.

Diverticulum
Diverticula can form in the absence of distal obstruction. They are associated with graft or flap-type hypospadias repairs which lack surrounding tissue support of native urethral tissue. They are treated by removal of redundant urethral tissue and urethral tapering.

Hair in the urethra
Hair-bearing skin is no longer used in hypospadias reconstruction, since it resulted in urinary tract infection or stone formation, particularly at puberty. In patients who now are adults, hairy skin may have been used. Attached stones and hairballs are occasionally seen.

Hypospadias in adults

Appearance
There is a wide range of size and appearance of the penis. Its growth with age has been documented and a centile growth chart is available.[16] The normal appearance has not been so well documented – like other human features there is a wide variation in that which is considered normal or beautiful.

It has been established, however, that the meatus is not always at the tip of the penis. Thirteen per cent of apparently normal men have a hypospadiac meatus and in a further 32% it is in the middle third of the glans. Most of these men thought they were normal, all voided normally and had sexual intercourse.[17] It could, therefore, be said that minor degrees of hypospadias, especially if there is no chordee, do not greatly matter to men or to their partners.

For men who have had surgery for hypospadias, there is often disagreement with the surgeon on the success of the operation. Up to 80% of adolescents are dissatisfied with their penile appearance although only 38–44% want further surgery.[18,19] There is a difference in results depending on the attitude of the community to circumcision: in countries where childhood circumcision is routine, results are perceived to be better than in those where it is uncommon.

When there is a direct comparison of the opinion of the patient and of the surgeon, there is almost no agreement. Mureau et al have introduced the helpful concept of the Genital Perception Score (GPS).[20] Eight features of the penis are scored from one to four, giving an overall range of eight to 32 with the highest score being the best result (Table 19.1). This allows a numerical comparison and helps to identify areas of concern for the patient. It is important to note, however, that

Table 19.1. *Features of the Genital Perception Score[21]*

Correctable features*	Uncorrectable features*
Glans shape	Penile size
Position of meatus	Penile thickness
Scars	Glans size
Scrotum	
General appearance	

*All the features are scored, but for the purposes of Fig. 19.4 they are divided into surgically correctable and uncorrectable items.

three of the eight features are concerned with penile size which cannot be altered by surgery.

Mureau et al asked patients and their surgeons to give a GPS for the surgical result. Surgeons gave a mean score of 29.1 and the patients gave a mean of 25.1, a difference which was statistically significant (Fig. 19.4a). For the uncorrectable size-related features, the patients gave a mean satisfaction score of 3.1 (out of four) while the surgeons gave a score of 3.9. For the features related to the surgery the patients' mean score was 3.2 and the surgeons' was 3.5 (Fig. 19.4b). Much of the dissatisfaction seems to have been related to the circumcised appearance in a society where circumcision is unusual and is perceived to shorten the penis.[20]

It seems likely, therefore, that surgeons can reliably correct those abnormal features of the hypospadiac penis that are amenable to reconstruction: chordee, the hooded prepuce (especially if the circumcised appearance is acceptable) and the position of the meatus. Features related to the size of the corpora or the glans are not correctable.

Voiding

Young men like to void standing up in a public urinal through their opened flies. Inability to perform in this way is a serious social impediment. The stream must be well formed and directable, a goal that is most easily achieved with a slit-like terminal meatus. In some series up to 40% of patients have a stream that sprays. There is a trend to improvement with newer repairs, but voiding problems remain common in adults especially when compared to controls (Fig. 19.5).[21]

Fortunately, the results achieved in childhood seem to be maintained or may even improve. In a large series of patients of all ages up to 66 years, the proportion of men with a normal peak flow rate increased with age (Fig. 19.6).[22] The implication of this finding is that the neo-urethra grows appropriately with age. The patients in this study seem to be a reasonable cross-section of the hypospadias population, though 87% originally had a glanular or coronal meatus. Seventeen per cent had a spraying stream. The results are particularly good

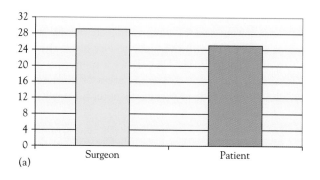

(a)

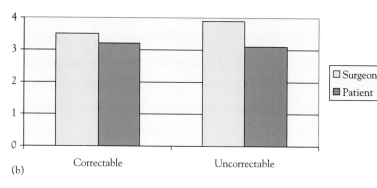

(b)

Figure 19.4. (a) Histogram showing the Genital Perception Score (GPS) for all eight features of the corrected hypospadiac penis by the surgeon and the patient. Maximum score is 32. The difference between the scores of the surgeon and the patient was significant (P≤0.001).[20] (b) Histogram showing mean GPS scores (maximum score 4) for features of hypospadias which are correctable and those that are not correctable by surgery. It is seen that there was little difference between patients and surgeons for the correctable features.[20]

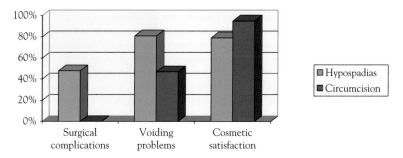

Figure 19.5. *This histogram compares the outcomes of surgery for hypospadias and circumcision for phimosis in adults. Hypospadias patients have more complications and more voiding problems. Nonetheless, cosmetic satisfaction is nearly equal and 47% of circumcision patients have some voiding problems. The survey was done in Finland where infants are rarely circumcised.*

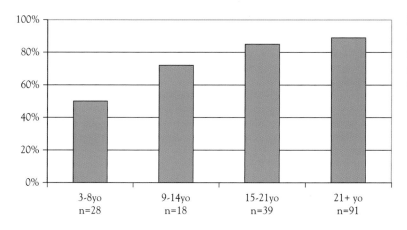

Figure 19.6. *Histogram showing the percentage of patients in each age group who had a valid flow rate between the fifth and 95th centiles for age.[22]*

as the more severe cases had the Byers-Denis Browne operation, which now is outmoded.

With severe penoscrotal hypospadias, it is particularly difficult to achieve normal voiding and a spraying stream is found in the majority of operated men.[23] Flow rates are on the low side of normal, but in the biggest long-term follow-up only nine of 42 patients (21%) were at or below the fifth centile.

An unknown number of men develop strictures, often as a result of balanitis xerotica obliterans (BXO). This chronic fibrosing process is of unknown etiology. Once the urethra is affected, it progresses proximally to produce particularly severe strictures. It may be seen both in men who have had hypospadias repair and in those whose hypospadias has never been corrected. Indeed, in previously unoperated hypospadiacs, meatal stricture due to

BXO is a relatively common reason for presentation to the surgeon. Because of the progressive nature of the condition, it is most important that all of the affected skin and urethra is excised before reconstruction, usually in a two-stage operation.[24,25] Some men who have never had hypospadias surgery and present with a BXO stricture may wish only to have the stricture excised and decline urethroplasty when they learn of the extent of surgery that is needed.

Chordee

Hypospadias repairs currently in use put great emphasis on correction of chordee, recommending frequent intraoperative artificial erections to check that the penis is straight. Older repairs were much less successful in this regard and at long-term follow-up 20% or more had residual chordee. As with strictures, it is very important to confirm that the man actually has significant symptoms from the chordee. The bend may be sufficient to prevent intercourse and therefore demand correction. There is also a group of men for whom the bent appearance, even if not a physical impediment to penetration, is an emotional cause of sexual dysfunction. It is interesting that in Summerlad's review 13 patients were thought, objectively, to have chordee of whom only eight had symptoms while two of 47 complained of curvature that was not confirmed on examination.[26] Later results have been better with only 18% of men having significant chordee.[18]

Chordee can occur many years after an apparently successful repair either at the site of the original operation or remote from the site of the hypospadias. In a group of 34 men referred for alleged recurrent chordee, 22 were identified who had adequate initial surgery confirmed by intraoperative erection and reported absence of chordee during follow-up. All had had proximal, or even penoscrotal, chordee and a tubularized free graft urethroplasty. The chordee developed during puberty from 12 to 18 years of age. The median age of presentation was 21 years and a mean of 17 years after the original surgery. Although in two-thirds of cases the urethra was shortened and fibrosed, its division did not correct the chordee in all cases. Disproportion of the corpora was present in 68% of men, with or without short urethra.[27] The cause of this late deterioration is unknown.

Residual chordee is a well-known and important cause of late morbidity. Even now many men are embarrassed to present themselves for treatment and sympathetic management is essential. The patient's description of the chordee is usually inadequate to plan surgery. Sometimes a Polaroid photograph is sufficient but direct inspection of the erection is invaluable (see Fig. 19.3). This can be achieved by injection of prostaglandin in the clinic. However, for an embarrassed patient with a difficult penile problem (often a hypospadias cripple, Fig. 19.7), an erection under anesthetic may be needed. It is most important to induce the erection by infusion of the corpora under pressure without a tourniquet: the chordee is sometimes more proximal than the site of the

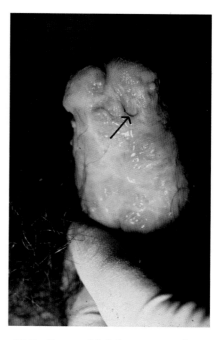

Figure 19.7. *Repeated failed surgery results in hypospadiac cripples. The tissues are grossly fibrotic and the probability of a good cosmetic outcome is poor. The arrow highlights the external urethral meatus.*

original hypospadias and may be disguised by a tourniquet.

Sexual function

Sexual activity

Problems with sexual intercourse, both physical and emotional have been reported. The 'physical causes' include soft glans, poor ejaculation, tight skin and pain. 'Emotional causes' include small size, poor appearance and the anxieties from the physical causes.[18]

The difficulties in assessing these 'causes' lie partly in the fact that similar problems are found in many adolescents (with or without genital anomalies) and partly that hypospadiac men appear to have intercourse in much the same way as everybody else. All reported series record that most men have sexual intercourse, even though the quality and quantity may be difficult to decipher from the data. Figures for successful intercourse range from 77 to 90%.[18,28,29] Curiously, frequency of sexual intercourse does not seem to be related to the success of the repair, although it is probably related to the degree of severity of the original hypospadias.

Nowhere in medicine is it more necessary to have control patients than in the assessment of adolescent sexual function. The greatest difficulty lies in the identification of a satisfactory control group with which to compare the hypospadiac patient with. Without controls it is impossible to know whether the myriad of sexual problems that have been identified are caused by the hypospadias. There is no group that mirrors all of the features of hypospadias but infant circumcision, herniorrhaphy and appendicectomy have all been used.

Two studies have shown that there was no difference in the number of sexual episodes or their perceived quality between hypospadiacs and controls (herniorrhaphy patients and circumcision patients, respectively).[19,21] This was despite the observation that the hypospadiacs had significantly more erectile problems such as curvature, shortness and pain, than the controls. There was no significant difference in the ages at which boys started masturbating, necking or having sexual intercourse. Hypospadiac men described themselves as more sexually inhibited than controls who had had a hernia repair (24% vs 1.8%).[19]

The quality of sexual satisfaction may be different when the hypospadiac man has suffered complications, as there is a correlation between more complications, dissatisfaction with the surgical outcome and dissatisfaction with sexual performance.[30] More complications are seen with the old Byers-Denis Browne operation which is no longer used and it may be reasonable to assume that the current surgical techniques with fewer complications may give a better sexual result.

Men with major postsurgical complications often have physical difficulty with intercourse. Apart from chordee, tight scarred skin makes penetration painful and may even tear with intercourse. Matters may be worsened if BXO has developed.

In the patients with most severe hypospadias there is a considerable overlap with intersex abnormalities especially androgen insensitivity syndromes.

In one series of posterior hypospadias 13 of 42 men had a major intersex anomaly. All had severe hypospadias (usually perineo-scrotal) and micropenis.[23] None of the 13 patients had sperm in their ejaculate. Even with hypospadias as severe as this intercourse still happens. In a series of 19 patients born with ambiguous genitalia, subsequently determined to be caused by perineal hypospadias, it was reported that 63% had had intercourse. However, only four had a regular partner. Fewer good figures were given in the series of Eberle et al. although 25 of 42 reported satisfactory erections, masturbation and ejaculation, few had sexual intercourse. Nine of 42 were married and three had children but only six had a stable relationship.[23]

Ejaculation

The first, or prostatic, phase of ejaculation is normal in men with hypospadias. The next stage is the expulsion of the semen by the bulbospongiosus muscle. In proximal hypospadias, this muscle is likely to be absent. It is, therefore, not surprising to find that ejaculation is unsatisfactory in 63% of severe hypospadiacs even though orgasm is normal in most.[31] Poor surgical results from a distal urethroplasty may cause a baggy urethra or even a diverticulum, further slowing the ejaculation. In more general reviews most authors state that ejaculation is normal though, by asking the right questions, Bracka found that 33% had 'dribbling ejaculation' and 4% were dry.[18]

Psychological aspects of intercourse

Emotional satisfaction with intercourse is particularly difficult to measure and series without controls are valueless. Most teenagers, exploring their sexuality, have anxieties that are unrelated to any penile abnormality although a penis that is perceived to be abnormal may get the blame.

Size may be a cause of dissatisfaction. The hypospadiac penis is often said to be short. In part this may be because of the circumcised appearance, especially in countries where infant circumcision is unusual. However, where a formal measurement has been made, 20% of hypospadiac penises were below the tenth centile. The finding was most marked in adolescents with four of seven being below the tenth centile (Fig. 19.8).[20]

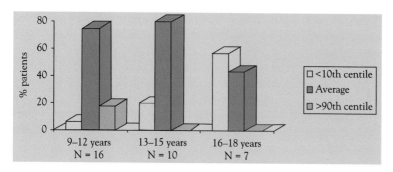

Figure 19.8. *Histogram showing the percentage of patients with stretched penile length by age compared to normal centiles.*[20]

Penile size is a source of considerable anxiety to many adolescents. Limited research is available on the relation of penile size to sexual satisfaction. Men with micropenis and with epispadias have intercourse that is satisfactory for them, although the opinions of their partners have not been investigated.[32] An investigation of women with multiple sexual partners has suggested that intercourse with an uncircumcised penis gives greater pleasure than a circumcised one.[33]

As there is no realistic means of enlarging the penis in hypospadias, it seems wise to help the patient to make the best use of what he has, rather than embark on surgery for lengthening which has a most uncertain outcome. The comparative trials of Mureau et al.[21] and Aho et al.[30] seem to indicate that hypospadiac boys are not greatly different from their peers in their sexual activity and enjoyment.

There is conflict over the effect of the success of the repair. Bracka made the interesting observation that those who were satisfied with the results of their repair had a sexual debut at a mean age of 15.6 years, while those who were dissatisfied had their debut at 19 years.[18] On the other hand, it has been reported that in a group of boys whose 'curative repair' was delayed beyond 12 years, 50% had their sexual debut before the definitive surgery.[34] It could be said that the experience of intercourse, acknowledged by the authors to be less satisfactory, drew attention to the shortcomings of the repair.

Fertility

It seems probable that boys with uncomplicated hypospadias are normally fertile. There have been no studies of a large cohort of hypospadiac patients. There is no excess of hypospadiacs in infertility clinics. In an apparently unselected group of 169 hypospadiac men, 50% were found to have a sperm count below 50 million/ml and 25% below 20 million/ml. More than half of those with the lowest sperm counts had associated anomalies such as undescended testes, which might have accounted for the poor result.[18] In a detailed study of 16 hypospadiacs, true oligo-astheno-teratozoospermia (OATS) was only found in the two patients with perineal hypospadias; low counts were seen in one of three with glanular and two of six with penile hypospadias but other parameters were normal. With two minor exceptions of slightly elevated luteinizing hormone, all the patients had normal hormone profiles.[35]

Psychological consequences

There is much debate about the psychological consequences of hypospadias and, again, there is a great need for control patients in the analyses. The problem is the selection of the controls. In the studies[26,28] quoted above, the control patients had had circumcision or a hernia repair, respectively. In the very extensive psychological reviews undertaken by Berg et al. the control patients had had appendicectomies.[36] Faults can obviously be found with all of these controls, none having undergone the same scale of surgery as hypospadiacs. On the other hand, there is no other condition that could be compared to hypospadias in terms of diagnosis and surgical trauma.

From the uncontrolled series, it seems that about 20% of adults remembered their surgery as traumatic. A third of men avoided changing in public.[26]

In the controlled studies, the main outcome has been sexual development as discussed above. There is no difference (compared to circumcision patients) in success of military conscripts in Finland, or in the number of men cohabiting.[28] Similarly, there were no differences in intelligence quotient, general health or socioeconomic background in the Swedish men reviewed by Berg et al. In the Dutch study, there was no evidence that hypospadiac men had less good psychosocial adjustment than the age-matched controls.[20]

New adult patients

From time to time a man will present with hypospadias who has had no previous surgery. Most often BXO will have caused a stricture. Occasionally, a man will present with an unconnected symptom and the hypospadias will be a chance finding. Even an uncomplicated hypospadiac meatus may not be large enough to accept a conventional cystoscope or resectoscope. The distal urethra is often fragile with no supporting corpus spongiosum and may easily be damaged by instrumentation (Fig. 19.9).

Before deciding on treatment, it is essential to establish what the patient hopes to achieve from surgery. For limited objectives, such as enlargement of the meatus, simple local surgery will suffice.

For complete reconstruction, the same techniques may be used as in children. Unfortunately, the complication rate of around 33% is much higher than that seen in younger patients.[37] Wound healing seems to be slower and the infection rate higher, than in children. Careful discussion with the patient about objectives and possible outcomes is essential.

The future

As the instruments, sutures, dressing materials and antibiotics have improved, so too have the

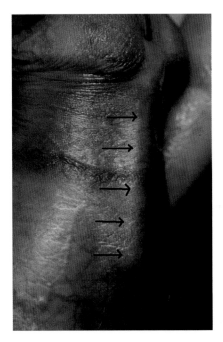

Figure 19.9. *The underdevelopment of the ventral aspect of the urethra is problematic for surgery as the tissues here are very thin (arrows). This paper-like tissue heals poorly, leading to urethro-cutaneous fistulae and failure of the reconstruction.*

outcomes. Newer technologies are being developed further to improve the results, such as tissue adherence techniques (glues and laser-activated soldering) that improve wound healing and reduce fistula formation, and urethral tissue substitutes (matrices impregnated with urethral epithelium and mesenchyme).[38] Prevention may become a reality as the understanding of the embryology of hypospadias improves.

As we await this exciting future, other important issues such as patient support and information need addressing. Several sources are currently available (see useful websites below).

Support websites

http://groups.msn.com/HypospadiasandEpispadias-Association

http://groups.yahoo.com/group/hypoepiassn/

http://groups.yahoo.com/group/hypospadias/

http://groups.yahoo.com/group/hypospadiasepis-
padiussnforum/

www.hypospadias.net

References

1. Paulozzi LJ, Erickson JD, Jackson RJ. Hypospadias trends in two US surveillance systems. Pediatrics 1997; 100: 831–4.
2. Baskin LS. Hypospadias and urethral development. J Urol 2000; 163: 951–6.
3. Aaronson IA, Cakmak MA, Key LL. Defects of the testosterone biosynthetic pathway in boys with hypospadias. J Urol 1997; 157: 1884–8.
4. Silver RI, Russell DW. 5alpha-reductase type 2 mutations are present in some boys with isolated hypospadias. J Urol 1999; 162: 1142–5.
5. Macnab AJ, Zouves C. Hypospadias after assisted reproduction incorporating in vitro fertilization and gamete intrafallopian transfer. Fertil Steril 1991; 56: 918–22.
6. Allen TD, Griffin JE. Endocrine studies in patients with advanced hypospadias. J Urol 1984; 131: 386–92.
7. Hadziselimovic F, Geneto R, Emmons LR. Elevated placental estradiol: a possible etiologic factor of human cryptorchidism. J Urol 2000; 164: 1694–5.
8. Aarskog D. Maternal progestins as a possible cause of hypospadias. N Engl J Med 1979; 300: 75–8.
9. Duckett JW. Hypospadias. In: Walsh PC, Retik AB, Vaughan ED et al. (eds). Campbell's Urology. 7th edn. Philadelphia: WB Saunders Co, 1998: 2093–119.
10. 10. Khuri FJ, Hardy BE, Churchill BM. Urologic anomalies associated with hypospadias. Urol Clin North Am 1981; 8: 565–71.
11. Kaefer M, Diamond D, Hendren WH et al. The incidence of intersexuality in children with cryptorchidism and hypospadias: stratification based on gonadal palpability and meatal position. J Urol 1999; 162: 1003–6.
12. Koff SA, Jayanthi VR. Preoperative treatment with human chorionic gonadotrophins in infancy decreases the severity of proximal hypospadias and chordee. J Urol 1999; 162: 1435–9.
13. Smith D. A de-epithelialised overlap flap technique in the repair of hypospadias. Br J Plast 1973; 26: 106–14.
14. Churchill BM, van Savage JG, Khoury AE et al. The dartos flap as an adjunct to preventing urethrocutaneous fistulas in repeat hypospadias surgery. J Urol 1996; 156: 2047–9.
15. Snodgrass W, Koyle L, Manzoni G et al. Tubularised incised plate hypospadias repair: Results of a multi-centre experience. J Urol 1996; 156: 839–41.
16. Schonfeld WA. Primary and secondary sexual characteristics. Am J Dis Child 1943; 65: 535–49.
17. Fichtner J, Filipas D, Mottrie AM, Voges GE, Hohenfellner R. Analysis of meatal location in 500 men: wide variation questions the need for meatal advancement in all pediatric anterior hypospadias cases. J Urol 1995; 154: 833–4.
18. Bracka AA. A long term view of hypospadias. Br J Plast Surg 1989; 42: 251–5.
19. Mureau MAM, Slijper FME, Nijman RJM et al. Psychosexual adjustment of children and adolescents after different types of hypospadias repair: a norm related study. J Urol 1995; 154: 1902–7.
20. Mureau MAM, Slijper FME, Koos Slob A, Verhulst FC, Nijman RJM. Satisfaction with penile appearance after hypospadias surgery: the patient and surgeon view. J Urol 1996; 155: 703–6.
21. Aho MO, Tammela OKT, Somppi EMJ, Tammela TLJ. A long term comparative follow up study of voiding, sexuality and satisfaction among men operated for hypospadias and phimosis during childhood. Eur J Urol 2000; 37: 95–101.
22. van der Werff JF, Boeve E, Brusse CA, van der Meulen JC. Urodynamic evaluation of hypospadias repair. J Urol 1997; 157: 1344–6.
23. Eberle J, Uberreiter S, Radmyr C et al. Posterior hypospadias: long term follow-up after reconstructive surgery in the male direction. J Urol 1993; 150: 1474–7.
24. Venn SN, Mundy AR. Urethroplasty for balanitis xerotica obliterans. Br J Urol 1998; 81: 735–7.
25. Kumar MV, Harris DL. Balanitis xerotica obliterans complicating hypospadias repair. Br J Plast Surg 1999; 52: 69–71.
26. Summerlad BC. A long term follow up of hypospadias patients. Br J Plast Surg 1975; 28: 324–30.
27. Vandersteen DR, Husmann DA. Late onset recurrent penile chordee after successful correction at hypospadias repair. J Urol 1998; 160: 1131–3.
28. Johanson B, Avellan L. Hypospadias: a review of 299 cases operated 1957–1969. Scand J Plast Reconstr Surg 1980; 14: 259–67.
29. Kenawi MM. Sexual function in hypospadiacs. Br J Urol 1976; 47: 883–90.

30. Aho MO, Tammela OKT, Tammela TLJ. Aspects of adult satisfaction with the result of surgery for hypospadias performed in childhood. Eur J Urol 1997; 32: 218–22.

31. Miller MAW, Grant DB. Severe hypospadias with genital ambiguity: adult outcome after staged hypospadias repair. Br J Urol 1997; 80: 485–8.

32. Woodhouse CRJ. Sexual function in boys born with exstrophy, myelomeningocoele and micropenis. Urology 1998; 52: 3–11.

33. O'Hara K, O'Hara J. The effect of male circumcision on the sexual enjoyment of the female partner. BJU Int 1999; 83(Suppl 1): 79–84.

34. Avellan L. Development of puberty, sexual debut and sexual function in hypospadiacs. Scand J Plast Reconstr Surg 1976; 10: 29–34.

35. Zubowska J, Jankowska J, Kula K, Owczarczyk I, Garbowska-Gorska A. Clinical, hormonal and semio-logical data in adult men operated in childhood for hypospadias. Endokrynologia Polsksa 1979; 30: 565–73.

36. Berg G, Berg R, Edman G, Svensson J, Astrom G. Androgens and personality in normal men and men operated for hypospadias in childhood. Acta Psychiatr Scand 1983; 68: 167–77.

37. Hensle TW, Tennenbaum SY, Reiley EA, Pollard J. Hypospadias repair in adults: adventures and misadventures. J Urol 2001; 165: 77–9.

38. Chen F, Yoo JJ, Atala A. Experimental and clinical experience using tissue regeneration for urethral reconstruction. World J Urol 2000; 18: 67–70.

Further reading

Thomas DFM, Rickwood AMK, Duffy PG (eds). Essentials of Paediatric Urology. London: Martin Dunitz, 2002.

Walsh PC, Retik AB, Vaughan ED, Wein AJ (eds). Campbell's Urology, 8th edn. Philadelphia: WB Saunders Co, 2002.

CHAPTER 20

HIV infection and AIDS

Andrew M Moon, John A Bartlett

Epidemiology

While remarkable therapeutic advances have prolonged the lives of many people infected with HIV, the HIV pandemic continues to expand, particularly in the most impoverished regions of the world. By the end of 2005, there were approximately 40 million people living with HIV or AIDS worldwide, of which 21.8 million were adult males (Fig. 20.1). In 2006 alone, 4.3 million adults were newly infected with HIV. In many regions, young people (15–24 years old) seem to be making up a larger proportion of these new infections. Young people accounted for 40% of all the new HIV infections in adults (older than 15) in 2006.[1] In 2006 there were an estimated 2.6 million deaths directly attributable to AIDS.[1]

According to the Joint United Nations Programme on HIV/AIDS (UNAIDS), in high-income countries in the West (including the USA, western Europe, and Japan), approximately 1.4 million people are now living with HIV/AIDS and an estimated 30 000 people died as a result of AIDS in 2006 alone. However, in the USA and western and central Europe, the introduction of antiretroviral therapy (ART) has dramatically reduced HIV–AIDS-related mortality (Fig. 20.2).[2] In a recent study performed on the impact of AIDS treatment, researchers concluded that per-person survival benefits in the USA had increased from 18.5 months in 1996, when combination ART was initially available, to 93.7 months in 2006.[1] Another study

concluded that ART has saved at least 3 million life years in the USA.[3] The impact of ART in the USA is also reflected in the number of AIDS deaths; in 1995, before widespread combination ART was available, there were over 50 000 estimated AIDS-related deaths, but in 2005 this number had dropped to 17 000.[2]

In recent years, the availability of these medications has also risen in low- and middle-income countries. The number of people receiving ART in low- and middle-income families increased from 240 000 to over 1.3 million between 2001 and 2005. This expanded access to medications has been estimated to have prevented between 250 000 and 350 000 AIDS deaths in the period 2003–2005.[1] Despite the reduction in the number of AIDS cases due to antiretroviral medications and opportunistic infection prophylaxis, the number of people living with HIV continues to rise steadily and ART is available to only one in five people who need it globally.

The demographics of the epidemic have changed dramatically in recent years, most notably in industrialized countries such as the USA and in western Europe. In the early years of the epidemic in these countries, the vast majority (as high as 78% in the USA) of HIV infections occurred in men who have sex with men (MSM).[4] The proportion of total cases occurring in MSM declined for a few years but recent evidence suggests that the MSM transmission has resurged in the USA. In 2001, MSM accounted for only 42% of new infections annually

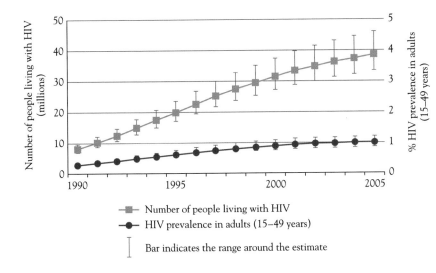

Figure 20.1. *Estimated global number of people living with HIV, and adult HIV prevalence, 1985–2005.*[1]

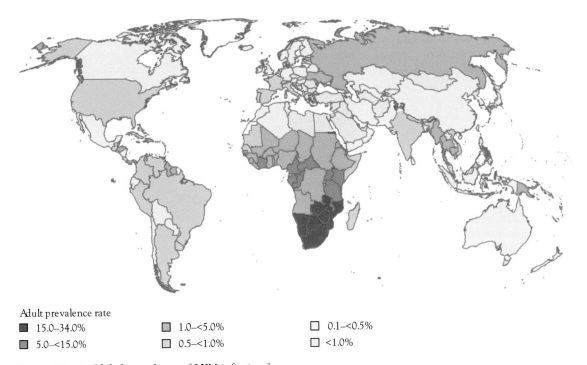

Figure 20.2. *Global prevalence of HIV infection.*[2]

but in 2004 MSM accounted for approximately half of all new HIV diagnoses in the US. In the population of men having unprotected sex with men in the United States, Canada and western Europe, HIV prevalence ranges between 10% and 20%.

Many studies have suggested that one factor contributing to this trend is a resurgence of risky behavior.[5,6] While the majority of cases in high-income countries still occur among men, women are assuming a larger proportion of the disease

253

burden. For example, in the USA, women now represent 25% of all AIDS diagnoses, whereas in 1992 they represented less than 10%.[7]

Other major epidemiological trends include the continuing shift of the epidemic into poorer and marginalized sections of society, especially among ethnic minorities. By 2005, African Americans, who make up 12% of the USA population (according to the 2000 US census), represented over 49% of new HIV–AIDS diagnoses.[8] In 2005, Hispanics accounted for 14% of the US population, but 18% of all new AIDS cases.[9] Furthermore, AIDS-related illnesses ranks in the top three causes of death for African–American men aged 25–54 years.[6] Relative to other groups, African–American men have reduced survival, perhaps related to less access to ART. African–Americans are half as likely to receive ART than other population groups, and AIDS deaths claimed twice as many African–Americans as whites.[6,9,10] Broader access to testing, evaluation, and treatment of HIV for this population may lead to a reduction in AIDS-related deaths.

Natural history

Progression
In untreated HIV-infected people, the median time from the acquisition of HIV infection to the development of symptomatic disease is approximately 10 years.[11] Therefore, HIV infection remains clinically silent for prolonged periods during which immunologic compromise may progress, and transmission of HIV may occur through risky behaviors. A number of factors have been elucidated which may influence the rate of progression of HIV disease, and they are discussed below. Of note, many of these observations on the progression of HIV disease were made in untreated HIV-infected people and progression may be profoundly impacted by successful antiretroviral therapy.

Laboratory markers of HIV progression
The laboratory assessment of HIV infection can provide important insight into an individual's risk of disease progression. A direct measurement of HIV replication is available through the determination of plasma HIV RNA levels with reverse

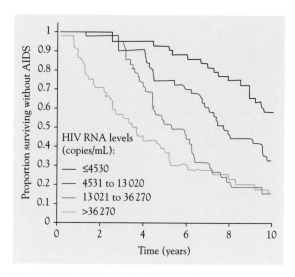

Figure 20.3. *Relationship between plasma HIV RNA levels and AIDS-free survival. Adapted from Mellors et al.[12]*

transcriptase polymerase chain reaction (RT-PCR) or branched-chain DNA techniques. Plasma HIV RNA levels correlate strongly with the risk of progression to symptomatic disease and survival (Fig. 20.3),[12] and also represent a sensitive method of following patients on ART. The immunologic competency of an HIV-infected patient can be assessed by measuring the absolute CD4+ lymphocyte count, and the opportunistic infections as complications of HIV disease typically occur when CD4+ lymphocyte counts fall below 200/mm.[3] Plasma HIV RNA levels and CD4+ lymphocyte counts offer complementary information in assessing HIV-infected persons, and are commonly used to guide ART.

Factors affecting progression
Observations on the relative roles of a variety of factors including HIV inoculum, host factors, viral factors, and co-infections may have a significant impact on the progression of HIV disease.

Inoculum
Early studies comparing patients who received HIV-infected transfusions with packed red blood cells or coagulation products suggested a more rapid progression to symptomatic HIV disease than

persons who acquired HIV infection through sexual transmission.[13] Beyond these early observations, an inoculum effect has not been well described as having an impact on the progression of HIV disease.

Host factors

An increasing number of host factors are being described which have an impact on the progression of HIV disease. Research has found that the viral levels in the plasma during asymptomatic HIV infection can vary by as much as 4 to 5 logs. Many of these factors involve specific human lymphocyte antigen (HLA) phenotypes, which may be important predictors of cell-mediated immune responses against HIV. Specific HLA phenotypes have been associated with long-term non-progression of HIV disease, and others with a more rapid progression to symptomatic HIV disease.[14] Recently HLA loci C and a RNA polymerase subunit have been linked to substantial changes in the progression of HIV.[15] Correlative studies have demonstrated that these HLA phenotypes result in relatively more or less vigorous cytotoxic T-lymphocyte responses against HIV antigens; the most successful responses are robust in magnitude and target a diversity of HIV antigens.[16] It also appears that mutations in HIV co-receptors, such as chemokine receptor-5 (CCR5), may have an important impact on the progression of HIV disease.[17] Persons with a homozygous 32 base pair deletion in the CCR5 receptor have an innate resistance to infection with macrophage-tropic HIV, the most commonly transmitted strains.[18] Therefore, they may be repeatedly exposed to HIV and have a low risk of acquiring the infection. Persons with a heterozygous 32 base pair deletion in their CCR5 receptors may have attenuated progression of their HIV disease and are more likely to be long-term non-progressors. It is very likely that additional host factors will continue to become elucidated and assist in predicting an individual's risk of progression to symptomatic HIV disease.

Viral factors

Viral characteristics may also affect progression of HIV disease. One HIV characteristic, the ability to form syncytia in virus cultures, has been associated with a more rapid progression to symptomatic HIV disease.[19] In contrast, when the prevalent HIV strains are non-syncytium-inducing, patients have a slower progression of HIV disease. When there is a shift from non-syncytium-inducing isolates to syncytium induction, patients may experience an acceleration of disease progression. A small number of people have been reported with a deletion in the *nef* gene of HIV that led to less rapid HIV progression, but these mutant strains are uncommon.[20] Finally, drug-resistant HIV isolates can be transmitted, including multidrug-resistant isolates.[21] Patients who acquire multidrug-resistant strains may not respond to treatment and therefore may be at greater risk for more rapid progression of their HIV disease.

Co-infections

Importantly, prevailing co-infections in resource-limited environments with organisms such as *Mycobacterium tuberculosis* and malaria may accelerate the progression of HIV disease. These infections may increase levels of tumor necrosis factor (TNF) and interleukin (IL)-2, cytokines known to enhance HIV replication.[22] Treatment of these co-infections can also result in lowered plasma HIV RNA levels and potentially attenuate HIV progression.[23] In the Western world, co-infection with other viruses such as hepatitis C may accelerate the course of HIV disease.[24] In some patient populations, the prevalence of co-infection with hepatitis C and HIV may exceed 50%.

Causes of death

Globally, 3 million persons with HIV disease die each year, and the majority of deaths are due to tuberculosis, malaria, or diarrhea and wasting. In the Western world, the causes of death of persons living with HIV disease have evolved over the past 10 years following the introduction of more effective ART. Increasingly the causes of death include end-stage liver disease due to hepatitis B and C, and end-stage renal disease.[25] In addition, in the Western world, the complications of long-term antiretroviral therapy are being identified as contributing factors in HIV-related deaths.[25]

Transmission and prevention

It has been more than 20 years after the advent of the HIV pandemic and the methods of transmission

> **Box 20.1.** *Factors associated with increased risk of HIV transmission*
>
> Presence of sexually transmitted infections (ulcerative or non-ulcerative) in insertive or receptive partner
>
> Higher viremia or more advanced immunodeficiency in infecting partner
>
> Sexual activity during menstruation
>
> Traumatic sexual practices (including dry sex, fisting, etc.)
>
> High number of sexual partners
>
> Repeated use of contaminated injecting equipment
>
> High number of needle-sharing partners
>
> Genital tract inflammation
>
> Acute HIV infection in infecting partner
>
> Lack of male circumcision
>
> Lack of barrier protection (male or female condom)
>
> Cervical ectopy in female partner
>
> High viral load in genital secretions
>
> Infection with syncytium-forming virus
>
> Use of nonoxynol-9 spermicide

are now well understood. While HIV is found in varying concentrations or amounts in blood, semen, vaginal fluid, breast milk, saliva, and tears, all clinical evidence supports three primary modes of transmission:

- sexual contact (responsible for >85% of all HIV transmission worldwide);
- exposure to blood and perinatal transmission; and
- breast feeding.

However, within these general categories different exposures and behaviors present a wide range of risk for HIV infection (Box 20.1).

High-risk exposures/behaviors

Vaginal intercourse

The risk per episode of receptive vaginal sexual exposure is estimated at 0.1–0.2%.[26] The risk to the insertive partner is lower, but still exists. Modeling suggests that HIV transmission rates per coital act are highest during the post-seroconversion period (0.8% per coital act), lower during asymptomatic HIV infection (0.07% per coital act), and then resurge with advancing disease (0.45% per coital act in the last 5–15 months of HIV-infected partner's life). This is supported by findings that peripheral blood viremia, which is highest during the initial and final stages of the disease, is the principal factor in heterosexual transmission.[27] Other factors linked to the rate of transmission during vaginal intercourse include ART use for the HIV-infected partner, which decreases transmission rates, the stage in the woman's menstrual cycle when vaginal intercourse occurs, and the presence of sexually transmitted diseases, which increase the chances of transmission.[28]

Studies have shown the HIV-1 virus is present in semen shortly after primary infection and at all stages of the disease. It is assumed that semen is the predominant vehicle for sexual transmission and it contains cell-associated or free virions (or both) or HIV-1-infected cells.[29] The exact location of HIV in semen has been investigated in recent studies, and both macrophages and T-lymphocytes in semen harbor HIV but there are no studies that convincingly show that the virus can be found in spermatozoa. A recent study demonstrated the presence of HIV-1 DNA in ejaculated abnormal spermatozoa of infected subjects. Although the spermatozoa were purified, it is possible that the presence of the virus was due to residual non-seminal cells or false-positive results caused by non-specific hybridization of *in situ* PCR. Researchers reported that DNA localization in the sperm head was seen only after sperm chromatin decondensation, suggesting that the virus could either be integrated into the sperm genome or trapped in the sperm nucleus.[29] Vasectomy studies suggest that the primary site of HIV production may be the male urethra, although further studies are needed to evaluate this suggestion.[30]

Studies have estimated that asymptomatic men transmit the virus five times more efficiently than asymptomatic women, but the transmission risks vary with plasma RNA levels and disease progression. In addition, having a sexually transmitted infection has been shown to increase transmission rates. Male circumcision has been shown to reduce male-to-female transmission rates. It has also been suggested that neutralizing antibody response in the host and replicative capacity of the virus may affect transmission rates.[31] There has been no transmission rate difference found between symptomatic men and women. It has been suggested that promising areas of future research will be immunoglobulin concentration changes with age, sex hormones, and natural genital mucosal defense systems in men and women.[28]

Anal intercourse

The baseline risk of transmission per episode of receptive penile–anal sexual exposure is estimated at 0.1–3%.[32] Any trauma to the anal region resulting in mucosal disruption or bleeding increases the risk of transmission.[33] While the risk to the insertive partner is lower than that of the receptive partner, it is still non-trivial.[26]

Exposure to blood via intravenous needles or syringes

The risk for HIV transmission per episode of exposure to an intravenous needle or syringe containing HIV-infected blood is estimated at 0.67%. The risk per episode of percutaneous exposure (e.g. a needlestick) to HIV-infected blood is estimated at 0.4%.[26,34] This risk may be increased when the injury penetrates deeply or involves a hollow bore needle or if the source patient has evidence of progressive HIV disease with higher plasma HIV RNA levels or low CD4+ lymphocyte counts. Acknowledging this low but measurable risk, post-exposure prophylaxis may be offered to healthcare providers who sustain a percutaneous injury. In general, three antiretroviral agents are started as soon as possible following the injury and are given for 4 weeks. HIV antibody testing of the exposed provider should be performed immediately following the injury, and then at 3 and 6 months.[34]

Transfusion of infected blood

The likelihood of a recipient becoming infected with HIV following the transfusion of an HIV-infected single donor blood product (whole blood, blood cellular components, plasma, clotting factors) is >95%. Fortunately, the screening of blood with HIV antibody testing has proved very effective in eliminating HIV-infected products; in the USA, the risk is estimated as 1 in 200 000–2 000 000.[35]

Lower-risk exposures/behaviors

Oral intercourse

No solid estimates of penile–oral transmission rates currently exist. One study reported a 0.04% seroconversion rate during unprotected receptive oral intercourse with ejaculation in MSM, although it has been suggested that the risk is highly dependent upon the type of exposure or contact involved.[36] A 2002 study involving 135 sexually active, serodiscordant heterosexual couples reported that no HIV transmission cases were found during over 19 000 instances of unprotected oral sex. Another study performed among MSM by the US Centers for Disease Control and Prevention (CDC) found that 8 of 102 (7.8%) recently infected men in the study were probably infected through oral sex.

Although more studies need to be performed to estimate transmission rates, instances of transmission have been reported for both the insertive and receptive partner, even in cases when insertive partners did not ejaculate. Researchers have suggested that the oral immune response factor that may be partially responsible for the lower transmission rate in the oral cavity compared with the anal or genital cavities is secretory leukocyte protease inhibitor (SLPI). SLPI, which is secreted primarily from the epithelial cells lining mucosal surfaces, has been shown to reduce inflammation, enhance wound healing, and block microbial growth. SLPI already present in the salivary fluids has been shown to protect target cells and tissues against transmission during initial infection. Additional SLPI expression occurs as a result of exposure to HIV-1, acting to limit virus spread throughout the tissues when initial oral defenses are overwhelmed and infection occurs.[37] In addition to oral intercourse, any other sexual activities involving contact with semen or blood contacting a non-intact surface carry a potential risk of transmission.[35]

Transplantation of organs or tissues

Documented cases of transmission have resulted from the liver, heart, kidney, pancreas, bone, and possibly skin transplantation, although such cases are rare, particularly in areas where routine screening is performed.[38,39]

Contact with healthcare providers

Transmission from a healthcare provider to patients has been documented, although very rarely, with only seven known cases out of over 22 000 patients of providers known to be HIV-infected.[40]

Exposure of mucous membranes or non-intact skin to blood

Although transmission through these routes has been documented, the risk is believed to be low and estimated at 0.09% or less per exposure.[34] Household contact HIV transmission has been documented between family members in a household setting, but this type of transmission is rare and is believed to have resulted from contact with infected blood or other secretions.[41]

Biting

A few cases of blood-to-blood transmission through a human bite exist, though these are extremely rare and are associated with severe tissue damage and the presence of blood.[42]

Kissing

The risk of acquiring HIV during open-mouth kissing is believed to be very low, although the CDC have investigated one case that may be attributed to contact with blood during open-mouth kissing.[42]

Tattooing and body piercing

There are no recorded cases of HIV transmission through tattooing or body piercing, although the theoretical risk does exist. Hepatitis B virus has been transmitted through these routes, and there has been one documented case of HIV transmission through acupuncture.[42]

Non-risky behaviors and exposures

Saliva, tears, and sweat

Contact with saliva, tears, or sweat has never been shown to result in transmission of HIV. Other body fluids (feces, nasal secretions, sputum, urine,

vomitus) are not considered infectious unless they contain blood.[35]

Insects

Numerous investigations have concluded that HIV is not transmitted by biting or bloodsucking insects.[42]

Business and social settings

There is no known risk of HIV transmission to coworkers, clients, or consumers from workers in the food service industry nor is there any evidence of transmission from personal-service workers (hairdressers, cosmetologists, massage therapists) to a client or vice versa.[42]

Environmental contact

HIV does not survive well in the environment, making the probability of environmental transmission remote. Evidence of high concentrations of virus being kept alive for weeks in laboratory settings has alarmed some people and has led to incorrect conclusions about the virus. Studies have shown that when high concentrations of the virus are dried, 90–99% of the infectious virus is gone within a few hours. Since these concentrations used in the laboratory are much higher than those actually found in blood or other bodily fluids, the theoretical risk of environmental transmission is essentially zero. No evidence has been found to support transmission through air or water.[42]

Sexually transmitted infections and HIV

Both epidemiological and biological studies have provided strong evidence that the presence of other sexually transmitted infections, both ulcerative and non-ulcerative, increase the risk of HIV transmission. For both men and women, concomitant sexually transmitted infections increase the susceptibility to, and the infectiousness of, HIV.

Several large epidemiological studies have established that ulcerative sexually transmitted infections (syphilis, genital herpes, and chancroid) are responsible for a 1.5- to 7-fold increased relative risk for acquiring HIV infection in both men and women.[43] This increase in risk is due to the presence of ulceration and mucosal disruption in the genital or anorectal regions caused by the infection as well as an increased number of HIV target cells (CD4[+] lymphocytes) at the ulcerative surfaces, owing to the inflammatory response.[43] Non-ulcerative sexually transmitted infections such as gonorrhea, chlamydia, and trichomoniasis are associated with an increase of 60–340% in the prevalence of HIV in both men and women through mucosal disruption of the genital and anorectal tracts.[43] Other non-ulcerative sexually transmitted infections (urethritis, cervicitis, balanitis, bacterial vaginitis, and genital warts) are also known to increase the risk for contracting HIV.[44] Co-infection of HIV with other sexually transmitted infections causes greater concentrations of HIV to be shed in genital secretions. In two African studies, co-infection with gonorrhea more than doubled the proportion of HIV-infected people with HIV RNA detectable in their genital secretions. The concentration of HIV RNA in semen dramatically increases in men with sexually transmitted infections and HIV compared with men infected with HIV alone.[45]

The most common genital co-infection when HIV is transmitted is human herpes simplex virus type 2 (HSV-2).[28] In addition to the disruption of epithelial barriers caused by HSV-2, an elevated risk of transmission may be caused by increased HIV shedding from HSV ulcers and biological modulation between the two infections. It has been suggested that co-infection with cytomegalovirus, chancroid, syphilis, gonorrhea, trichomonas, and chlamydia also all increase the level of HIV in semen. In addition, studies have found an association between both symptomatic and asymptomatic urethritis and HIV shedding in semen. The proposed reason for this association is that cellular inflammation increases both HIV replication and HIV shedding.[28]

The proper diagnosis and treatment of sexually transmitted infections thus becomes an extremely important component of HIV prevention. The majority of STIs are readily treatable with a variety of antibiotic regimens, and can have dramatic effects on HIV transmission. For example, the treatment of gonorrhea in HIV-infected men results in a reduction in the number of men shedding HIV in semen as well as a lower concentration of HIV RNA.[43] In a more dramatic example, a community-based, randomized trial in rural Tanzania demonstrated a 42% decrease in the rate of new HIV infections in communities utilizing more rigorous STI diagnosis and treatment guidelines.[46]

Other preventative measures

Safer sex

The term 'safer sex' refers to a set of risk-reduction strategies intended to reduce the risk of HIV transmission through sexual contact. Safer sex encompasses both behavior modification strategies and the proper use of barrier protection. Among the behavioral modification strategies that are known to decrease the risk of acquiring HIV are:

- reducing the number of sexual partners;
- reducing the frequency of anal sex;
- reducing (or eliminating) the frequency of sexual activities that traumatize the genital or anorectal epithelium (such as 'fisting' and 'dry sex');
- encouraging sexual activities that do not involve direct contact with body fluids (such as mutual masturbation and fantasization); and
- avoiding sexual contact during menstruation.

Efforts to encourage delayed initiation of sexual activity, monogamy, and sexual abstinence have contributed to the reduction of HIV incidence rates in several countries, most notably Uganda.[1]

The use of barrier methods such as the male or female condom is an elemental component of all safer sex strategies. Numerous epidemiological studies and large-scale public health interventions have demonstrated the impact of condom promotion programs on the reduction of HIV incidence rates in every region of the world.[1] Aside from sexual abstinence, monogamous sex with a seronegative partner, or sexual behaviors not involving contact with body fluids, the use of barrier methods such as the male latex condom are the most effective means for preventing the sexual transmission of HIV. Recent meta-analyses by a CDC expert panel concluded that consistent use of the male latex condom decreases the risk of HIV transmission by approximately 85%.[47] Additionally, while still a relatively new and underutilized technology, the female or vaginal condom provides similar rates of protection against HIV as the male latex condom if used properly and consistently.[48]

Antiretroviral therapy

It has been suggested that ART use by the HIV-infected partner reduces HIV RNA levels in blood, seminal plasma, female genital tract secretions, and rectal secretions.[49] Several studies (but not all) have shown that ART is associated with decreased detection and concentration of HIV in semen, but the penetration of these medications is drug-specific.[43] Recent studies have reported that concentrations of protease inhibitors, with the exception of indinavir, are less than 10% in the blood plasma of the male genital tract, providing an explanation for reports of protease inhibitor resistance in HIV isolates found in the seminal plasma.[49] A large non-randomized, observational study of serodiscordant heterosexual couples in Italy demonstrated that ART was associated with a nearly 50% reduction in the sexual transmission of HIV.[50]

No randomized, controlled trial has ever been conducted on this association although the National Institutes of Health Prevention Trials Network plans to open a 5-year study enrolling 1750 serodiscordant couples to investigate this association. Recent research has shown that combination ART decreases HIV RNA shedding in the genital tract, and that serodiscordant couples in whom the infected partner is using ART have fewer seroconversions in the HIV-negative partners.[51] In addition, ART may be given to HIV-negative partners as a post-exposure prophylaxis. In 2005, the CDC recommended triple-drug ART to be taken as post-exposure prophylaxis 72 hours or sooner after non-occupational, high-risk exposure to known or suspected HIV.

However, despite the use of ART and suppression of HIV RNA levels in plasma, HIV may be persistently detected in the genital secretions of both men and women.[52,53] This observation indicates that the protective effect provided by even highly effective ART on the sexual transmission of HIV is likely to be incomplete and is dependent upon sensitivity of the virus to the medications selected, patient adherence, and the patient's long-term commitment to therapy. Therefore, even

patients with non-detectable plasma HIV RNA levels are not completely non-infectious and must continue to follow safer sex precautions.[54] Furthermore, one recent study suggested that ART is unlikely to reduce the spread of HIV because of the limited protection of ART on HIV transmission, the associated emergence of HIV-resistant variants, and an increase in risk-taking behavior, which offset the biological benefits of ART.[49]

Recent studies have concluded that infection with HIV does not protect against re-infection with another HIV strain. Infection with more than one HIV strain, known as superinfection, is associated with higher viral HIV RNA plasma levels than single strain infection and may lead to more rapid clinical progression of HIV disease. Based on the association between elevated HIV RNA plasma levels and higher transmission rates, superinfecting forms are likely to be more pathogenic.[55] Therefore it is also very important to stress safe sex practices among sexual partners when both partners are HIV-infected.

An important result of wide availability of ART is resistant HIV strains. The mechanisms of viral resistance related to ART therapy include problems with patient adherence, poor pharmokinetics of the medication, and inadequate cellular uptake. These situations all result in low drug concentrations and an associated increase of viral replication.[56] The virus has been shown to have the ability to develop resistance to all currently used ART, owing to its high replication rate combined with the low fidelity of viral reverse transcripterase.[57] Transmission of resistant strains has been observed through the different transmission routes.[58] To reduce the dissemination of these resistant strains it is critical to counsel patients on the importance of safer sex precautions.

The best strategy to reduce resistant strains is to suppress virus replication fully with high-adherence, potent regimens, and encouragement of safer sex.

Circumcision

The majority of studies (both cross-sectional and prospective) support the finding that uncircumcised men are at increased risk for HIV infection compared with their circumcised counterparts.

Over 30 studies have found statistically significant associations between HIV infection and circumcision status, with relative risks two to eight times higher for uncircumcised men.[59] Although a definitive biological mechanism has yet to be established, several researchers have hypothesized that the intact foreskin provides a vulnerable portal of entry to HIV and other pathogens, owing to a high density of CD4-receptor-bearing Langerhans cells (the primary target cells in the sexual transmission of HIV) and have noted the susceptibility of foreskin epithelium to traumatic disruption during sexual activity. Other suggested direct factors for the protective effects of male circumcision are keratinization of the glans when not protected by the foreskin, short drying after sexual contact (reducing the life expectancy of HIV on the penis after sexual contact with a seropositive partner), and the increased chance of epithelial tears in the foreskin. An indirect factor may be that male circumcision reduces acquisition of other sexually transmitted infections which, as a result, reduces the chance of HIV transmission.[60–63]

In 2005, randomized, controlled, blindly evaluated intervention trials were performed in South Africa, Kenya, and Uganda to determine if male circumcision provides protection against HIV-1 infection. The researchers concluded that after controlling for important behavioral factors such as increased sexual contacts in the circumcision group, condom use, and health-seeking behavior, female-to-male HIV transmission was reduced by up to 60% for newly circumcised subjects (Table 20.1).[60–62] According to modeling studies, this type of protection could prevent 5.7 million new HIV cases and 3 million deaths over 20 years.[64]

The protective effect of circumcision for men could probably be indirectly passed on to women, and therefore children. Some have suggested that male circumcision may also be protective against male-to-female transmission. A study of serodiscordant couples in Uganda showed that for HIV-infected males with a plasma HIV RNA level <50 000 copies/mL, there was no transmission in circumcised patients while uncircumcised patients had a transmission rate of 9.6 per 100 person-years.[62] Although these findings suggest some protection from male-to-female transmission when HIV RNA levels are

Table 20.1. *Combined findings of randomized circumcision trials in South Africa,[60] Kenya,[61] and Uganda[62]*

	Circumcision group	Control group
Number of participants	6132	6162
Number of HIV infections	64	141
Prevalence rate of HIV infection	1.04%	2.29%

*South African trial had 21 months' follow-up,[61] Kenya and Uganda trials had 24 months' follow-up.[61,62]

low, the study found no significant association between circumcision and male-to-female transmission in all HIV-infected subjects. More extensive studies need to be performed to examine the potential association between circumcision and both male-to-female and male-to-male transmission.

Several factors need to be taken into account before large-scale circumcision programs are implemented. The procedure may be performed under poor hygienic conditions, which lead to infection, bleeding, permanent injury, and even HIV infection from non-sterilized instruments. Inappropriate treatment of sequelae may also occasionally cause death. Complication rates reported range from 0.2% to 2.0% in the USA.[65] The randomized trial in South Africa found a complication rate of 3.8% with the most common reported problems being pain, followed by swelling or hematoma, bleeding, and problems with appearance. There were also a few instances of damage to the penis, infection, and delayed wound healing, although these complications were rare. There were no reported deaths or problems with urination.[60]

Besides the health risk, there is a danger that patients will engage in sexual activity during the healing period, when there may be a higher risk of HIV infection. In addition, circumcision may be perceived as full protection and lead to a decrease of condom use or increase in risky sexual behavior.

261

During the South African trial, the group receiving new circumcisions was, in fact, found to have significantly more sexual contacts.[60]

Currently 665 million men (30%) are estimated to be circumcised worldwide. According to a probability sample of adults conducted by the Social Life Survey in 1992, 77% of men in the USA are circumcised.[63]

Undoubtedly, wherever the procedure is offered, certification and training of providers and close evaluation of programs will be required. Based on findings from studies in Malawi, Kenya, and Zambia there is a need for facilities, training, certification, surgical instruments, and expendable supplies before safety and quality control can be assured. Currently government health centers in these areas do not have the resources necessary to perform circumcision safely.[66]

Many people have practiced circumcision as a cultural rite of passage or for religious reasons. It is common in the Jewish and Muslim faith to circumcise males within the first few weeks of life, although a Muslim may be circumcised at any time between birth and puberty. Some sects of Christianity practice large-scale circumcision although it varies among locations and denominations. In a recent study investigating acceptability of circumcision in Malawi, many boys cited religious reasons for not wanting to be circumcised, mentioning that it was not meant for Christians.[67]

Recent studies investigating the acceptability of circumcision, which were primarily conducted in sub-Saharan Africa where a large-scale program would probably make the most impact, have highlighted many of the local men's reasons for and against getting circumcised. The most common reasons for circumcision are religion and tradition, medical conditions (such as penile ulcerations), increased genital hygiene, protective effects against HIV and other sexually transmitted infections, peer pressure, and sexual pleasure and satisfaction. Reasons against circumcision included infections and other complications from the procedure, pain, cost, and religious reasons. The study concluded that many men and women would welcome the availability of male circumcision services that were affordable, safe, and confidential. Acceptability of male circumcision was found to be higher among women and young men than among older men.[67]

In a study performed in Zambia nearly all the men participating were willing to be circumcised themselves or have their son circumcised as long as the benefits were clear and the procedure was affordable or free.[67] A study in Botswana found that 60–80% of the local population definitely or probably favored circumcision. The majority of participants favored circumcision before the age of 6 years and virtually all believed it should be performed in a hospital setting.[68] Studies in areas of western Kenya, Zimbabwe, South Africa, and Tanzania where circumcision is currently not performed, found that approximately 45–70% of uncircumcised men would be circumcised or seriously consider it if the procedure was proven to reduce transmission of sexual infections. In addition, these studies concluded that participants in communities where circumcision is traditionally practiced desired having circumcision services moved to health facilities, suggesting that circumcision services should not be restricted to areas where the practice is rare.[66]

Microbicides

One of the most commonly held misconceptions in HIV prevention is that the widely distributed spermicide nonoxynol-9 (N-9) is protective against HIV infection. This has been conclusively proved *not* to be the case – in 2001, the World Health Organization released a consensus statement citing research concluding that N-9 is not only ineffective in reducing the risk of HIV infection through vaginal intercourse, but actually increases the risk of infection when used frequently.[69] A study has shown that N-9 used in combination with water-based lubricant is toxic and when diluted to non-toxic concentrations is ineffective at preventing infection of immune cells or blocking transfer of virus from epithelial cells to activated peripheral blood mononuclear cells.[70] In addition, under no circumstances should N-9 be used rectally – several studies have found that N-9 severely damages rectal epithelium, thereby greatly increasing the probability of HIV transmission.[71] That said, efforts are under way to develop a microbicide that is effective and safe for vaginal and rectal application. At least one candidate product has entered phase III efficacy trials, and upwards of 20 other candidates are in earlier stages of development.

Vaccines

Although HIV vaccine research has taken some important steps forward since 2000, and promising vaccine candidates have been developed, it is likely that it will still be some time before even a partially effective vaccine is widely available. Owing to the struggles with HIV vaccine trials for prevention, investigators have identified a secondary goal of lowering the plateau HIV RNA levels (the stable level after primary infection) to delay disease progression if vaccine recipients become HIV-infected.[72] To date, there have been more than 35 candidate vaccines tested in over 65 phase I–II clinical trials.[73] Currently there are five phase II trials, four phase I–II trials, and 31 phase I trials in progress. There have been two phase III trials completed and one is currently in progress in Thailand. The first few efficacy trials of a candidate vaccine were recently completed and the results failed to show any protection against HIV infection.[74] These early vaccines will probably confer only partial immunity to HIV at best. In 2005, vaccine development for HIV entered the era of cytotoxic T-lymphocyte (CTL)-mediated vaccine efficacy trials to determine whether the available viral vector vaccines are capable of eliciting the quality and quantity of T-lymphocyte responses necessary to alter the course of HIV infection on both an individual and global level.

Studies performed on non-human primates have shown vaccine-elicited cellular immune response that lowers HIV viremia and CD4+ lymphocyte loss, suggesting it should be possible to create an effective HIV vaccine.[75] Current vaccine trials have shown that an effective HIV vaccine or vaccine regimen may need to induce both cell-mediated immunity and humoral immunity to more than one HIV epitope, as a mechanism to address the high genetic variability of HIV. Many questions remain before the feasibility and timeline for vaccine development can be estimated. Researchers have not yet solved the challenges of the high variability of the virus and its ability to evade immune responses, on the specific protective immune mechanisms of HIV

and how to elicit potent virus-neutralizing antibodies with broad specificity against primary HIV isolates. A truly effective vaccine should be capable of raising immunity at the major virus transmission routes such as the genital, rectal, and intestinal mucosa.[73]

Treatment

Successful treatment of HIV infection with antiretroviral drugs has resulted in a dramatic decrease in the reporting of AIDS and AIDS-related deaths in countries where treatment is available. The success of these interventions has led to keen interest in extending the benefits of treatment to all countries of the world. Although treatment has clearly provided unprecedented improvements in survival and quality of life, it is not a panacea. ART requires close monitoring to assess its success and potential toxicities and a firm commitment to adherence with the medication schedule, and it may result in drug-resistant HIV. Therefore, a strategic approach to the management of treatment is necessary.

Strategies

Identification of patients in need of treatment

In acknowledgement of limitations of ART, a guiding principle is the identification of persons at highest risk for HIV progression as candidates for therapy. The identification of highest-risk persons with HIV infection relies on the results of natural history studies for extrapolation to therapeutic guidelines, and will probably never be supported by a randomized intervention trial to identify the most appropriate point of initiation. Guidelines are currently published by the International AIDS Society, the US Public Health Service, and the World Health Organization Global Programme on AIDS. In general, these guidelines focus on HIV-related symptoms, CD4+ lymphocyte counts, and plasma HIV RNA levels as the indicators for intervention. The presence of symptoms suggests that treatment should be started. For HIV-infected people with CD4+ lymphocyte counts above 350/mm^3, a delay in treatment is recommended. For those with CD4$^+$ lymphocytes of 200–350/mm^3, treatment should be considered. Finally, for those with CD4$^+$ lymphocyte counts below 200/mm^3, treatment should be strongly recommended. When plasma HIV RNA levels are available, current guidelines emphasize 55 000 copies/mL in RT-PCR assays as a threshold for the initiation of treatment. These guidelines are constantly updated, and in general these have evolved in a more conservative strategy of deferring treatment over the past 5 years.

A patient population for whom ART is more universally recommended is HIV-infected pregnant women. Suppression of maternal plasma HIV RNA to the greatest possible extent is the guiding strategy. When plasma HIV RNA levels are successfully suppressed below the limits of detection, less than 2% of infants become HIV-infected.[76] Owing to potential teratogenicity, efavirenz should be avoided as a component of ART regimen in an HIV-infected pregnant woman. ART may also be recommended for post-exposure prophylaxis following sexual contact with a partner known to have HIV infection, in high-risk circumstances including rape, and in healthcare workers following a blood or body fluid exposure.

Suppression of viral replication

The ideal aim of ART is suppression of plasma HIV RNA levels below the limit of detection. The lower limits of detection for plasma HIV RNA may vary between 50 and 400 copies/mL, depending on the assay used. This strategic target is crucial for the durability of ART response because when HIV replication is suppressed to the lowest possible level, the emergence of drug-resistant isolates is substantially delayed.[77] For patients who achieve a plasma HIV RNA of <50 copies/mL, the annual relapse rate is 2–3% per year for the next 3 years. To achieve this level of potent suppression of HIV replication, it is necessary to use multiple antiretroviral drugs, usually three different agents.

Adherence

Crucial to the successful suppression of plasma HIV RNA and the achievement of a durable response is the need for strict medication adherence. Owing to the persistence of HIV despite suppression, and its ability to reinitiate replication when drug levels become inadequate, failure to maintain adherence will rekindle virus replication in the presence of subtherapeutic drug levels. Inevitably this results in antiretroviral drug resistance. Clinical studies have demonstrated that a minimum of 95% adherence is required to achieve the best virologic outcomes,[78] and achievement of such a high level of adherence is formidable given the indefinite need for treatment. Adherence cannot be predicted on the basis of a patient's socioeconomic status, sex, race, or risk behavior. However, depression and active substance abuse with either alcohol or cocaine do predict poor adherence.[79] The identification of simpler antiretroviral regimens, adherence education, and adherence reinforcement mechanisms have substantially aided in improving adherence in clinical practice.

Minimizing toxicities

Each antiretroviral agent carries the potential risk of drug-related toxicities. The patterns of drug-related toxicities are summarized in Box 20.2.

The assessments of toxicities related to these agents have dramatically evolved with time. For example, the lipodystrophy syndrome, related to ART interventions and to HIV disease itself, was described after several years of drug utilization in clinical practice. An important strategy for minimizing drug-related toxicities is to individualize the choice of a therapeutic regimen based upon a patient's medical history, response to specific agents, and preferences. The expanding number of ART drugs supports the use of this individually oriented strategy.

Resistance testing

Resistance testing is now commonly employed in clinical practice. Owing to the staggered introduction of antiretroviral drugs over the past 15 years, and incomplete suppression of viral replication, up to 56% of HIV-infected persons in the USA may harbor drug-resistant isolates.[80] Drug resistance may be assessed through the use of genotypic techniques that look for characteristic mutations, or through the use of phenotypic resistance tests that directly observe virus replication in the presence of drug. These assays can be an important guide for the choice of specific ART regimens.

Box 20.2. *Pattern of drug-related toxicities with antiretroviral agents*

Nucleoside reverse transcriptase inhibitors

Anemia, leukopenia (zidovudine)

Peripheral neuropathy (didanosine, stavudine, and zalcitabine)

Pancreatitis (didanosine, stavudine, and zalcitabine)

Hypersensitivity (abacavir)

Lactic acidosis (all)

Hepatic steatosis (all)

Peripheral fat loss (all, perhaps greater with didanosine, stavudine, and zalcitabine)

Elevated lipids (mild but all)

Non-nucleoside reverse transcriptase inhibitors

Rash (all)

Central nervous system symptoms (efavirenz)

Early hepatic abnormalities (nevirapine)

Elevated lipids (all)

Peripheral fat loss (efavirenz)

Protease inhibitors

Centripedal fat accumulation (all)

Elevated lipids (all)

Nephrolithiasis (indinavir)

Glucose intolerance (all)

Fusion inhibitors
Injection site reactions (enfuvirtide)

Antiretroviral agents

There are currently a total of 25 approved agents that inhibit four targets in the HIV lifecycle: two enzymatic steps, the binding of HIV to the co-receptor CCR5, and the fusion of HIV into the host cell membrane. The two enzymatic targets are reverse transcriptase (the enzyme that catalyzes the formation of DNA from viral RNA) and HIV protease (which cleaves large precursor polyproteins into their functional components). Within the category of reverse transcriptase inhibitors there are nucleoside, non-nucleoside, and nucleotide inhibitors. Within the protease inhibitor class, the agents share the common characteristics of relatively more difficult drug delivery, and the potential need for enhancement of drug levels. The currently approved antiretroviral agents are listed in Table 20.2. The fusion inhibitors were approved in 2003. Careful consideration of potential interactions should be used when prescribing these agents.

Two new drug classes were approved recently, CCR5 antagonists (also called entry inhibitors) and integrase inhibitors. CCR5 antagonists were developed on the basis of the findings that chemokine receptors are primordial virus receptors, that chemokines have the capacity to block HIV entry, and that host defects in CCR5 expression severely reduce acute HIV infection. The first approved CCR5 antagonist, maraviroc, has been shown to be effective against all CCR5-tropic HIV-1 viruses tested but not viruses targeting a second co-receptor, CXC chemokine receptor-4. Vicriviroc, another CCR5 antagonist, specifically binds to CCR5 and blocks CCR5-dependent intracellular signaling and cell migration depending on the C–C motif ligands CCL3, CCL4, and CCL5.[81] The newest class of drugs, integrase inhibitors, works by blocking integration of the HIV DNA into host DNA. This new class of drug is especially promising for HIV-infected patients who have developed resistance to reverse transcriptase and protease inhibitors. Recent clinical trials testing the safety and efficacy of raltegravir, the first approved integrase inhibitor, reported that plasma HIV RNA levels were lowered to below 50 copies/mL within 24 months in 90% of the subjects using raltegravir in combination with tenofovir and lamivudine. The safety profile of raltegravir was not significantly different from that of placebo and there were no apparent dose-related toxicities.[82]

Genitourinary complications of treatment

The principal genitourinary complication of treatment has been crystallization of the protease

Table 20.2. *Antiretroviral agents and their dosing*

Agent	Dose
Nucleoside reverse transcriptase inhibitors	
Zidovudine	300 mg twice daily
Didanosine	400 mg every day or 250 mg every day if <60 kg
Zalcitabine	0.75 mg thrice daily
Stavudine	40 mg twice daily or 30 mg twice daily if <60 kg
Lamivudine	150 mg twice daily
Abacavir	300 mg twice daily
Emtricitabine	200 mg once daily
Zidovudine – lamivudine – abacavir	1 pill twice daily
Zidovudine – lamivudine	1 pill twice daily
Efavirenz – tenofovir – emtricitabine	1 pill once daily
Abacavir – lamivudine	1 pill once daily
Tenofovir – emtricitabine	1 pill once daily
Non-nucleoside reverse transcriptase inhibitors	
Nevirapine (Viramune)	200 mg once daily for 2 weeks, then 200 mg twice daily
Delavirdine (Rescriptor)	400 mg three times daily or 600 mg twice daily
Etavirenz (Sustiva, Stocrin)	600 mg once daily
Nucleotide reverse transcriptase inhibitors	
Tenofovir	300 mg once daily
Protease inhibitors	
Saquinavir	1200 mg three times daily

(Continued)

Table 20.2. *(Continued)*

Agent	Dose
Ritonavir	600 mg three times daily
Indinavir	800 mg every 8 hours
Nelfinavir	1250 mg twice daily
Amprenavir	1200 mg twice daily
Lopinavir/ritonavir	2 pills twice daily
Atazanavir	400 mg once daily
Fosamprenavir	1400 mg twice daily
Darunavir	3 pills twice daily (2 darunavir pills + 1 ritonavir pill twice daily)
Tipranavir	3 pills twice daily (2 tipranavir pills + 1 ritonavir pill twice daily)
Fusion inhibitors	
Enfuvirtide	90 mg subcutaneously twice daily
CCR-5 antagonists or entry inhibitors	
Maraviroc	150 mg twice daily, 300 mg twice daily, or 600 mg twice daily, depending on other medications
Vicriviroc	No dosage recommended yet
Integrase inhibitors	
Raltegravir	400 mg twice daily

inhibitor indinavir within the urinary tract. Owing to the need for strict every-8-hour dosing and avoidance of food with each dose, the use of indinavir in HIV clinical practice has substantially declined. Two recent trials have combined indinavir with the pharmacokinetic enhancer ritonavir in an attempt to reduce dosing frequency and eliminate the need to avoid food.[83,84] Unfortunately both trials had high rates of drug discontinuation because of crystallization of indinavir in the urinary tract.

Sexuality and HIV

A diagnosis of HIV does not signal the end of a person's sex life or sexual identity. The majority of HIV-infected people are young or middle-aged adults who are now living longer and healthier lives as a result of advances in ART and prophylaxis of opportunistic infections, and it is important for clinicians to acknowledge that sexual functioning remains of great importance with significant impact on quality of life.[85,86] Furthermore, for patients on ART, sexual dysfunction may be associated with reduced adherence and therefore may be a factor in a patient's clinical outcome.[87]

Clinicians caring for HIV-infected patients should also be aware that a substantial number of people with HIV infection complain of sexual dysfunction, and since the advent of combination ART this number has been steadily increasing. Several types of sexual dysfunction are common, and while multiple possible etiologies have been suggested, no definitive cause has been identified. It has been well documented, however, that the prevalence of sexual dysfunction is more common in symptomatic HIV patients, particularly those carrying an AIDS diagnosis, than in asymptomatic people.[88]

Prevalence of sexual dysfunction

To date, the prevalence of sexual dysfunction in HIV–AIDS has been poorly studied, making epidemiological estimates difficult. In general, however, three types of sexual dysfunction have been documented in this population: erectile dysfunction (ED), loss of interest in sex, and delayed orgasm. An early study by Brown et al. reported the presence of sexual dysfunction in more than 20% of a cohort of asymptomatic, healthy HIV-infected men.[89] Several later studies reported substantially higher proportions in cases of symptomatic HIV infection, usually in excess of 50% among AIDS patients,[90] suggesting that the prevalence of sexual dysfunction increases with increasing disease severity.

Since the advent of combination ART, several investigators have reported increasing rates of sexual dysfunction in their patient populations. Recent studies, performed in the era of combination ART,

have found that 9–74% of HIV-infected men report ED.[91] A large multi-site trial demonstrated that protease inhibitor-experienced patients (male and female) were 3.5 times more likely to report a decrease in sexual interest and libido than protease inhibitor-naïve patients. Further, protease inhibitor-experienced men were over 2.5 times more likely to report a decrease in sexual potency compared with protease inhibitor-naïve men. Among these inhibitors, indinavir and ritonavir were found to be most strongly associated with decrease in both sexual interest and sexual potency.[90] These results may be partially explained by more progressive underlying HIV disease in patients selected to receive protease inhibitors rather than the effect of the medications themselves. More recent studies have found no link between past or present ART use and sexual dysfunction, suggesting further investigation is needed on this subject.

Etiology of sexual dysfunction

The etiology of sexual dysfunction is often multi-factorial, and may be attributed to any combination of endocrine, psychogenic, neurogenic, arteriogenic, or iatrogenic factors.[92] However, in HIV-infected patients the list of possible etiologies is further expanded to include fatigue, psychological and emotional reactions to HIV infection and its consequences, endocrine dysfunction, low testosterone levels, HIV-related neurologic disease including autonomic neuropathy, and ART side effects.[88]

In a recent study in the UK of HIV-infected MSM complaining of ED, 44% were diagnosed with a primarily psychogenic dysfunction, 22% with primarily organic dysfunction, and 34% with mixed dysfunction.[88] However, other studies have suggested that organic etiologies, rather than situational or psychogenic factors, are primarily responsible for sexual dysfunction in such a patient population.[85,86,90]

Before combination ART was widely available, sexual dysfunction was more common among those patients who had progressed to AIDS. The prevalence of ED among those with AIDS was found to be 62% compared with 42% in those men with HIV whose disease had not progressed to AIDS.[91] In this era prior to the availability of more effective combination ART, androgen deficiency, particularly of testosterone, was considered to be the primary organic cause of sexual dysfunction, especially in those with advanced HIV disease. More recent research has found no association between past or current use of ART and development of ED, suggesting that these medications should not be withdrawn to alleviate sexual dysfunction. This is especially true since recent studies have found a significant link between low CD4[+] lymphocyte counts and ED, and discontinuing ART may lead to a decline in CD4[+] lymphocyte counts.[91]

Treatment of sexual dysfunction

In patients with documented low levels of testosterone, supplementation may help to relieve the symptoms. In a small study, Rabkin et al. demonstrated that testosterone supplementation improved ED and increased libido in patients with hypogonadism.[93] Testosterone supplementation may also have additional beneficial effects. It has been shown to increase hemoglobin levels by 3–19%, which may be helpful for HIV-infected patients who are anemic. Furthermore, there is no evidence to suggest that testosterone use is linked with immunosuppression, any effects on CD4[+] lymphocyte count or plasma HIV RNA levels, or progression of Kaposi's sarcoma. However, supplementation has been linked to reduced spermatogenesis and a reduction in testicular volume, but both of these effects are reversible if therapy is discontinued.[91] As low levels of testosterone are more common in patients with symptomatic HIV disease or AIDS, it is reasonable to measure serum testosterone levels in such patients who complain of low sexual drive or other forms of sexual dysfunction.

For cases not linked to hypotestosteronism, however, psychological and physical methods of treatment have both been found to be effective, particularly the physical methods. Psychological methods have included cognitive behavioral therapy, while the physical methods have consisted of alprostadil administered either by intrapenile injection or transurethrally, vacuum constriction devices, or insertion of a penile prosthesis. Another treatment option is phosphodiesterase types 5 (PDE-5) inhibitors, including sildenafil, vardenafil and tadalafil. Care should be taken when using PDE-5 inhibitors as a treatment option given their association with unsafe sexual behavior and sexually transmitted diseases, and their drug interactions with protease inhibitors. Adverse events such as visual disturbances, decreased blood pressure, syncope, and prolonged erection are more common in those receiving ritonavir (a protease inhibitor causing profound inhibition of the CYP3A4 isoenzyme of the P450 system) with high serum levels of sildenafil. A decreased dosage of sildenafil is recommended in patients also taking ritonavir, and current pharmacokinetic data suggest a maximum single dose of 25 mg over a 48-hour period.[94] Overall, treatment for sexual dysfunction in HIV-infected patients has been quite successful. In one study, the combination of psychological and medical therapy was shown to be effective in 90% of cases.[91]

Recent research has shown that most cases of ED in HIV-infected patients go unrecognized because of patients' failure to notify their provider or physicians' failure to ask about sexual dysfunction. These findings suggest that ED is underdiagnosed in the HIV-infected population of men and will become more prevalent as successful ART treatment increases longevity for HIV-infected people.[91] Finally, any physician treating an HIV-infected patient for sexual dysfunction should be sensitive to the importance of sexual functioning in these patients, and should be supportive of the needs and concerns of the patients while simultaneously stressing the importance of safer sex practices. Recent research suggests that placing HIV-infected men on treatment for ED leads to an increase in unsafe sexual behavior. A study performed by Cachay et al. found a significant association between sildenafil prescription and risky sexual behavior. The study reported that 13% of HIV-infected men with a sildenafil prescription had two or more sexual partners during the prior month compared with only 5% if no prescription was documented.[95] Therefore, any patient visit about sexual dysfunction due to HIV serves as an excellent opportunity to emphasize the importance of practicing safe sex.

References

1. Joint United Nations Programme on HIV/AIDS. Report on the Global AIDS Epidemic a UNAIDS 10th Anniversary Special Edition, 2006 [available at: http://www.unaids.org/en/HIV_data/2006Global Report/default.asp].

2. Centers for Disease Control and Prevention. HIV/AIDS Surveillance: General Epidemiology. (Through 2006) Atlanta: Centers for Disease Control and Prevention, 2006 [available at: http://www.cdc.gov/hiv/topics/surveillance/resources/slides/epidemiology/index.htm].

3. Freedberg KA, Welensky RP, Paltiel D, Losina E. Survival benefits of AIDS treatment in the United States. Infect Dis 2006; 194: 11–19.

4. Centers for Disease Control and Prevention. AIDS Weekly Surveillance Report: 31 December, 1984. Atlanta: Centers for Disease Control and Prevention, 1984 [available at: http://www.cdc.gov/hiv/topics/surveillance/resources/reports/pdf/surveillance84.pdf].

5. Centers for Disease Control and Prevention. A glance at HIV/AIDS among men who have sex with men. Atlanta: Centers for Disease Control and Prevention, 2007 [available at: http://www.cdc.gov/hiv/resources/factsheets/msm_glance.html].

6. Centers for Disease Control and Prevention. HIV/AIDS surveillance report, 15. Atlanta: Centers for Disease Control and Prevention, 2004 [available at: http://www.cdc.gov/hiv/topics/surveillance/resources/reports/2006report/default.htm].

7. Centers for Disease Control and Prevention. CDC Fact Sheet: HIV/AIDS Among US Women: Minority and Young Women at Continuing Risk. Atlanta: Centers for Disease Control and Prevention [available at: http://www.cdc.gov/hiv/pubs/facts/women.html].

8. Centers for Disease Control and Prevention. HIV/AIDS Among African Americans. Atlanta: Centers for Disease Control and Prevention [available at: http://www.cdc.gov/hiv/topics/aa/resources/factsheets/aa.html].

9. Centers for Disease Control and Prevention. HIV/AIDS Surveillance Report. Atlanta: Centers for Disease Control and Prevention, 2004; 11: 46 [available at: http://www.cdc.gov/hiv/topics/surveillance/resources/reports/2004report/pdf/2004 surveillanceReport.pdf].

10. Walensky R, Weinstein M, Kimmel A, Seage G. Routine human immunodeficiency virus testing: an economic evaluation of current guidelines. Am J Med 2005; 118: 292–300.

11. Lifson AR, Rutherford GW, Jaffe HW. The natural history of human immunodeficiency virus infection. J Infect Dis 1988; 158: 1360–7.

12. Mellors JW, Rinaldo CR Jr, Gupta P et al. Prognosis in HIV-1 infection predicted by the quantity of virus in plasma. Science 1996; 272: 1167–70.

13. Ward JW, Bush TJ, Perkins HA et al. The natural history of transfusion-associated infection with human immunodeficiency virus. Factors influencing the rate of progression to disease. N Engl J Med 1989; 321: 947–52.

14. Clotet B, Ruiz L, Ibanez A. Long-term survivors of human immunodeficiency virus type 1 infection. N Engl J Med 1995; 332: 1646–8.

15. Fellay J, Shianna KV, Ge D, Colombo S. A whole-genome association study of major determinants for host control of HIV-1. Science 2007; 317: 944–7.

16. Gao X, Nelson GW, Karacki P et al. Effect of a single amino acid change in MHC class I molecules on the rate of progression to AIDS. N Engl J Med 2001; 344: 1668–75.

17. Dean M, Carrington M, Winkler C et al. Genetic restriction of HIV-1 infection and progression to AIDS by a deletion allele of the CKR5 structural gene. Science 1996; 273: 1856.

18. Liu R, Paxton WA, Choe S et al. Homozygous defect in HIV-1 coreceptor accounts for resistance of some multiply-exposed individuals to HIV-1 infection. Cell 1996; 86: 367–77.

19. Schuitemaker H, Koot M, Kootstra NA et al. Biological phenotype of human immunodeficiency virus type 1 clones at different stages of infection: progression of disease is associated with a shift from monocytotropic to T-cell-tropic virus population. J Virol 1992; 66: 1354–60.

20. Learmont JC, Geczy AF, Mills J et al. Immunologic and virologic status after 14 to 18 years of infection with an attenuated strain of HIV-1 – a report from the Sydney blood bank cohort. N Engl J Med 1999; 340: 1715–22.

21. Hecht FM, Grant RM, Petropoulos CJ et al. Sexual transmission of an HIV-1 variant resistant to multiple reverse-transcriptase and protease inhibitors. N Engl J Med 1998; 339: 307–11.

22. Del Amo J, Malin AS, Pozniak A, De Cock KM. Does tuberculosis accelerate the progression of HIV disease? Evidence from basic science and epidemiology. AIDS 1999; 13: 1151–8.

23. Goletti D, Weissman D, Jackson RW et al. Effect of Mycobacterium tuberculosis on HIV replication. Role of immune activation. J Immunol 1996; 157: 1271–8.

24. Greub G, Ledergerber B, Battegay M et al. Clinical progression, survival, and immune recovery during antiretroviral therapy in patients with HIV-1 and hepatitis C virus coinfection: the Swiss HIV Cohort Study. Lancet 2000; 356: 1800–5.

25. Reisler R, Han C, Burnab W, Tedaldi E, Neaton J. Incidence of grade IV events, AIDS and mortality in a large multicenter cohort receiving HAART. Presented at Ninth Conference on Retroviruses and Opportunistic Infections, Seattle, WA 24–28 February 2002 (abstract 36).

26. Management of possible sexual, injecting-drug-use, or other nonoccupational exposure to HIV, including considerations related to antiretroviral therapy. MMWR Morb Mortal Wkly Rep 1998; 47: 1–14.

27. Wawer MJ, Gray RH, Nelson SK, Serwadda D. HIV transmission by stage of infection. J Infect Dis 2005; 191: 1403–9.

28. Coombs RW, Reichelderfer PS, Landay AL. Recent observations on HIV type-1 infection in the genital tract of men and women. AIDS 2003; 17: 455–80.

29. Muciaccia B, Corallini S, Vicini E, Padula F. HIV-1 viral DNA is present in ejaculated abnormal spermatozoa of seropositive subjects. Hum Reprod 2007; 22: 2868–78.

30. Krieger JN, Nirapathpongporn A, Chaiyaporn M et al. Vasectomy and human immunodeficiency virus type 1 in semen. J Urol 1998; 159: 820–5; discussion 825–6.

31. Fiore JR, Zhang YJ, Bjorndal A et al. Biological correlates of HIV-1 heterosexual transmission. AIDS 1997; 11: 1089–94.

32. Mastro TD, de Vincenzi I. Probabilities of sexual HIV-1 transmission. AIDS 1996; 10: S75–82.

33. Darrow WW, Echenberg DF, Jaffe HW et al. Risk factors for human immunodeficiency virus (HIV) infections in homosexual men. Am J Public Health 1987; 77: 479–83.

34. Updated US Public Health Service Guidelines for the management of occupational exposures to HBV, HCV, and HIV and recommendations for postexposure prophylaxis. MMWR Morb Mortal Wkly Rep 2001; 50: 1–42.

35. Schreiber GB, Bush MP, Kleinman SH, Korelitz JJ. The risk of transfusion-transmitted viral infections. N Engl J Med 1996; 334: 1635–90.

36. Vittinghoff E, Bucbinder SP, Judson F et al. Per contact risk for transmission of HIV associated with four types of homosexual contact. Presented at 5th Conference on Retrovirus and Opportunistic Infections, Chicago, February 1–5, 1998.

37. Jana NK, Gray LR, Shugars DC. Human immunodeficiency virus type 1 stimulates the expression and production of secretory leukocyte protease inhibitor (SLPI) in oral epthelial cells: a role for SLPI in innate mucosal immunity. J Virol 2005; 79: 6432–40.

38. Erice A, Rhame FS, Heussner RC, Dunn DL, Balfour HH Jr. Human immunodeficiency virus infection in patients with solid-organ transplants: Report of five cases and review. Rev Infect Dis 1991; 13: 537–47.

39. Clarke JA. HIV transmission and skin grafts. Lancet 1987; 1: 983.

40. Robert LM, Chamberland ME, Cleveland JL et al. Investigations of patients of health care workers infected with HIV: the Centers for Disease Control prevention database. Ann Intern Med 1995; 122: 653–7.

41. Human immunodeficiency virus transmission in household settings – United States. MMWR Morb Mortal Wkly Rep 1994; 43: 347, 353–6.

42. Centers for Disease Control and Prevention. HIV and its transmission. Atlanta: Centers for Disease Control and Prevention, 1999 [available at: http://www.cdc.gov/hiv/resources/factsheets/transmission.html].

43. Royce RA, Sena A, Cates WJr, Cohen MS. Sexual transmission of HIV. N Engl J Med 1997; 336: 1072–8.

44. Laga M, Manoka A, Kivuvu M et al. Non-ulcerative sexually transmitted diseases as risk factors for HIV-1 transmission in women: results from a cohort study. AIDS 1993; 7: 95–102.

45. Centers for Disease Control and Prevention. HIV Prevention Through Early Detection and Treatment of Other Sexually Transmitted Diseases. Atlanta: Centers for Disease Control and Prevention, 1998 [available at: http://www.cdc.gov/mmwr/preview/mmwrhtml/00054174.htm].

46. Gilson L, Mkanje R, Grosskurth H et al. Cost effectiveness of improved treatment services for sexually transmitted diseases in preventing HIV-1 infection in Mwanza Region, Tanzania. Lancet 1997; 350: 1805–9.

47. National Institute of Allergy and Infectious Diseases. Scientific Evidence on Condom Effectiveness for Sexually Transmitted Disease (STD) Prevention

Herndon, VA: 2000 [available at: www.ccv.org/downloads/pdf/CDC_condom_study.pdf]

48. Trussell J, Sturgen K, Strickler J, Dominik R. Comparative contraceptive efficacy of the female condom and other barrier methods. Fam Plann Perspect 1994; 26: 66–72.

49. Cohen MS, Gay C, Kashuba AD, Blower S. Antiretroviral therapy for preventing the sexual transmission of HIV-1. Ann Intern Med 2007; 146: 591–601.

50. Musicco M, Lazzarin A, Nicolasi A et al. Antiretroviral treatment of men infected with human immunodeficiency virus type 1 reduces the incidence of heterosexual transmission: Italian Study Group on HIV Heterosexual Transmission. Arch Intern Med 1994; 154: 1971–6.

51. Lalani T, Hicks C. Does antiretroviral therapy prevent HIV transmission to sexual partner. Curr HIV/AIDS Rep 2007; 4: 80–5.

52. Debiaggi M, Zara F, Spinillo A et al. Viral excretion in cervicovaginal secretions of HIV-1-infected women receiving antiretroviral therapy. Eur J Clin Microbiol Infect Dis 2001; 20: 91–6.

53. Si-Mohamed A, Kazatchkine MD, Heard I et al. Selection of drug-resistant variants in the female genital tract of human immunodeficiency virus type 1-infected women receiving antiretroviral therapy. J Infect Dis 2000; 82: 112–22.

54. Haase AT, Schacker TW. Potential for transmission of HIV-1 despite highly active antiretroviral therapy. N Engl J Med 1998; 339: 1846–8.

55. McCutchan FE, Hoelscher M, Tovanabutra S, Piyasirisilp S. In-depth analysis of heterosexually acquired human immunodeficiency virus type 1 superinfection: evolution, temporal fluctuation, and intercompartment dynamics from the seronegative window period through 30 months postinfection. J Virol 2005; 79: 1693–704.

56. Clotet B. 2004. Strategies for Overcoming Resistance in HIV-1 Infected Patients Receiving HAART. AIDS Rev 6: 123–30.

57. Van Vaerenbergh K. Study of the impact of HIV genotypic drug resistance testing on therapy efficacy. Verh K Acad Geneeskd Belg 2001; 63: 447–73.

58. Blackard JT, Cohen DE, Mayer KH. Human immunodeficiency virus superinfection and recombination: Current state of knowledge and potential clinical consequences. Clin Infect Dis 2002; 34: 1108–14.

59. Halperin DT, Bailey RC. Male circumcision and HIV infection: 10 years and counting. Lancet 1999; 354: 1813–15.

60. Auvert B, Taljaard D, Lagarde E et al. Randomized, controlled intervention trial of male circumcision for reduction of HIV infection risk: The ANRS 1265 trial. PLoS Med 2005; 2: e298.

61. Bailey RC, Moses S, Parker CB, Agot K. Male circumcision for HIV prevention in young men in Kisumu, Kenya: a randomised controlled trial. Lancet 2007; 369: 643–56.

62. Gray RH, Kigozi G, Serwadda D, Makumbi F. Male circumcision for HIV prevention in men in Rakai, Uganda: A randomised trial. Lancet 2007; 369: 657–66.

63. Centers for Disease Control and Prevention. Male circumcision and risk for HIV transmission: implications for the United States. Atlanta: Centers for Disease Control and Prevention [available at: http://www.cdc.gov/hiv/resources/factsheets/circumcision.htm].

64. Male Circumcision is Important Additional Step in Cutting HIV Infection. New York: United Nations Press Conference, 28 March 2007 [available at: http://www.un.org/apps/news/story.asp?NewsID=22036&Cr=HIV&Cr1=AIDS/].

65. Alanis MC, Lucidi RS. Neonatal circumcision: a review of the world's oldest and most controversial operation. Obstet Gynecol Surv 2004; 59: 379–95.

66. Lukobo MD, Bailey RC. Acceptability of male circumcision for prevention of HIV infection in Zambia. AIDS Care 2007; 19: 471–7.

67. Ngalande RC, Levy J, Kapondo CP, Bailey RC. Acceptability of male circumcision for prevention of HIV infection in Malawi. AIDS Behav 2006; 10: 377–85.

68. Shapiro RL, Kebaabetswe P, Lockman S, Mogwe S. Male circumcision: An acceptable strategy for HIV prevention in Botswana. Sex Transm Infect 2003; 79: 214–19.

69. Vandebosch A, Goetghebeur E, Ramjee G, Alary M. Acceptability of COL-1492, a vaginal gel, among sex workers in one Asian and three African cities. Sex Transm Infect 2004; 80: 241–3.

70. Dezzutti CS, James VN, Ramos A, Sullivan ST. In vitro comparison of topical microbicides for prevention of human immunodeficiency virus type 1 transmission. Antimicrob Agents Chemother 2004; 48: 3834–44.

71. Phillips DM, Taylor CL, Zacharopoulos VR, Maguire RA. Nonoxynol-9 causes rapid exfoliation of sheets of rectal epithelium. Contraception 2000; 63: 149–54.

72. Berkley SF, Koff WC. Scientific and policy challenges to development of an AIDS vaccine. Lancet 2007; 370: 94–101.

73. Girard MP, Osmanov SK, Kieny M. A review of vaccine research and development: The human

immunodeficiency virus (HIV). Vaccine 2006; 24: 4062–81.

74. International AIDS Vaccine Initiative. When will an AIDS vaccine be found? The state of global research. New York: 2002 [available at: http://www. iavireport.org/].

75. Letvin NL. Progress and obstacles in the development of an AIDS vaccine. Nature Rev Immunol 2002; 6: 930–9.

76. Shapiro D, Tuomala R, Samuelson R. MTCT rates according to ART, mode of delivery and viral load. Abstract 114 presented at Ninth Conference on Retroviruses and Opportunistic Infections, Seattle, WA 24–28, February 2002.

77. Kempf DJ, Rode RA, Xu Y et al. The duration of viral suppression during protease inhibitor therapy for HIV-1 infection is predicted by plasma HIV-1 RNA at the nadir. AIDS 1998; 12: F9–14.

78. Paterson DL, Swindells S, Mohr J et al. Adherence to protease inhibitor therapy and outcomes in patients with HIV infection. Ann Intern Med 2000; 133: 21–30.

79. Bartlett JA. Addressing the challenges of adherence. J Acquir Immune Defic Syndr 2002; 29(Suppl 1): S2–10.

80. Richman D, Bozzette S, Morton S et al. The prevalence of antietroviral drug resistance in the US. [Abstract LB-17] 41st Interscience Conference on Antimicrobial Agents and Chemotherapy. Chicago, 16–19 December 2001.

81. Este JA, Telenti A. HIV entry inhibitors. Lancet 2007; 370: 81–8.

82. Grinsztejn B, Nguyen B, Katlama C, Gatell J. Safety and efficacy of the HIV-1 integrase inhibitor raltegravir (MK-0518) in treatment-experienced patients with multidrug-resistant virus: A phase II randomised controlled trial. Lancet 2007; 369: 1261–9.

83. Gatell J, Lundgren J, Gerstaft J. A randomized study comparing continued indinavir (800 mg TID) vs switching indinavir/ritonavir (800/100 mg BID) in HIV patients having achieved viral load suppression with indinavir plus 2 nucleoside analogues. The BID efficacy and safety trial. Presented at 8th European Conference on Clinical Aspects and Treatment of HIV-Infection, Athens, Greece 28–31 October 2001. (abstract 8).

84. Castagna A, Dragsted U, Chave JP. The interim analysis of a phase IV, randomized, open-label, multicenter trial to evaluate safety and efficacy of IDV/RTV (800/100 mg BID) vs S Q/RTV (800/100 mg BID) in adult HIV-1 infection. Presented at Ninth Conference on Retroviruses and Opportunistic Infections, Seattle, WA 24–28 February 2002 (abstract 450W).

85. Tindall B, Forde S, Goldstein D, Ross MW, Cooper DA. Sexual dysfunction in advanced HIV disease. AIDS Care 1994; 6: 105–7.

86. Newshan G, Taylor B, Gold R. Sexual functioning in ambulatory men with HIV/AIDS. Int J STD AIDS 1998; 9: 672–6.

87. Ammassari A, Antinori A, Aloisi MS, Trotta MP. Depressive symptoms, neurocognitive impairment, and adherence to highly active antiretroviral therapy among HIV-infected persons. Psychosomatics 2004; 45: 394–402.

88. Catalan J, Meadows J. Sexual dysfunction in gay and bisexual men with HIV infection: evaluation, treatment and implications. AIDS Care 2000; 12: 279–86.

89. Brown GR, Rundell JR, McManis SE et al. Prevalence of psychiatric disorders in early stages of HIV infection. Psychosom Med 1992; 54: 588–601.

90. Schrooten W, Colebunders R, Youle M et al. Sexual dysfunction associated with protease inhibitor containing highly active antiretroviral treatment. AIDS 2001; 15: 1019–23.

91. Crum NF, Furtek KJ, Olson PE, Amling CL. A review of hypogonadism and erectile dysfunction among HIV-infected men during the pre- and post-HAART eras: diagnosis, pathogenesis, and management. AIDS Patient Care STDs 2005; 19: 655–71.

92. Broderick GA, Lue TF. Evaluation and nonsurgical management of erectile dysfunction and priapism. In: Walsh PC, Retik AB, Vaughan ED Jr et al., eds. Campbell's Urology, 8th edn. Philadelphia: Elsevier, 2002; 1619–71.

93. Rabkin J, Rabkin R, Wagner J. Testosterone treatment of clinical hypogonadism in patients with HIV/AIDS. Int J STD AIDS 1997; 8: 537–45.

94. Viagra.com. Full Prescribing Information New York: 2007 [available at: http://www.viagra.com/content/viagra-prescribing-information-professional.jsp?setShowOn=../content/viagra-prescribing-information-professional.jsp&setShowHighlightOn=../content/viagra-prescribing-information-professional.jsp].

95. Cachay E, Mar-Tang M, Matthews C. Screening for potentially transmitting sexual risk behaviors, urethral sexually transmitted infection, and sildenafil use among males entering care for HIV infection. AIDS Patient Care STDs 2004; 18: 349–54.

CHAPTER 21

Sexually transmitted infections

Katherine M Coyne, Simon E Barton

Introduction

Sexually transmitted infections (STIs) are a threat to health worldwide. An estimated 340 million people are infected each year with chlamydia, gonorrhea, trichomoniasis, or syphilis.[1] In the poorest countries, unsafe sex is second only to malnutrition as the leading risk factor for disease, disability, and death, and in the developed world unsafe sex is the ninth most important risk factor.[2]

Symptomatic men present to a range of settings including general practice, genitourinary medicine (GUM) clinics, emergency departments, and urology services. Urethritis (dysuria or urethral discharge) is most often caused by *Chlamydia trachomatis*, *Neisseria gonorrhea*, or *Mycoplasma genitalium*, but also by viruses such as herpes simplex virus (HSV) or adenovirus. Epididymo-orchitis can develop from ascending spread of bacteria and is associated with infertility. Genital ulceration is mostly due to HSV, less commonly to syphilis or lymphogranuloma venereum (LGV), and rarely to chancroid or donovanosis in returning travellers. Genital lumps may be warts or molluscum contagiosum. Itching in the pubic area occurs with scabies or lice.

Asymptomatic men may be infected with *C. trachomatis*, *N. gonorrhea*, M. *genitalium*, HSV, human papilloma viruses, syphilis, or HIV. The dual purpose of screening is to detect latent disease requiring treatment, in the case of syphilis or HIV, and to prevent transmission to sexual partners. It has long been recognized that other STIs facilitate both acquisition and transmission of HIV.[3] Treatment of STIs can reduce the incidence of HIV[4] and is of paramount importance in those at risk. HIV and hepatitis B and C are discussed in separate chapters.

Clinical assessment

Assessment involves history taking, examination, and investigations. The history should be tailored to aid appropriate management but not cause embarrassment by eliciting unnecessary details. Questions should probe symptoms of dysuria, urethral discharge, testicular pain, rectal symptoms, skin rashes, lumps and itching, and previous STIs. Risk assessment includes recent sexual partners (e.g. in the past 3 months), whether they were female or male, and if condoms were worn for vaginal or anal sex. Men who have sex with men (MSM) should be asked whether they were the active (insertive) or passive (receptive) partner for anal sex.

Examination of the genitalia includes inspection of the pubic hair, penis, urethral meatus, scrotum, and perineal and perianal skin, and palpation of the inguinal lymph nodes and testicles. In an uncircumcised man the prepuce should be retracted to reveal the glans. Men with rectal symptoms should have a proctoscopy. Examination may include the mouth and skin.

Investigations include swabs and urine and blood tests. Urethral swabs can either sample visible discharge expressed from the meatus or can be inserted 1–2 cm into the meatus and rotated. Rectal swabs are best taken at proctoscopy, but can be taken 'blind' in asymptomatic men. Throat swabs are taken from the posterior pharynx. Ulcers can be swabbed for viral culture or for polymerase chain reaction for herpes simplex, syphilis, or chancroid. First-void urine samples are suitable for chlamydia or gonorrhea testing. Serology for HIV, syphilis, hepatitis B, and hepatitis C are offered as appropriate.

Genital chlamydia

Genital chlamydial infection is the most common bacterial STI in the developed world. In the UK the number of diagnoses has been increasing each year, and reached over 113 000 in 2006, double the number in 1996.[5] Risk factors include young age, previous chlamydia, change in sexual partner in the past 3 months, and two or more sexual partners in the past 12 months.[6] The UK National Chlamydia Screening Programme aims to offer annual testing to all men and women aged 16–25. The highest rates in men are in those aged 20–24, with a prevalence of up to 10%. Screening is occurring at a wide variety of venues, including general practices, schools, colleges, prisons, youth centers, pharmacies, drug user clinics, and accident and emergency departments. In some areas postal kits are available.

C. *trachomatis* is an obligate intracellular parasite that infects only humans. Serovars D–K cause genital infections, whereas serovar L causes invasive disease and the clinical syndrome of LGV (see below). The most common sites of infection are the male urethra and the cervix. Urethral infection is asymptomatic in at least 50% of men, but it can cause dysuria and urethral discharge.[7] Infection may spread to the testis or epididymis and reduce fertility.[8] Rectal infection is usually asymptomatic. Proctitis may occur with serovars D–K, but does so more commonly with LGV. Chlamydia can also cause conjunctivitis and pharyngitis.

Reactive arthritis is an uncommon complication of chlamydia, gonorrhea, or enteropathic bacterial infection. It is a pathological immunological response and classically presents with a large-joint oligoarthritis, which may be severe and relapsing.

The standard diagnostic tests for chlamydia are now nucleic acid amplification tests (NAATs), which are sensitive and specific. First-void urine samples are as good as urethral swabs in men,[9] and are more practical in many settings. Urethral swabs are useful where microscopy can be performed, as in GUM clinics. If the urethral smear shows urethritis then antibiotics that cover chlamydia can be given immediately. Swabs can also be taken from the rectum and pharynx as appropriate.

Uncomplicated chlamydia is treated with a single oral dose of azithromycin 1 g or 1-week course of doxycyline 100 mg twice daily. Both regimens have cure rates of approximately 97%,[10] and resistance is not yet an issue. Men should abstain from sex, even with a condom, for a week after treatment is initiated. Sexual partners need to be tested, and then treated for chlamydia while awaiting results. Since chlamydia is so often asymptomatic, all partners in the preceding 6 months should be notified. Follow-up is necessary to ensure adherence to treatment and to check partner notification. A test of cure is not recommended since NAATs may be falsely positive for weeks after treatment because of dead organisms. However, re-infection rates are high, and re-screening after 3–4 months may be advisable.

Gonorrhea

N. *gonorrhea* infects mucous membranes and causes a similar spectrum of disease to chlamydia. It has a global distribution with higher rates in the developing world. In the UK gonorrhea is much less common than chlamydia and is concentrated among groups with high rates of partner change, including in urban areas and among young people and MSM.[11]

Urethral infection is symptomatic in 80% of men, causing dysuria and urethral discharge, which may be clear or purulent. Complications include epididymo-orchitis and reactive arthritis. Pharyngeal and rectal infections are frequently asymptomatic. Septicemia, septic arthritis, meningitis, and endocarditis are rare but serious sequelae.

Gonorrhea can be diagnosed by visualizing Gram-negative intracellular diplococci on microscopy of a urethral or rectal smear, allowing immediate treatment. This result needs to be confirmed, since N. meningitidis appears identical under the microscope. Swabs can be taken for culture. NAATs can be performed on swabs or urine samples but will not provide antibiotic sensitivities. Antibiotic choice has been complicated worldwide by extensive antimicrobial resistance. Antibiotics that cover at least 95% of local isolates should be chosen. In the UK, the recommended first-line drug is a single dose of cefixime 400 mg orally.[12] If pharyngeal penetrance is required, then ceftriaxone 250 mg intramuscularly is preferred. In cases of allergy to cefalosporins an alternative is spectinomycin 2 g intramuscularly. Co-infection with chlamydia occurs in 20–40% of cases[13] and so azithromycin is often co-prescribed. As with chlamydia, people diagnosed with gonorrhea need to abstain from sex for 1 week and ensure that partners are treated.

Non-specific urethritis

Non-specific urethritis (NSU) describes urethritis in which neither chlamydia nor gonorrhea has been isolated. Urethritis is diagnosed on microscopy if ≥5 white blood cells (WBCs) per oil-immersion field are detected on the Gram staining of urethral secretions, or if ≥10 WBCs are seen per high-power field with first-void urine. NSU may be associated with dysuria and urethral discharge, or it may be asymptomatic. Infectious causes of NSU include M. genitalium, Ureaplasma urealyticum, Trichomonas vaginalis, HSV, warts, adenovirus, and candida. Non-infectious etiologies include complications of urethral stricture, urinary calculi, and topical irritants.

NSU diagnosed on microscopy often proves to be chlamydia when test results are available, and therefore NSU is treated with azithromycin 1 g orally or 1 week of doxycycline. M. genitalium

responds less well to single dose azithromycin and very poorly to doxycycline. In men with persistent NSU, an extended course of azithromycin (500 mg on the first day, followed by 250 mg daily for 4 days) can be considered, since it is 96% effective at eradicating M. genitalium.[14] As with chlamydia, men should abstain from sex for 1 week. Sexual partners should be tested and treated, since a high proportion will be diagnosed with chlamydia.[15]

Epididymo-orchitis

Infection of the testis or epididymis causes pain and swelling, sometimes associated with scrotal erythema, hydrocele, or fever. The differential diagnosis includes the surgical emergency of torsion of the testis, suggested by a sudden onset of pain. Clinical examination and often ultrasound scanning are used to differentiate these conditions. Testicular cancer should be considered if symptoms and signs do not settle completely with antibiotics.

In young, sexually active men the most important pathogens are C. trachomatis and N. gonorrhea. In older men epididymo-orchitis is more often caused by bacterial spread from the urinary tract, particularly when prostatic hypertrophy results in incomplete bladder emptying. Urine cultures may identify the organism and provide antibiotic sensitivities. A suitable choice of antibiotic would be ofloxacin 200 mg twice daily for 2 weeks, with gonococcal cover if appropriate. Orchitis can also be caused by mumps and other viruses, and by Mycobacterium tuberculosis.

Lymphogranuloma venereum

LGV is a genital ulcer disease; it was rare outside tropical regions until outbreaks occurred among MSM in Europe in 2003. It is caused by C. trachomatis serovar L1–3, which is capable of tissue invasion and destruction. The primary ulcer occurs at the site of inoculation, followed by spread to local lymphatics. A penile ulcer is accompanied by inguinal lymphadenopathy, and untreated disease may progress to urethral stricture or genital elephantiasis. Rectal inoculation can cause proctitis, rectal strictures, and fistulae. A high index of suspicion is required in MSM who present with proctitis,[16] since LGV can be mistaken for inflammatory bowel disease. The diagnosis is made by positive chlamydia NAAT with serovar identification at a reference laboratory. LGV can be treated with doxycyline 100 mg twice daily for 3 weeks.[17] Alternative regimens with weekly azithromycin have been tried successfully.

Trichomoniasis

T. vaginalis is a flagellated protozoan transmitted through vaginal sex.[18] It is important worldwide as a cause of pre-term birth and a facilitator of HIV transmission. Although women may have an odorous vaginal discharge, men are usually asymptomatic. Urethritis can occur and persist despite standard treatment for NSU. The diagnosis is made by wet-preparation microscopy or culture in specialized medium, neither of which is routinely performed in men. Most men become aware of infection when the diagnosis is made in a female partner. Treatment is with metronidazole 400 mg twice daily for 5 days or a single dose of metronidazole 2 g.[19]

Genital herpes

HSV-1 and HSV-2 cause most genital ulcers.[20] Historically HSV-1 caused orolabial herpes and HSV-2 genital herpes, but recent data show that genital herpes is now caused by HSV-1 as often as by HSV-2.[21] Lesions are classically painful, and evolve from red papules to vesicles to shallow ulcers that heal within 1–3 weeks (see Fig. 21.1). There is a wide spectrum of disease, from asymptomatic to severe ulceration accompanied by systemic symptoms.[22] Atypical presentations are common, including itching. Urinary retention can result from sacral nerve involvement.

Primary episodes are usually the most painful. The virus migrates to the dorsal root ganglion, where it lies dormant but may reactivate. Symptomatic recurrences occur in approximately 50% of people and may be preceded by tingling in the skin. HIV-

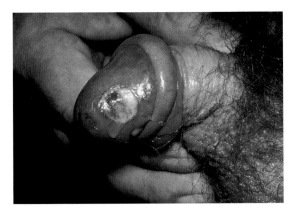

Figure 21.1. *Primary HSV.*

positive adults may have more severe and prolonged attacks.

HSV can be diagnosed on culture or PCR from a swab of the vesicle or ulcer, the sensitivity being highest from new lesions. A negative swab does not exclude HSV. Determination of type 1 or 2 can inform prognosis since type 1 recurrences are generally milder and less frequent.

Outbreaks can be treated with antiviral drugs. Treatment should start immediately prodromal symptoms appear, and may abort the attack. Standard regimens include acyclovir 200 mg five times a day for 5 days, but shorter courses are effective, such as acyclovir 800 mg three times a day for 2 days.[23] If recurrences are frequent (e.g. six per year) or distressing, then acyclovir 400 mg twice daily is effective as prophylaxis. Valacyclovir and famciclovir are alternatives with less-frequent dosing regimens.

HSV is shed from lesions and those affected individuals should abstain from sex during an outbreak. Asymptomatic shedding of virus also occurs frequently[24] and can infect partners. Condoms reduce transmission, but not completely, since genital skin contact still occurs. There is evidence that onward transmission is reduced by daily antiviral prophylaxis with valaciclovir[25] but also presumably with other effective antiviral therapies.

HSV causes considerable anxiety because of its chronicity, unpredictability, and infectiousness. Serological tests for antibodies to HSV-1 and -2 can help with advising couples. For example, if a man has genital HSV-1, and his female partner tests negative for IgM or IgG to HSV-1 then she is susceptible to acquiring infection. This information may be particularly important when the woman is pregnant, since primary infection can cause life-threatening neonatal herpes.

Syphilis

Syphilis causes a chronic infection that can affect almost every organ of the body, leading the 19th century physician Sir William Osler to write that to know syphilis is to know medicine. The stages of syphilis are primary, secondary, latent, and tertiary. Primary syphilis involves an ulcer at the site of inoculation after 2–3 weeks, which is classically single and painless, heals spontaneously in a few weeks, and may be unnoticed (see Fig. 21.2). The secondary stage is of bacteremia 4–8 weeks later, which may present with fever, malaise, widespread rash, wart-like condylomata lata, headache, meningitis, arthritis, periostitis, hepatitis, nephritis, or iritis. Latent (asymptomatic) syphilis is divided into early (less than 2 years since infection) and late stages. Primary, secondary, and early latent syphilis are infectious. Tertiary syphilis follows after more than 5 years and includes gumma and cardiovascular and neurological complications. Congenital syphilis occurs if a pregnant woman has infectious syphilis, but it is fortunately rare where syphilis serology is performed antenatally.

In the UK, syphilis had almost disappeared by the 1980s but has re-emerged since 1997, with 2766 diagnoses of infectious syphilis in 2006. Many new infections are in MSM, but heterosexual clusters have appeared in several cities, with some linked to commercial sex work.

Since syphilis can mimic so many conditions, a high index of suspicion is warranted. In GUM clinics, dark ground microscopy of a scrape from ulcer base can visualize spirochetes and allow immediate diagnosis. Syphilis serology should be a standard component of STI screening although interpretation can be complex.

Parenteral penicillin is the mainstay of treatment, but dosages and duration depend on disease stage.[26] It is advised that men with syphilis are referred to GUM specialists for management and follow-up.

Genital human papilloma virus infections

HPV infections are common and often subclinical.[27] Genital warts (condylomata acuminata) are mostly caused by 'low-risk' HPV-6 and HPV-11. Infection usually results from genital contact with an infected partner, the risk increasing with number of sexual partners and other STIs.[28] The incubation period before appearance of warts is up to 2 years, with a median of 3 months.[29] HPV DNA persists for months or even years after warts have disappeared. Warts are commonly found on the penis, but also in hair-bearing areas. Perianal and anal warts frequently occur in MSM, but are not uncommon in men who never have anal sex, probably caused by transfer of virus via fingers or genital secretions.

Warts can be treated with creams, physical destructive techniques such as cryotherapy, or surgery.[30] Podophyllotoxin cream 0.5% is most effective against non-keratinized warts, and is relatively inexpensive. Keratinized warts respond better to imiquimod cream 5%, which also reduces the risk of recurrence. Warts in the urethral meatus may need to be removed surgically (see Fig. 21.3).

Cervical, anal, and penile cancers are associated with oncogenic HPV-16 and HPV-18, which are also sexually transmitted. Recent interest has focussed on the development of promising vaccines. A vaccine (Gardasil, Merck) against HPV-6, -11, -16, and -18 has shown dramatic reductions in the risk of genital warts and cervical cancer in women.[31]

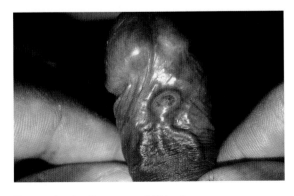

Figure 21.2. *Primary syphilitic chancre.*

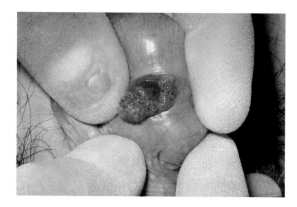

Figure 21.3. *Urethral wart.*

Large trials have not been performed in men, but it would be expected to reduce incidence of warts and anal cancer. A bivalent vaccine (Cervarix, GlaxoSmithKline) targets only HPV-16 and -18. Many countries are debating the arguments for widespread vaccination programs, and whether to vaccinate girls only, or also boys.

Molluscum contagiosum

Molluscum contagiosum presents as small pearly pink papules with a central depression. It is caused by a pox virus that is contagious through skin contact. Children often acquire infection from social contact, and widespread lesions develop, followed by protective immunity. Some people are first exposed to the virus as adults from a sexual partner, and lesions predominate in the genital area. They are generally asymptomatic and resolve without treatment in a few months. If the cosmetic appearance is distressing, they can be treated with cryotherapy, expression of the core, or by podophyllotoxin 0.5% or imiquimod 5% (unlicensed indication).

Scabies and pubic lice

Scabies is an infestation caused by the mite *Sarcoptes scabiei*, which spreads through skin-to-skin contact. The main symptom is itch resulting from a hypersensitivity reaction to mite excrement. The silvery tracks of mite burrows may be visible in the

interdigital folds, wrist, and elbows. On the genitals there may be papules or nodules. The diagnosis is usually clinical but mites can be visualized under light microscopy of scrapings from the burrows.

Pubic lice are properly known as *Phthirus pubis* and are transmitted by close body contact. Adult lice lay eggs (nits) on pubic hair or other thick body hair. They may be asymptomatic or cause itch. Lice and eggs can be seen by the naked eye.

Treatment of both scabies and lice is with permethrin 5% cream or malathion 0.5% lotion. Sexual and household contacts also need treatment.

Health promotion

A consultation about sexual health is an opportunity for health promotion. Men should be aware of the risks inherent in protected and unprotected sex. Condom use reduces risk of HIV,[32] chlamydia, and gonorrhea.[33] HSV, HPV, and syphilis are easily transmitted from genital skin not covered by a condom. Men at risk of hepatitis B, including all MSM, should be vaccinated. Men who are exposed to HIV need to be aware of post-exposure prophylaxis and how to access it promptly.

References

1. World Health Organization. Global prevalence and incidence of selected curable sexually transmitted infections: overview and estimates. Geneva: World Health Organization, 2001.
2. Ezzati M, Lopez AD, Rodgers A et al. Selected major risk factors and global and regional burden of disease. Lancet 2002; 360: 1347–60.
3. Fleming DT, Wasserheit JN. From epidemiological synergy to public health policy and practice: the contribution of other sexually transmitted diseases to sexual transmission of HIV infection. Sex Transm Infect 1999; 75: 3–17.
4. Korenromp EL, White RG, Orroth KK et al. Determinants of the impact of sexually transmitted infection treatment on prevention of HIV infection: a synthesis of evidence from the Mwanza, Rakai, and Masaka intervention trials. J Infect Dis 2005; 191: S168–78.

5. Health Protection Agency. Testing Times. HIV and other Sexually Transmitted Infections in the United Kingdom. London, 2007.

6. Department of Health. New Frontiers: Annual Report of the National Chlamydia Screening Programme in England 2005/06 London: Department of Health, 2006.

7. Peipert JF. Genital chlamydial infections. N Engl J Med 2003; 349: 2424–30.

8. Idahl A, Boman J, Kumlin U, Olofsson JI. Demonstration of *Chlamydia trachomatis* IgG antibodies in the male partner of the infertile couple is correlated with a reduced likelihood of achieving pregnancy. Hum Reprod 2004; 19: 1121–6.

9. Cook RL, Hutchinson SL, Ostergaard L, Braithwaite S, Ness RB. Systematic review: noninvasive testing for *Chlamydia trachomatis* and *Neisseria gonorrhoeae*. Ann Intern Med 2005; 142: 914–25.

10. Lau CY, Qureshi AK. Azithromycin versus doxycycline for genital chlamydia infections: a meta-analysis of randomized clinical trials. Sex Transm Dis 2002; 29: 497–502.

11. Fenton K, Lowndes CM. Recent trends in the epidemiology of sexually transmitted infections in the European Union. Sex Transm Infect 2004; 80: 255–63.

12. BASHH Guidelines. National Guideline on the Diagnosis and Treatment of Gonorrhoea in Adults 2005 [accessible at http://www.bashh.org/guidelines/2005/gc_final_0805.pdf, Accessed 31: March, 2008].

13. Dicker LW, Mosure DJ, Berman SM, Levine WC. Gonorrhea prevalence and coinfection with chlamydia in women in the United States, 2000. Sex Transm Dis 2003; 30: 472–6.

14. Bjornelius E, Anagrius C, Bojs G et al. Antibiotic treatment of symptomatic *Mycoplasma genitalium* infection in Scandinavia: a controlled clinical trial. Sex Transm Infect 2008; 84: 72–6.

15. McCathie RP, Carlin EM. Does partner notification of men with asymptomatic non-gonococcal non-chlamydial urethritis identify chlamydia-positive women? Int J STD AIDS 2007; 18: 606–9.

16. Richardson D, Goldmeier D. Lymphogranuloma venereum: an emerging cause of proctitis in men who have sex with men. Int J STD AIDS 2007; 18: 11–5.

17. BASHH Guidelines. 2006 National Guideline for the Management of Lymphogranuloma Venereum (LGV) [accessible at: http://www.bashh.org/guidelines/2007/lgv_gdl_revised_final2_1106.pdf accessed 31 March, 2008].

18. Schwebke JR, Burgess D. Trichomoniasis. Clin Microbiol Rev 2004; 17: 794–803.

19. Thin RN, Symonds MAE, Booker R, Cook S, Langlet F. Double-blind comparison of a single dose and a five-day course of metronidazole in the treatment of trichomoniasis. Brit J Vener Dis 1979; 55: 354–6.

20. Gupta R, Warren T, Wald A. Genital herpes. Lancet 2007; 370: 2127–37.

21. Haddow LJ, Dave B, Mindel A et al. Increase in rates of herpes simplex virus type 1 as a cause of anogenital herpes in western Sydney, Australia, between 1979 and 2003. Sex Transm Infect 2006; 82: 255–9.

22. Kimberlin DW, Rouse DJ. Genital herpes. N Engl J Med 2004; 350: 1970–7.

23. Wald A, Carrell D, Remington M, Kexel E, Corey L. Two-day regimen of acyclovir for treatment of recurrent genital herpes simplex virus type 2 infection. Clin Infect Dis 2002; 34: 944–8.

24. Wald A, Zeh J, Selke S et al. Reactivation of genital herpes simplex virus type 2 infection in asymptomatic seropositive persons. N Engl J Med 2000; 342: 844–50.

25. Barton SE. Reducing the transmission of genital herpes. BMJ 2005; 330: 157–8.

26. French P. Syphilis. BMJ 2007; 334: 143–7.

27. Partridge JM, Koutsky LA. Genital human papilloma virus infection in men. Lancet Infect Dis 2006; 6: 21–31.

28. Ault KA. Epidemiology and natural history of human papillomavirus infections in the female genital tract. Infect Dis Obstet Gynecol 2006; 14: 404–7.

29. Winer RL, Kiviat NB, Hughes JP et al. Development and duration of human papilloma virus lesions after initial infection. J Infect Dis 2005; 191: 731–8.

30. Maw R. Critical appraisal of commonly used treatment for genital warts. Int J STD AIDS 2004; 15: 357–64.

31. Garland SM, Hernandez AM, Wheeler CM et al. Quadrivalent vaccine against human papillomavirus to prevent anogenital diseases. N Engl J Med 2007; 356: 1928–43.

32. Cayley WE. Effectiveness of condoms in reducing heterosexual transmission of HIV. Am Fam Physician 2004; 70: 1268–9.

33. Warner L, Stone KM, Macaluso M, Buehler JW, Austin HD. Condom use and risk of gonorrhea and Chlamydia: a systematic review of design and measurement factors assessed in epidemiologic studies. Sex Transm Dis 2006; 33: 36–51.

CHAPTER 22

Circumcision

Angus HN Whitfield, Hugh N Whitfield

Introduction

It is estimated that there are currently in the world 650 million males who have been circumcised. Despite being one of the oldest and most common surgical procedures worldwide, circumcision is unique in that the majority of procedures are not performed for medical reasons or by qualified medical practitioners. The historical origins of circumcision are unclear, but the practice is found throughout the world – in Native Americans, Australian Aboriginals, African and Middle Eastern tribesmen, and in the earliest Egyptian mummies. Almost all of these circumcisions were carried out for cultural or religious reasons, and in much of the world this continues to the present day, with circumcision a part of defining religious or tribal identity. A wonderful example of this can be found in the autobiography of Nelson Mandela,[1] in which he describes his own circumcision as part of his rite of passage to adulthood. In the USA, circumcision remains the cultural norm, and 70–90% of all male babies are circumcised.

In this chapter we detail the medical indications for circumcision and the complications of surgery. Some of the issues that govern circumcision for religious purposes are discussed, and we examine the ethical and legal implications that are pertinent to the circumcision of minors. Medical practitioners need to be familiar with all these aspects of circumcision, to be able to advise on the wide range of questions that can arise when counselling parents and patients.

Religious circumcision

Amongst the major religions of the world, only in Judaism and Islam is circumcision an accepted religious rite. The origins of Christianity are found in Judaism and there are many similarities in the rites and laws of both religions, but there is no mandatory circumcision in Christianity. Similarly, there is no obligation for circumcision in the Buddhist, Sikh and Hindu religions.

Judaism
The circumcision of newborn males is a central feature of Judaism, and takes its roots in the Torah as part of the covenant between God and Abraham.

> This is my covenant that you shall keep between Me and you and your descendants after you: every male among you shall be circumcised . . . . . At the age of eight days every male among you shall be circumcised throughout your generation.
>
> (Genesis 17: 10–14)

This practice is further reinforced within the laws given to Moses on Mt Sinai, as recorded within the Book of Leviticus.

Circumcision of a male neonate is therefore an essential undertaking within the Jewish religion, and is performed by a specifically trained *mohel* (pl. *mohelim*). In the United Kingdom (UK), *mohelim* are trained according to strict guidelines under the auspices of the Initiation Society. It is a requirement that a *mohel* is a practising Jew himself (it is generally accepted that a *mohel* has been circumcised, thus precluding women), attends around 50 circumcisions before actually performing one, and is examined through both written and practical assessments. Although the Torah states that circumcision occurs on the eighth day, the *mohel* visits the family a few days prior to this to ensure that the child is healthy. Jewish law allows for a delay in circumcision should the child be suffering from any ailment, since the welfare of the child is paramount. For the procedure itself the use of local anesthetics, though not routine, is not prohibited within the Jewish Talmud (an explanatory commentary and debate on the various biblical laws) and may occur at the request of the family. The cut edge of the prepuce is not sutured and hemostasis is achieved by means of bandaging. The *mohel* is required to visit at least once after the procedure to check the wound, and leaves aftercare instructions. Although no precise figures are available, the complication rates of Jewish circumcisions in the UK are thought to be low.

Given its place as part of the covenant of Abraham, it is likely that circumcision will remain a central part of Judaism and, as such, it may be of the utmost importance to a Jewish parent that their son be circumcised, even if the other parent is not a Jew.

Islam

Islam is a much younger religion than Judaism, and it is not surprising that circumcision predates the religion's founding within the Arab world. Within the Sunnah (the sayings of the Prophet Muhammad), it is recognized that circumcision is a feature of pre-Islamic cultural traditions. However, the circumcision of males is not mentioned within the Koran itself and is considered instead to be Hadith (the Prophet's tradition – derived from consensus within the Muslim community). Of the many Islamic schools of thought (sects), circumcision is only required by the Shafiite sect; for the others, it is merely recommended. Despite the almost universal

circumcision of males within the Muslim community, a male is not excluded from Islam if he is uncircumcised, and it is not essential for a convert to Islam to undergo circumcision. Female circumcision (now more commonly known as female genital mutilation) – although widely practised within Muslim countries in different forms – does not receive a mention in the Koran either, and is similarly considered to be a practice from the Hadith.

Although Muhammad recommended that circumcision should be performed early, the exact age at which males are circumcised varies within the Muslim community and can occur within the first week of life or as old as 5–10 years in parts of the Middle East and Pakistan. Similarly, there is considerable variation concerning who performs circumcisions. Whereas doctors or health technicians perform 90–95% of circumcisions within the Gulf States, the figure is no more than 5–10% in rural areas of the Middle East and Pakistan. Unsurprisingly, there is a corresponding variation in complication rates although these are rarely reported and in most cases it is likely that the child is never brought to the attention of a qualified medical practitioner.[2]

With the seemingly ambivalent attitude towards circumcision that is found in Islamic law, it is most likely that the religious founders sought a way in which to allow a continuation of a cultural practice rather than using it to define a religious identity.

Medical considerations in circumcision

Embryology and functional anatomy of the prepuce

The prepuce develops from ectoderm, neuroectoderm and mesenchyme to form a structure that is comprised of an inner epithelial-lined mucosa, a lamina propria, dartos muscle, with dermis and glabrous skin on the outer surface. The prepuce first appears at 8 weeks' gestation as an epithelial thickening that grows forward over the developing glans, covering the glans completely by 16 weeks.

During development, there is no plane of separation between the epithelium of the glans and that of the under-surface of the prepuce, and at birth the

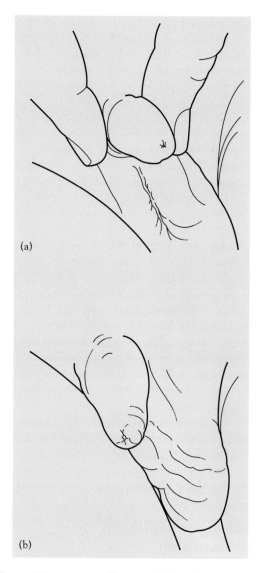

Figure 22.1 *A normally retractile foreskin.*

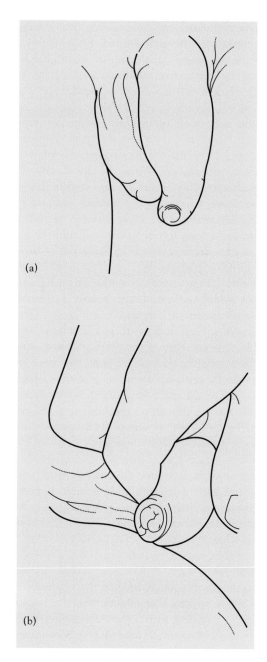

Figure 22.2 *A partially retractile foreskin; this condition will usually respond to conservative management.*

prepuce is almost always non-retractile. Separation of the two layers occurs as a result of spontaneous desquamation that commences in the distal prepuce at the end of gestation and proceeds proximally at varying rates. Hence, there is a considerable variation in the age at which the prepuce is fully retractile in different individuals with 90% having a non-retractile prepuce at birth and 98% having a fully retractile prepuce at puberty. Importantly,

even though a child may not have a fully retractle foreskin, partial retraction of the foreskin to its limit produces a characteristic 'flowering' appearance around the prepuce. The importance and significance of this are discussed later. The somatosenory innervation of the prepuce is by the dorsal nerve of the penis and branches of the perineal nerve. Additionally, the prepuce receives an autonomic innervation – parasympathetic visceral efferents and afferents from the sacral plexus and sympathetic visceral afferents from the lateral horns of T11–L2. Thus, neither a block of the dorsal penile nerve nor topical EMLA cream (AstraZeneca, Luton, UK) completely relieve the pain of circumcision. Microscopically, the prepuce has a dense population of fine touch nerve endings (mainly Meissner's corpuscles). Conversely, the glans has very few such nerve endings and is instead innervated by those associated with pain and temperature sensation, with the exception of the corona and frenulum. During intercourse, the glans glides over the prepuce whereas in the circumcised male it slides directly against the vaginal wall resulting in considerably more friction. Interestingly, there is some suggestion that women having experience of intercourse with both circumcised and uncircumcised find the latter to be preferable.[3]

The prepuce is therefore a specialized erogenous tissue, and surgical removal of the normal prepuce results in the loss of most of the fine touch receptors of the penis, and the glans itself becomes thickened and keratinized.

Medical indications for circumcision

The pathology that provokes the need for circumcision is different in infants and adults.

In infants there is often a dilemma whether a non-retractile prepuce is truly phimosed. The appearance of ballooning of the prepuce during micturition is often thought to indicate a significant degree of phimosis, but this is not so. The only absolute evidence in an infant that circumcision is essential is when, on attempted retraction, the prepuce takes on the appearance of a helmet. If the prepuce begins to open and to take on the appearance of a flower, then no true phimosis exists. There is seldom any contraindication to pursuing a conservative management policy, and reviewing the child after an interval of 6–12 months.

In an adult the only absolute indication for circumcision is true pathological phimosis, which is almost invariably due to balanitis xerotica obliterans (BXO, diagnosed on histological examination). This condition is essentially genital lichen sclerosis in males. It is characterized by hyperkeratinization, collagen deposition within the papillary dermis and lymphocyte infiltration into the inner dermis. Macroscopically, there is scarring of the preputial opening (with or without narrowing of the urethral meatus). Affected areas appear white, scarred and indurated. Attempts to retract the foreskin do not produce the normal 'flowering' of a developmentally incompletely retractile foreskin. The most florid cases of BXO affect the whole of the preputial sac, resulting in a scarred prepuce that is densely adherent to the underlying glans. Although there has been the suggestion that BXO is a premalignant condition, this is not a universally accepted belief and a full consideration of this topic is beyond the scope of this chapter.

Other conditions such as balanoposthitis (inflammation of the prepuce) and paraphimosis can usually be managed without resorting to circumcision, which should be reserved for frequent troublesome recurrences (although circumcision does offer permanent cure).

Surgical technique and complications

The operative procedure is similar in all age groups. Some form of topical analgesia is necessary, but without a general anesthetic the procedure will always be very uncomfortable. A dorsal penile block can be used to provide worthwhile postoperative analgesia. The adhesions between the glans and the inner layer of the prepuce must be broken down. This may leave the glans raw if there is a severe extent of BXO. The penile skin at the level of the corona should be marked circumferentially and incised cleanly. The two layers of the prepuce should be divided dorsally in the midline longitudinally between artery forceps from the preputial opening to 5 mm proximal to the corona. The inner layer of the prepuce should then be incised circumferentially, maintaining the 5 mm distance from the corona. Ventrally the frenular artery will be divided and must be ligated with a stitch ligature. The subcutaneous tissue by which the prepuce then remains attached should be divided, and any veins encountered should either be coagulated with diathermy or ligated with a fine absorbable ligature. If diathermy is used it is essential to use bipolar and not monopolar diathermy (see below). The penile and inner preputial layers of skin are then approximated with a fine absorbable suture material. Ventrally the inner layer of the prepuce should be closed longitudinally for a distance of a few millimeters, before commencing a circumferential closure. This will ensure that there is no tight band ventrally, which can be uncomfortable on erection and intercourse.

Recognized complications occur both early and late. If the frenular artery or a significant penile vein is not secured, significant bleeding can occur, necessitating ligation of the vessel under general anesthesia. Infection can develop, most commonly at the level of the corona, particularly if there has been balanitis at the time of the circumcision. Systemic antibiotics and cleaning the infected area with saline will usually result in an acceptable cosmetic and functional result, though this may take several weeks. In patients with BXO the external urethral meatus may be affected, resulting in meatal stenosis, which can be a difficult problem to resolve. Erections may be impaired if too much penile skin is removed. The most devastating complication of all can occur if the 'guillotine' technique is used for circumcision. The practitioner pulls on the end of the prepuce and with a swift motion cuts across what is thought to be prepuce, but which in reality is glans and prepuce. The resulting distal penile amputation is an irretrievable disaster.

Uncircumcision

Some men who were circumcised soon after birth request an operative procedure to reverse their circumcision. This is not at all easy to do. Some men attempt to lengthen the penile skin by attaching small weights to tapes attached to the skin of the penis. The lengthening process may take more than a year and the end result is often disappointing. Reconstructive surgical procedures have been described,[4] but are risky. Descriptions of surgical technique have usually been anecdotal, and results of long-term follow-up are virtually non-existent in the literature, but are probably poor.[5]

Sexually transmitted disease and circumcision

Although Islam and Judaism account for only a small proportion of religious identities within the USA, up to 90% of all newborn males are circumcised. One of the reasons for this practice is the long-held conviction that circumcision significantly lowers the risk of the development in adult life of a number of disorders of the penis, and of contracting sexually transmitted diseases.

There is variable evidence for such a 'protective' role for circumcision, but with little consistency in either the quality of different reports, or in the degree of attention given to different disorders. It is beyond the scope of this chapter to provide the reader with a full analysis of the merits and weaknesses of the evidence pertaining to each condition, and so a summary is presented.

A large population-based study from the USA[6] found no clear association between circumcision status and hepatitis B, syphilis, gonorrhea or nongonococcal urethritis. In addition, there has been no consistent difference between circumcised and uncircumcised men for herpes simplex.[7] Because of its association with penile and cervical carcinomas, the differing incidences of human papilloma virus (HPV) in circumcised and uncircumcised men have been closely examined. Although in the USA penile cancer has been reported to be more common in uncircumcised men, more recent evidence suggests that HPV infection is equally common.[8] However, the results of population studies of circumcised and uncircumcised men are awaited to see if there is a corresponding change in the incidence of penile cancer.

Perhaps most interesting, and certainly most topical, is the suggestion that circumcision protects against human immunodeficiency virus (HIV) infection. Although large meta-analyses of this issue have reached vastly differing conclusions, in one study a very strong suggestion that circumcision is indeed protective against HIV has been shown. As part of a study on HIV infection in Africa in couples with disparate HIV status[9] it was noted that, of the 60 couples where the male was HIV negative and the female HIV positive, none of the circumcised males became infected whereas 17% of the uncircumcised males contracted HIV.

Legal and ethical issues surrounding circumcision

It is widely recognized internationally that circumcision (medically irreversible removal of a specialized erogenous tissue which confers no unequivocal prophylactic medical benefit and carries potential risks and long-term consequences) is still accepted as a right within certain religious groups, is encouraged in many other societies, and is the norm in the USA. More recently, some have challenged the idea that circumcision is a pre-requisite for a newborn male to be accepted into Jewish religion and culture, and this has come from within the Jewish community – both in the USA and in Israel itself.

To fully examine this complex and highly sensitive issue, two concepts have to be considered: the right of an individual (adult or child) to be circumcised, and the right of a child to be protected from being circumcised until he is adequately competent to make a decision for himself.

The right to be circumcised

It would be difficult to argue that a competent adult requesting circumcision for religious, cultural or perceived medical reasons does not have the right to the procedure. Although UK law has found that consent from a competent adult does not guard against prosecution for extreme acts of sadomasochism through torture or genital mutilation, circumcision does not at present fall into this category and it would require a direct legal challenge to change this. The distinction as to when it becomes a matter for the individual concerned or for the parents of a minor depends on, in the UK, the child being 'Gillick competent'. This means that the child must have the mental capacity to make a decision for himself based on an analysis of the risk and benefits.

Where a child lacks this ability, the decision rests with the parents and thus it is essential to be sure that they are acting in the child's best interests.

The argument that a child has the legal right to be circumcised for cultural or religious reasons, or put differently that the parents have a right to circumcise *their* child for *their* religious or cultural beliefs, relies on the assumption that not to do so would be to the detriment of the child's welfare. Whilst arguably not in the interests of the child's physical welfare at the time, ritual circumcision is part of long-established practice and it is argued that denying this to a child excludes him from fully participating in his community or religious life. Thus it can be argued that failure by Jewish or Muslim parents to circumcise their child constitutes abuse as this would result in psychological harm from exclusion at school or in the community. The International Convention on the Rights of the Child states in Article 8 that 'States Parties undertake to respect the right of the child to preserve his or her identity', although the Article does not assist by defining or elucidating on the term 'identity'. Furthermore, Article 14 gives further support to a parent's right to bring up their child according to established ritual practices since States 'shall respect the rights of and duties of parents . . . to provide direction to the child in the exercise of his or her right in a manner consistent with the evolving capacities of the child', and thus circumcision can be argued to be consistent with 'direction'. Hence, when viewed in the long term, the best interests of Jewish and Muslim children and children from cultures where childhood circumcision forms a rite of passage require that parents allow them to undergo circumcision.

A child's right to protection from circumcision

As noted earlier, an adult has the capacity to give consent for circumcision for religious or cultural reasons, and certainly it cannot be argued that an adult cannot consent for circumcision for medical reasons. Thus it follows that in such situations, a medical practitioner has a legal defense against malpractice and a religious circumciser against actual bodily harm.

The legal position of involuntary circumcision (of children) is controversial, especially when considering religious circumcision. The argument by opponents of circumcision is that it is tantamount to child abuse. Such a claim potentially carries very serious consequences and its validity must be examined closely. Given that a child cannot give consent for circumcision, this must be obtained from a parent acting on behalf of the child. But for parents to give informed consent for a medical procedure, it is required that the child must be suffering from an illness or trauma that would result in injury, deformity, disability or death were treatment withheld. For non-emergency conditions, where delay would not endanger the child, it is now considered that treatment should be delayed until the child can make his or her own informed decision. Courts in both the USA and elsewhere have consistently ruled to uphold the bodily integrity of incompetent people, minors and adults. Likewise, the ability of parents to secure medical interventions for their children has been limited if the intervention could pose a risk to the health or safety of the child. A court in Texas prevented an incompetent girl from being put forward as a kidney donor, ruling that consent for surgical intrusions is limited to 'treatment'. All similar rulings have upheld that the removal of normal tissue or organs is not treatment.

Article 24.3 of the International Convention on the Rights of the Child, which has been ratified by all countries of the United Nations except Somalia and the USA, requires that all practices prejudicial to the health of the child be abolished. Article 19.1 requires that states ensure that no abuse or harm come to a child whilst in the care of parents or guardians. Article 16 requires that there be no unlawful or arbitrary interference with the privacy of children. Because of the persisting legality of corporal punishment, the UK has been found to be in breach of the Convention. Thus, the over importance of the child's best interest limits parental power. Parents must be seen to act in accordance with what children would wish for themselves. In a survey of American men circumcised as neonates, only 0.3% responded that they would

have undergone the procedure later in life if given the choice. Hence, parental consent can only be valid if circumcision is required as the immediate treatment for a medical pathology, and it is hard to defend it on the dubious grounds of being a preventative measure.

It is further argued by some that involuntary circumcision cannot constitute child abuse because it is only a 'minor procedure' and, in neonates, causes only mild discomfort. Compare this with the observation that, although frequently a day case procedure in adults, circumcision is seldom performed under regional or local anesthesia. Although neonates exhibit reactions to painful stimuli that are different from those expressed by children or adults, there is no doubt that circumcision is a highly noxious stimulus. Certainly, the DSM-IV definition of trauma (an experience outside normal experience including torture, assault or threat to physical integrity) certainly applies to circumcision when looked at from the infant's point of view. Studies have in fact shown that there is a considerable rise in heart rate[10] and serum cortisol,[11] and that children circumcised as neonates demonstrate a grossly exaggerated response to routine vaccinations compared to uncircumcised children.[12] Additionally, there are many cases of mothers whose babies are circumcised in their presence (especially Jewish women) who report considerable psychological trauma arising from the experience.[13]

Of the different cultural and religious groups that promote or require circumcision, Judaism has a very strong basis for the practice. It is perhaps significant therefore that there is growing cultural practice of 'anti-circumcision' arising from Jewish groups within both the USA and Israel. Their contention is that the sole requirement to a Jewish identity is to be born of a Jewish mother[14] and that, contrary to popular belief, circumcision is not a necessity for this identity. They also contend that there is very little understanding within the Jewish authorities concerning the psychological harm arising from circumcision and that, despite the above evidence to the contrary, it is standard belief amongst mohelim and rabbis that neonatal circumcision is entirely harmless and pain free (or that there is 'mild discomfort' only). Whilst it is certainly not our intention to challenge thousands of years of religious practice, it is important to be fully aware of changing beliefs regarding circumcision, and to be able to advise and support parents accordingly.

Conclusion

Traditions dictate much of the behavior that occurs in society. Whether circumcision should remain a tradition will be strongly debated and any medical practitioner who has dealings with such patients or parents must be fully aware of the how ethical and social trends are changing. The operation, when performed for medical reasons, requires skill, care and time and patients should be aware of the need to arrange a period of convalescence. Complications can occur following any surgery, and circumcision is no exception.

Useful organizations and websites

Organizations and websites promoting genital integrity:

Attorneys for the Rights of the Child, 2961

Ashby Ave., Berkeley, CA 94705, USA – http://www.noharmm.org/ARC.htm

Circumcision Resource Centre/Jewish Associates of CRC, PO Box 232, Boston, MA 02133 USA – http://www.circumcision.org

References

1. Mandela NR. Long Walk To Freedom. London: Abacus, 2002: 36–41.

2. Ozdemir E. Significantly increased complications with mass circumcisions. Br J Urol 1997; 80: 136–9.

3. O'Hara K, O'Hara J. The effect of male circumcision on the sexual enjoyment of the female partner. BJU Int 1999; Suppl 1: 79–84.

4. Lynch MJ, Pryor JP. Uncircumcision: a one-stage procedure. Br J Urol 1993; 72: 257–8.

5. Brandes SB, McAninch JW. Surgical methods for restoring the prepuce: a critical review. BJU Int 1999; (Suppl 1): 109–13.

6. Laumann EO, Masi CM, Zuckerman EW. Circumcision in the United States: prevalence, prophylactic effects, and sexual practice. JAMA 1997; 277: 1053–7.

7. Taylor PK, Rodin P. Herpes genitalis and circumcision. Br J Vener Dis 1975; 51: 274–7.

8. Aynaud O, Ionesco M, Barrasso R. Penile intraepithelial neoplasia. Specific clinical features correlate with histological and virological findings. Cancer 1994; 74: 1762–7.

9. Gray RH, Kiwanuka N, Quinn TC et al. Male circumcision and HIV acquisition and transmission: cohort studies in Rakai, Uganda. Rakai Project Team. AIDS 2000; 14: 2371–81.

10. Benini F, Johnston CC, Faucher D, Aranda JV. Topical anaesthesia during circumcision in newborn infants. JAMA 1993; 270: 850–3.

11. Gunnar MR, Malone S, Vance G, Fisch RO. Coping with aversive stimulation in the neonatal period; quiet sleep and plasma cortisol levels during recovery from circumcision. Child Dev 1985; 56: 824–34.

12. Taddio A, Katz J, Illersich AL, Koren G. Effect of neonatal circumcision on pain response during subsequent routine vaccination. Lancet 1997; 349: 599–603.

13. Goodman J. Jewish circumcision: an alternative perspective. BJU Int 1999; (Suppl 1): 22–7.

14. Encyclopedia Judaica. Circumcision. Jerusalem: Keter Publishing, 1971.

CHAPTER **23**

Genital piercing

William R Anderson, Simon AV Holmes

Introduction

We would like to offer a quick insight into the rather bizarre, but increasingly popular, practice of genital piercing. There is surprisingly little written on this subject in the nursing and medical literature. However, it could be argued that within medicine, we should have a good working knowledge of this so-called 'body art': as its popularity increases, so does the likelihood that we will have to deal with the complications.

In recent years, there has been a significant increase in the number of people inflicting themselves with body piercings. Much of this is due to the work of three men, namely Alan Oversby (Mr Sebastian), Jim Ward and Doug Malloy. They are generally regarded as being the father figures of modern, Western piercing as they have done a great deal to develop the terminology and many of the techniques that are currently used worldwide.

It would be wrong to say however, that piercing is an invention of the late twentieth century, as it has been described for millennia and even features in several monumental texts. For example in the Bible, within Genesis alone, there are three separate references to the term 'earring.' For instance, Abraham is looking for a wife for his son Isaac, so he sends out his eldest and most trusted servant, who brings back Rebekah. Abraham presents Rebekah with a golden earring. (Some biblical translations describe this as a nose-ring.)

The *Kama Sutra* was written at some point between the first and sixth centuries AD by the Sanskrit scholar Vatsayana. In the second chapter, he states that

> The people of the southern countries think that true sexual pleasure cannot be obtained without perforating the Lingam*, and they therefore cause it to be pierced like the lobes of the ears of an infant pierced for earrings

although it is not clear from this excerpt which part of the penis is pierced.

In addition, anthropologists have found mummified remains of the Dyak tribe from Borneo dating back to 2000 BC: within the remains of these bodies have been found bony piercings of the penis.

At the present time in the United Kingdom (UK), there is minimal legislation relating to body piercing. If an individual wishes to establish a piercing clinic, he or she can do so without any formal training or certification. The clinic does not require a special licence as would be requisite for a medical clinic, but public and employer liability insurance is essential.

Indeed, the clinic only has to be registered with its local authority in one of three situations:

---

* Hindu term for phallus.

(i) if the clinic is in London,* (ii) if the clinic is in Edinburgh,* or (iii) if there is ear piercing offered as part of the service.

Ideally, all piercing clinics should be registered with their local Department of Environmental Health (DEH), but local DEH rules vary throughout the UK. This would help regulate equipment hygiene, sterilization of tools and piercings, as well as increase the awareness of human immunodeficiency virus (HIV) and viral hepatitis. There is no necessity for a doctor or nurse to be associated with the clinic.

Although most clinics are reluctant to perform piercing of children under the age of 16 years, it is not illegal to pierce a child with or without parental consent. Piercing of the genitals is usually not performed under the age of 18 years, and only after adequate counselling. The Piercing Association of the UK (PAUK) and the European Professional Piercing Association (EPPA) offer non-compulsory guidance to piercers regarding such issues as techniques, training and establishing clinics. The Chartered Institute of Environmental Health has made numerous calls for improved legislation of the piercing industry in the UK, and these calls were repeated in September 2002. It is likely that there will be new legislation introduced in the UK in the near future: the first Parliamentary reading of a new Local Government Bill relating to body piercing was made in September 2003.

Techniques

A full medical enquiry should be completed prior to any piercing, with issues such as needle phobias, fainting tendencies, allergies and the possibility of pregnancy being addressed. Ideally, a person competent in first-aid should be at hand, and any serious concerns should result in the piercing being refused.

Many piercing techniques are learned as a 'hands-on' apprenticeship, with some piercers even practising upon themselves or entrusting 'a pound of their flesh' to a worthy friend. Courses are available

---

*Edinburgh and London offer local authority legislation, possibly due to increased concerns over HIV and hepatitis B and C.

through magazines and piercing organizations but these options are entirely voluntary.

Local anesthetic should be offered to the patient, usually in the form of a spray, such as xylocaine or ethyl chloride, or a topical cream, e.g. Ametop® (Smith and Nephew Healthcare Ltd, Hull, UK) or Emla® (AstraZeneca, Luton, UK). The piercing is usually a spike, rod, barbell or ring. Certain piercings may be more prone to infection or 'cutting-out' than others, and the patient should therefore be guided by the experience of the piercer.

An antiseptic should be applied to the area that is to be pierced. Forceps may be used on the skin, and the piercing motion should be quick and confident. Relaxation of the patient is important throughout. Dressings may be required afterwards for protection of clothes, and also for hygiene and reassurance. An aftercare information sheet should be available, and follow-up offered to anyone experiencing any concerns or problems.

Types of genital piercing

Although many body piercings are exotically named, the renowned piercer Jim Ward accepted that most of the names were contrived.

The 'Pubic piercing' is a piercing at the base of the penis (Fig. 23.1), which can take from 4 to 8 months to heal fully. We would hope that this is time well spent, as this piercing is said to improve clitoral sensation during intercourse when the woman is astride her partner. A piercing of the coronal ridge is known as a dydoe (Fig. 23.2). It is possibly Jewish in origin and heals within 6–8 weeks. Not uncommonly, it is arranged as a double or multiple dydoe. Foreskin rings are relatively common and usually heal within 6–10 weeks (Fig. 23.3). The piercing can sometimes be used as a 'chastity belt' to link one lateral side of the foreskin to the other. The foreskin is therefore difficult and painful to retract, so the female can rest fairly well assured that her partner is not indulging in extracurricular activities.

The Ampallang (palang or pallang) is a transverse piercing of the glans whereby the barbell goes either dorsal to, or through, the urethra (Fig. 23.4).

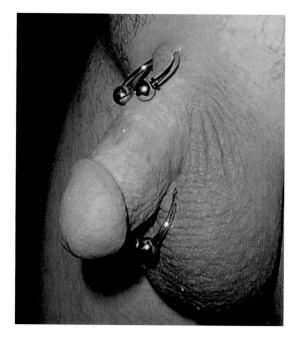

Figure 23.1. *Pubic piercing.*

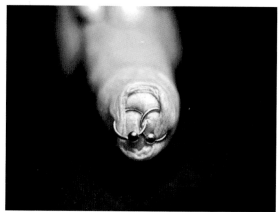

Figure 23.3. *Foreskin rings as chastity rings.*

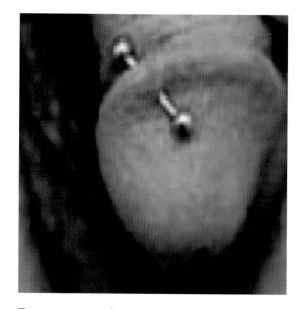

Figure 23.2. *Dydoe.*

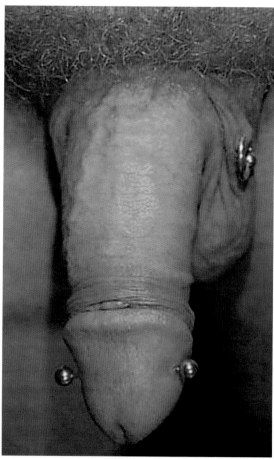

Figure 23.4. *Ampallang.*

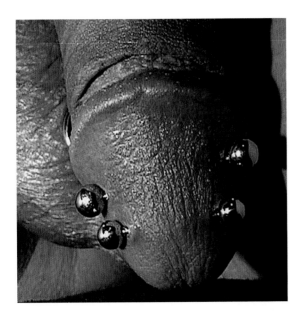

Figure 23.5. *Double ampallang.*

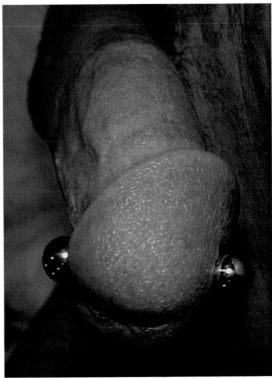

Figure 23.6. *Apadravya.*

It possibly originated in Borneo, as a bony piercing, where it is associated with the Dyak tribe. Perhaps optimistically, it will avoid the corpora, but despite this consideration, it has a reputation for blood loss. Indeed, it can bleed for up to a fortnight after the piercing has been performed, and can take up to 9 months to heal fully. This should allow sufficient time to consider the possibility of having a double ampallang (Fig. 23.5). The Apadravya (*apad*, *apa-davya* or *apadavrya*) is the vertical equivalent of the ampallang (Fig. 23.6). It pierces from dorsum to ventrum by way of the urethra, and usually heals in 2–5 months. It can be placed more proximally in the shaft of the penis, at which point it is named a Shaft or Deep Apadravya.

The term 'Frenum' is given to piercings of the frenulum (Fig. 23.7). This piercing is not recommended in men who are circumcised, as it is technically more difficult to place, and is more likely to cut-out or become infected due to the decreased vascularity. It will usually heal within 6–8 weeks and can be repeated along the length of the frenulum and midline raphe as a Frenum Ladder (Fig. 23.8). Many piercers do not place more than two or three 'rungs' at a time, partly for reasons of comfort and also because of increased

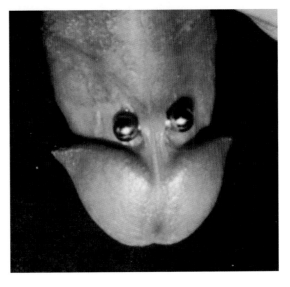

Figure 23.7. *Frenum.*

291

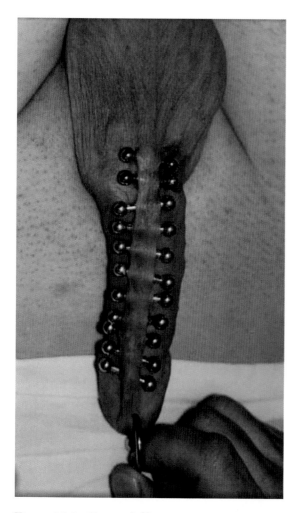

Figure 23.8. *Frenum ladder.*

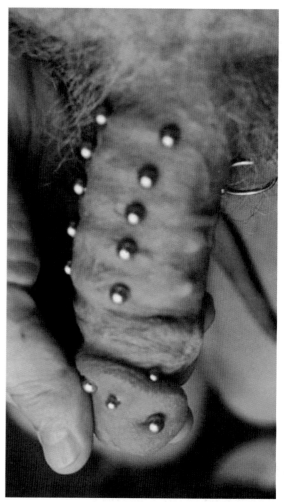

Figure 23.9. *Jacob's ladder.*

concerns over infections and cutting-out. However, there is no generally agreed limit to the number of piercings that can be placed at any one sitting. Jacob's Ladder is the term given to a stepped piercing of the dorsum of the penis (Fig 23.9), although many enthusiasts use the term interchangeably for piercings of the dorsum *and* ventrum of the penile shaft.

The Prince Albert consists of a ring through the urethral meatus that exits on the ventral aspect of the penis (Fig. 23.10). It is the most renowned of the genital piercings and is said to offer 'an intense urethral stimulation during intercourse'. The Prince Albert heals relatively quickly, in 2–4 weeks, and

this may contribute to its popularity. Some of the more considerate owners choose to attach various objects to their Prince Albert. One such device is the 'Dragonfly', which consists of six plastic, flexible barbells arranged like the wings of a dragonfly. This attachment possibly increases vaginal stimulation during sex. Two variations on this theme are the 'Reverse Prince Albert', where the ring exits on the dorsum of the glans (Fig. 23.11), and the barbaric looking Prince's wand, which consists of two bars arranged in a T-shape (Fig. 23.12). The ventral bar of the Prince's wand goes through the ventral opening of the Prince Albert, and threads into the urethral bar. The origin of the name

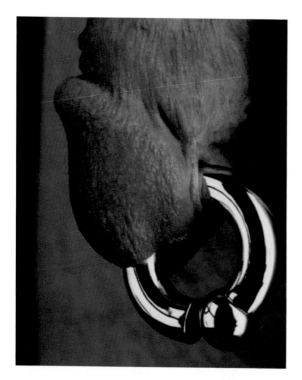

Figure 23.10. *Prince Albert.*

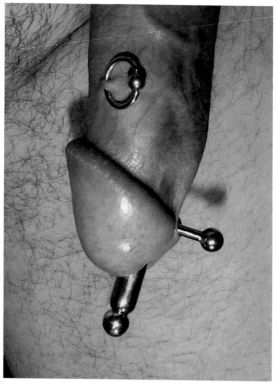

Figure 23.12. *Prince's Wand.*

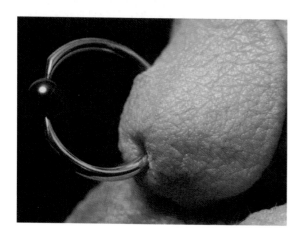

Figure 23.11. *Reverse Prince Albert.*

Prince Albert is debatable. It has been suggested that Queen Victoria's husband, the Prince Consort, had an angulated manhood due to the ravages of Peyronie's disease. This ring possibly represented a noble attempt at straightening out his apparatus.

However, the most widely accepted notion is that Prince Albert had such a piercing when he was a young man. These rings were known as *dress rings*, and were designed to assist the hang of one's genitals in relatively tight trousers, which were considered to be the height of fashion in mid-nineteenth century England. Once the royal connection became publicly known, the ring earned its nickname of 'Prince Albert'. Nevertheless, it is also worth noting that the legendary piercer Jim Ward has dismissed the name's origin as being a modern myth, designed to romanticize genital piercing.

The term Hafada (or Hafad) is given to a scrotal piercing with a ring or barbell, placed high and laterally (Fig. 23.13). Single scrotal piercings usually heal within 2–3 months, and can be configured in a step-wise arrangement (Fig. 23.14), usually along the midline raphe.

The term Guiche (pronounced 'geesh') refers to a piercing of the perineum (Fig. 23.15), usually in the midline. It can also be placed lateral to

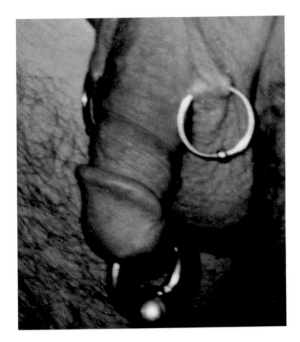

Figure 23.13. *Hafada.*

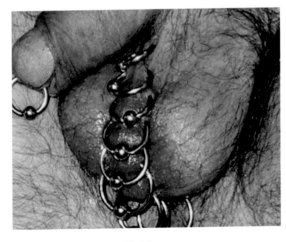

Figure 23.14. *Scrotal ladder.*

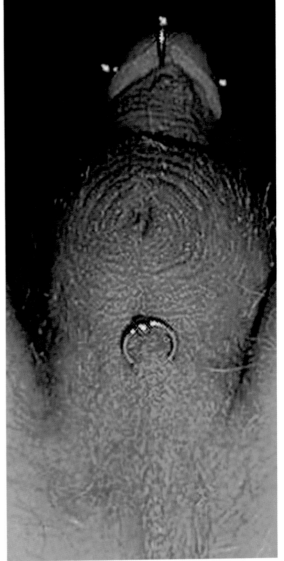

Figure 23.15. *Guiche.*

the midline, or through the anus as an Anal Ring (Fig. 23.16).

The focus of this chapter is upon *male* genital piercing, and the authors will therefore only briefly outline genital piercings that are available to women. Possible legalities to consider with female genital piercing include breaching the terms of the Prohibition of Female Circumcision Act 1985 (UK), and the World Health Organization's definition of type IV female genital mutilation (FGM). Piercings of the labia (majora and minora) and clitoral hood are the most commonly performed female

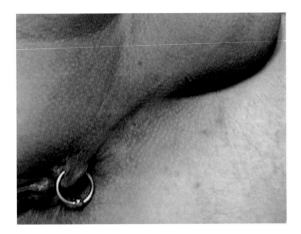

Figure 23.16. *Anal ring.*

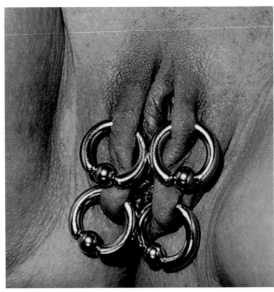

Figure 23.17. *Outer labial piercings.*

genital piercings (Fig. 23.17). Less commonly, one might encounter piercings of the clitoral body, and The Christina, which is a vertical piercing through the clitoral body which exits suprapubically (Fig. 23.18).

The Princess Albertina and labial chastity rings (Fig. 23.19) are the female equivalents of the Prince Albert and foreskin chastity rings, respectively.

Complications

There are no current official figures on complication rates for body piercings that would stand thorough scrutiny. Precautionary measures over the possibility of hepatitis B and C and HIV transmission from body piercing are to be welcomed. However, many of the patients who have possibly contracted these infections from body piercing have more than one risk factor for these conditions, and it is therefore difficult to fully implicate piercing as the cause of transmission.

As with most surgical procedures, the possibility of bleeding and infection must be considered. Localized cellulitis should be treated with wound hygiene, and possibly antibiotic cream or oral antibiotics. Removing a piercing from an early cellulitis is to be discouraged, as it may promote abscess formation.

Bivalving of the urethra from a Prince Albert piercing 'cutting-out' has been described, and termed 'Prince Albert's revenge'. The authors of

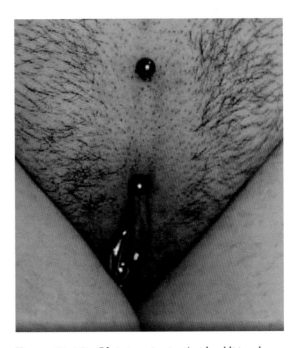

Figure 23.18. *Christina piercing (with additional labial piercing).*

295

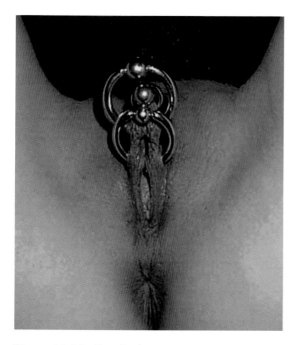

Figure 23.19. *Female chastity rings.*

this review have recently encountered a young man who became bored with his Prince Albert, which he decided to remove. Unfortunately, this left a permanent urethral fistula that required a two-stage repair.

Other possible complications include priapism, paraphimosis and recurrent condylomata. Many complications may be underreported, but consideration should be given to the possibilities of allergic reactions and difficulty with hygiene, although it

has been argued that pierced individuals have cleaner genitals than those who prefer 'the natural look', due to increased care and attention, keloid and hypertrophic scarring and urethral stricture. In addition, a review of some of the 'piercing websites' reveals anecdotal complications to the *partner* of the pierced individual, including trapping of piercings between the partner's teeth, teeth-chipping, choking on swallowed piercings and trauma to the vagina or anus.

Conclusions

Amongst members of the public, there seems to be a general acceptance towards piercings of the ears and nose. This hospitality does not appear to extend to our humble but well-meaning genitals. Sometimes 'art' is creative to one person, but vulgar to the next. This body art appears to be a case in point. The law regarding body piercing is currently lacking and recently proposed legislation in this area is well overdue.

Acknowledgements

The authors sincerely thank Shannon Larratt at www.bmezine.com. for their permission in providing pictures for this chapter.

Further reading

WR Anderson, DJ Summerton, DM Sharma, SA Holmes. The urologist's guide to genital piercing. BJU Int 2003; 91: 245–51.

Men and chronic conditions

CHAPTER 24

Osteoporosis in men

Lionel S Lim

Introduction

Osteoporosis is a condition characterized by a reduction in bone mineralization and bone mass, leading to skeletal fragility and an increased predisposition to fractures. Osteoporosis has traditionally been considered a disease of women, owing to the higher prevalence of osteoporosis in women. However, 20% of osteoporosis cases are in men,[1] and, as the proportion of older people in the population increases, there will be a concurrent increase in the number of men with osteoporosis and related fractures.

This chapter addresses the epidemiology and etiology of osteoporosis in men, including secondary causes of osteoporosis. Osteoporosis evaluation, including laboratory work-up and bone mineral density (BMD) testing are discussed, followed by non-pharmacologic and pharmacologic treatment options.

Definition of osteoporosis

The World Health Organization has defined osteoporosis as a BMD measurement that is 2.5 standard deviations (SD) below the young adult mean.[2] This is referred to as the T-score. When this criterion was established, it was based on studies performed in postmenopausal women. However, the same cut-off is now being applied for diagnosing osteoporosis in men over 50 years of age. In men younger than

50 years of age, using the z-score is recommended instead. The z-score gives the standard deviation of the measured bone density relative to the normal population of the same age range; Z-scores less than −2.0 are below the expected range. The Clinical Society for Clinical Densitometry and Osteoporosis Canada have recommended a unique set of criteria for diagnosing osteoporosis and reduced bone density in men (Table 24.1).[3]

Epidemiology of osteoporosis and osteoporotic fractures

Data collected from NHANES III in the USA suggest that between 1 and 2 million men aged 50 and above have osteoporosis.[4] This number is expected to increase to almost 3 million in 2010. The number of men aged 50 and over with reduced bone density or osteopenia, defined as a BMD between 1.0 and 2.5 SD below the mean for young adult males, is between 8 and 13 million, or 28–47% of that population. The prevalence of osteoporosis and osteopenia is higher in white men than in black or Hispanic men (Fig. 24.1).

It is estimated that one in four men over the age of 50 will have an osteoporosis-related fracture during his lifetime.[1] Osteoporosis causes 1.5 million fractures annually, including 300 000 hip fractures and 700 000 vertebral fractures. Approximately 30% of hip fractures and 20% of vertebral fractures occur in men. Although vertebral fractures tend to occur earlier on in life, hip fracture incidence accelerates after age 70, and overtakes vertebral fracture incidence in men in their mid 70s (Fig. 24.2). Some notable sex differences in fracture incidence include fracture onset later on in life, and fewer distal forearm (Colles') fractures in men than in women. Healthcare expenditure for osteoporotic fractures in men was US$2.7 billion in 1995.[5] In 2002, the total expenditure for all osteoporotic fractures (in both men and women) was US$18 billion,

and this number is expected to increase.[1] Compared with women, men with vertebral or hip fractures have a higher mortality.[6,7] Compared with 17% in women, 31% of men with a hip fracture do not survive more than 1 year.[8] Furthermore, men who sustain vertebral or hip fracture have an increased risk of developing additional fractures.[9,10] Despite the morbidity and mortality associated with osteoporotic fractures, osteoporosis remains underdiagnosed and inadequately treated in men.

Table 24.1. *Interpretation of bone mineral density in men*	
Age group and score	**Diagnostic classification**
Men ≥50 years T-score	
≤−2.5	Osteoporosis
−1.5 to −2.5	Reduced bone density
Men <50 years Z-score	
<−2.0	Below the expected range for age
≥−2.0	Within the expected range for age

Etiology of osteporosis

Age-related bone loss is influenced by peak bone mass, bone geometry, hormonal influences, calcium and vitamin D sufficiency, and physical activity level.

Determinants of peak bone mass
Peak bone mass is determined by endogenous factors (race, genetics, and hormonal influences) and exogenous factors (e.g. lifestyle).[11] There are notable racial differences in bone mass in men. For example, African–Americans have a higher BMD and fewer fractures than Caucasians.

Genetic predisposition plays a significant role in peak bone mass and fracture risk. Genetic factors

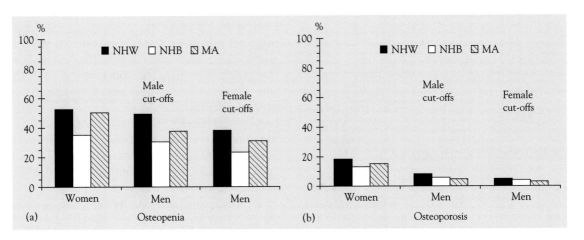

Figure 24.1. *Age-adjusted prevalence of low femur neck bone mineral density (osteopenia, graph a or osteoporosis, graph b) by race or ethnicity, ages ≥50 years.[4] Data are graphed to indicate the percentage of the male population with (a) osteopenia or (b) osteoporosis using a T-score cut-off from male or female databases. NHW, Non-Hispanic white; NHB, Non-Hispanic black; MA, Mexican American.*

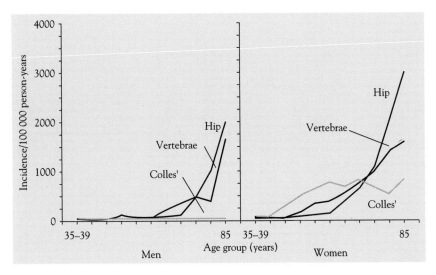

Figure 24.2. *Age-specific incidence rates for hip, vertebral, and distal forearm (Colles') fracture in Rochester, MN, for men and women. From Cooper C and Melton LJ III. Epidemiology of osteoporosis. Trends Endocrinol Metab 1992; 3: 224–229.*

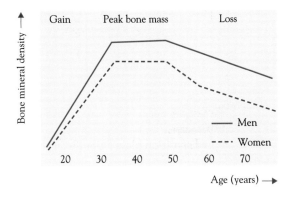

Figure 24.3. *Age-related changes in bone mass in men and women.*

account for about 75% of the variation in peak bone mass in twin and family studies.[12] Several genes associated with BMD have been identified, including the vitamin D receptor, estrogen receptor, collagen type-α1, insulin-like growth factor (ILF)-1 and the aromatase genes.[11–14] Polymorphisms of these and other genes lead to variations in BMD and determine the rate of bone loss in men.[13]

Hormonal changes during adolescent sexual development influence peak bone mass in both men and women. Peak bone mass is generally achieved by the third decade (Fig. 24.3). Women tend to achieve peak bone mass at an earlier age than men, owing to the earlier onset of puberty. However, men have a higher peak bone mass than

women, owing to their body size. The age of puberty in men plays a role in determining peak bone mass. Males with a constitutional delay in puberty have a lower BMD than those with normal pubertal development. Exogenous influences such as dietary calcium intake and physical activity are also positively correlated with BMD.[15–17]

Sex differences in bone geometry

There are several sex-related differences in bone structure that have an impact on fracture rates. Fracture is less common in men than in women and part of the reason is that the accumulation of skeletal mass during growth, particularly in puberty, is greater in men. Sex-related changes in bone geometry also account for differences in fracture rates among men and women. Compared with females, males have a greater resistance to fracture, owing to greater cortical thickness and bone diameter. A larger cross-sectional area in the male vertebra confers a greater mechanical advantage than in women. Continuous periosteal growth observed in aging male vertebrae but not in aging female vertebrae may also blunt the inevitable bone loss associated with aging.[18] With aging, the girth of the femur and other long bones increases in men at a greater rate than in women. All of these differences in skeletal geometry result in a greater biomechanical advantage and lower fracture rates in men.

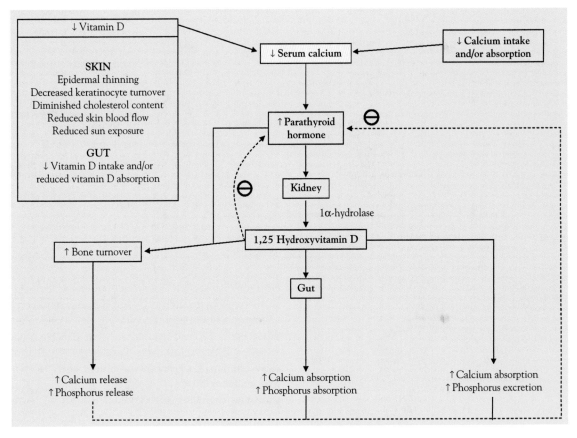

Figure 24.4. *Schematic representation of mineral metabolism in the elderly.*

Hormonal influences on bone loss

Bone loss in the elderly is the net result of increased bone turnover and decreased bone formation. Explanations for this include increased parathyroid hormone (PTH) levels, declining renal function, calcium and vitamin D deficiency, decreased physical activity, and decline in sex hormone, growth hormone (GH), and IGF-1 levels.

Although currently still in debate, several studies have shown that serum concentration of parathyroid hormone (PTH) increases with age. This mechanism is not entirely understood. It has been postulated that episodic decreases in serum calcium levels from inadequate calcium intake, poor intestinal calcium absorption, and impaired renal calcium conservation increases PTH secretion in the elderly (Fig. 24.4).[19] Renal insufficiency leads to decreased

1,25-hydroxyvitamin D production, which contributes to secondary hyperparathyroidism by reduced inhibitory feedback on the parathyroid gland. Vitamin D deficiency also results from reduced cutaneous synthesis and decreased oral intake and intestinal absorption.[20] Cutaneous production of vitamin D declines with increasing age as a result of changes in the epidermis and reduced sun exposure.[19] The resulting increase in PTH activity leads to greater bone resorption and net bone loss. Decreased physical activity and immobility also contribute to bone loss.[21]

Testosterone deficiency negatively affects bone and calcium homeostasis. Apart from maintaining bone formation, testosterone also acts as the substrate for aromatization to estrogen in the testis, peripheral tissue, and bone. The age-related decline

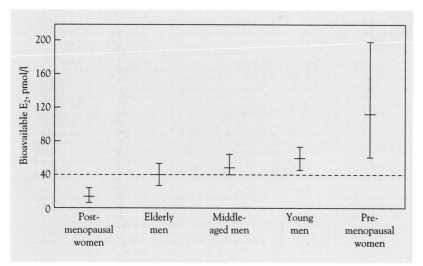

Figure 24.5. *Medians and interquartile ranges of bioavailable estradiol levels in three age groups of men and women. Reproduced with permission from Khosla et al. The Endocrine Society. Jelin Endocrinol Metab 2007; 86: 3555–61.*

in free testosterone levels may also have a negative effect on vitamin D metabolism.[22] In normal aging, men experience a decline in serum total testosterone by 25%, owing to reduced gonadal synthesis and an increase in sex hormone binding globulin.[23] As a result of the latter, the bioavailable fractions of testosterone and estrogen also decline by approximately 70% and 50%, respectively.[24] Even though skeletal development in men is influenced by the actions of both testosterone and estradiol, recent studies have demonstrated a stronger relationship between bone density and serum estradiol than serum testosterone. In elderly men, estrogen and testosterone account for approximately 70% and 30% of the total effect of sex steroids on bone resorption, respectively.[25]

Aging men do not experience the equivalent of the female menopause leading to an accelerated phase of bone loss (see Fig. 24.5). Nonetheless, the age-related decrease in estrogen levels in both sexes results in a bone remodeling imbalance in which bone resorption outpaces bone formation, resulting in net bone loss. This starts to occur around middle age. Aging men experience a greater increase in bone loss when the level of bioavailable estradiol falls below 40 pmol/L, a level found in most postmenopausal women.[26] Subsets of middle-aged men and up to 50% of elderly men have estradiol levels below this threshold (Fig. 24.5).

Serum concentrations of GH and IGF-1, hormones that are essential for the acquisition and maintenance of bone mass, decrease with advancing age. GH stimulates the production of IGF-1 in the skeleton, and the latter is often used as a marker of GH status. Apart from promoting chondrocyte and osteoblast differentiation and growth, IGF-1 also stimulates renal 1α-hydroxylase activity to produce 1,25 hydroxyvitamin D.

Secondary causes of osteoporosis in men

The three major causes of secondary osteoporosis in men are long-term glucocorticosteroid use, hypogonadism, and chronic alcohol use. These causes account for 40–50% of all cases of osteoporosis in men.[27] Other causes of secondary osteoporosis are listed in Table 24.2.

Glucocorticosteroid excess is a frequent cause of bone loss in men and accounts for 20% of all cases.[28] Glucocorticosteroid excess includes both endogenous and exogenous causes, such as Cushing's disease and glucocorticosteroid therapy, respectively. There are several mechanisms by which glucocorticosteroids cause bone loss. They directly influence the pituitary, gonads, and adrenal glands to suppress

Table 24.2. *Causes of secondary osteoporosis in men*

Medical conditions

Chronic inflammatory diseases
(e.g. rheumatoid arthritis)

Chronic liver disease

Chronic obstructive pulmonary disease

Chronic renal failure

Endocrinopathies

  Diabetes mellitus (type 1 or 2)

  Hypercortisolism (Cushing's syndrome)

  Hyperparathyroidism

  Hyperthyroidism

  Hypogonadism*

Gastrointestinal malabsorption

  Celiac disease

  Gastrectomy

  Inflammatory bowel disease

  Jejunoileal bypass

  Pancreatic insufficiency

  Primary biliary cirrhosis

Genetic (osteogenesis imperfecta,
homocystinuria)

Idiopathic hypercalciuria

Inadequate vitamin D levels

Malignancy (multiple myeloma, lymphoma)

Neuromuscular disorders (stroke, Parkinson's
disease)

Organ transplantation

Systemic mastocytosis

Drugs and exogenous substances

Long-term systemic corticosteroid use*†

High alcohol intake*

Cigarette smoking

Androgen deprivation therapy
(gonadotropin-releasing hormone agonists)

(Continued)

Table 24.2. *(Continued)*

Acid suppression therapy

  Aluminum-containing antacids

  Proton pump inhibitors

Anticoagulation

Anticonvulsants

Immunosuppressants

Loop diuretics

Psychotropic drugs

  Traditional neuroleptics

  Serotonin reuptake inhibitors

Thyroid hormone replacement

Vitamin A excess

*Mayor cause of secondary osteoporosis in men
†Equivalent to greater than 7.5 mg prednisone daily
for at least 3 months.

gonadal hormone production. They also decrease bone formation by inhibiting osteoblast recruitment and reducing collagen synthesis. Glucocorticosteroids reduce calcium absorption in the renal tubules and impair intestinal calcium absorption.

The Rancho Bernado study highlighted the prevalence of hypogonadism in older men by estimating that 70% of men in their 70s have low free testosterone levels.[29] The prevalence of hypogonadism in osteoporotic men is 30%.[30] In addition, up to 20% of men with symptomatic vertebral fractures and 50% of elderly men with hip fractures have hypogonadism.[23] Causes of hypogonadism include orchiectomy, hyperprolactinemia, hypogonadotrophic hypogonadism, pituitary tumors, and medications. Traditional neuroleptics may induce hyperprolactinemia, which can result in secondary hypogonadism. Over 40% of patients taking antipsychotics that raise prolactin levels have osteopenia associated with hypogonadism.[31] The use of gonadotropin analogs in the treatment of prostate cancer can also induce hypogonadism.

Alcohol abuse is associated with osteoporosis and increased fracture risk. Axial BMD decreases proportionally to the duration of alcohol consumption.[32] Alcohol directly suppresses osteoblast activity, and chronic alcoholism can cause testicular atrophy and hypogonadism. Poor nutrition resulting from alcoholism and reduced hepatic vitamin D production results in calcium and vitamin D deficiency. Furthermore, alcohol intoxication increases the risk of falls and fractures. Although moderate alcohol intake does not appear to be detrimental to bone,[33] the threshold level of alcohol intake associated with bone loss is unclear.

Drug-induced osteoporosis

Anticonvulsants, such as phenytoin, phenobarbital, sodium valproate, and carbamazepine, lower BMD by altering vitamin D metabolism, intestinal calcium absorption, or collagen synthesis in bone. The effect of anticonvulsants on BMD is dependent on the number of medications used, daily dose, and duration of use.[34] There is evidence to suggest that chronic use of oral anticoagulants may have a detrimental effect on BMD and leads to a higher risk of fracture.[35,36] Non-steroid immuno-suppressants, including cyclosporine, tacrolimus, and methotrexate, are also detrimental to bone metabolism, and are associated with increased bone loss.[37-41] Excessive thyroid hormone replacement not only decreases BMD, but chronic use may be a predictor of fracture occurrence in males.[42] Aluminum-containing antacids can also cause bone loss by altering bone remodeling through intestinal calcium loss and inhibition of calcium absorption.[43] Long-term use of proton-pump inhibitors, and to a lesser extent histamine-2-receptor blockers, has been associated with an increased risk of hip fractures.[44]

Psychotropic medications, especially the traditional neuroleptics, may cause hyperprolactinemia-induced hypogonadism and osteoporosis.[45-47] Selective serotonin reuptake inhibitors (SSRIs) have also been associated with reduced bone density, plausibly because of the disruption of serotonin transporters in osteoblasts, osteoclasts, and osteocytes.[48,49] In addition, SSRIs and tricyclic antidepressants have the potential to increase the risk of falls and fractures in older people.[50,51] Loop diuretic use in men has also recently been associated with hip bone loss.[52]

Evaluation of men with osteoporosis

It is essential to rule out pathologic fractures and secondary causes of osteoporosis in men who present with fragility fractures. Men who present with height loss, back pain, or kyphosis should undergo spine radiography to exclude vertebral fractures. The prevalence of secondary causes of osteoporosis is high in male osteoporotics, with one study showing a prevalence as high as 64%.[53] Appropriate investigations for secondary causes of osteoporosis are listed in Table 24.3. Vitamin D insufficiency is an important cause of osteoporosis. It has been estimated that the wintertime prevalence of vitamin D insufficiency in the USA is 44%, 30%, and 17% among African American, Hispanic, and white men, respectively.[54] Vitamin D insufficiency should be considered in all men with osteopenia or osteoporosis

Table 24.3. *Laboratory work-up for secondary osteoporosis in men*

Recommended

Basic chemistry profile (serum electrolytes, creatinine, glucose)

Complete blood count

Erythrocyte sedimentation rate

Liver function tests

Sensitive thyroid stimulating hormone level

Serum calcium, phosphorus, and alkaline phosphatase

Serum 25-hydroxyvitamin D (1,25-hydroxyvitamin D if renal impairment is present)

Serum testosterone, total and free

Urine calcium and creatinine excretion (24-hour or spot urine calcium–creatinine ratio*)

Additional (if indicated)

Parathyroid hormone level

Serum and urine protein electrophoresis

24-hour urine free cortisol

*Spot urine calcium–creatinine ratio ≥0.30 diagnostic for hypercalciuria.

and should be measured by serum 25-hydroxyvitamin D assay. A level of less than 30 mg/mL is considered suboptimal, while a level of less than 20 ng/mL is considered deficient.[55]

Dual-energy X-ray absorptiometry (DXA) is the most universally used method of measuring BMD. Obtaining a DXA scan of the hip is preferred over one of the spine, especially in older people, owing to false elevations from vertebral osteoarthritic changes and aortic calcifications. BMD measurements can help to identify candidates for intervention. A general rule of thumb is that every decrease of 1 SD in T-score increases the fracture risk by 1.5–2.0-fold. BMD testing should be obtained in older men with risk factors for osteoporosis,

Table 24.4. *International Society for Clinical Densitometry indications for measurement of bone mineral density in men*

Age 70 and older

Adults with fragility fracture

Adults with a disease or condition associated with low bone mass or bone loss

Adults taking medications associated with low bone mass or bone loss

Anyone being considered for pharmacologic therapy

Anyone being treated, to monitor treatment effect

Anyone not receiving treatment in whom evidence of bone loss would lead to treatment

including low body mass index (<20 kg/m²), presence of vertebral deformities, low trauma fracture, radiographic evidence of osteopenia, and other conditions associated with osteoporosis (Table 24.4).[56] Monitoring of BMD may be performed every 1 or 2 years to assess response to osteoporosis therapy or in high-risk untreated people. Universal densitometry screening of men aged 80 years and older, or men aged 65 years and older with a prior fracture, followed by bisphosphonate treatment may even be cost-effective.[57] It is anticipated that the introduction of generic alendronate may enable cost-effective screening to occur in men as young as 70 years of age. Recently updated guidelines from the National Osteoporosis Foundation (NOF) and the American College of Physicians recommend osteoporosis screening in men aged 70 years and older.[58,59]

However, there are limitations to using BMD solely to predict fracture risk. For instance, men with reduced bone density may not necessarily be at risk of fracture, and other risk factors need to be considered as well. To overcome some of the limitations of relying on BMD alone, Osteoporosis Canada has recommended that absolute fracture risk be quantified by using additional risk factors of age, prior fracture, and glucocorticoid use.[3] By using BMD and age, a patient is stratified into three 10-year absolute fracture risk categories of low ($<10\%$), moderate (10–20%), and high ($>20\%$) (Fig. 24.6). The presence of a prior fragility fracture or glucocorticoid use increases the fracture risk into the next risk category. For example, a 60-year-old man with a T-score of -3.0 would be considered at moderately high risk of osteoporotic fracture.

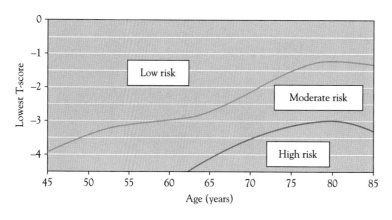

Figure 24.6. *Ten-year absolute risk of fracture for low-, moderate-, and high-risk groups.*

The additional presence of a previous fragility fracture or glucocorticoid use would push this man into the high-risk category. The NOF also proposes the calculation of the 10-year absolute risk of hip or major osteoporotic fracture (clinical spine, wrist, hip or shoulder fracture) based using the WHO FRAX tool.[60]

Biochemical markers of bone turnover can be measured in the serum and urine. These include bone formation markers such as serum osteocalcin and bone-specific alkaline phosphatase, as well as bone resorption markers, including collagen degradation products, that can be measured in the urine (e.g., Type 1 collagen N-telopeptide and Type 1 collagen C-telopeptide). They can be useful in assessing response to osteoporosis treatment, but because of individual biologic variability, they are not currently recommended for diagnosing osteoporosis.

Treatment of osteoporosis in men

Non-pharmacologic management

Addressing the risk factors of low bone mass and falls is key to osteoporotic fracture prevention. Lifestyle modifications should be implemented once osteoporosis has been identified. These include smoking cessation, reduction of alcohol consumption, and regular weight-bearing exercise. Exercise has been shown to increase BMD at the femur, lumbar, and os calcis, particularly in older men.[61] Regular physical activity may even protect against hip fracture in men.[62,63] Other benefits of exercise include improved muscle strength and balance.

Fall intervention strategies should be implemented for those at risk or with a prior history of falls. People with gait instability should be assessed for appropriate gait aids. A program of balance and muscle-strengthening exercises can also reduce falls in the elderly.[64] Household hazards such as throw rugs and loose wires should be removed. Safety equipment like hand rails on stairs and grab bars in bathrooms should be installed. Adequate lighting in the home and the use of night-lights should be encouraged. Hip protectors should be considered for those at risk for osteoporotic fractures. However, the hip fracture reduction efficacy of this intervention is questionable in community-dwelling older adults, and adherence may be an issue.[65]

Pharmacologic management

Pharmacologic intervention is recommended in men who have osteoporosis or who are at increased risk of fragility fracture. The first objective of pharmacological management of osteoporosis is medication review. Medications that worsen osteoporosis should be discontinued if possible. Medications that cause sedation or increase falls should also be reviewed and discontinued, especially psychotrophic medications (e.g. benzodiazepines, sedatives, and tricyclic antidepressants).[66] The second objective is to increase bone strength. This is achieved by calcium and vitamin D supplementation and the use of bisphosphonates and other therapies described below.

Calcium and vitamin D

Calcium and vitamin D supplementation can improve BMD and reduce the risk of fractures in older people and should be given routinely to men with risk factors or established osteoporosis.[67] In addition, vitamin D helps to maintain muscle strength and function, and appropriate supplementation has been shown to decrease the risk of falls.[68] Calcium intake in elderly men should be at least 1200 mg daily. The results of a recent meta-analysis suggest that a minimum intake of 700–800 international units (IU) of vitamin D is superior in reducing hip and non-vertebral fractures compared to 400 IU daily.[69] The National Osteoporosis Foundation increased the recommended daily intake of vitamin D to 800–1000 IU daily in adults aged 50 years and over.[70] People suffering from vitamin D deficiency require appropriate vitamin D repletion therapy with vitamin D_2 (ergocalciferol), 50 000 IU weekly for 8 weeks followed by maintenance therapy with vitamin D_2, 50 000 IU every 2–4 weeks or vitamin D_3 (cholecalciferol), 1000 IU daily.[55] Those with malabsorption syndromes or chronic kidney disease may require higher amounts of vitamin D therapy or active vitamin D analogs. Oral supplementation with 100 000 IU of cholecalciferol every 4 months has been shown to reduce the risk of wrist, hip, or vertebral fracture by one-third in older community-dwelling adults.[71]

However, high-dose cholecalciferol is not available in the USA.

Testosterone replacement therapy

In hypogonadal men, replacement of sex steroids can help to prevent further bone loss. However, testosterone replacement has not been proven to reduce fractures.[72] Men with a total testosterone level of less than 200 ng/dL and who have symptomatic hypogonadism (lethargy, fatigue, decreased libido and mood, reduced muscle and bone mass, increased visceral fat, impotence, and mild cognitive impairment) are potential candidates for testosterone replacement therapy.[73] However, testosterone is not recommended solely for increasing BMD, and the treatment benefit is greater in men who are more severely hypogonadal. Testosterone treatment is contraindicated in men with a history of breast or prostate cancer. Some of the potential adverse effects of testosterone are polycythemia, dyslipidemia, increasing prostate-specific antigen (PSA) level, and the possible risk of unmasking indolent prostate cancers. Testosterone should be initiated only after examination of the prostate and evaluation of serum hematocrit, PSA level, and lipid levels. Further clinical trials are needed before testosterone therapy can be recommended in eugonadal men with low normal serum levels of testosterone for osteoporosis prevention or treatment. Currently, testosterone should only be used for treating clinical hypogonadism with the addition of a bisphosphonate if osteoporosis is present.

Bisphosphonates

Antiresorptives, such as the bisphosphonates, decrease the rate of bone remodeling so that the bone matrix can complete a course of secondary mineralization. Alendronate and risedronate are the only two approved bisphosphonates for treating male osteoporosis in the USA. Alendronate has been shown to increase spine, hip, and total body BMD. In a landmark study there was an absolute increase in the BMD of 1.6 to 5.3% in men who took 10 mg of alendronate daily over a 2-year period. This dose also reduced the risk of vertebral fractures by almost 90%.[28] In an open-label study of men with primary or secondary osteoporosis, daily risedronate

treatment (5 mg) increased BMD at the lumbar spine, femoral neck, and total hip, and decreased new vertebral fractures by 60%.[74] Overall, alendronate and risedronate are well tolerated, although gastrointestinal and musculoskeletal side effects may occur. Both the once-weekly alendronate (70 mg) and risedronate (35 mg) are as effective as daily dosing in maintaining BMD.

Bisphosphonate therapy is indicated in corticosteroid-induced osteoporosis, and should be initiated at the start of long-term corticosteroid therapy. Bisphosphonate therapy should also be considered in men on antiandrogen treatment for prostate cancer or other conditions associated with reduced BMD and osteoporotic fractures. Intravenous pamidronate and zoledronic acid have been shown to prevent bone loss in the hip and lumbar spine in men receiving androgen-blocking therapy for non-metastatic prostate cancer.[75,76] Treatment with risedronate has been shown to increase BMD and reduce hip fractures in elderly men suffering from neurologic conditions such as Parkinson's disease and stroke.[77,78]

Calcitonin

Calcitonin, a weaker antiresorptive agent than the bisphosphonates, has fracture-reduction efficacy in the spine but not the hip. Although controlled trials in men are lacking, calcitonin may be useful when bisphosphonates are contraindicated or not tolerated. Its analgesic properties in osteoporotic vertebral fractures make it a useful treatment adjunct.[79]

Recombinant human parathyroid hormone

Anabolic agents stimulate bone formation and turn on bone remodeling to increase bone mass and strength. Human PTH (hPTH) increases bone formation by increasing osteoblast lifespan via decreased osteoblast apoptosis and stimulation of preosteoblasts to osteoblasts. PTH also stimulates IGF-1 and induces the synthesis of cytokines that target osteoclast recruitment, such as interleukin-6. The combined effect allows for the coupling of bone resorption to formation, in favor of bone formation. Recombinant hPTH(1-34), the first available anabolic osteoporosis medicine, has been shown to increase BMD at the spine and hip and to decrease vertebral and non-vertebral fracture rates in postmenopausal women with previous vertebral fracture.[80] Trials of recombinant hPTH(1-34) in osteoporotic men also showed favorable increases in spine and hip BMD.[81–83] However, anti-fracture efficacy has yet to be proven in men. Another form of hPTH, hPTH(1-84), which is unavailable in the USA, has been shown to have favorable BMD results in post-menopausal women.

Combined antiresorptive and anabolic therapy

Although concomitant antiresorptive and anabolic therapy is generally not recommended,[84] there may be sufficient rationale for sequential anabolic and antiresorptive treatments. An anabolic agent such as PTH will stimulate bone turnover and enhance bone formation over bone resorption. By adding an antiresorptive agent after PTH treatment, overall bone formation is further enhanced, owing to the reduction in bone resorption.[85]

Other therapies

Several other agents are under investigation for treating osteoporosis. The use of GH for treating osteoporosis has provided mixed results and is not recommended. IGF-1 is being explored as an alternative to GH because it has fewer side effects and is a direct stimulus to bone formation.[86] The use of HMG coenzyme A inhibitors has been associated with a modest increase in BMD and reduced fracture risk, making it potentially useful beyond its lipid-reducing properties.[87] However, further controlled studies are needed to confirm the findings from these observational studies.

A potent intravenous bisphosphonate, zoledronic acid, administered once a year showed similar efficacy to that of oral daily bisphosphonates in postmenopausal women in terms of bone turnover and BMD. There was also a 77% and 41% reduction in clinical spine and hip fractures, respectively.[88] In the HORIZON recurrent fracture trial, intravenous zoledronic acid given to older men and women within 3 months of hip fracture surgery reduced new vertebral and non-vertebral fractures as well as mortality.[89] Strontium, which has both anabolic and antiresorptive properties, has modest vertebral and

non-vertebral fracture-reducing efficacy in postmenopausal women.[90] Osteoprotegerin, a decoy receptor for Receptor Activator for Nuclear Factor κ B Ligand (RANKL) that inhibits osteoclast recruitment and differentiation, is currently being studied for use in osteoporotic women. RANKL inhibition with a monoclonal antibody, denosumab, has been shown to increase BMD and decrease bone turnover in postmenopausal women.[91] Clinical trials exploring the use of these novel agents in men are pending. The development of specific androgen receptor modulators, similar to selective estrogen receptor modulators, may be another novel antiresorption therapy in male osteoporosis.[92]

Conclusion

Osteoporosis is a disease that is associated with a significant morbidity and mortality. It remains underdiagnosed and undertreated in men, posing a major public health problem. Men with osteoporosis or existing fractures are at risk for future fractures. Hence, it is paramount that evaluation and appropriate treatment be implemented. A large proportion of men have reversible causes of osteoporosis. The major risk factors for secondary osteoporosis are corticosteroid use, excessive alcohol ingestion, and hypogonadism. The presence of these and other risk factors should prompt BMD testing with DXA. The presence of additional risk factors such as previous fragility fracture and the use of glucocorticoids increase the absolute fracture risk beyond that suggested by DXA. BMD testing should be obtained at baseline and at subsequent regular intervals to monitor osteoporosis progression or treatment response. Treatment of established osteoporosis in men involves non-pharmacologic measures such as lifestyle changes (smoking cessation, reducing alcoholism, exercise) and fall prevention strategies, as well as pharmacologic interventions, including discontinuation (if possible) of osteoporosis- and fall-inducing medications, ensuring adequate calcium and vitamin D intake, and antiresorptive therapies (e.g. bisphosphonates) or anabolic therapies (e.g. hPTH (1-34)) as indicated. Bisphosphonate and hPTH should not be given concurrently, owing to the absence of additive benefit. Testosterone treatment should only be used for clinical hypogonadism and not as sole osteoporosis therapy. Promising new therapies that are under evaluation may rapidly reverse bone loss.

References

1. Anonymous. Osteoporosis disease facts. Vol. 2007: National Osteoporosis Foundation; 2007.
2. Anonymous. (World Health Organization). Assessment of fracture risk and its application to screening for postmenopausal osteoporosis. Technical report series. Geneva; 1994.
3. Khan AA, Hodsman AB, Papaioannou A et al. Management of osteoporosis in men: an update and case example. Can Med Assoc J 2007; 176: 345–8.
4. Looker AC, Orwoll ES, Johnston CC Jr et al. Prevalence of low femoral bone density in older U.S. adults from NHANES III. J Bone Min Res 1997; 12: 1761–8.
5. Ray NF, Chan JK, Thamer M, Melton 3rd LJ. Medical expenditures for the treatment of osteoporotic fractures in the United States in 1995: report from the National Osteoporosis Foundation. J Bone Min Res 1997; 12: 24–35.
6. Center JR, Nguyen TV, Schneider D, Sambrook PN, Eisman JA. Mortality after all major types of osteoporotic fracture in men and women: an observational study. Lancet 1999; 353: 878–82.
7. Cooper C, Atkinson EJ, Jacobsen SJ, O'Fallon WM, Melton 3rd LJ. Population-based study of survival after osteoporotic fractures. Am J Epidemiol 1993; 137: 1001–5.
8. Forsen L, Sogaard AJ, Meyer HE, Edna T, Kopjar B. Survival after hip fracture: short- and long-term excess mortality according to age and gender. Osteoporos Int 1999; 10: 73–8.
9. Colon-Emeric CS, Sloane R, Hawkes WG et al. The risk of subsequent fractures in community-dwelling men and male veterans with hip fracture. A J Med 2000; 109: 324–6.
10. Melton 3rd LJ, Atkinson EJ, Cooper C, O'Fallon WM, Riggs BL. Vertebral fractures predict subsequent fractures. Osteoporos Int 1999; 10: 214–21.
11. Gilsanz V. Accumulation of bone mass during childhood and adolescence. In: Orwoll ES, ed. Osteoporosis in Men. 1st ed. San Diego: Academic Press: 1999; 65–86.
12. Boyden LM, Mao J, Belsky J et al. High bone density due to a mutation in LDL-receptor-related protein 5. N Engl J Med 2002; 346: 1513–21.
13. Gennari L, Brandi ML. Genetics of male osteoporosis. Calcif Tissue Int 2001; 69: 200–4.
14. Stewart TL, Ralston SH. Role of genetic factors in the pathogenesis of osteoporosis. J Endocrinol 2000; 166: 235–45.
15. Rubin LA, Hawker GA, Peltekova VD et al. Determinants of peak bone mass: clinical and genetic analyses in a young female Canadian cohort. J Bone Min Res 1999; 14: 633–43.
16. Salamone LM, Glynn NW, Black DM et al. Determinants of premenopausal bone mineral density: the interplay of genetic and lifestyle factors. J Bone Min Res 1996; 11: 1557–65.
17. Pollitzer WS, Anderson JJ. Ethnic and genetic differences in bone mass: a review with a hereditary vs environmental perspective. Am J Clin Nutr 1989; 50: 1244–59.
18. Mosekilde L, Mosekilde L. Sex differences in age-related changes in vertebral body size, density and biomechanical competence in normal individuals. Bone 1990; 11: 67–73.
19. Halloran BP, Bikle DD. Age-related changes in mineral metabolism. In: Orwoll ES ed. Osteoporosis in Men. 1st ed. San Diego: Academic Press 1999; 179–96.
20. Sahota O, Hosking DJ. The contribution of nutritional factors to osteopenia in the elderly. Curr Opin Clin Nutr Metab Care 2001; 4: 15–20.
21. Krolner B, Toft B. Vertebral bone loss: an unheeded side effect of therapeutic bed rest. Clin Sci (Lond) 1983; 64: 537–40.
22. Hagenfeldt Y, Linde K, Sjoberg HE, Zumkeller W, Arver S. Testosterone increases serum 1,25-dihydroxyvitamin D and insulin–like growth factor-I in hypogonadal men. Int J Androl 1992; 15: 93–102.
23. Francis RM. Androgen replacement in aging men. Calcif Tissue Int 2001; 69: 235–8.
24. Riggs BL, Khosla S, Melton 3rd LJ. Primary osteoporosis in men: role of sex steroid deficiency. Mayo Clin Proc 2000; 75: S46–50.
25. Falahati-Nini A, Riggs BL, Atkinson EJ et al. Relative contributions of testosterone and estrogen in regulating bone resorption and formation in normal elderly men. J Clin Invest 2000; 106: 1553–60.
26. Khosla S, Melton 3rd LJ, Riggs BL. Clinical review 144: Estrogen and the male skeleton. J Clin Endocrinol Metab 2002; 87: 1443–50.
27. Bilezikian JP. Osteoporosis in men. J Clin Endocrinol Metab. 1999; 84: 3431–4.
28. Orwoll E, Ettinger M, Weiss S et al. Alendronate for the treatment of osteoporosis in men. N Engl J Med 2000; 343: 604–10.

29. Greendale GA, Edelstein S, Barrett-Connor E. Endogenous sex steroids and bone mineral density in older women and men: the Rancho Bernardo study. J Bone Min Res 1997; 12: 1833–43.

30. Grossman JM, MacLean CH. Quality indicators for the management of osteoporosis in vulnerable elders. Ann Intern Med 2001; 135: 722–30.

31. Howes O, Smith S, Winning S. Hyperprolactinaemia caused by antipsychotic drugs. BMJ 2002; 324: 1278.

32. Laitinen K, Tahtela R, Valimaki M. The dose-dependency of alcohol-induced hypoparathyroidism, hypercalciuria, and hypermagnesuria. Bone Min 1992; 19: 75–83.

33. Rico H. Alcohol and bone disease. Alcohol Alcohol 1990; 25: 345–52.

34. Wolinsky-Friedland M. Drug-induced metabolic bone disease. Endocrinol Metab Clin North Am 1995; 24: 395–420.

35. Caraballo PJ, Gabriel SE, Castro MR, Atkinson EJ, Melton 3rd LJ. Changes in bone density after exposure to oral anticoagulants: a meta-analysis. Osteoporos Int 1999; 9: 441–8.

36. Caraballo PJ, Heit JA, Atkinson EJ et al. Long-term use of oral anticoagulants and the risk of fracture. Arch Intern Med 1999; 159: 1750–6.

37. Epstein S, Shane E, Bilezikian JP. Organ transplantation and osteoporosis. Curr Opin Rheumatol 1995; 7: 255–61.

38. Cheung AM. Post-liver transplantation osteoporosis. J Hepatol 2001; 34: 337–8.

39. Sambrook P. Alfacalcidol and calcitriol in the prevention of bone loss after organ transplantation. Calcif Tissue Int 1999; 65: 341–3.

40. Rodino MA, Shane E. Osteoporosis after organ transplantation. Am J Med 1998; 104: 459–69.

41. Mazanec DJ, Grisanti JM. Drug-induced osteoporosis. Cleve Clin J Med 1989; 56: 297–303.

42. Sheppard MC, Holder R, Franklyn JA. Levothyroxine treatment and occurrence of fracture of the hip. Arch Intern Med 2002; 162: 338–43.

43. Spencer H, Kramer L. Osteoporosis: calcium, fluoride, and aluminum interactions. Am Coll Nutr 1985; 4: 121–8.

44. Yang YX, Lewis JD, Epstein S, Metz DC. Long-term proton pump inhibitor therapy and risk of hip fracture. JAMA 2006; 296: 2947–53.

45. Haddad PM, Wieck A. Antipsychotic-induced hyperprolactinaemia: mechanisms, clinical features and management. Drugs. 2004; 64: 2291–314.

46. Misra M, Papakostas GI, Klibanski A. Effects of psychiatric disorders and psychotropic medications on prolactin and bone metabolism. J Clin Psychiatry 2004; 65: 1607–18; quiz 1590, 1760–1.

47. Meyer JM, Lehman D. Bone mineral density in male schizophrenia patients: a review. Ann Clin Psychiatry 2006; 18: 43–8.

48. Haney EM, Chan BK, Diem SJ et al. Association of low bone mineral density with selective serotonin reuptake inhibitor use by older men. Arch Intern Med 2007; 167: 1246–51.

49. Diem SJ, Blackwell TL, Stone KL et al. Use of antidepressants and rates of hip bone loss in older women: the study of osteoporotic fractures. Arch Intern Med 2007; 167: 1240–5.

50. Liu B, Anderson G, Mittmann N et al. Use of selective serotonin-reuptake inhibitors of tricyclic antidepressants and risk of hip fractures in elderly people. Lancet 1998; 351: 1303–7.

51. Richards JB, Papaioannou A, Adachi JD et al. Effect of selective serotonin reuptake inhibitors on the risk of fracture. Arch Intern Med 2007; 167: 188–94.

52. Lim LS, Fink HA, Kuskowski MA et al. Loop diuretic use and increased rates of hip bone loss in older men: the osteoporotic fractures in men study. Arch Intern Med 2008; 14; 168: 735–40.

53. Kelepouris N, Harper KD, Gannon F, Kaplan FS, Haddad JG. Severe osteoporosis in men. Ann Intern Med 1995; 123: 452–60.

54. Gruntmanis U. Male osteoporosis: deadly, but ignored. Am J Med Sci 2007; 333: 85–92.

55. Holick MF. Vitamin D deficiency. N Engl J Med 2007; 357: 266–81.

56. Indications for bone mineral density testing. Vol. 2007: The International Society for Clinical Densitometry; 2005. [available at http://www.iscd.org/Visitors/positions/OfficialPositionsText.cfm]

57. Schousboe JT, Taylor BC, Fink HA et al. Cost-effectiveness of bone densitometry followed by treatment of osteoporosis in older men. JAMA 2007; 298: 629–37.

58. National Osteoporosis Foundation. Clinician's Guide to Prevention and Treatment of Osteoporosis [Internet] 2008 [cited 2008 September 10]; Available from: http://www.nof.org/professionals/Clinicians_Guide.htm.

59. Qaseem A, Snow V, Shekelle P et al. Screening for osteoporosis in men: a clinical practice guideline from the American College of Physicians. Ann Intern Med 2008; 148: 680–4. Erratum in: Ann Intern Med 2008; 148: 888.

60. World Health Organization Collaborating Centre for Metabolic Bone Diseases. FRAX WHO Fracture

Risk Assessment Tool. [Internet] 2008 [cited 2008 March 23]; Available from: http://www.shef.ac.uk/FRAX/index.htm.

61. Kelley GA, Kelley KS, Tran ZV. Exercise and bone mineral density in men: a meta-analysis. J Appl Physiol 2000; 88: 1730–6.

62. Grisso JA, Kelsey JL, O'Brien LA et al. Risk factors for hip fracture in men. Hip Fracture Study Group. Am J Epidemiol 1997; 145: 786–93.

63. Kujala UM, Kaprio J, Kannus P, Sarna S, Koskenvuo M. Physical activity and osteoporotic hip fracture risk in men. Arch Intern Med 2000; 160: 705–8.

64. Robertson MC, Devlin N, Gardner MM, Campbell AJ. Effectiveness and economic evaluation of a nurse delivered home exercise programme to prevent falls. 1: Randomised controlled trial. BMJ 2001; 322: 697–701.

65. Parker MJ, Gillespie WJ, Gillespie LD. Effectiveness of hip protectors for preventing hip fractures in elderly people: systematic review. BMJ 2006; 332: 571–4.

66. Campbell AJ, Robertson MC, Gardner MM, Norton RN, Buchner DM. Psychotropic medication withdrawal and a home-based exercise program to prevent falls: a randomized, controlled trial. J Am Geriatr Soc 1999; 47: 850–3.

67. Dawson-Hughes B, Harris SS, Krall EA, Dallal GE. Effect of calcium and vitamin D supplementation on bone density in men and women 65 years of age or older. N Engl J Med 1997; 337: 670–6.

68. Bischoff-Ferrari HA, Dawson-Hughes B, Willett WC et al. Effect of Vitamin D on falls: a meta-analysis. JAMA 2004; 291: 1999–2006.

69. Bischoff-Ferrari HA, Willett WC, Wong JB et al. Fracture prevention with vitamin D supplementation: a meta-analysis of randomized controlled trials. JAMA 2005; 293: 2257–64.

70. Anonymous. National Osteoporosis Foundation's Updated Recommendations for Calcium and Vitamin D Intake. National Osteoporosis Foundation; 2007.

71. Trivedi DP, Doll R, Khaw KT. Effect of four monthly oral vitamin D3 (cholecalciferol) supplementation on fractures and mortality in men and women living in the community: randomised double blind controlled trial. BMJ 2003; 326: 469.

72. Kamel HK, Perry 3rd HM, Morley JE. Hormone replacement therapy and fractures in older adults. J Am Geriatr Soc 2001; 49: 179–87.

73. Liu PY, Swerdloff RS, Veldhuis JD. Clinical review 171: The rationale, efficacy and safety of androgen

therapy in older men: future research and current practice recommendations. J Clin Endocrinol Metab 2004; 89: 4789–96.

74. Ringe JD, Faber H, Farahmand P, Dorst A. Efficacy of risedronate in men with primary and secondary osteoporosis: results of a 1-year study. Rheumatol Int 2006; 26: 427–31.

75. Smith MR, McGovern FJ, Zietman AL et al. Pamidronate to prevent bone loss during androgen-deprivation therapy for prostate cancer. N Engl J Med 2001; 345: 948–55.

76. Smith MR, Eastham J, Gleason DM et al. Randomized controlled trial of zoledronic acid to prevent bone loss in men receiving androgen deprivation therapy for nonmetastatic prostate cancer. J Urol 2003; 169: 2008–12.

77. Sato Y, Honda Y, Iwamoto J. Risedronate and ergocalciferol prevent hip fracture in elderly men with Parkinson disease. Neurology 2007; 68: 911–15.

78. Sato Y, Iwamoto J, Kanoko T, Satoh K. Risedronate sodium therapy for prevention of hip fracture in men 65 years or older after stroke. Arch Intern Med 2005; 165: 1743–8.

79. Lyritis GP, Paspati I, Karachalios T et al. Pain relief from nasal salmon calcitonin in osteoporotic vertebral crush fractures. A double blind, placebo-controlled clinical study. Acta Orthop Scand Suppl 1997; 275: 112–14.

80. Cranney A, Papaioannou A, Zytaruk N et al. Parathyroid hormone for the treatment of osteoporosis: a systematic review. Can Med Assoc J 2006; 175: 52–9.

81. Kurland ES, Cosman F, McMahon DJ et al. Parathyroid hormone as a therapy for idiopathic osteoporosis in men: effects on bone mineral density and bone markers. J Clin Endocrinol Metab 2000; 85: 3069–76.

82. Orwoll ES, Scheele WH, Paul S et al. The effect of teriparatide [human parathyroid hormone (1–34)] therapy on bone density in men with osteoporosis. J Bone Min Res 2003; 18: 9–17.

83. Slovik DM, Rosenthal DI, Doppelt SH et al. Restoration of spinal bone in osteoporotic men by treatment with human parathyroid hormone (1-34) and 1,25-dihydroxyvitamin D. J Bone Min Res 1986; 1: 377–81.

84. Finkelstein JS, Hayes A, Hunzelman JL et al. The effects of parathyroid hormone, alendronate, or both in men with osteoporosis. N Engl J Med 2003; 349: 1216–26.

85. Kurland ES, Heller SL, Diamond B et al. The importance of bisphosphonate therapy in maintaining bone mass in men after therapy with

teriparatide [human parathyroid hormone (1-34)]. Osteoporos Int 2004; 15: 992–7.

86. Rosen CJ, Bilezikian JP. Clinical review 123: Anabolic therapy for osteoporosis. J Clin Endocrinol Metab 2001; 86: 957–64.

87. Hatzigeorgiou C, Jackson JL. Hydroxymethyl-glutaryl-coenzyme A reductase inhibitors and osteoporosis: a meta-analysis. Osteoporos Int 2005; 16: 990–8.

88. Black DM, Delmas PD, Eastell R et al. Once-yearly zoledronic acid for treatment of postmenopausal osteoporosis. N Engl J Med 2007; 356: 1809–22.

89. Lyles KW, Colón-Emeric CS, Magaziner JS et al.; HORIZON Recurrent Fracture Trial. Zoledronic acid and clinical fractures and mortality after hip fracture. N Engl J Med 2007; 357: 1799–809.

90. O'Donnell S, Cranney A, Wells GA, Adachi JD, Reginster JY. Strontium ranelate for preventing and treating postmenopausal osteoporosis. Cochrane Database Syst Rev 2006; 3: CD005326.

91. McClung MR, Lewiecki EM, Cohen SB et al. Denosumab in postmenopausal women with low bone mineral density. N Engl J Med 2006; 354: 821–31.

92. Vermeulen A. Androgen replacement therapy in the aging male – a critical evaluation. J Clin Endocrinol Metab 2001; 86: 2380–90.

CHAPTER 25

Overactive bladder in men

Karen E Smith, Karl J Kreder

Introduction

Multiple factors have resulted in an increase in the median age of the world's population. A decrease in fertility rate as well as an increase in the average lifespan, in part due to advances in public health interventions, will result in an increase in both the number and the proportion of older adults in the years to come.[1] The US population is also aging, and by the year 2030 it is estimated that those aged 65 years or older will make up almost 20% of the nation's population. In the year 2000, there were 13.1 million men over the age of 65 and 1.2 million men over the age of 85 in the US. It is estimated that by the year 2050, there will be 29 million men over the age of 65 and 7 million men over the age of 85 in the US (Fig. 25.1).[2] As the population ages, we will witness a concomitant increase in the prevalence of chronic diseases and comorbidities. Urologic problems seen with increased frequency in aging men are benign prostatic hyperplasia (BPH), bladder outlet obstruction (BOO), and overactive bladder (OAB). The focus of this chapter is discussion of the prevalence and impact of OAB in men, potential etiologies of OAB and lower urinary tract symptoms (LUTS) in men, and treatment options for refractory OAB. The evaluation and treatment of BPH is beyond the scope of this chapter.

Background

The definition of OAB was revised by the International Continence Society in 2002; it was redefined as a syndrome characterized by 'urgency, with or without urge incontinence, usually with frequency and nocturia', in the absence of other etiology.[3] Previously, the definition had been based on the existence solely of urge urinary incontinence. The definition was subsequently revised in order to characterize it as a syndrome based on the main symptom of urgency, as it was recognized that approximately two-thirds of patients with OAB do not have urge urinary incontinence.[4]

Based on epidemiologic studies, it is estimated that approximately 34 million people in the US have OAB.[5] The National Overactive Bladder Evaluation (NOBLE) Program was the first epidemiologic study to report the prevalence of OAB in adult men and women across a large sample of the US population using validated symptom-based criteria. According to this study, the overall prevalence of OAB was estimated at 16.5% (Fig. 25.2),[6] and it was found to be more prevalent than either hypertension or heart disease.[7] The prevalence of OAB was also shown to increase with age in both sexes. The more recent European Prospective Investigation into Cancer and Nutrition (EPIC) study

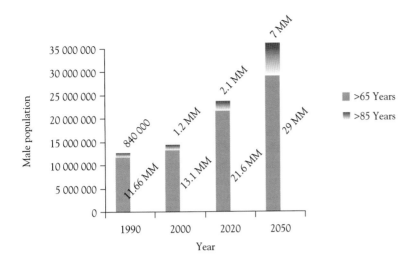

Figure 25.1. *Male population trend in the US. US Census Bureau.*

■ >65 Years
■ >85 Years

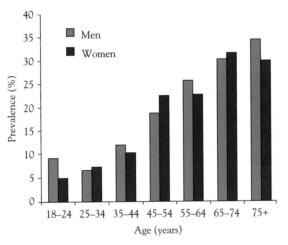

Figure 25.2. *Prevalence of overactive bladder (OAB) in the US. From Stewart et al.[6]*

- Overall, 16.5% had symptoms of OAB

- Prevalence of OAB increased with age

surveyed 19 165 adult men and women in four European countries and Canada, and estimated the prevalence of OAB symptoms at 11.8%, with an increase in prevalence with age as well.[8] OAB appears to affect both men and women to a similar degree, with a prevalence of 16.9% in women and 16.0% in men as reported by the NOBLE study. OAB has been further divided into 'OAB wet', which accounts for approximately one-third of patients, and 'OAB dry', which accounts for the remaining two-thirds.[9] In men, the prevalence of OAB dry was shown to be considerably higher than that of OAB wet (13.4% vs 2.6%), in contrast to women, who displayed an almost equal prevalence.[9]

OAB has been linked to significant economic cost both to society and to the individual. According to the NOBLE study, the overall cost of OAB in the US was estimated to be $12.2 billion in the year 2000, with $9.17 billion spent in the community setting. It was estimated that the cost of OAB for men specifically in the community setting was $1.79 billion in 2000. This included not only direct treatment and care costs, but also indirect costs such as lost productivity, which were estimated at $431.84 million.[5] OAB has significant personal costs as well, as illustrated by quality of life (QOL) data. Depression, low self-esteem, and social avoidance have been directly linked to this condition in both sexes.[9]

315

In short, OAB is a prevalent condition in both men and women, with significant negative economic and personal impact. Despite these statistics, OAB in both sexes remains largely untreated, since it has been shown that many people still do not seek medical attention for this condition. According to the NOBLE study, only 25% of people with OAB visited their physician for this complaint.[9]

Confusing terminologies and potential etiologies

A discussion of OAB would not be complete without addressing the potential role of the prostate in this symptom complex in men. However, first we must attempt to define the often confusing litany of associated terms. One term frequently and often interchangeably used to describe a similar constellation of symptoms is the term 'lower urinary tract symptoms', or LUTS. LUTS includes both voiding or obstructive symptoms, as well as storage or irritative symptoms, the last-named of which may be indistinguishable from OAB symptoms.[10] LUTS is a non-specific, descriptive term, and the symptoms can arise from a myriad of pathologic conditions, such as infection and bladder outlet obstruction caused by prostatic enlargement.

Some authors support the purist view of OAB, maintaining that 'the definition of OAB requires that there is "no proven infection or other pathology"', which implies that if there is an underlying pathologic etiology of these symptoms, the condition is technically not OAB.[11] For example, men with prostatic obstruction and symptoms as described for OAB would therefore not truly have OAB, since 'other pathology' exists.[11] While it may be easy to attribute LUTS in young males with otherwise non-obstructive voiding to OAB, it becomes more challenging to determine the exact cause of these symptoms in men as they age, especially in those patients with documentation of only borderline BOO. In fact, multiple factors may make this determination impossible in some cases. For example, given the fact that the prevalence of both OAB and BOO increase with age independently of each other, the presence of symptoms alone in the absence of documented BOO does not help to determine the exact etiology. Furthermore, even if obstruction is present, the most bothersome symptoms may be ones of storage, and require treatment as if 'pure OAB' in nature. In short, it may be difficult and even impractical in some cases to determine the true etiology of LUTS in men.

In the past, it had been widely held that BPH, BPE (benign prostatic enlargement), BOO, and LUTS were causally related. However, increasing evidence supports the notion that correlation may not necessarily equal causation. One large multinational study demonstrated that 90% of men aged 50–80 years reported bothersome LUTS,[12] illustrating the prevalence of LUTS in this age group. However, another study estimated that only 25–50% of patients with BPH report LUTS, suggesting that not all patients with BPH indeed complain of LUTS.[10] Furthermore, other studies have demonstrated that prostate size is not an important predictor of LUTS,[13] and also that urodynamically proven BOO is found in only 48% of men referred for LUTS.[10] Thus, not all patients with BPH or documented BOO have LUTS, and vice versa. Finally, LUTS in men, which had previously been termed 'prostatism' and attributed to an enlarged prostate, has been shown to occur with the same frequency in age-matched women.[13] Given the facts that the prevalence of these entities increase independently with age and that this symptom complex is just as common in aging females, it is likely that the majority of storage LUTS in males is multifactorial in nature.

In men with both storage LUTS and documented BOO, the presence of detrusor overactivity (DO) is frequently seen on urodynamic studies.[14] Several potential mechanisms have been proposed for the development of DO in both animal and human models of BOO. For example, animal studies have demonstrated reductions in detrusor blood flow in obstructed bladders compared with unobstructed bladders, which has been thought to lead to ultrastructural changes within the bladder and subsequently to DO.[15] Human bladder specimens from patients with DO show 'patchy denervation', suggesting that ischemia and subsequent neuronal death might predispose to overactivity through what is termed 'post-junctional supersensitivity'.[15] Unfortunately, similar detrusor changes can be seen as a result of normal aging, making them potentially indistinguishable from those seen in BOO.[16] Others suggest that DO can result from abnormal sensory stimuli caused by an anatomically altered prostatic urethra, as seen in cases of prostatic enlargement.[15]

In the absence of obstruction, other potential risk factors likely exist for the development of OAB symptoms in men. While these have been extensively studied in women, such studies in men are few. For example, studies in women have demonstrated that OAB has an association with metabolic factors, specifically obesity.[17] In a study of men with BPH by Hammarsten et al., an association between the metabolic syndrome and LUTS caused by BPH was also demonstrated.[18]

In short, the exact etiology of storage LUTS or OAB in men may be difficult to ascertain. It is clear that not all cases are due to BPH or BOO. Further investigation is needed to uncover other potential causes of OAB in males, since this will help to guide potential therapies better.

Management

Pharmacologic treatment

In the past, many practitioners have been reluctant to treat men complaining of LUTS with anticholinergics or antimuscarinics, owing to a fear of precipitating urinary retention, which is certainly a rational concern. Therefore, medical therapy for LUTS has relied on medications aimed at the bladder outlet (i.e. alpha-blockers and 5-alpha-reductase inhibitors), despite the fact that the most bothersome symptoms associated with BOO have been shown to be those of OAB.[19] However, recent studies have shown that treating LUTS in men with antimuscarinics is both safe and efficacious.

A recent study using antimuscarinic monotherapy in men with LUTS demonstrated safety of this therapy. Abrams et al. compared the use of antimuscarinic monotherapy versus placebo in a study of 222 men aged 40 years or older, with urinary frequency, urgency, and DO documented on urodynamics.[20] The study included men with mild to severe outlet obstruction, although it excluded those with a post-void residual volume (PVR) >40% of the maximum cystometric bladder capacity or >200 ml, and those with history of urinary retention within the past 12 months. The men were randomized to treatment with tolterodine 2 mg twice daily or to placebo, and they were followed over a 12-week period. One episode of urinary retention occurred during the study period in the placebo group, and although none occurred in the tolterodine group, two patients in this group were withdrawn because of high PVR. While this therapy was noted to be safe, the authors suggested close monitoring of PVR in certain patients.

Studies done with combination alpha-blocker therapy and antimuscarinics demonstrated both safety and efficacy of antimuscarinic use in men with LUTS and evidence of mild-to-moderate BOO. Athanasopoulos et al. reported a 3-month study of 50 men aged 52–80 years with mild-to-moderate BOO and documented DO on urodynamics, comparing tamsulosin monotherapy 0.4 mg once daily to combination therapy with tamsulosin plus tolterodine 2 mg twice daily.[21] Pre- and post-treatment urodynamics were done on all patients. The study showed no significant difference in maximum flow rate between groups, and there were no episodes of urinary retention in either group. Using changes in the UROLIFE QOL score as the only measure of subjective symptom improvement, the study demonstrated significant improvement from baseline in the combination group but not in the tamsulosin-only group (Fig. 25.3).

Lee et al. reported a non-blinded, non-randomized study of 144 men with BOO, which compared the use of doxazosin monotherapy to combination therapy with doxazosin plus tolterodine. The patients were divided into two groups based on their urodynamic findings, specifically into a group with isolated BOO, and one with evidence of BOO and DO.[22] Men with evidence of severe obstruction on screening were excluded. For those who did not improve on a 3-month course of alpha-blockers alone, tolterodine 2 mg twice daily was added for an additional 2 months. Sixty patients in total went on to combined treatment, owing to unsatisfactory results with alpha-blockade alone. Clinical response was assessed by changes in International Prostate Symptom Score (IPSS). Urinary retention occurred in 2 of 60 men on combination therapy, which resolved with short-term catheterization and cessation of the antimuscarinic. In this study, 79% of

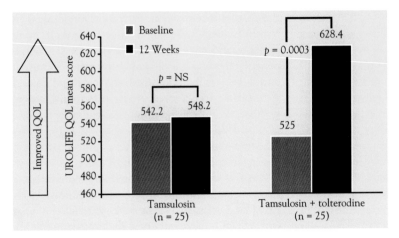

Figure 25.3. *Quality of life (QOL) improvements with tolterodine and tamsulosin combination therapy. From Athanasopoulos et al.[21]*

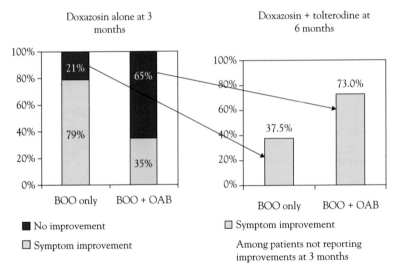

Figure 25.4. *Symptom improvement with doxazosin, with and without tolterodine. BOO, bladder outlet obstruction; OAB, overactive bladder. From Lee et al.[22]*

patients with BOO alone improved clinically with alpha-blockers alone, compared with only 35% of those with BOO and documented DO. In those patients not responding to alpha-blockers alone, the addition of tolterodine was associated with clinical improvement in 38% in the BOO-only group, compared with 73% of patients in the BOO and DO group (Fig. 25.4). The authors therefore suggested that the presence of DO in patients with BOO may predict whether alpha-blockers alone will improve LUTS.

Two other studies that evaluated the use of combination therapy using alpha-blockers and the antimuscarinic propiverine also demonstrated improvements in LUTS, without any episodes of

overt retention. In a study by Lee et al., voiding diary data showed a favorable response to the combination treatment with respect to daytime frequency, total voiding frequency, and mean voided volume.[23] There was also improvement in IPSS storage symptom and urgency scores, as well as global satisfaction scores in the combination group. Okada's group also demonstrated improvement of the storage symptom component of the IPSS, and in maximum flow, voided volume, and QOL scores as well.[24]

A more recent study of antimuscarinic monotherapy, with the longest follow-up to date, was done by Kaplan et al., who studied 43 men aged 50–83 years with LUTS and BPH.[25] Patients in whom alpha-blockade had failed, either because of intolerable side effects or lack of efficacy, were given tolterodine 4 mg extended release (ER) for a total of 6 months. No episodes of urinary retention occurred during this 6-month period. In fact, patients demonstrated an improvement in maximum urinary flow and a decrease in PVR (Fig. 25.5). This study also demonstrated a significant improvement in American Urological Association (AUA) symptom score (–6.1 points), as well as a decrease in daytime and nighttime urinary frequency (Fig. 25.6).

New data support the notion that men with OAB symptoms who do not respond to either alpha-blockers or antimuscarinic monotherapy may respond better to combination therapy. Kaplan

et al. conducted a large-scale randomized, double-blind, placebo-controlled trial of 879 men with both OAB and BPH, who were recruited from 95 urology centers across the US.[26] They were assigned to receive either placebo, tolterodine ER 4 mg, tamsulosin 0.4 mg, or tolterodine ER plus tamsulosin for a total of 12 weeks. IPSS and bladder diaries were used to assess outcome. There were no statistically significant differences among the treatment groups with respect to change in maximum urinary flow rate or PVR. Two patients in the placebo group, 1 patient in the tolterodine ER group, and 1 patient in the combination group withdrew because of urinary retention or decreased urinary flow. A significantly greater proportion of patients in the combination group reported treatment benefit compared to the other three groups, specifically with respect to urgency, urge incontinence, 24-hour frequency, and nocturnal frequency. The treatment benefits seen in the monotherapy groups were also not significantly different from placebo. This study not only further supports the safety of treating men in this group with antimuscarinics, but also suggests that maximum treatment benefit in men with OAB may be obtained with therapy aimed at both the bladder and the bladder outlet.

The resistance to the idea of treating men who have LUTS with anticholinergic medications aimed at relaxing the detrusor muscle is slowly changing, as more data supporting the safety of this approach are reported. It is likely to take time for urologists to overcome concerns about causing urinary retention by using antimuscarinic agents in these patients,

	N	Q_{max} (ml/s)	PVR (ml)
Baseline	43	9.8	97
1 month	43	11.4	79
3 months	39	10.9	72
6 months	39	11.7	75

Figure 25.5. *Tolterodine extended release monotherapy in men with lower urinary tract symptoms in whom alpha-blocker therapy has failed: maximal urinary flow rate (Q_{max}) and post-void residual volume (PVR) at baseline and at 1 month, 3 months, and 6 months. From Kaplan et al.[25]*

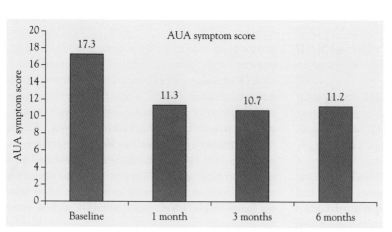

Figure 25.6. *Tolterodine extended release monotherapy in men with lower urinary tract symptoms in whom alpha-blocker therapy has failed: American Urological Association (AUA) symptom score. From Kaplan et al.[25]*

and most authors do agree that close monitoring of high-risk patients is advisable. As this practice becomes more frequent, men with LUTS are likely to be better served, since we will be addressing their more bothersome symptoms more directly.

LUTS and transurethral resection of the prostate: persistence of symptoms after surgical therapy

When medical therapy for BPH fails, surgical therapy such as transurethral resection of the prostate (TURP) is often the next step. However, not all patients experience symptomatic improvement with respect to their LUTS after surgery. In fact, it has been reported that 5–35% of patients may report recurrent or persistent LUTS after TURP.[27] Patients may complain of persistent or *de novo* urgency, frequency, urinary incontinence, or a combination of these symptoms. Persistent or recurrent LUTS after TURP can present a challenging scenario for the urologist. Unfortunately, it is often difficult to predict resolution of symptoms after surgical therapy, and persistent LUTS may be difficult to treat successfully.

There are currently few diagnostic methods that allow us to predict successfully whether LUTS will resolve after TURP. It has been demonstrated that LUTS related to BOO is more likely to resolve after TURP than LUTS without BOO. For example, one study demonstrated that LUTS resolved in 70% of those with BOO compared with 40% of those patients with equivocal obstruction.[28] Therefore, the performance of preoperative urodynamic studies, specifically pressure flow studies, is strongly suggested in those patients with LUTS for whom we are considering invasive treatment. Since not all patients with LUTS have BOO,[29] it is likely that persistent postoperative voiding symptoms may be related to other etiologies, including OAB.

Several series have demonstrated that symptoms alone are an unreliable predictor of the underlying etiology of LUTS after TURP.[27,29] Patients with persistent voiding symptoms are frequently thought to have persistent obstruction, and may even undergo a second surgical procedure to address these symptoms. In fact, true BOO has been demonstrated in only 4–11% of patients with persistent LUTS after TURP.[27] Urodynamic studies are therefore

imperative in patients with persistent bothersome voiding symptoms after TURP in order to guide therapy correctly, especially if another invasive therapy is being considered.

Urinary incontinence is one of the most bothersome outcomes following TURP, and has been noted to occur in 10% of patients.[27] Although stress urinary incontinence resulting from damage to the sphincter can occur, DO has been documented on postoperative urodynamic studies in the majority of patients with post-TURP incontinence.[27] As stated previously, DO is frequently seen on urodynamics in men with both LUTS and BOO,[14] and in one study was documented in 50% of patients undergoing TURP.[30] It is therefore imperative to recognize that the patient with LUTS and DO but without incontinence may in fact develop incontinence after bladder outlet resistance is surgically altered with TURP. This further illustrates the importance of preoperative urodynamics in patients with LUTS, specifically to identify presence of DO. Such information may thereby allow us to better counsel these patients as to the potential risk of postoperative incontinence.

A recent study demonstrated that those patients who have persistent LUTS after TURP may actually have evidence of decreased bladder perfusion, which could potentially result in persistence of these symptoms. Mitterberger et al. studied 50 men with urodynamically confirmed DO and BPH undergoing TURP, of whom 15 (30%) had persistent DO documented on urodynamics postoperatively. Evaluation of the detrusor blood vessels in this latter group demonstrated significantly higher resistive indices, suggesting decreased blood flow and hypoxia or ischemia.[15] This finding supports previous data, suggesting that ischemia may be linked to the development of OAB symptoms or LUTS in general.

In summary, persistent or recurrent LUTS may occur after TURP, a frustrating situation for both patient and physician. There is no absolute way to predict this, and treatment is often difficult with conservative therapy. Studies suggest that ischemia may be related to the persistence of these symptoms after surgery. Finally, we emphasize that it is essential to attempt to define objectively the etiology of LUTS both preoperatively and in those patients with persistent symptoms postoperatively.

We recommend the use of multichannel urodynamic studies, specifically pressure flow studies, since symptoms alone are non-specific.

Other therapies

Botulinum toxin

Other therapies are emerging to address refractory OAB symptoms. For example, botulinum toxin (BTX), a known potent skeletal and smooth muscle neurotoxin, has been used with success in patients with neurogenic detrusor overactivity (NDO), although the benefits of therapy are not durable.[31] The use of BTX has been expanded to include its use with idiopathic OAB patients who are refractory to more conservative treatments. However, at this time, BTX is not approved in the US by the Food and Drug Administration for this indication.

Studies have demonstrated favorable results in both men and women with refractory OAB who had undergone injections of BTX into the detrusor muscle. In a prospective, non-randomized study by Schmid et al., 23 men and 77 women (mean age, 63 years) with non-neurogenic overactive bladder were treated with cystoscopic injections of BTX into the detrusor muscle.[32] Those patients with obstructive voiding, an acontractile bladder or an elevated post-void residual were excluded. The study showed improvement in both subjective symptoms and in urodynamic parameters in 88% of patients after 4 and 12 weeks. Specifically, urgency resolved in 82% and incontinence resolved in 86% within 1–2 weeks after injections; mean urinary frequency decreased by half, and nocturia decreased from an average of 4 micturitions per night to 1.5. Urodynamically, mean maximum cystometric capacity increased 56% (from 246 ml to 381 ml), pretreatment DO resolved in 74% of patients, and mean volume at first desire to void increased (from 126 ml to 212 ml). Temporary urinary retention occurred in 4 patients, and there were no other severe adverse effects. Mean duration of efficacy was approximately 6±2 months, at which point symptoms began to increase.

BTX has also been used in men with BPH and LUTS, with several studies documenting the efficacy of injection directly into the prostate. BTX has been shown to reduce prostatic volume in both animals and humans and to increase urinary flow, presumably through induction of prostate apoptosis.[33–35] In 2003, Maria et al. reported on intraprostatic injection of BTX in 15 men with BPH and voiding dysfunction.[35] Thirteen of the 15 men reported symptomatic improvement, with AUA symptom score improving from 23.2 to 8.0 (65%). The maximal urinary flow rate (Qmax) also increased from 8.1 ml/s to 16.8 ml/s, and prostate volume decreased from 52.6 ml to 16.8 ml. Intraprostatic injection of BTX has also been shown to increase Qmax and to improve LUTS even in cases where prostatic volume does not change, suggesting additional potential mechanisms of action in men with BPH.[36] Chuang et al. studied 41 men with symptomatic BPH to determine the efficacy of intraprostatic BTX injection on LUTS and QOL, and evaluated them at baseline and at 1 month, 3 months, and 6 months postoperatively.[36] No local or systemic side effects were documented. LUTS improved by >30% in 31 of 41 patients, and efficacy and improvements in QOL were sustained at 12 months. Furthermore, 4 of 5 men with retention could void spontaneously after injection. Finally, although 12 of 41 patients did not demonstrate change in prostate volume, 7 of those patients still demonstrated >30% improvement in Qmax, LUTS, and QOL. The authors therefore proposed that improvement in LUTS and Qmax resulting from intraprostatic injection of BTX may be due to factors other than decrease in prostatic volume.

In short, BTX has been demonstrated to be a safe and efficacious alternative treatment for men with refractory OAB symptoms. The effect of intraprostatic injection currently appears to be more durable than injection into the detrusor muscle. Intraprostatic injection has been demonstrated to improve Qmax and improve LUTS, even in the absence of a decrease in prostatic volume. Some propose that this may be due to other factors, such as a decrease in smooth muscle tone at the bladder outlet or inhibitory effects on sensory pathways.[36,37]

Sacral neuromodulation

Another therapy that is gaining more widespread use for voiding dysfunction in both men and women is sacral nerve stimulation, or sacral neuromodulation (SNM). Studies have demonstrated the safety and long-term efficacy of this therapy in both men and women with refractory urgency–frequency syndrome, urge incontinence, and non-obstructive urinary retention.[38] However, there are currently no studies addressing the use of SNM specifically in men with OAB. The majority of patients treated with SNM to date have been women, and most studies report on the combined results of both men and women.

Van Kerrebroek et al. published the most recent large study on SNM, reporting a 5-year, prospective, worldwide multicenter trial that evaluated the long-term safety and efficacy of this therapy in patients with refractory urge incontinence, urgency–frequency syndrome, and urinary retention.[39] A total of 17 centers worldwide enrolled 163 patients, of which 87% were female. Of those treated with implantation, 96 (63.2%) had urge incontinence and 25 (16.4%) had urgency–frequency. For patients with urge incontinence, mean leaking episodes per day decreased from an average 9.6 to 3.9 at 5 years. For patients with urgency–frequency, mean voids per day decreased from an average 19.3 to 14.8, and mean volume voided per void increased from an average 92.3 ml to 165.2 ml. At 5 years after implantation, 68% of patients with urge incontinence and 56% with urgency–frequency still demonstrated successful clinical response. This recent long-term study supports the findings of previous studies, demonstrating that SNM is safe and effective for refractory cases of OAB. While the majority of patients treated with this modality have been women, studies reporting the results of SNM in men with OAB are forthcoming.

Conclusions

OAB in men is a major health issue, with significant cost to society and to the individual. The impact will become even more substantial as the proportion of our elderly population increases. While OAB in men may not be a preventable entity, early recognition and symptomatic treatment may significantly improve QOL. However, many patients do not seek medical attention for this problem, because they are embarrassed or attribute their symptoms to a normal aging process. Previous assumptions relating OAB

symptoms in men to the prostate, and fear of causing urinary retention, have often caused us to dwell on treating the bladder outlet and not the actual symptoms. Newer data supporting the safety and efficacy of treating men complaining of LUTS with antimuscarinics will certainly change the way urologists address one of the most common complaints seen in our practice. Finally, newer, less invasive therapies, such as SNM and BTX injection, are likely to improve QOL without compromising patient safety.

References

1. United Nations. Report of the Second World Assembly on Aging. Madrid, Spain: United Nations, 8–12 April, 2002.
2. US Census Bureau. International database. Table 094. Midyear population, by age and sex [http://www.census.gov/population/www/projections/natdet-D1A.html].
3. Abrams P, Cardozo L, Fall M et al. The standardisation of terminology in lower urinary tract function: report from the standardisation sub-committee of the International Continence Society. Urology 2003; 61: 37–49.
4. Milsom I, Abrams P, Cardozo L et al. How widespread are the symptoms of an overactive bladder and how are they managed? A population-based prevalence study. BJU Int 2001; 87: 760–6.
5. Hu TW, Wagner TH, Bentkover JD et al. Costs of urinary incontinence and overactive bladder in the US. A comparative study. Urology 2004; 63: 461–5.
6. Stewart WF, Van Rooyen JB, Cundiff GW et al. Prevalence and burden of overactive bladder in the United States. World J Urol 2003; 20: 327–36.
7. Hu TW, Wagner TH, Bentkover JD et al. Estimated economic costs of overactive bladder in the United States. Urology 2003; 61: 1123–8.
8. Irwin DE, Milsom I, Hunskaar S et al. Population-based survey of urinary incontinence, overactive bladder, and other lower urinary tract symptoms in five countries: results of the EPIC study. Eur Urol 2006; 50; 1306–15.
9. Tubaro A. Defining overactive bladder: epidemiology and burden of disease. Urology 2004; 64 (Suppl 6A): 2–6.
10. Chapple CR, Roehrborn CG. A shifted paradigm for the further understanding evaluation, and treatment

of lower urinary tract symptoms in men: focus on the bladder. European Urology 2006; 49: 651–9.

11. Blavais J. Nomenclature. In: Kreder K, Dmochowski R, eds. The Overactive Bladder: Evaluation and Management. London: Informa, 2007: 3–9.

12. Rosen R, Altwein J, Boyle P et al. Lower urinary tract symptoms and male sexual dysfunction: the Multinational Survey of the Ageing Male (MSAM-7). Eur Urol 2003; 44: 637–49.

13. Lepor H. Pathophysiology of lower urinary tract symptoms in the aging male population. Rev Urol 2005; 7 (Suppl 7): S3–11.

14. Knutson T, Edlund C, Fall M, Dahlstrand C. BPH with coexisting overactive bladder dysfunction: an everyday urological dilemma. Neurourol Urodynam 2001; 20: 237–47.

15. Mitterberger M, Pallwein L, Gradl J et al. Persistent detrusor overactivity after transurethral resection of the prostate is associated with reduced perfusion of the urinary bladder. BJU Int 2007; 99: 831–5.

16. Holm NR, Horn T, Hald T. Detrusor in ageing and obstruction. Scand J Urol Nephrol 1995; 29: 45–9.

17. Teleman PT, Lidfeldt J, Nerbrand C et al. Overactive bladder: prevalence, risk factors and relation to stress incontinence in middle-aged women. Br J Obstet Gynaecol 2004; 111: 600–4.

18. Hammarsten J, Hogstedt B, Holthuis N, Mellstrom D. Components of the metabolic syndrome: risk factors for the development of benign prostatic hyperplasia. Prostate Cancer Prostatic Dis 1998; 1: 157–62.

19. Peter TJ, Donovan JL, Kay HE et al. The International Continence Society Benign Prostatic Hyperplasia Study: the bothersomeness of urinary symptoms. J Urol 1997; 157: 885–9.

20. Abrams P, Kaplan SA, De Koning Gans HJ, Millard R. Safety and tolerability of tolterodine for the treatment of overactive bladder in men with bladder outlet obstruction. J Urol 2006; 175: 999–1004.

21. Athanasopoulos A, Gyftopoulos K, Giannitsas K et al. Combination treatment with an alpha-blocker plus an anticholinergic for bladder outlet obstruction: a prospective, randomized, controlled study. J Urol 2003; 169: 2253–6.

22. Lee JY, Kim HW, Lee SJ et al. Comparison of doxazosin with or without tolterodine in men with symptomatic bladder outlet obstruction and an overactive bladder. BJU Int 2004; 94: 817–20.

23. Lee KS, Choo MS, Kim DY et al. Combination treatment with propiverine hydrochloride plus doxazosin controlled release gastrointestinal therapeutic system formulation for overactive bladder

and coexisting benign prostatic obstruction: a prospective, randomized, controlled multicenter study. J Urol 2005; 174: 1334–8.

24. Okada H, Shirakawa T, Muto S et al. Propiverine hydrochloride relieves irritative symptoms of benign prostatic hyperplasia. J Urol 2004; 171 (Suppl 4): 357–8.

25. Kaplan SA, Walmsley K, Te AE. Tolterodine extended release attenuates lower urinary tract symptoms in men with benign prostatic hyperplasia. J Urol 2005; 174: 2273–6.

26. Kaplan SA, Roehrborn CG, Rovner ES et al. Tolterodine and tamsulosin for treatment of men with lower urinary tract symptoms and overactive bladder: a randomized controlled trial. JAMA 2006; 296: 2319–28.

27. Nitti VW, Kim Y, Combs AJ. Voiding dysfunction following transurethral resection of the prostate: symptoms and urodynamic findings. J Urol 1997: 157: 600–3.

28. Machino R, Kakizaki H, Ameda K et al. Detrusor instability with equivocal obstruction: a predictor of unfavorable symptomatic outcomes after transurethral prostatectomy. Neurourol Urodyn 2002; 21: 444–9.

29. Kuo HC. Analysis of the pathophysiology of lower urinary tract symptoms in patients after prostatectomy. Urol Int 2002: 68: 99–104.

30. Brading A, Pessina F, Esposito L, Symes S. Effects of metabolic stress and ischaemia on the bladder, and the relationship with bladder overactivity. Scand J Urol Nephrol Suppl 2004; 215: 84–92.

31. Reitz A, Stohrer M, Kramer G et al. European experience of 200 cases treated with botulinum-A toxin injections into the detrusor muscle for neurogenic incontinence due to neurogenic detrusor overactivity. Eur Urol 2004: 45: 510–15.

32. Schmid DM, Sauermann P, Werner M et al. Experience with 100 cases treated with botulinum-A toxin injections in the detrusor muscle for idiopathic overactive bladder syndrome refractory to anticholinergics. J Urol 2006; 176: 177–85.

33. Doggweiler R, Zermann DH, Ishigooka M, Schmidt RA. Botox-induced prostatic involution. Prostate 1998; 37: 44–50.

34. Chuang YC, Tu CH, Huang CC et al. Intraprostatic injection of botulinum toxin type-A relieves bladder outlet obstruction in humans and induces prostate apoptosis in dogs. BMC Urol 2006; 6: 12.

35. Maria G, Brisinda G, Civello IM et al. Relief by botulinum toxin of voiding dysfunction due to benign prostatic hyperplasia: results of a

randomized, placebo-controlled study. Urology 2003; 62: 259–65.

36. Chuang YC, Chiang PH, Yoshimura N et al. Sustained beneficial effects of intraprostatic botulinum toxin type A on lower urinary tract symptoms and quality of life in men with benign prostatic hypertrophy. BJU Int 2006; 98: 1033–7.

37. Yao-Chi C, Giannantoni A, Chancellor M. The potential and promise of using botulinum toxin in the prostate gland. BJU Int 2006; 98: 28–32.

38. Siegel SW, Catanzaro F, Dijkema HE et al. Long-term results of a multicenter study on sacral nerve stimulation for treatment of urinary urge incontinence, urgency–frequency, and retention. Urology 2000; 56 (6 Supp 1): 87–91.

39. van Kerrebroeck PE, van Voskuilen AC, Heesakkers JP et al. Results of sacral neuromodulation therapy for urinary voiding dysfunction: outcomes of a prospective, worldwide clinical study. J Urol 2007; 178: 2029–34.

CHAPTER 26

Benign prostatic hyperplasia

Tom McNicholas, Charlotte Foley

Introduction

Men rarely complain of a big prostate, but usually present with lower urinary tract symptoms (LUTS) or a complication from unrelieved bladder outflow obstruction (BOO) (Table 26.1). The cause of their symptoms is not always the prostate! Females develop similar symptoms as they age. Bladder neuromuscular changes associated with aging lead to over-activity of the bladder, and endocrine, cardiac, renal, dietary (especially fluid), and pharmacological effects can all lead to LUTS, especially passing urine frequently, urgently, and at night (frequency, urgency, and nocturia), which are the most bothersome symptoms and most likely to bring a patient to see a doctor. A range of conditions may therefore precipitate a consultation for advice and treatment, and the advisor will need to work through them to determine the primary causes.

The term benign prostatic hyperplasia (BPH) was used almost synonymously with LUTS but the 5th International Consultation of 2000 recommended 'LUTS suggestive of BOO' (or LUTS/BOO) as the preferable term to use for this condition since 'BPH' is a purely descriptive term for the microscopic enlargement of epithelial and stromal prostate tissue developing in some of these men. Nevertheless, increasing LUTS is common in men as they age and in approximately 50% is associated with measurable and endoscopically visible enlargement of the prostate (Fig. 26.1).[1] In other men obstruction to bladder emptying caused by bladder neck muscular tissue (Fig. 26.2) or scarring of the urethral passage (urethral stricture) may lead to similar symptoms.

Anatomy and function of the prostate gland

In the post-pubertal adult male the prostate is approximately the size of a walnut ($20\,cm^3$), and it gradually enlarges from around the age of 40 years onwards as a result of BPH.[2] It sits deep in the bowl of the pelvis, behind the pubic bone and below the bladder, with the urethra passing through it into the penis (Figs. 26.3 and 26.4). The posterior aspect of the prostate can be readily examined by a finger or ultrasound probe in the rectum, which lies immediately behind.

The function of the prostate gland is primarily related to fertility. Prostatic secretions contribute most of the ejaculate, and are rich in fructose, providing energy for sperm metabolism, and also prostatic specific antigen (PSA), a serine protease in the human kallikrein family, which is thought to liquefy the viscous seminal fluid, facilitating motility of spermatozoa. PSA has become an easily measured serum marker; it is prostate-specific, *not* cancer-specific. PSA increases with age, prostate enlargement, and inflammation or injury to the prostate as well as with cancer.

Table 26.1. *Symptoms and signs of benign prostate hyperplasia, and complications*

Obstructive, voiding or flow symptoms	Irritative or storage symptoms
Hesitancy	Urgency
Intermittent stream	Frequency
Weak urinary stream	Nocturia
Prolonged voiding time	
Straining to void	
Terminal dribble	
Incomplete emptying	

Complications	Symptoms
Urinary tract infection	Fever, dysuria, irritative symptoms, general confusion
Bladder calculi	Pain, intermittent stream, urinary tract infection, hematuria, irritative symptoms
Acute urinary retention	Pain, urgency
Chronic urinary retention	Overflow incontinence, obstructive symptoms
Chronic renal failure	Malaise, nausea, vomiting
Hematuria	Microscopic or visible hematuria
Bladder diverticula	Urinary tract infection, double voiding, bladder calculi

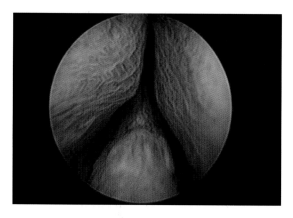

Figure 26.1. *Endoscopic view of the prostate showing lateral lobes of enlarged prostatic tissue to each side and the bladder neck muscle directly ahead.*

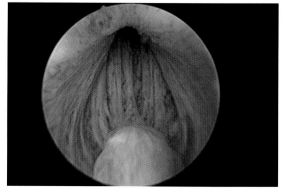

Figure 26.2. *Endoscopic view of the prostate and bladder neck showing the bladder neck muscle directly ahead and only minimal enlargement of the lateral lobes of prostatic tissue.*

Population prevalence

Several large population studies have shown that progressive prostate enlargement is extremely common and is seen in the majority of men aged over 70. Perhaps the most studied populations are those of Baltimore, the Forth Valley in Scotland, and Olmsted County in Minnesota, which have provided a great deal of information about the complex interactions between BPH, LUTS, serum PSA, risk of acute urinary retention (AUR), urinary flow rate, and risk of surgery over time.[3-5]

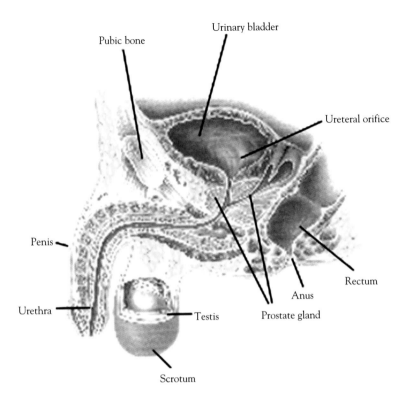

Figure 26.3. *Color diagram of the lower urinary tract in the male.*

Pubic bone

Urinary bladder

Ureteral orifice

Penis

Rectum

Urethra

Anus

Testis

Prostate gland

Scrotum

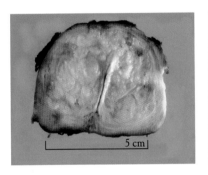

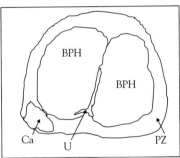

5 cm

BPH

BPH

Ca

U

PZ

Figure 26.4. *Cross-section through a surgically removed prostate specimen, showing benign prostatic hyperplasia compressing the urethra (U) and the peripheral zone (PZ). A focus of cancer (Ca) is present in the right posterior peripheral zone.*

In Scotland there was a 25% overall incidence of a combination of reduced urinary flow, urinary symptoms, and 'measurable BPH', rising to 43% in men aged over 60.[4] In Olmsted County, median urinary flow rate dropped by approximately 2% per year, and more rapidly in those presenting with a restricted flow and in those over 70 years of age.[5] The Baltimore Longitudinal Study of Aging showed that men with prostatic enlargement and symptoms were eight times more likely to undergo prostatectomy within 10 years than those of the same age without.[3]

Risk factors

Age
Increasing prostate size is strongly associated with age. Approximately 40% of men in their 50s, and over 90% of men in their 80s have microscopic evidence of BPH.[2]

Genetic factors
Studies of twins and men with early-onset BPH have identified family history of BPH as a risk factor for clinical BPH and suggest the presence of

a predisposing gene.[6] Candidate genetic polymorphisms are the androgen receptor and the SRD5A2 gene coding for the 5-α reductase enzymes responsible for the conversion of testosterone to dihydrotestosterone (DHT).[7] DHT is necessary for BPH to develop.

Race

Differences in cellular composition of BPH have been shown in Caucasian–American, African–American, and Japanese men.[8] This may account for previously observed racial differences in PSA, PSA density, and the incidence of clinical BPH. The prevalence of and surgery rates for BPH are lower in Asian men than in Caucasian men. A higher prevalence of moderate to severe LUTS has been reported in Afro–Caribbean men than in Caucasians. Other studies, however, have shown a similar rate of diagnosis of BPH and similar hospitalization rate for BPH-related surgery in Afro–Caribbean and Caucasian men suggesting that differences in symptom tolerance may be important.[9]

Diet

A 'Western' diet and reduced exercise levels are risk factors for BPH. Elevated total energy and total animal protein intake increases the risk of BPH even in Asian men.[10] Processes that predispose to the development of diabetes and obesity appear to be risk factors, possibly through mechanisms that activate the sympathetic nervous system and alter hormonal balance.[11,12] Obesity seems to increase the risk of men going on to prostate surgery.[13] Overall, obesity and diabetes increases the risk and physical activity and moderate alcohol intake reduces the risk of BPH and LUTS in older men.[14]

Cellular and molecular pathology

The pathogenesis of BPH remains incompletely understood. Detailed reviews are available.[15] A multifactorial pathogenesis is likely given the great variation in macroscopic, microscopic and molecular changes seen in BPH.[16]

Hyperplasia of the epithelial component of BPH is at least partly related to age-related changes in stem cell-driven tissue renewal. Gradually cells accumulate that show age-related changes in their behavior resulting in abnormal cellular responses to peptide growth factors and other cellular signaling, thus allowing the development of BPH. The rate of apoptosis within BPH epithelium is reduced, possibly in relation to increased expression of bcl-2, a well known antiapoptotic proto-oncogene, which is switched on in many cancers.

Secretion of peptide growth factors under the control of circulating androgens is fundamental to the development and maintenance of typical prostatic morphology, and in BPH it seems that this feedback control becomes abnormal, stimulating the growth of both epithelial and stromal components. The prostatic stroma produces growth factors that stimulate epithelial growth.

With aging, the epithelial cell may lose the ability to respond to negative growth signaling such as transforming growth factor (TGF)-β. Increased levels of TGF-β as seen in BPH tissue promotes differentiation of stromal cells, which partly accounts for the increased amount of smooth muscle seen in BPH. This tends to increase the resting muscular tone of the prostate, which is one of the factors causing urinary outflow obstruction.

Diagnosis and assessment of men with benign prostatic hyperplasia and lower urinary tract symptoms

Diagnosis requires a clinical history, a focused examination, and special tests. In practice many men are anxious that they may have prostate cancer or that they might be going into renal failure, and they are often worried about AUR. A history of symptoms, comorbidity, and age combined with a careful examination with measurement of serum creatinine, PSA, and the urinary flow rate can allow one to estimate these risks very rapidly. Severe life-threatening urinary tract infection (UTI) and renal failure are now extremely unusual in Western countries in men with BPH.[17]

A history of dietary fluid intake is useful. The use of frequency–volume charts and input–ouput charts can be very revealing and can identify simple lifestyle changes that may help symptoms substantially at very little risk. A drug history may identify vasoactive agents as found in many proprietary cough and cold remedies, which can lead to deterioration of urinary function by increasing α-adrenoceptor stimulation. A history of cardiovascular disease, particularly congestive cardiac failure, and a history of falling may contraindicate vasodilating α-blocker drug therapy.[18] The history should also encompass sexual function and social factors such as the need for outward ejaculation or fertility in relatively younger men (or those with younger partners).

It is worth trying to divide men into categories of severity. The most widely used symptom score is the American Urological Association's seven-question Symptom Score, which with the addition of a question on quality of life becomes the International Prostate Symptom Score (IPSS) (Fig. 26.5).[19] Others include the interviewer-administered Boyarsky Index and Madsen-Iversen Index and the self-administered Maine Medical Assessment Program Index and the Danish Prostatic Symptom Score (DAN-PSS-1).[20–23] The International Continence Society BPH study used a questionnaire with three components to assess symptoms, impact on quality of life, and impact on sexual function.[24]

The IPSS score segregates men into those with mild (score 0–7), moderate (score 8–19), or severe (score 20–35) symptoms. The IPSS may undervalue storage symptoms (urgency, frequency) that are generally more bothersome. The single quality of life question is also useful for determining how bothered men are by their symptoms, since many men will accept a surprising degree of urinary symptoms if reassured that there is nothing more serious going on.[24,25]

Examination should include a urine dipstick to exclude infection and hematuria, examination for a palpable bladder, signs of renal impairment, and a digital rectal examination (DRE) of the pelvis to assess prostate size, consistency, and pelvic tone. A simple assessment of 'normal', 'big', or 'very big' is sufficient and is useful for choosing therapy and for operation list planning. Assess whether the prostate feels regular in shape and consistency or whether there are hard nodules suggesting prostate cancer, remembering that 22% of men with PSA of 2.6–4 ng/mL will harbor a prostate cancer.[26]

Measuring PSA is sensible, together with serum creatinine. Simple uroflowmetry by asking the man to void with a comfortably full bladder into a flow rate meter will be helpful as long as he can void 150 mL or more. A flow rate above 15 mL/second suggests the cause is unlikely to be BOO (though 30% of patients will indeed be obstructed), and a flow rate below 10 mL/second is highly likely to be due to BOO.[27] More complex pressure flow studies (PFS) can be kept in reserve for when the clinical picture is unclear or when there is predominance of 'irritable' or 'storage' symptoms or following previously failed invasive treatment. Most urologists offer surgery if there is a convincing pattern of symptoms and measurements. Since men with relatively poorly functioning bladder detrusor muscle do not do well with surgical treatment it appears that the only way to prove BOO and a functioning bladder muscle prior to surgery is by PFS.[28,29] PFS prior to any repeat surgery seems sensible.[30] Difficulty performing PFS can often be the first indication of a stricture causing the obstruction, although this may also be suspected from the history or the flow rate traces.

There is little scientific evidence supporting examination of the kidneys by ultrasound unless there is a large residual urine volume, a palpable bladder, or raised creatinine levels. Transrectal ultrasound (TRUS) of the prostate to measure prostate volume accurately is valuable if the DRE or PSA are abnormal, but it is most important for guiding prostate biopsies.

Treatment

Active treatment options include pharmacotherapy, minimally invasive therapies (MITs), and more traditional surgical options, though with modern improvements. Even with strong evidence for efficacy and safety, there has been a profound 'flight from surgery' (Fig. 26.6) since the 1980s to MITs (despite a relative lack of efficacy data) and to drug treatment (with good-quality data).[31] Interestingly, after adjusting for inflation, overall costs of BPH treatment in the US have decreased as a result of less operations despite many more men seeking treatment.[31]

International Prostate Symptom Score (I-PSS)	Not at all	Less than 1 time in 5	Less than half the time	About half the time	More than half the time	Almost always	Your score
1. Incomplete emptying Over the past month, how often have you had a sensation of not emptying your bladder completely after you have finished urinating?	0	1	2	3	4	5	
2. Frequency Over the past month, how often have you had to urinate again less than two hours after you finished urinating?	0	1	2	3	4	5	
3. Intermittency Over the past month, how often have you found you stopped and started again severel times when you urinated?	0	1	2	3	4	5	
4. Urgency Over the past month, how often have you found it difficult to postpone urination?	0	1	2	3	4	5	
5. Weak stream Over the past month, how often have you had a weak urinary stream?	0	1	2	3	4	5	
6. Straining Over the past month, how often have you had to push or strain to begin urination?	0	1	2	3	4	5	
	None	1 time	2 times	3 times	4 times	5 times or more	
7. Nocturia Over the past month, how many times did you most typically get up to urinate from the time you went to bed until the time you got up in the morning?	0	1	2	3	4	5	
TOTAL I-PSS							
Quality of life due to urinary symptoms	Delighted	Pleased	Mostly satisfied	Mixed-equally satisfied	Mostly dissatisfied	Unhappy	Terrible
If you were to spend the rest of your life with your urinary condition just the way it is now, how would you feel about it? (circle number)	0	1	2	3	4	5	6

Figure 26.5. *Urinary symptom score sheet (IPSS).*

Pharmacotherapy relieves excessive smooth muscle tone within the lower urinary tract by using compounds designed to block α-adrenoceptors at the bladder neck and trigone and within the prostate [α-receptor blockers (ARBs)] or by blocking hormonal mechanisms responsible for promoting BPH [5-α reductase inhibitors (5-ARIs)]. Most experts would agree with the statement by Clifford and Farmer that 'neither finasteride (a 5-ARI) nor α-blockers approach the efficacy of prostatic surgery in terms of improvement in either symptoms or flow rates'.[32]

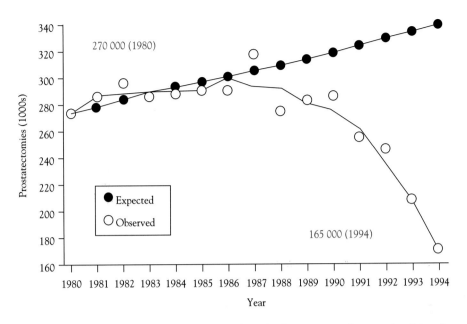

Figure 26.6. *The flight from surgery: data from the US show far fewer men undergoing 'traditional' surgery (usually transurethral resection of the prostate) for benign prostatic hyperplasia since the peak in the mid 1980s. European data are similar but the shift occurred a few years later. There has been a migration to medical therapy and the use of 'minimally invasive' treatments.*

α-receptor blockers

ARBs work quickly and on all prostate sizes. They are usually well tolerated but can affect blood pressure and cause dizziness with a risk of falling. Care is needed in the presence of cardiac failure. Younger men often report interference with ejaculation, nasal stuffiness, and 'asthenia' despite the low rates recorded in good clinical trials. The risk of treatment failure seems to be related to baseline prostate volume, occurring in 48% with prostate volumes under 40 cm³, but in 72% with glands over this size. Overall re-treatment rates due to ARB treatment failure were reported as 38% at 3 years and 54% at 5 years.[33]

5-α reductase inhibitors

5-ARIs work over 4–6 months to achieve moderate symptom improvement by blocking the enzymes metabolizing testosterone to the more potent intracellular DHT. An approximate 30% shrinkage and a halving of PSA levels can be expected. These are safe agents with side effects of altered libido and sexual function.

The MTOPS study highlighted important differences in long-term outcomes between 5-ARIs and ARBs. Only the 5-ARIs demonstrated reduced risk of AUR and BPH-related surgery.[17] 5-ARIs therefore offer an opportunity to prevent progression of BPH on a long-term prophylactic basis as well as for the management of established BPH. Currently they are being explored as possible modifiers of prostate cancer risk.[34,35]

Combination therapy

The MTOPS and COMBAT studies showed an overall advantage for treatment with a 5-ARI (finasteride or dutasteride) and an ARB (doxazosin or tamsulosin) compared with either drug singly, although at extra cost (economically and in side effects).[17,36] It seems possible to withdraw the ARB after 9–12 months of combination therapy.[37] Finally, anticholinergic drugs in combination with ABs may also be helpful for urinary frequency and urgency without increasing risks of AUR.[38]

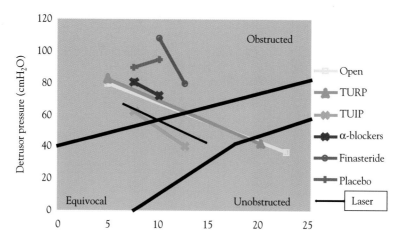

Figure 26.7. *Effects of treatments on urethral resistance. Shown here is a graphical representation of the Abrams–Griffiths nomogram in which patient urodynamic variables are computed to produce a number. If the number falls in the upper zone they are 'obstructed' and if in the lower zone then they are 'unobstructed'. There is an 'equivocal' zone lying between these two. As can be seen, only open surgery and transurethral resection of the prostate have been clearly shown to transfer the treated man from the obstructed into the unobstructed zone. Modified by the authors, after Bosch 1997.[43] Copyright Elsevier, New York, 1997; used with permission, Elsevier 2008.*

Minimally invasive therapies

MITs usually involve heating the prostate using electrical, microwave or laser energy sources, either inserted directly into the substance of the prostate as a needle or via the urethra. Heating can be relatively low energy when the effects are thought to be due to α-adrenoceptor blockade or damage (with similar outcomes to ARB use) or high energy, usually requiring anesthesia, when obstructing tissue is coagulated or vaporized directly (with less bleeding than conventional surgery). Long-term data and large-scale studies are hard to come by. Such vital studies are expensive and rarely supported by healthcare systems. Re-treatment rates appear higher than with conventional surgery, which will reduce cost effectiveness.[39,40]

'Greenlight' laser vaporization with the potassium-titanyl-phosphate (KTP) laser has attracted much attention and appears relatively simple and safe, with good short-term efficacy.[41] The Holmium laser can be used for simple vaporization or incision of obstructing tissue. There is no evidence that Holmium incision or KTP vaporization are more effective or safer than transurethral incision of the prostate (TUIP), and they are more expensive.

Proper comparative trials are needed. The Holmium laser can be used to 'resect' or 'enucleate' obstructing prostatic adenoma tissue akin to TURP or open removal of the adenoma.[42] The quality and length of follow-up data are encouraging but the uptake of the technique is less than expected, probably owing to significant equipment costs and the considerable learning curve involved.

Surgical options

Surgical procedures characteristically incise or remove obstructing tissue, require anesthesia, and require a short hospital stay with a catheter. Surgery relieves obstruction while other therapies do not appear to do so entirely (Fig. 26.7) but do relieve symptoms 'enough' for many men's purposes.[43] We do not know the long-term effects of relieving symptoms but not obstruction. Flanigan et al. suggested a less good response to delayed surgery.[44]

Transurethral resection of the prostate

TURP removes tissue using diathermy current through a fine metal cutting loop and remains the 'gold standard' in BPH therapy. Efficacy is proven in terms of symptom relief, removal of obstruction, and low re-operation rates. In 10-year follow-up series, repeat operation was performed for bladder neck contracture in 2.4%, for recurrent BPH in 1.9% and urethral strictures in 1.7%. Major complications will rarely occur. Modern improvements to the energy source used, refinements to the loops and sheaths delivering the energy to the target, and advances in anesthesia have dramatically reduced the morbidity and mortality of surgery for BPH. More recent large studies have shown very low or no mortality.[45,46]

Transurethral incision of the prostate

With better assessment, TUIP, also known as bladder neck incision (BNI), deserves to be more widely used for potentially up to 40% of Western men with symptoms, and most men with small prostates (20–40 cm³) and primarily a bladder neck muscular obstruction. In sexually active men, TUIP can be performed by adjusting the endoscopic incision to reduce the 15–30% incidence of retrograde ejaculation. However, this cannot be guaranteed and if fertility or outward ejaculation is essential then surgery should be avoided and drug therapy (which has reversible effects) can be maintained. With DRE or transrectal ultrasound scanning or by the use of PSA as a further surrogate for size we can select out men with small prostates and primarily a bladder neck muscular obstruction for drug therapy with ABs or surgery by TUIP.[47]

Randomized controlled trials suggest that the risks of impotence and incontinence are low with surgery and similar to or better than with conservative management.[48] Ejaculatory function may be altered (90% of men have retrograde ejaculation after TURP), but there is no good level 1 evidence that TUIP and TURP damage erectile function.

The challenge of acute urinary retention

AUR is a sudden and painful complication of BPH. It may occur spontaneously in patients with a history of gradually worsening LUTS or be precipitated in men with more blameless urological pasts by UTI, general anesthetics, immobility, pain, bladder over-distention, excess fluid intake (especially alcohol), constipation, and drugs with sympathomimetic or anticholinergic properties (as found in cold remedies).

Typically patients present in pain, with a palpable bladder from which at least 300 mL of urine is drained upon catheterization, with immediate relief. Where pain is not a prominent feature, chronic retention of urine is more likely, suggesting a degree of underlying detrusor failure. Such patients often present with overflow incontinence and residual urine volumes over 1 L. All patients need a serum creatinine measured, recognition of any post-obstructive diuresis (urine output >200 mL for 2 hours or longer), and any precipitants corrected. In most straightforward cases an ARB is commenced and a trial without catheter (TWOC) undertaken after 2–3 days, with 53% of such patients successfully returning to spontaneous voiding.[49] Alfuzosin is the only ARB that has been shown to improve the likelihood of passing a TWOC, from 48% without it to 62% with it.[50] Patients that fail a TWOC may undergo a second TWOC, with a 25% chance of success, or proceed to TURP. Currently, 42% of all TURPs in the UK and 24% of all TURPs in the US are on men catheterized after AUR.[51]

Given the high incidence of LUTS, AUR is a relatively rare complication. The Olmstead County Study reported a cumulative incidence of AUR of 2.7% over 4 years, while predicting that 10% of men in their 70s and 33% of those in their 80s would experience it over the next 5 years.[52] However, one episode of retention predisposes to another, with the risk increased six-fold.[53] Being admitted to hospital with AUR is also associated with a worse life expectancy. The 1-year mortality rate for patients aged 75–84 admitted with spontaneous AUR was 12.5% without comorbidities and 28.8% with comorbidities.[54] Furthermore, undergoing TURP after AUR increases morbidity and mortality compared with having surgery for symptoms only. Intra-operative bleeding and postoperative complications such as catheter-related UTI all contribute to a 3.3-fold increased mortality rate.[51]

AUR is therefore best avoided, and a number of baseline and dynamic risk factors have been defined to help identify those at high risk.[52,54,55] For those men with such risk factors, both dutasteride and finasteride have been shown to halve the risk of AUR. Conversely, ARBs can only delay AUR but not prevent it.[17,56] They are useful though to help men void after TWOC and identify those non-responders who are likely to need surgical treatment.[57]

What therapy for which man?

BOO secondary to bladder neck obstruction is often seen in younger men with a low PSA (≤1.4 ng/mL) and a small prostate. Choices lie between lifestyle changes, ARBs, MITs, and TUIP for severe symptoms.

BOO secondary to BPH is seen characteristically in older men with obvious palpable prostatic enlargement or PSA levels >1.4 ng/mL. The choices are lifestyle changes, ARBs, 5-ARIs (finasteride or dutasteride), MITs, and TURP.

For the very large prostate (over 100 cm³), open retropubic prostatectomy or Holmium laser enucleation appear the best long-term options. In older, sicker men a judicious combination of a limited but adequate TURP or laser vaporization and then long-term 5-ARI therapy may be sufficient.

Conclusions

Men in Western society or those who are increasingly exposed to Western diets and who do less exercise will develop microscopic BPH. Approximately 50% will develop macroscopic BPH and measurable enlargement of the prostate. Their response to this and whether they develop symptoms depends on a complex interplay of factors and, in particular, bladder function.

Men without symptoms will rarely present and can be left alone. Men with symptoms or complications may wish treatment. Lifestyle changes can reduce mild to moderate symptoms. Those who wish to avoid or defer surgery will generally show symptomatic improvement with ARB therapy or 5-ARI therapy (particularly if the prostate is measurably enlarged) or both in combination. 5-ARIs reduce

the progressive development of BPH, both as an alternative to surgery and as a supplement to it to prevent or minimize recurrence.

Men who are very bothered do best with surgical therapy. Surgery should remove any obstruction, which generally relieves symptoms and effectively cures the condition. However there will be a rate of complications and a tendency to further growth of the prostate that means even successful surgery may need repeating years in the future.

We can now begin to predict those men most at risk of progression to worse symptoms, to needing surgery, or to developing AUR. For the first time, 5-ARI therapy allows the possibility of reducing those risks.

References

1. Blanker MH, Groeneveld FP, Prins A et al. Strong effects of definition and nonresponse bias on prevalence rates of clinical benign prostatic hyperplasia: the Krimpen study of male urogenital tract problems and general health status. BJU Int 2000; 85: 665–71.
2. Berry SJ, Coffey DS, Walsh PC, Ewing LL. The development of human benign prostatic hyperplasia with age. J Urol 1984; 132: 474–9.
3. Arrighi HM, Metter EJ, Guess HA, Fozzard JL. Natural history of benign prostatic hyperplasia and risk of prostatectomy. The Baltimore Longitudinal Study of Aging. Urology 1991; 38: 4–8.
4. Garraway WM, Collins GN, Lee RJ. High prevalence of benign prostatic hypertrophy in the community. Lancet 1991; 338: 469–71.
5. Jacobsen SJ, Girman CJ, Guess HA et al. Natural history of prostatism: longitudinal changes in voiding symptoms in community dwelling men. J Urol 1996; 155: 595–600.
6. Sanda MG, Beaty TH, Stutzman RE, Childs B, Walsh PC. Genetic susceptibility of benign prostatic hyperplasia. J Urol 1994; 152: 115–19.
7. Roberts RO, Bergstralh EJ, Farmer SA et al. Polymorphisms in the 5 alpha reductase type 2 gene and urologic measures of BPH. Prostate 2005; 62: 380–7.
8. Aoki Y, Arai Y, Maeda H, Okubo K, Shinohara K. Racial differences in cellular composition of benign prostatic hyperplasia. Prostate 2001; 49: 243–50.
9. Platz EA, Kawachi I, Rimm EB, Willett WC, Giovannucci E. Race, ethnicity and benign prostatic

hyperplasia in the health professionals follow-up study. J Urol 2000; 163: 490–5.

10. Gu F. Changes in the prevalence of benign prostatic hyperplasia in China. Chin Med J (Engl) 1997; 110: 163–6.

11. Steers WD, Clemow DB, Persson K et al. The spontaneously hypertensive rat: insight into the pathogenesis of irritative symptoms in benign prostatic hyperplasia and young anxious males. Exp Physiol 1999; 84: 137–47.

12. Hautanen A. Synthesis and regulation of sex hormone-binding globulin in obesity. Int J Obes Relat Metab Disord 2000; 24(Suppl 2): S64–70.

13. Giovannucci E, Rimm EB, Chute CG et al. Obesity and benign prostatic hyperplasia. Am J Epidemiol 1994; 140: 989–1002.

14. Parsons JK. Modifiable risk factors for benign prostatic hyperplasia and lower urinary tract symptoms: new approaches to old problems. J Urol 2007; 178: 395–401.

15. Shariat S, Canto E, Slawin K. Molecular genetics of benign prostatic hyperplasia. In: Kirby R, McConnell J, FitzPatrick J, Roehrborn C, Boyle P, eds. Textbook of Benign Prostatic Hyperplasia. Abingdon, UK: Taylor and Francis, 2004: 119–37.

16. McNeal JE. Origin and evolution of benign prostatic enlargement. Invest Urol 1978; 15: 340–5.

17. McConnell JD, Roehrborn CG, Bautista OM et al. The long-term effect of doxazosin, finasteride, and combination therapy on the clinical progression of benign prostatic hyperplasia. N Engl J Med 2003; 349: 2387–98.

18. Messerli FH. Implications of discontinuation of doxazosin arm of ALLHAT. Antihypertensive and Lipid-Lowering Treatment to Prevent Heart Attack Trial. Lancet 2000; 355: 863–4.

19. Barry M, Fowler F, O'Leary M et al. The American Urological Association symptom index for benign prostatic hyperplasia. J Urol 1992; 148: 1549–57.

20. Boyarsky S, Jones G, Paulson DF, Prout GR Jr. A new look at bladder neck obstruction by the Food and Drug Administration regulators: guidelines for investigation of benign prostatic hypertrophy. Trans Am Assoc Genitourin Surg 1976; 68: 29–32.

21. Madsen P, Iversen P. A point system for selecting operative candidates. In: Hinman E, ed. Benign Prostatic Hypertrophy. New York: Springer-Verlag, 1983: 763–5.

22. Fowler FJ Jr, Wennberg JE, Timothy RP et al. Symptom status and quality of life following prostatectomy. JAMA 1988; 259: 3018–22.

23. Hald T, Nordling J, Andersen JT et al. A patient weighted symptom score system in the evaluation of uncomplicated benign prostatic hyperplasia. Scand J Urol Nephrol Suppl 1991; 138: 59–62.

24. Peters TJ, Donovan JL, Kay HE et al. The International Continence Society 'Benign Prostatic Hyperplasia' Study: the bothersomeness of urinary symptoms. J Urol 1997; 157: 885–9.

25. Treagust J, Morkane T, Speakman M. Estimating a population's needs for the treatment of lower urinary tract symptoms in men: what is the extent of the unmet need? J Public Health Med 2001; 23: 141–7.

26. Catalona WJ, Smith DS, Ornstein DK. Prostate cancer detection in men with serum PSA concentrations of 2.6 to 4.0 ng/mL and benign prostate examination. Enhancement of specificity with free PSA measurements. JAMA 1997; 277: 1452–5.

27. Reynard JM, Yang Q, Donovan JL et al. The ICS-'BPH' Study: uroflowmetry, lower urinary tract symptoms and bladder outlet obstruction. Br J Urol 1998; 82: 619–23.

28. Thomas AW, Cannon A, Bartlett E, Ellis-Jones J, Abrams P. The natural history of lower urinary tract dysfunction in men: the influence of detrusor underactivity on the outcome after transurethral resection of the prostate with a minimum 10-year urodynamic follow-up. BJU Int 2004; 93: 745–50.

29. de la Rosette JJ, Witjes WP, Schafer W et al. Relationships between lower urinary tract symptoms and bladder outlet obstruction: results from the ICS-'BPH' study. Neurourol Urodyn 1998; 17: 99–108.

30. Brown CT, Yap T, Cromwell DA et al. Self management for men with lower urinary tract symptoms: randomised controlled trial. BMJ 2007; 334: 25.

31. Wei J, Calhoun E, Jacobsen S. Benign prostatic hyperplasia. In: Litwin M, Saigal C, eds. Urologic Disease in America. Washington, DC: US Department of Health and Human Sciences, Public Health Service, National Institutes of Health, 2007: 45–69.

32. Clifford GM, Farmer RD. Medical therapy for benign prostatic hyperplasia: a review of the literature. Eur Urol 2000; 38: 2–19.

33. de la Rosette JJ, Kortmann BB, Rossi C et al. Long-term risk of re-treatment of patients using alpha-blockers for lower urinary tract symptoms. J Urol 2002; 167: 1734–9.

34. Thompson I, Goodman P, Tangen C et al. The influence of finasteride on the development of prostate cancer. N Engl J Med 2003; 349: 215–24.

35. Andriole G, Roehrborn C, Schulman C et al. Effect of dutasteride on the detection of prostate cancer in

men with benign prostatic hyperplasia. Urology 2004; 64: 537–41; discussion 542–3.

36. Roehrborn CG, Siami P, Barkin J et al. The effects of dutasteride, tamsulosin and combination therapy on lower urinary tract symptoms in men with benign prostatic hyperplasia and prostatic enlargement: 2-year results from the CombAT study. J Urol 2008; 179: 616–21; discussion 621.

37. Baldwin KC, Ginsberg PC, Roehrborn CG, Harkaway RC. Discontinuation of alpha-blockade after initial treatment with finasteride and doxazosin in men with lower urinary tract symptoms and clinical evidence of benign prostatic hyperplasia. Urology 2001; 58: 203–9.

38. Kaplan SA, Roehrborn CG, Rovner ES et al. Tolterodine and tamsulosin for treatment of men with lower urinary tract symptoms and overactive bladder: a randomized controlled trial. JAMA 2006; 296: 2319–28.

39. Madersbacher S, Schatzl G, Djavan B, Stulnig T, Marberger M. Long-term outcome of transrectal high-intensity focused ultrasound therapy for benign prostatic hyperplasia. Eur Urol 2000; 37: 687–94.

40. Schatzl G, Madersbacher S, Djavan B, Lang T, Marberger M. Two-year results of transurethral resection of the prostate versus four 'less invasive' treatment options. Eur Urol 2000; 37: 695–701.

41. Te AE, Malloy TR, Stein BS et al. Impact of prostate-specific antigen level and prostate volume as predictors of efficacy in photoselective vaporization prostatectomy: analysis and results of an ongoing prospective multicentre study at 3 years. BJU Int 2006; 97: 1229–33.

42. Tan AH, Gilling PJ, Kennett KM et al. A randomized trial comparing holmium laser enucleation of the prostate with transurethral resection of the prostate for the treatment of bladder outlet obstruction secondary to benign prostatic hyperplasia in large glands (40 to 200 grams). J Urol 2003; 170: 1270–4.

43. Bosch JL. Urodynamic effects of various treatment modalities for benign prostatic hyperplasia. J Urol 1997; 158: 2034–44.

44. Flanigan R, Reda D, Wasson J et al. 5-year outcome of surgical resection and watchful waiting for men with moderately symptomatic benign prostatic hyperplasia: a Department of Veterans Affairs cooperative study. J Urol 1998; 160: 12–17.

45. Varkarakis J, Bartsch G, Horninger W. Long-term morbidity and mortality of transurethral prostatectomy: a 10-year follow-up. Prostate 2004; 58: 248–51.

46. Zwergel U, Wullich B, Lindenmeir U, Rohde V, Zwergel T. Long-term results following transurethral resection of the prostate. Eur Urol 1998; 33: 476–80.

47. Roehrborn C. The potential of serum prostate-specific antigen as a predictor of clinical response in patients with lower urinary tract symptoms and benign prostatic hyperplasia. BJU Int 2004; 93: 21–6.

48. Wasson JH, Reda DJ, Bruskewitz RC et al. A comparison of transurethral surgery with watchful waiting for moderate symptoms of benign prostatic hyperplasia. The Veterans Affairs Cooperative Study Group on Transurethral Resection of the Prostate. N Engl J Med 1995; 332: 75–9.

49. Desgrandchamps F, De La Taille A, Doublet JD. The management of acute urinary retention in France: a cross-sectional survey in 2618 men with benign prostatic hyperplasia. BJU Int 2006; 97: 727–33.

50. McNeill SA, Hargreave TB. Alfuzosin once daily facilitates return to voiding in patients in acute urinary retention. J Urol 2004; 171: 2316–20.

51. Pickard R, Emberton M, Neal DE. The management of men with acute urinary retention. National Prostatectomy Audit Steering Group. Br J Urol 1998; 81: 712–20.

52. Jacobsen SJ, Jacobson DJ, Girman CJ et al. Natural history of prostatism: risk factors for acute urinary retention. J Urol 1997; 158: 481–7.

53. Emberton M, Elhilali M, Matzkin H et al. Symptom deterioration during treatment and history of AUR are the strongest predictors for AUR and BPH-related surgery in men with LUTS treated with alfuzosin 10 mg once daily. Urology 2005; 66: 316–22.

54. Armitage JN, Sibanda N, Cathcart PJ, Emberton M, van der Meulen JH. Mortality in men admitted to hospital with acute urinary retention: database analysis. BMJ 2007; 335: 1199–202.

55. Slawin KM, Kattan MW, Roehrborn CG, Wilson TH. Development of nomogram to predict acute urinary retention or surgical intervention, with or without dutasteride therapy, in men with benign prostatic hyperplasia. Urology 2006; 67: 84–8.

56. Roehrborn C, Boyle P, Nickel J, Hoefner K, Andriole G. Efficacy and safety of a dual inhibitor of 5-alpha-reductase types 1 and 2 (dutasteride) in men with benign prostatic hyperplasia. Urology 2002; 60: 434–41.

57. Emberton M, Lukacs B, Matzkin H et al. Response to daily 10 mg alfuzosin predicts acute urinary retention and benign prostatic hyperplasia related surgery in men with lower urinary tract symptoms. J Urol 2006; 176: 1051–6.

CHAPTER 27

Prostatitis and chronic pelvic pain

J Curtis Nickel

Introduction

Prostatitis is a significant and prevalent male healthcare issue, a fact that is not generally recognized by either physicians or the lay community. As a prostate-related condition, it does not have the respect that is associated with prostate cancer nor the perceived importance of benign prostatic hyperplasia. However, a community-based survey of family physicians' offices in Olmsted County (a county in Minnesota serviced by the Mayo Clinic) noted that 11% of men had a physician diagnosis of prostatitis.[1] In Finland, 14% of fit men in the Oulu district had a current or previous diagnosis of prostatitis.[2] In the US health professional epidemiological study, 14% of male health professionals surveyed recollected a diagnosis of prostatitis.[3] It has been estimated from population-based studies in Canada and the USA that 2–6% of men in the community are experiencing at least mild to moderate prostatitis-like symptoms at any particular time.[4-6] In fact, the diagnosis of prostatitis is the most common diagnosis in urology outpatient practice in the USA in men under 50 years of age (and the third most common diagnosis in men over 50 years of age), representing approximately 8% of a urologist's outpatient visits. In family practice, the diagnosis of prostatitis represents 1% of outpatient visits.[7]

Prostatitis, either acute or chronic, is characterized by a constellation of symptoms, which include pain (genitourinary or pelvic, or both), variable voiding, and sexual dysfunction, which have significant impacts on patients' quality of life. Employing standard quality-of-life assessment tools, patients with prostatitis have a quality of life similar to that of patients who have just had an acute myocardial infarction or suffer from unstable angina, active Crohn's disease, congestive heart failure, or severe diabetes mellitus.[8,9] Patients with prostatitis do not have an enviable quality of life, and many find it impossible to do the mental and physical activities they would like to do or accomplish goals that they have set for themselves. Many of these patients become disabled in the age category that should represent the time of their major contribution to society. Physician visits, diagnostic testing, long-term medical therapy, alternative minimal invasive therapies, and surgery in some instances are expensive. The economic costs of prostatitis have been found to be enormous and based on the estimated number of patients in the USA alone, it could reach hundreds of millions of dollars a year.[10]

Etiology

Prostatitis can present clinically as an acute or chronic syndrome and etiologically as an infectious or non-infectious process. The etiology of acute prostatitis is almost invariably infectious and the agents implicated are usually *Enterobacteriaceae* spp. (particularly *Escherichia coli* but also *Klebsiella pseudomonas* and other *Enterobacteriaceae* spp.) and occasionally Gram-positive *Enterococci* spp. A small percentage (estimated to be between 5% and 10%) of cases of chronic prostatitis appear to have either an etiology or an association with chronic infection of the prostate gland (with similar organisms as acute bacterial prostatitis). Patients with an infectious chronic prostatitis suffer acute exacerbations, which usually resolve with appropriate antibiotic therapy. However, because the bacteria can persist as a nidus in the prostate gland, patients with chronic bacterial prostatitis are characterized by recurrent episodes of infection. Patients may be asymptomatic between these acute infectious episodes while the bacteria lie dormant in the prostate gland. The *Enterobacteriaceae* (*E. coli*, *Klebsiella* spp., *Pseudomonas* spp.) and *Enterococcus* spp. remain the most common organisms isolated but many investigators believe that *Chlamydia* spp., *Mycoplasma* spp., and perhaps even anaerobic bacteria such as *Corynebacterium* spp. and in some specific cases (such as immunocompromised patients) fungi, viruses, and other atypical pathogens may also be involved.[11]

Significant controversy exists in the research community in relation to patients who suffer from chronic prostatitis symptoms and who have no history of urinary tract infection (UTI) but in whom bacteria are localized to the prostate gland. The controversy exists because recent studies, employing standard clinical microbiological techniques,[12] have indicated that asymptomatic men who do not suffer from prostatitis have the same prevalence of uropathogenic and non-uropathogenic bacteria localized to the prostate.

The majority of patients with a chronic prostatitis syndrome do not have recurrent UTI and do not have bacteria localized to the prostate gland. A number of inter-related factors are thought to play a role in the multifactorial etiology of the syndrome. It is believed that the process begins by various initiators (different for each individual) starting a cascade of events in a patient who is anatomically or perhaps genetically susceptible to develop the syndrome. The initiators include infection, immunogens, trauma, and dysfunctional voiding. The anatomic abnormalities include lower urinary tract obstruction (bladder neck stenosis, detrusor sphincter incoordination, urethral stricture, and meatal

stenosis) and intra-prostatic ductal reflux (perhaps due to prostatic ducts entering the prostatic urethra at a less acute angle).[13] High-pressure dysfunctional voiding causes turbulence, which further exacerbates the problem, and urine with potentially harmful and toxic constituents (such as potassium and immunogenic proteins) or micro-organisms can reflux in the prostatic ducts and the acini, causing prostatic inflammation.[14]

There is no doubt that some patients presenting with a chronic prostatitis syndrome directly develop the symptom complex from trauma, usually repetitive perineal trauma (such as from bicycle riding, horse riding, and poorly designed and suspended heavy equipment and vehicle seats).

Other investigators feel that prostatitis results from a primary immunologic problem, perhaps even an autoimmune process. In this hypothesis, the chronic inflammation can be propagated by autoimmune mechanisms even when the initiating agent has been eradicated or resolved or has disappeared. Many investigators and clinicians believe that patients who suffer from chronic prostatitis for many months or many years eventually develop a typical neuropathic pain pattern, associated with local muscular dysfunction.[15]

In summary then, this author believes that chronic prostatitis and its associated chronic pelvic pain syndrome is not secondary to a single defined etiologic agent but is rather a syndrome consisting of a continuous spectrum, initiated and propagated by multiple and probably inter-related factors. The initiators could be infection, high-pressure dysfunctional voiding, trauma, or some unknown toxin. This initiating event results in either injury or inflammation, or both. The initial neuropathy, muscular dysfunction, or immunologic reaction can progress because of persisting initiating factors (persistence of bacteria, dysfunctional voiding, or perineal trauma), or the pathology could persist even with eradication or amelioration of these factors through self-perpetuating stimulatory loops (inflammation by autoimmune mechanism, while peripheral neuropathy can progress because of upregulation of the local pelvic neuroloop and 'wind up' of the spinal cord – in other words, central nervous system sensitization). The symptom complex and particularly its impact on quality of life and activities is modulated by psychosocial parameters such as depression, stress, anxiety and coping mechanisms (both beneficial and maladaptive).

Classification

Classification of the prostatitis syndromes relies on history, physical examination, and microbiological and cytological evaluation of lower urinary tract specimens. Traditionally the classification system consisted of acute bacterial prostatitis, chronic bacterial prostatitis, chronic non-bacterial prostatitis, and prostatodynia.[16] Many investigators and clinicians have long realized that the prostate gland may not be involved at all in many patients presenting with a 'chronic prostatitis syndrome'.

The National Institutes of Health (NIH) classification system,[17] which is now accepted both in North America and internationally as the accepted system to differentiate patients for research and clinical trials but also clinical practice, consists of four categories. Category I is similar to acute bacterial prostatitis and is associated with acute infection of the prostate gland. Category II is similar to chronic bacterial prostatitis and is associated with chronic infection of the prostate gland. Category III, chronic pelvic pain syndrome (CPPS), is diagnosed when patients present with pain or discomfort in the pelvic region for longer than 3 months and no uropathogenic bacteria localized to prostate-specific specimens (expressed prostatic secretion, post-prostatic massage urine, or semen) on standard culture. This category was further subdivided into an inflammatory group (category IIIA CPPS), which is very similar to the previous categorization of chronic non-bacterial prostatitis, and a non-inflammatory group (category IIIB CPPS), which is very similar to the old traditional classification of prostatodynia. Category IIIA was differentiated from category IIIB based on the degree of leukocytosis (the number of white blood cells) in the prostate-specific specimens (prostatic fluid, semen, or urine sediment after prostate massage). Unfortunately, no study to date has validated this sub-categorization of category III as an important clinical differentiation. The NIH classification also includes a unique and very interesting new category, category IV, or asymptomatic inflammatory prostatitis (AIP). Patients with category IV AIP are asymptomatic; the inflammation is noted on prostate-specific specimens or even histological preparations and is usually an incidental finding in patients being assessed for elevated prostate-specific antigen (PSA), benign prostatic hyperplasia, or infertility. Table 27.1 describes the NIH classification system.

Clinical presentation

Category I: acute bacterial prostatitis
Patients in category I (acute bacterial prostatitis) present with acute local and systemic symptoms. These include severe perineal and suprapubic pain, irritative and obstructive voiding symptoms associated with dysuria, and in most cases generalized symptoms such as fever, aches, and pains.

Category II: chronic bacterial prostatitis
Patients in category II (chronic bacterial prostatitis) may not be symptomatic between flare-ups and they are clinically characterized by UTI usually with the same organisms. Following successful antibiotic therapy many patients, but not all, become asymptomatic. Some patients continue to have symptoms that are indistinguishable from patients who present with category III CPPS.

Category III: chronic pelvic pain syndrome
CPPS is characterized by a characteristic constellation of symptoms in patients with no clinical evidence or history of urinary tract infection. These patients usually have a long history (by definition longer than 3 months) of genitourinary and pelvic pain and of irritative and obstructive voiding symptoms, and perhaps symptoms of sexual dysfunction; many have other associated generalized symptoms such as fatigue or 'aches and pains'. Pain or discomfort is usually localized to the perineum, suprapubic area, penis, testicles, or scrotum and the patient may complain of pain during or after ejaculation and discomfort or dysuria during and after voiding. Symptoms tend to wax and wane (hourly, daily, weekly, and monthly).

Table 27.1. *National Institutes of Health classification system for the prostatitis syndromes[17]*

Category	Description	Presentation
Category I	Acute infection of the prostate gland	Acute febrile illness associated with perineal and suprapubic pain, dysuria, and obstructive voiding symptoms
Category II	Chronic infection of the prostate	Recurrent urinary tract infections (usually with the same organism) associated frequently with voiding disturbances
Category III Chronic pelvic pain syndrome	Chronic genital urinary pain in the absence of uropathogenic bacteria localized to the prostate gland employing standard methodology	Chronic perineal, suprapubic, groin, testicular, penile, ejaculatory pain associated with variable dysuria and obstructive and irritative voiding symptoms
Category IIIA Inflammatory chronic pelvic pain syndrome	Significant number of white blood cells in expressed prostatic secretions, post-prostatic massage urine sediment, or semen	
Category IIIB Non-inflammatory chronic pelvic pain syndrome	Insignificant number of white blood cells in expressed prostatic secretions, post-prostatic massage urine sediment, or semen	
Category IV Asymptomatic inflammatory prostatitis	White blood cells (and/or bacteria) in expressed prostatic secretions, post-prostatic massage urine sediment, semen, or histological specimens of the prostate gland	Asymptomatic

Diagnosis and evaluation

Category I: acute bacterial prostatitis

Assessment of a patient suspected of having acute bacterial prostatitis includes a history of the relevant symptoms and a physical examination, with examination of the abdomen, external genitalia, and perineum and a digital rectal examination. The prostate is usually boggy and exquisitely tender on examination as is the perineum and suprapubic area on palpation. Before any treatment is instituted, a midstream urine collection for culture is mandatory. If the patient is septic, blood cultures are indicated as well.

Category II: chronic bacterial prostatitis

If patients present with an acute episode of cystourethritis, antibiotic treatment after midstream urine cultures is appropriate. If patients continue to have recurrent UTI or persistent symptoms, a thorough history, physical examination, urinalysis and urine culture are mandatory.

Traditionally, the Meares–Stamey four-glass test (Fig. 27.1) has been recommended to localize bacteria to the prostate gland, thus justifying long-term antibiotic therapy.[18] Bacteria or leukocytosis in the initial first voided specimen (VB1) indicates urethritis. Uropathogenic bacteria in a midstream urine specimen (VB2) would indicate that the

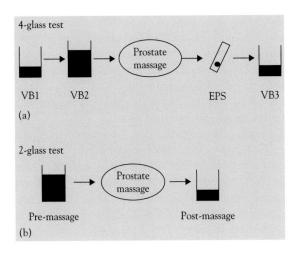

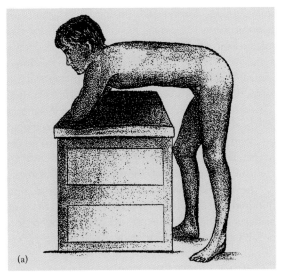

Figure 27.1. (a) Meares–Stamey four-glass test[18] and (b) pre- and post-massage two-glass test.[20]

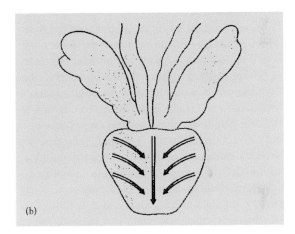

patient has either a primary or associated cystitis. Prostate-specific specimens are obtained after first obtaining VB1 and VB2 and carefully performing a digital rectal examination. The technique for prostatic massage is described in Fig. 27.2. This technique may also be used for treatment in patients who discover amelioration of their symptoms with this technique. Uropathogenic bacteria in the expressed prostatic secretion or post-prostatic massage urine specimen (VB3) would lead to a diagnosis of bacterial prostatitis, if the same bacteria were not present (or cultured in a one hundred-fold less concentration) in the VB1 and VB2. However, many physicians, including urologists, do not perform this test unless the patients have been selected to participate in clinical research trials. The tests are cumbersome, expensive, and difficult and many clinicians believe that the results do not change their therapeutic decision-making.[19]

It does not appear to be justified to prescribe treatment without any type of lower urinary tract evaluation and therefore, the pre- and post-massage two-glass test was introduced so the physicians could perform an adequate, simple evaluation of the culture and inflammatory status of the lower urinary tract (see Fig. 28.1).[20] A midstream urine specimen (pre-prostatic massage urine) is taken and sent to the laboratory for culture and microscopy of the sediment. Following vigorous prostatic massage, the

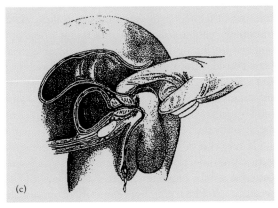

Figure 27.2. Technique of doing a (a) correct digital rectal examination and a (b) diagnostic and (c) therapeutic prostatic massage.[54]

initial stream of urine (post-prostatic massage urine) is also sent as a separate specimen for culture and microscopic examination of the sediment. Uropathogenic bacteria localized to the pre-massage specimen indicate bacterial presence within the prostate gland and a subsequent diagnosis of category II prostatitis. This test provides a very useful screen and if bacteria are localized to the post-massage specimen, it would be ideal (but not necessary in most cases) to go on to perform the Meares–Stamey four-glass test to confirm absolutely that the bacteria are localized to the prostate gland by noting at least a one hundred-fold increase in concentration of that bacteria in either the expressed prostatic secretion or VB3 compared with VB1 or VB2.

Category III: chronic pelvic pain syndrome

There are no objective signs or laboratory tests that would definitely differentiate a man with CPPS from a normal man without asymptomatic prostatitis. The evaluation consists of a careful history, since a syndrome is best diagnosed by the constellation of symptoms with which it is associated. Except for eliciting pain and various painful trigger points in the pelvis, perineum, or external genitalia, the physical examination does not contribute much information. The prostate can feel normal, firm, or soft (boggy) while in most cases palpation of the prostate does elicit tenderness and it is difficult to use this as a diagnostic tool. The primary importance of the history and physical examination is to rule out other causes of pain and discomfort. As a minimum, patients require a midstream urinalysis and culture, but in these patients it is advisable to at least consider the pre- and post-massage screening test (see Fig. 27.1). As in category II, it may be important to proceed to the more complicated and difficult four-glass test (see Fig. 27.1) if bacteria are localized to the post-massage specimen.

It has always been advocated that in patients with a non-infectious, chronic prostatitis syndrome (non-bacterial prostatitis, prostatodynia, or – recently – CPPS) it is important to determine if it falls into an inflammatory or non-inflammatory category by examining the number of white blood cells in prostate-specific specimens. While this is still an interesting exercise, studies have not indicated any clinical value in differentiating patients into these inflammatory or non-inflammatory categories at this time.[12] In the future, however, clinical studies evaluating various treatment modalities may determine that some patients with inflammatory or non-inflammatory status react differently to different treatment modalities.

In an attempt to develop a consensus in regard to evaluation of the man presenting with chronic prostatitis or CPPS, prostatitis experts have attempted to provide a best evidence-based approach to the clinical workup of patients presenting with a prostatitis syndrome. Table 27.2 describes one such suggested evaluation based on a North American consensus meeting.[21] Mandatory evaluations include the history and physical examination, urinalysis, and midstream urine specimen, as outlined above. Optional investigations include the previously described Meares–Stamey four-glass test (or the simpler pre- and post-massage screening test), a urine cytology (to rule out the possibility of cancer or carcinoma in situ of the bladder) using standardized symptom assessment index (see below), and a flow rate and residual urine determination (usually done in the urologist's office). Optional evaluations include a urethral swab for culture, semen analysis, cystoscopy, transrectal ultrasound, abdominal and pelvic radiologic evaluations (ultrasound, computed tomography scan, magnetic resonance imaging), sophisticated urodynamics, and serum PSA determination. Except for the serum PSA, which should be performed only in men who would normally be screened for prostate cancer, these optional evaluations will probably be entertained only by specialists or urologists that are assessing difficult prostatitis cases that have not been adequately addressed (either diagnostically or therapeutically) with the mandatory and recommended tests noted above.

The NIH chronic prostatitis symptom index (NIH-CPSI)[22] was developed as a practical, validated, and reliable symptom assessment tool for research in chronic prostatitis. During the validation of this index, it was discovered that the prostatitis experience could be adequately explored by examining the pain and discomfort symptoms (location, frequency, and severity), the irritative and obstructive voiding symptoms, and the impact of these symptoms on the patient's quality of life. Nine separate items

Table 27.2. *Evaluation of a man with chronic pelvic pain syndrome*

A consensus meeting of the National Institutes of Health Chronic Prostatitis Collaborative Research Network met during a 1-day symposium in Chantilly, Virginia, USA, 26 March, 2002, to develop a working consensus regarding the appropriate management of chronic prostatitis and chronic pelvic pain syndrome.[21]

Mandatory

History

Physical examination, including digital rectal examination

Urinalysis and urine culture

Recommended

Lower urinary tract localization test

Symptom inventory or index (NIH-CPSI)

Flow rate

Residual urine determination

Urine cytology

Optional

Semen analysis and culture

Urethral swab for culture

Pressure flow studies

Video urodynamics (including flow electromyography)

Cystoscopy

Transrectal ultrasound

Pelvic imaging (ultrasound, computed tomography scan, magnetic resonance imaging)

Prostate-specific antigen

NIH-CPSI, National Institutes of Health Chronic Prostatitis Symptom Index.

that could be answered by most patients in about 5 minutes addressed all these important issues. The six major locations or type of pain or discomfort, the frequency of pain or discomfort, and the severity of pain or discomfort were rated on a scale of 0–21.

The irritative and obstructive voiding symptoms were rated on a score of 0–10, while the impact on quality of life was rated on a score of 0–12. Each of these domains could be assessed independently or the three could be added together for a total NIH-CPSI score of 0–43. The NIH-CPSI not only proved to be invaluable in prostatitis research (in epidemiologic studies, longitudinal natural history studies, and treatment trials) but even more importantly, the NIH-CPSI has proved itself as a valuable tool for the practicing physician to evaluate a patient at initial presentation and to follow him over time to assess treatment outcomes.[23] The NIH-CPSI is presented in Appendix 27.1.

Therapy

Category I: acute bacterial prostatitis

The objectives of treatment of this acute bacterial infection are simple, once the clinical diagnosis has been made and the appropriate cultures have been taken.[24] Urinary drainage must be optimized and this may entail insertion of a small-caliber urethral catheter. (If that can't be tolerated, a small-caliber suprapubic tube must be considered.)

The patient should be started initially on intravenous, broad-spectrum antibiotic therapy. The best drugs are either (1) a combination of a penicillin (e.g. ampicillin) and an aminoglycoside (e.g. gentamicin), (2) a second- or third-generation cephalosporin, or (3) one of the fluoroquinolones. The patient is then switched to a specific oral antibiotic, based on culture and sensitivity data, as soon as the acute infection has settled down. The best oral antibiotics are one of the fluoroquinolones, trimethoprim, or trimethoprim–sulfamethoxazole. The fluoroquinolone class of antibiotics appears to be superior. Antibiotics are continued for 2–4 weeks.

General supportive care includes anti-pyrexial analgesics and, if required, intravenous fluid replacement. Close follow-up in the first 36–48 hours is required since the occasional patient may develop an abscess. These patients are characterized by failure to respond to appropriate therapy within 36–48 hours. Prostatic abscesses are best drained (usually transurethrally) by a urologic specialist.

Category II: chronic bacterial prostatitis

In patients who have recurrent UTI (whether they are symptomatic or not between infections) and in whom the bacteria are localized to the prostate gland require long-term antimicrobial therapy.[25] Optimal antibiotic therapy includes trimethroprim (or trimethoprim–sulfamethoxazole) and the fluoroquinolones. Although trimethroprim–sulfamethoxazole is the most studied antibiotic in prostatitis, the penetration of the fluoroquinolones into the prostate gland and the increased bacterial susceptibility to this class of drug makes them superior to trimethoprim or trimethoprim–sulfamethoxazole. Clinical studies have confirmed the improved efficacy of fluoroquinolones over trimethroprim or trimethoprim–sulfamethoxazole.[26] The duration of therapy is controversial and suggestions have ranged from 4 weeks to 12 weeks.[27] Since there is the very real possibility of persistence, the physician should err on the side of too much antibiotic rather than too little.

Even with appropriate antibiotic therapy some patients have either recurrence of UTI or persistence of lower urinary tract symptoms. In such patients, it appears justified to change the class of antibiotics and perhaps even change the antibiotic within the class (for instance, ciprofloxacin appears to be superior to norfloxacin). There is some theoretical and anecdotal evidence and even some clinical trial experience showing that adding tetracycline (doxycycline) or a macrolide (azithromycin or clarithromycin) may be of benefit. In patients who continue to have recurrent UTI or in whom symptoms recur when the antibiotics are discontinued, low-dose, long-term suppressive therapy may have to be considered.

A number of investigators have advocated the combination of prostatic massage and antibiotic therapy.[28,29] Theoretically prostatic massage may improve prostatic ductal drainage and improve antibiotic penetration. Up to this point, the evidence remains anecdotal but this approach should be considered in refractory patients. There is weak evidence that the addition of an α-blocker to antibiotic therapy may reduce the recurrence rate of patients with chronic bacterial prostatitis.[30] Surgery should be considered only as a last resort to treat chronic bacterial prostatitis. There are a few studies in the literature (primarily case reports) employing radical transurethral resection of the prostate gland or open prostatectomy.[31] This treatment should be entertained only in patients with documented chronic bacterial prostatitis who have recurrent lower UTI with the same organism despite prolonged courses of antibiotics, in whom the organism can be localized to the prostate between documented infections, and in whom prostatic calculi are present. Another indication would be an incidental diagnosis of concurrent prostate cancer.

Category III: chronic pelvic pain syndrome

Patients who are diagnosed with CPPS complain of long-term pain and voiding disturbances as well as sexual disturbances, all of which have a severe impact on their quality of life. These patients do not have documented infection but may have demonstrable inflammation. Physicians must individualize a therapeutic plan according to the patient's presenting symptoms, clinical findings, and the course over time. Both physicians and patients must have a realistic expectation of treatment goals in this syndrome, especially since patients' symptoms wax and wane and often cannot be completely eradicted by a physician's intervention. The physician's job is to ameliorate symptoms, decrease the impact the condition has on the patient's daily activities, and consequently improve the patient's quality of life. The goal of therapy may be only amelioration of symptoms rather than a complete cure. A 25% improvement in the NIH-CPSI symptom score is a perceptible and even acceptable improvement in some patients with CPPS. A 50% improvement in this score should be considered an excellent response to therapy. These types of realistic therapy goals are achievable.

Tables 27.3 and 27.4 outline the various therapies, drugs and interventions that have been reported to help some patients with CPPS. The most important and empowering intervention a physician could provide is an empathic discussion of the diagnosis and realistic therapeutic expectations for CPPS. The patient must be reassured that the condition does not usually progress over time and in fact tends to wax and wane and eventually improve over time. He should be counseled that prostatitis is not

Table 27.3. *Medical therapy for chronic prostatitis and chronic pelvic pain syndrome (categories II and III)*

Medication	Dose
Antibiotics	
Trimethoprim–sulfamethoxazole	800/160 mg twice daily
Norfloxacin	400 mg twice daily
Ciprofloxacin	500 mg twice daily
Ofloxacin	300 mg twice daily
Lomefloxacin	400 mg once daily
Levofloxacin	500 mg once daily
Gatifloxacin	400 mg once daily
Moxifloxacin	400 mg once daily
Doxycycline	100 mg twice daily
Erythromycin	500 mg four times daily
Azithromycin	250–500 mg once daily
Clarithromycin	500 mg twice daily
α-blockers	
Terazosin	5–10 mg daily
Doxazosin	4–8 mg daily
Tamsulosin	0.4–0.8 mg daily
Alfusozin	10 mg daily
Anti-inflammatory agents	
Ibuprofen	400–600 mg four to six times daily
Diclofenac	25–50 mg three times daily
Indomethacin	25–50 mg three times daily
Rofecoxib	25–50 mg three times daily
Celecoxib	100–200 mg twice daily
Pentosan polysulfate	100–300 mg three times daily

(Continued)

Table 27.3. *(Continued)*

Medication	Dose
Hormonal agents	
Finasteride	5 mg daily
Muscle relaxants	
Diazepam	5–10 mg daily
Baclofen	5–20 mg three times daily
Cyclobenzaprine	10 mg three times daily
Phytotherapeutic agents	
Quercetin	500 mg twice daily
Saw palmetto	160 mg twice daily
Pollen extract	1 tablet three times daily
Tricyclic antidepressants	
Amitriptyline	10–100 mg daily
Neuromodulatory agents	
Gabapentin	300–600 mg three times daily
Pregabalin	50–100 mg three times daily

associated with prostate cancer (but he has the same risk of developing prostate cancer as asymptomatic men). The patient should avoid stress and anxiety and physical activity that aggravates the situation (such as bicycle riding), long periods of sitting (or should at least modify the seat with a donut or air cushion) and should consider the use of gentle local heat application (with, for instance, hot sitz baths, heating pads, heated car seats). Advice regarding diet should be based on the patient's experience – occasionally avoiding caffeine, alcohol, and spicy or acidic foods and drinks may help to control the symptoms in particular patients.

Almost every patient diagnosed with chronic prostatitis is eventually treated with antibiotics; despite no documented infection. Theoretically they should not be treated with antibiotics, however,

Table 27.4. *Other therapies employed in the treatment of chronic pelvic pain syndrome*

Physical therapies

Repetitive prostate massage

Myofascial trigger point release therapy

Relaxation exercise

Biofeedback

Neuromodulation therapies

Acupuncture

Cognitive behavioral therapies

Minimally invasive therapies

Transurethral microwave thermal therapy

Transrectal hyperthermia

Other heat therapies

Transurethral balloon dilatation

Transurethral needle ablation of the prostate

Prostatic laser therapies

Invasive neuromodulation

Surgery

Circumcision (phimosis causing obstruction, chronic balanitis or recurrent urinary tract infection)

Urethral stricture surgery

Drainage of prostatic abscesses, large prostatic cysts, or obstructive ejaculatory ducts

Seminal vesicular surgery for documented seminal vesicular pathology

Transurethral incision of the bladder neck

Radical transurethral resection of the prostate

Radical prostatectomy

many patients do seem to improve with antibiotics. Studies consistently show that approximately 40% of patients treated with antibiotics show significant clinical improvement.[27,32] Studies, however, have indicated that if patients don't respond to a 4-week trial of antibiotic therapy, they will probably not respond to further antibiotic therapy. Based on theoretical grounds only, the fluoroquinolone class of antibiotics would appear to be the best choice of therapy. Some clinicians justify a trial of either a tetracycline (doxycycline) or a macrolide (azithromycin, clarithromycin) because of the possibility of a chlamydial or mycoplasmal infection. Two large multi-center, randomized, controlled trials comparing antibiotic therapy (in one case levofloxacin and the other ciprofloxacin) versus placebo have been recently reported.[33,34] These trials indicate that antibiotic therapy may not be much more successful than placebo therapy in CPPS patients with disease of long duration.

Prospective placebo-controlled studies have indicated that α-blocker therapy may benefit patients presenting with CPPS, but the data are conflicting.[34-37] A look at the evidence from these four prospective treatment studies would indicate that the therapy works best in α-blocker naïve patients who have become recently symptomatic or have been recently diagnosed and that the therapy must be prolonged for much longer than 6 weeks to be successful.

Anti-inflammatory agents also appear to benefit some patients with CPPS but they must be given in high doses and for reasonably long durations (at a minimum, 6 weeks). One large multi-center study has shown that the use of a cyclo-oxygenase-2 inhibitor results in minor amelioration of symptoms compared with placebo following 6 weeks of therapy.[38] Another anti-inflammatory agent, pentosan polysulfate, has been used to ameliorate the symptoms of interstitial cystitis (an inflammatory CPPS of the bladder, which occurs primarily in females). An uncontrolled pilot study[39] and one recently reported multi-center placebo controlled trial[40] would indicate that pentosan polysulfate may benefit some men with CPPS as well.

Finasteride, a 5-α-reductase inhibitor that has been employed in the treatment of benign prostatic hyperplasia, has also been evaluated for the treatment of CPPS. Trials have suggested that there may be some treatment benefit in using finasteride,[41] but the treatment effect is very modest when compared to placebo.[42,43]

Phytotherapeutic agents (plant extract or herbal remedies) have been tested in small clinical trials.[44] Quercetin (a natural bioflavinoid) and pollen extract (cernilton) have demonstrated clinical evidence of benefit in patients with chronic prostatitis.[45,46] Larger multi-center, randomized, placebo-controlled trials are needed to assess the real effect of these herbal extracts.

Many other medical therapies have been advocated for the treatment of CPPS but many of these have not been adequately tested. Certainly many patients are successfully treated with skeletal muscle relaxants (diazepam, baclofen, or cyclobenzaprine), tricyclic antidepressants (amitriptyline), and neuromodulatory agents (gabapentin or pregabalin).[15]

Physical therapies have always been important in the treatment of CPPS. For most of the last century, repetitive prostate massage has been the therapy of choice (and before antibiotic therapy was introduced it was the only therapy available). Anecdotally, many patients felt that they obtained significant relief of symptoms (at least enough to submit repeatedly to this uncomfortable procedure). Prostatic massage fell out of fashion with physicians in the 1970s and 1980s only to re-emerge as a potential therapy in the 1990s following a number of international reports of success. Anecdotal evidence would suggest that as many as one-third and perhaps as many as two-thirds of patients may respond to some degree of repetitive prostate massage.[29] (See Fig. 27.2 for details of how prostatic massage should be done.) Others[47-51] have reported treatment of trigger points associated with the development of myofascial pain with heat therapy, physiotherapy massage, ischemic compression, stretching and progressive relaxation exercise, anesthetic injections, electroneuromodulation, yoga, biofeedback, and acupuncture.

Almost every minimally invasive therapeutic procedure evaluated for benign prostatic hyperplasia has been advocated for the treatment of prostatitis. Transurethral balloon dilatation, transurethral needle ablation of the prostate, transurethral laser therapy, and localized heat application employing transrectal hyperthermia or transurethral thermal therapy have all been tested in small uncontrolled pilot studies.[15] These therapies cannot be generally advocated until randomized, sham-controlled trials are available.

Surgery does not have an important role in the treatment of most cases of CPPS unless a specific indication is discovered during the evaluation of the patient.[14] Severe obstructive phimosis,

meatal stenosis, urethral stricture, documented seminal vesicle pathology, obstructed ejaculatory ducts, prostatic cysts, and bladder neck obstructions are all potential conditions that may be associated with refractory CPPS. These conditions are amenable to surgical treatment and such treatment may result in improvement of voiding symptoms and subsequent amelioration of pain and discomfort associated with CPPS. Radical transurethral resection of the prostate or even radical prostatectomy should not be advocated in patients with CPPS who do not have localized infection or prostate cancer.

Our increasing understanding of the 'biopsychosocial' aspects that influence a patient's life has demonstrated that pain, disability, and quality of life are predicted by depression, degree of social support, and various maladaptive pain coping techniques (such as catastrophizing).[52,53] Cognitive behavioral treatment protocols for CPPS, which aim at increasing tolerance of chronic pain, decreasing disability, and improving quality of life, are presently being developed and evaluated. This therapeutic alternative will be attractive for patients who do not respond to traditional medical therapy.

Category IV: asymptomatic inflammatory prostatitis

Patients diagnosed with category IV disease (asymptomatic inflammatory prostatitis) are asymptomatic, and most do not require any therapy. Antibiotic therapy (and perhaps anti-inflammatory therapy) may be contemplated in some men with mildly elevated PSA, particularly if prostatic inflammation is noted on biopsies, and perhaps in selected infertile men with leukospermia.

Conclusions

Our understanding of the prostatitis syndromes and their classification, etiology, diagnosis, and treatment has undergone more dramatic changes in the past decade than in the previous hundred years. While we still do not understand the exact etiology for most cases of CPPS, the standardized clinical definitions and classification systems, and the development of validated outcome parameters and a consensus on diagnostic algorithms have significantly improved our initial evaluation of the patient presenting with a prostatitis syndrome. Many large multi-center, randomized, placebo-controlled trials have been initiated and supported by peer-reviewed and pharmaceutical funding agencies, to evaluate the treatment modalities available. In the coming years, we will be able to manage patients using an evidence-based management strategy.

References

1. Roberts RO, Lieber MM, Rhodes T et al. Prevalence of a physician-assigned diagnosis of prostatitis: the Olmsted County study of urinary symptoms and health status among men. Urology 1998; 51: 578–84.

2. Mehik A, Hellstrom P, Lukkarinen O et al. Epidemiology of prostatitis in Finnish men: a population-based cross-sectional study. BJU Int 2001; 86: 443–8.

3. McNaughton-Collins M, Meigs JB, Barry MJ et al. Prevalence and correlates of prostatitis in the health professionals follow-up study cohort. J Urol 2002; 167: 1363–6.

4. Nickel JC, Downey J, Hunter D, Clark J. Prevalance of prostatitis-like symptoms in a population based study employing the NIH-chronic prostatitis symptom index (NIH-CPSI). J Urol 2001; 165: 842–5.

5. Moon TD. Questionnaire survey of urologists and primary care physicians' diagnostic and treatment practices for prostatitis. Urology 1997; 50: 543–7.

6. Roberts RO, Jacobson DJ, Girman CJ et al. Prevalence of prostatitis-like symptoms in a community based cohort of older men. J Urol 2002; 168: 2467–71.

7. McNaughton-Collins M, Stafford RS, O'Leary MP, Barry MJ. How common is prostatitis? A national survey of physician visits. J Urol 1998; 159: 1224–8.

8. Wenninger K, Heiman JR, Rothman I et al. Sickness impact of chronic nonbacterial prostatitis and its correlates. J Urol 1996; 155: 965–8.

9. McNaughton-Collins M, Pontari MA, O'Leary MP et al. Quality of life is impaired in men with chronic prostatitis: the Chronic Prostatitis Collaborative Research Network. J Gen Intern Med 2001; 16: 565–662.

10. Calhoun EA, McNaughton Collins M, Pontari MA et al. Chronic Prostatitis Collaborative Research Network. The economic impact of chronic prostatitis. Arch Intern Med 2004; 164: 1231–6.

11. Nickel JC, Moon T. Chronic bacterial prostatitis: an evolving clinical enigma. Urology 2005; 66: 2–8.

12. Nickel JC, Alexander RB, Schaeffer AJ et al. Leukocytes and bacteria in men with chronic prostatitis/chronic pelvic pain syndrome compared to asymptomatic controls. J Urol 2003; 170: 818–22.

13. Blacklock NJ. Anatomical factors in prostatitis. Br J Urol 1974; 46: 47–54.

14. Kirby RS, Lowe D, Bultitude MI, Shuttleworth KED. Intraprostatic urinary reflux: an aetiological factor in abacterial prostatitis. Br J Urol 1982; 54: 729–31.

15. Nickel JC. Inflammatory conditions of the male genitourinary tract: prostatitis and related conditions, orchitis, and epididymitis. In Wein AJ et al., eds. Campbell–Walsh Urology, 9th edn. Philadelphia: WB Saunders, 2007; 304–29.

16. Drach GW, Fair WR, Meares EM, Stamey TA. Classification of benign diseases associated with prostatic pain: prostatitis or prostatodynia? J Urol 1978; 120: 266.

17. Krieger JN, Nyberg LJ, Nickel JC. NIH consensus definition and classification of prostatitis. JAMA 1999; 282: 36.

18. Meares EM Jr, Stamey TA Bacteriologic localization patterns in bacterial prostatitis and urethritis. Invest Urol 1968; 5: 492–518.

19. McNaughton-Collins M, Fowler EH, Elliott DB et al. Diagnosing and treating chronic prostatitis: do urologists use the 4-glass test? Urology 2000; 55: 403–7.

20. Nickel JC. The Pre and Post Massage Test (PPMT): a simple screen for prostatitis. Tech Urol 1997; 3: 38–43.

21. Nickel JC. Clinical evaluation of the man with chronic prostatitis/chronic pelvic pain syndrome. Urology 2002; 60: 20–3.

22. Litwin MS, McNaughton-Collins M, Fowler FJJ et al. The National Institutes of Health Chronic Prostatitis Symptoms Index: development and validation of a new outcome measure. J Urol 1999; 162: 369–75.

23. Nickel JC, McNaughton-Collins M, Litwin SM. Development and use of a validated outcome measure for prostatitis. J Clin Outcomes Manage 2001; 8: 30–7.

24. Neal DE Jr. Treatment of acute prostatitis. In: Nickel JC, ed. Textbook of Prostatitis. Oxford: Isis Medical Media, 1999: 279–84.

25. Nickel JC, Weidner W. Chronic prostatitis: current concepts in antimicrobial therapy. Infect Urol 2000; 13: S22–9.

26. Naber KJ. Antibiotic treatment of chronic bacterial prostatitis. In: Nickel JC, ed. Textbook of Prostatitis. Oxford: Isis Medical Media, 1999: 283–92.

27. Bjerklund Johansen T, Gruneberg RN, Guibert J et al. The role of antibiotics in the treatment of chronic prostatitis: a consensus statement. Eur Urol 1998; 34: 457–66.

28. Shoskes DA, Zeitlin SI. Use of prostatic massage in combination with antibiotics in the treatment of chronic prostatitis. Prostate Cancer Prostatic Dis 1999; 2: 159–62.

29. Nickel JC, Alexander R, Anderson R et al. Prostatitis Unplugged: Prostate massage revisited. Tech Urol 1999; 5: 1–7.

30. Barbalias GA, Nikiforidis G, Liatsikos EN. Alpha-blockers for the treatment of chronic prostatitis in combination with antibiotics. J Urol 1998; 159: 883–7.

31. Kirby RS. Surgical considerations in the mangement of prostatitis. In: Nickel JC, ed. Oxford: Isis Medical Media, 1999: 346–64.

32. Nickel JC, Downey J, Johnston B, Clark J, the Canadian Prostatitis Research Group. Predictors of patient response to antibiotic therapy for chronic prostatitis/chronic pelvic pain syndrome: a prospective muliticenter clinical trial. J Urol 2001; 165: 1539–44.

33. Nickel JC, Downey J, Clark J et al. Levofloxacin for chronic prostatitis/chronic pelvic pain syndrome in men: A randomized placebo-controlled multicenter trial. Urology 2003; 62: 614–17.

34. Alexander RB, Propert KJ, Schaeffer AJ et al. Ciprofloxacin or tamsulosin in men with chronic prostatitis/chronic pelvic pain syndrome. Ann Intern Med 2004; 141: 581–9.

35. Cheah PY, Liong ML, Yuen KH et al. Terazosin therapy for chronic prostatitis/chronic pelvic pain syndrome: a randomized, placebo controlled trial. J Urol 2003; 169: 592–6.

36. Mehik A, Alas P, Nickel JC, Sarpola A, Helstrom PJ. Alfuzosin treatment for chronic prostatitis/chronic pelvic pain syndrome: A prospective, randomized, double-blind, placebo-controlled, pilot study. Urology 2003; 63: 425–9.

37. Nickel JC, Narayan P, McKay J, Doyle C. Treatment of chronic prostatitis/chronic pelvic pain syndrome with tamsulosin: a randomized double-blind trial. J Urol 2004; 171: 1594–7.

38. Nickel JC, Pontari M, Moon T et al. A randomized, placebo-controlled, multicenter study to evaluate the safety and efficacy of rofecoxib in the treatment of chronic nonbacterial prostatitis. J Urol 2003; 169: 1401–5.

39. Nickel JC, Johnston Downey J et al. Pentosan poly-sulfate therapy for chronic nonbacterial prostatitis (chronic plevic pain syndrome category IIIA): A prospective multicenter clinical trial. Urology 2000; 56: 413–7.

40. Nickel JC, Forrest JB, Tomera K et al. Pentosan polysulfate sodium therapy for men with chronic pelvic pain syndrome: a multicenter, randomized, placebo-controlled study. J Urol 2005; 173: 1252–5.

41. Nickel JC. 5 alpha reductase therapy for chronic prostatitis. In: Nickel JC, ed. Textbook of Prostatitis. Oxford: Isis Medical Media, 1999: 333–7.

42. Leskinen M, Lukkarinen O, Marttila T. Effects of finasteride in patients with inflammatory chronic pelvic pain syndrome: a double-blind, placebo controlled, pilot study. Urology 1999; 53: 502–5.

43. Nickel JC, Downey J, Pontari MA, Shoskes DA, Zeitlin ZI. Randomized placebo-controlled, multi-center study to evaluate the safety and efficacy of finasteride in the treatment of male chronic pelvic pain syndrome: category IIIA CPPS (chronic nonbacterial prostatitis). BJU Int 2004; 93: 991–5.

44. Lowe FC, Fagelman E. Phytotherapeutic agents in the treatment of chronic prostatitis. In: Nickel JC, ed. Textbook of Prostatitis. Oxford: Isis Medical Media, 1999: 329–31.

45. Rugendorff EW, Weidner W, Ebeling L. Results of treatment with pollen extract (Cernilton N) in chronic prostatitis and prostatodynia. Br J Urol 1993; 71: 433–8.

46. Shoskes DA, Zeitlin SI, Shahed A, Rajfer J. Quercetin in men with category III chronic prostatitis: a preliminary prospsective, double-blind, placebo control trial. Urology 1999; 34: 960–3.

47. Anderson RU. Treatment of prostatodynia (pelvic floor myalgia or chronic non-inflammatory pelvic pain syndrome). In: Nickel JC, ed. Textbook of Prostatitis. Oxford: Isis Medical Media, 1999: 357–64.

48. Anderson RU, Wise D, Sawyer T et al. Integration of myofascial trigger point release and paradoxical relaxation training treatment of chronic pelvic pain in men. J Urol 2005; 174: 155.

49. Kaplan SA, Santarosa RP, D'Alisera PM et al. Pseudodyssynergia (contraction of the external

sphincter during voiding) misdiagnosed as chronic nonbacterial prostatitis and the role of biofeedback as a therapeutic option. J Urol 1997; 157: 2234–7.

50. Cornel EB, van Haarst EP, Schaarsberg RW et al. The effect of biofeedback physical therapy in men with chronic pelvic pain syndrome type III. Eur Urol 2005; 47: 607.

51. Chen R, Nickel JC. Acupuncture ameliorates symptoms in men with chronic prostatitis/chronic pelvic pain syndrome (CP/CPPS). Urology 2003; 61: 1156–9.

52. Tripp DA, Nickel JC, Landis JR et al. Predictors of quality of life and pain in chronic prostatitis/chronic pelvic pain syndrome: findings from the National Institutes of Health Chronic Prostatitis Cohort Study. BJU Int 2004; 94: 1279–82.

53. Tripp DA, Nickel JC, Wang Y et al. Catastrophizing and pain-contingent rest predict patient adjustment in men with chronic prostatitis/chronic pelvic pain syndrome. J Pain 2006; 710: 697–708.

54. Feliciano AE Jr.. Repetitive prostate massage. In: Nickel JC. Textbook of Prostatitis. Oxford: Isis Medical Media, 1999: 311–18.

Appendix 27.1.

The National Institutes of Health Chronic Prostatitis Symptom Index (NIH-CPSI) captures the three most important domains of the prostatitis experience: pain (location, frequency and severity), voiding (irritative and obstructive symptoms), and quality of life (including impact). This index is useful in research studies and clinical practice. (Reprinted with permission from MS Litwin et al. J Urol 1999; 162: 369–75.[22])

NIH-Chronic Prostatitis Symptom Index
Pain or Discomfort

1. In the last week, have you experienced any pain or discomfort in the following areas?

		Yes	No
a.	Area between rectum and testicles (perineum)	☐1	☐0
b.	Testicles	☐1	☐0
c.	Tip of the penis (not related to urination)	☐1	☐0
d.	Below your waist, in your pubic or bladder area	☐1	☐0

2. In the last week, have you experienced:

		Yes	No
a.	Pain or burning during urination?	☐1	☐0
b.	Pain or discomfort during or after sexual climax (ejaculation)?	☐1	☐0

3. How often have you had pain or discomfort in any of these areas over the last week?
   - ☐0 Never
   - ☐1 Rarely
   - ☐2 Sometimes
   - ☐3 Often
   - ☐4 Usually
   - ☐5 Always

4. Which number best describes your AVERAGE pain or discomfort on the days that you had it, over the last week?

☐ ☐ ☐ ☐ ☐ ☐ ☐ ☐ ☐ ☐ ☐
0 1 2 3 4 5 6 7 8 9 10

NO   PAIN AS
PAIN   BAD AS
                  YOU CAN
                  IMAGINE

Urination

5. How often have you had a sensation of not emptying your bladder completely after you finished urinating, over the last week?
   - ☐0 Not at all
   - ☐1 Less than 1 time in 5
   - ☐2 Less than half the time
   - ☐3 About half the time
   - ☐4 More than half the time
   - ☐5 Almost always

(NIH-CPSI)

6. How often have you had to urinate again less than two hours after you finished urinating, over the last week?
   - ☐0 Not at all
   - ☐1 Less than 1 time in 5
   - ☐2 Less than half the time
   - ☐3 About half the time
   - ☐4 More than half the time
   - ☐5 Almost always

Impact of Symptoms

7. How much have your symptoms kept you from doing the kinds of things you would usually do, over the last week?
   - ☐0 None
   - ☐1 Only a little
   - ☐2 Some
   - ☐3 A lot

8. How much did you think about your symptoms, over the last week?
   - ☐0 None
   - ☐1 Only a little
   - ☐2 Some
   - ☐3 A lot

Quality of Life

9. If you were to spend the rest of your life with your symptoms just the way they have been during the last week, how would you feel about that?
   - ☐0 Delighted
   - ☐1 Pleased
   - ☐2 Mostly satisfied
   - ☐3 Mixed (about equally satisfied and dissatisfied)
   - ☐4 Mostly dissatisfied
   - ☐5 Unhappy
   - ☐6 Terrible

Scoring the NIH-Chronic Prostatitis Symptom Index Domains

Pain: Total of items 1a, 1b, 1c, 1d, 2a, 2b, 3, and 4   = ___

Urinary Symptoms: Total of items 5 and 6   = ___

Quality of Life Impact: Total of items 7, 8, and 9   = ___

CHAPTER 28

Androgenetic alopecia

Desmond Chia Chin Gan, Rodney Sinclair

Introduction

Androgenetic alopecia (AGA), also known as common baldness or male-pattern hair loss, is the most common cause of hair loss in men. In its most classic form, it follows a distinctive pattern of hair loss, starting from bitemporal recession and going on to diffuse frontal and vertex loss, with preservation of occipital hair. A variant also exists which presents as a general diffuse hair loss, more commonly found among Asians. The pathogenesis involves androgen-induced miniaturization of terminal hairs into vellus hairs in affected regions of the scalp. Some degree of follicular miniaturization and consequential hair loss is universal and is considered to be a physiological secondary sexual characteristic. AGA is generally regarded as an aging process and only becomes a medical problem when the hair loss is excessive, premature, and distressing to the patient.

Pathogenesis

Alteration of hair cycle dynamics and follicular miniaturization under the influence of androgens are key features of AGA.

Hair cycle dynamics

A normal hair cycle is composed of three stages (Fig. 28.1). Hair grows in the anagen phase (lasting 3–5 years), followed by a transitional catagen phase (2 weeks), and goes into a resting telogen phase (3 months).[1] During the telogen phase, hair shedding occurs (exogen), and a latent phase exists before hair resumes the anagen growth phase.[2] The normal ratio of anagen to telogen hairs is 12:1.

In AGA, the duration of anagen decreases with each cycle, whilst the length of telogen remains the same or becomes prolonged.[3,4] The maximum length that a hair can grow therefore decreases with each cycle. Ultimately, the anagen growth phase is so short that hair stops growing before it reaches the skin surface, leaving an empty follicular pore.

This change in hair cycle dynamics produces a relative increase in telogen hair count. As telogen hair is more easily plucked, men with AGA commonly experience increased hair shedding, especially during washing and combing of hair.

In addition, the latent phase becomes progressively longer, further leading to a decrease in number of hairs seen in the scalp.[2]

Hair follicle miniaturization

The basic structure of hair follicles consists of hair shaft (which ultimately becomes visible hair), the inner and outer root sheath, the sebaceous gland, and the hair bulb. The hair bulb, situated at the base of the hair follicle, consists of matrix cells, which are a living, actively proliferating group of cells that produce the hair shaft. Beneath this is a pear-like structure called the dermal papilla, which is a small collection of specialized fibroblasts. The dermal papilla is fed by capillaries, and is responsible for

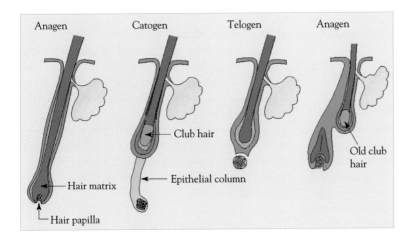

Figure 28.1. *The normal human hair cycle.*

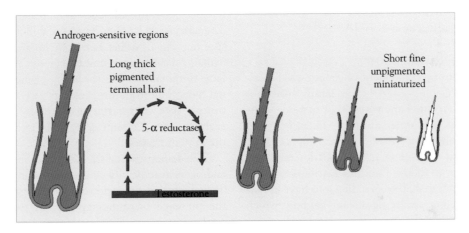

Figure 28.2. *The process of hair miniaturization in androgenetic alopecia.*

inducing follicle development and production of hair fiber.

Hair follicle miniaturization produces smaller follicles that produce finer hairs (Fig. 28.2). The caliber of hair shafts reduces from $\geq 80\ \mu m$ to $<60\ \mu m$. This is accompanied by decreased pigmentation.

The dermal papilla, being central in the control of hair growth, is the most likely target of androgen-mediated events leading to miniaturization and hair cycle changes.[5–7] The constant geometric relationship between the dermal papilla size and the size of the hair matrix[3] suggests that the size of the dermal papilla determines the size of the hair bulb and ultimately the hair shaft produced.[4] The exact mechanism by which this occurs is not known.

Several possibilities include apoptotic cell death; decreased proliferation of keratinocytes; cell displacement with loss of cellular adhesion, leading to dermal papilla fibroblasts dropping off into the dermis; and migration of dermal papilla cells into the dermal sheath associated with the outer root sheath of the hair follicle.[4]

As the cross-sectional area of the growing hair remains constant throughout the anagen phase, it can be surmised that miniaturization occurs in between hair cycles in a stepwise fashion, rather than as a continuous process. Recent modeling suggests that the transition from terminal to vellus hair occurs in a few, large steps rather than multiple small steps.[8] The lengthy delay between the commencement of treatment and the clinical response[9] is because any pharmacological intervention will affect hairs only during a small window in the growth cycle – at the point of miniaturization.

Inflammation

From findings of scalp biopsies, 40% of cases of AGA are observed to have moderate perifollicular, lymphohistiocytic infiltrate, perhaps with concentric layers of perifollicular collagen deposition, compared with 10% of normal controls.[10] Occasional eosinophils and mast cells can be seen. The cellular inflammatory changes also occur around lower follicles in some cases and occasionally involve follicular stellae. It is unknown to what degree the inflammation affects the pathogenesis of AGA.[10]

Genetic predisposition

There is a strong component of genetic predisposition to developing AGA.[11,12] A family history is common from either the paternal or maternal side. The genetics is complex and most likely follows a polygenic inheritance model. This is supported by the fact that a range of phenotypes for men and women seem to follow a normal distribution,[13] and also by the fact that 80% of balding sons have fathers who have cosmetically significant balding, which greatly exceeds the proportion expected of an autosomal-dominant pattern.[12] Current modeling suggests involvement of at least four genes that combine to modify the age of onset, the pattern of loss, and the rate of progression of AGA.[11]

The androgen receptor gene has been heavily investigated. An association of male AGA with a polymorphism of the androgen receptor gene has been described in an Australian study.[14] The androgen receptor gene *StuI* restriction fragment length polymorphism (RFLP) was found in almost all (98.1%) young bald men and most older bald men (92.3%), but in only 77% of non-bald men. This polymorphism therefore appears to be necessary in cases of premature balding, but not sufficient on its own to cause balding in all age groups. The same study also demonstrated a triplet repeat polymorphism on the androgen receptor gene. The combination of shorter CAG and GGC triplet repeat lengths was more prevalent in young bald men

(50%) than controls (29.5%). In another recent study, patients affected by Kennedy's disease, who have a functional abnormality of the androgen receptor gene, have a reduced risk of AGA.[15] Of note, the androgen receptor gene is located on the X chromosome, which is passed on from the mother to a male child.

To date, none of the other candidate genes, including the 5α-reductase enzymes,[14] the insulin gene,[16] and the aromatase gene,[11] has been demonstrated to be directly associated with the tendency to go bald.

The effects of androgen

At puberty, males develop secondary sexual characteristics under the influence of increased androgens. The effects androgens have on follicles are site-specific. Small vellus hair follicles in the pubic, axillary, beard, and chest regions enlarge into large terminal hairs. In the scalp, pigmented terminal hairs from frontal region and vertex are miniaturized into non-pigmented vellus hairs. The eyebrow and occipital scalp hair is spared from the miniaturization.[17]

The demonstration that eunuchs,[18] patients with androgen-insensitivity syndrome,[19] and those with 5α-reductase deficiency[20] do not bald suggests that the presence of androgen and, in particular, its active metabolite dihydrotestosterone (DHT) are the prerequisite for developing AGA.

DHT is formed primarily in the prostate, testes, adrenals, and hair follicles, through the enzyme 5α-reductase. Compared with testosterone, DHT has five times the avidity to bind with androgen receptors, and is more potent in its ability to cause downstream activation.[21] Two isoenzymes of 5α-reductase have been characterized. Type 1 isoenzyme is found in scalp and skin, with its activity more concentrated in sebaceous glands. The physiological role of type 1 enzyme in AGA is relatively unknown. The type 2 isoenzyme is found in the prostate, hair follicles, and other androgen-sensitive organs, and accounts for 80% of circulating DHT.[16] Increased levels of DHT have been found in balding scalp compared with non-balding scalp.

The exact effects of androgens on hair follicles are not yet known. Intrafollicular over-activity may be the result of systemic or local factors. Possible systemic factors are increased circulating androgens providing increased substrate for the conversion to DHT, and increased systemic production of DHT at distant sites such as the prostate gland. Possible local factors include an increased number of androgen receptors, functional polymorphisms of the androgen receptor, increased local production of DHT, and reduced local degradation of DHT.

There is little evidence in supporting the systemic factors as the causation of AGA. There is no demonstrable correlation between degree of baldness and hair density in trunks and limbs, bone, skin and muscle thickness, sebum excretion rate, and libido.[22] In addition, there have been few studies demonstrating associations between levels of circulating androgens with severity of AGA.[23–25] Thus it is likely that normal level of systemic androgens is adequate for maximal production of DHT.

The paradoxical effect of androgens in inducing growth in the beard area and of body hair and in causing hair loss in vertex scalp is dependent on the intrinsic factors within each hair follicle. It has been shown that dermal papilla cells in beard secrete growth-inducing autocrine growth factors in response to testosterone. Occipital scalp follicles do not produce the same effect.[26] The response of the balding vertex scalp is unknown, although experiments on stump-tailed macaque show that testosterone inhibits growth and proliferation of keratinocytes in balding scalp.[27]

This intrinsic auto-regulatory function of hair follicles is probably the main mechanism producing the patterned hair distribution seen in AGA. Increased levels of 5α-reductase and androgen receptors are found in balding scalp compared to non-balding scalp.[28] In vitro experiments have shown that dermal papillae are able to regulate their own response to androgens by upregulating expression of both 5α-reductase and androgen receptors.[29–31] This intrinsic auto-regulation is retained when hair follicles are transplanted: occipital hairs maintain their resistance to AGA when transplanted to vertex, and scalp hairs from vertex transplanted to the forearm miniaturize at the same rate as those neighboring follicles on the donor scalp.[4] This forms the basis of hair transplantation surgery.

Epidemiology

Prevalence of androgenetic alopecia in the community

Normal pre-pubertal males do not develop AGA.[32] The prevalence and severity of AGA increase with age. Around 20% of Caucasians start to develop cosmetically significant AGA (diffuse frontal, vertex, or full baldness) in their 20s, and this goes up to 50% by the age of 50 and 75% by the age of 80 (Fig. 28.3).[32,33] Men of Asian, native American, and African background have a lower incidence.[34]

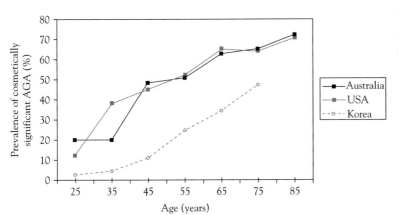

Figure 28.3. *The prevalence of cosmetically significant androgenetic alopecia (AGA) among males in the community. Adapted from: Gan and Sinclair.[32]*

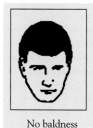 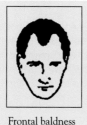 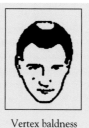 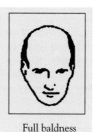

No baldness   Frontal baldness   Vertex baldness   Full baldness

Figure 28.4. *Patterns of androgenetic alopecia in men.*

Recession of the bitemporal hairline does not occur in pre-pubertal males of normal development, but is present in more than half of the males after the age of 30 (Fig. 28.4).[32]

Association of androgenetic alopecia with other diseases

AGA has been found to be associated with an increased incidence in both benign prostatic hyperplasia and prostate cancer.[35–38] With regard to specific hair patterns, vertex balding was associated with a 50% increase in the risk of prostate cancer.[38] Frontal balding or frontal concurrent with vertex balding confers no increased risk. However, significant associations with high-grade prostate cancer were found in all patterns of AGA, especially in men aged 60–69 years.

Ischemic heart disease has also been found to be associated with AGA.[39–42] This statistically significant, though weak, association was discovered by epidemiological, cohort, and case control studies. In general, severe early onset of AGA before the age of 30 may suggest a higher risk for ischemic heart disease. Interestingly, vertex balding is also associated with an increased risk of myocardial infarction.[43] A recent prospective study (in 2007) also demonstrated an association of AGA with hypertension.[44]

No clear mechanistic link between these diseases has been found. High androgen levels have been postulated to cause AGA as well as atherosclerosis and thrombosis; however other data have shown no association between baldness and established coronary risk factors.[45] A pathophysiological mechanism for the link between AGA and prostate cancer also remains to be established but it may involve the dual dependence of these conditions on dihydrotestosterone.[46]

Diagnosis

Clinical diagnosis

Diagnosis of AGA relies mainly on the basis of history and physical examination. A history of episodic hair shedding is common but not universal. Affected patients describe progressive hair loss over time. A family history of AGA on either the maternal or paternal side of the family is obtainable in 80% of the cases.

The clinical appearance of AGA is easily recognizable in most cases. In its classical form, hair loss occurs in an orderly manner and has been well documented by the seven categories of the Hamilton–Norwood scale (Fig. 28.5).[33,47] Not all cases of hair loss conform to this progression. A variant called the Ludwig pattern exists, especially among Asians. This Ludwig pattern is similar to the common pattern observed in women; it presents as a diffuse frontal and vertex hair thinning. Hair density thinning can be assessed with wider central parting over the vertex and is useful for monitoring of treatment response. The scalp is generally normal. A positive hair pull test may exist, signifying a relative increase in telogen hair count, although its reliability is questionable.

The differential diagnoses include alopecia areata (an autoimmune disease characterized typically by recurrent circumscribed asymmetrical baldness with findings of exclamation-mark hairs), chronic telogen effluvium (increased shedding of normal hairs), and cicatricial alopecia (destruction

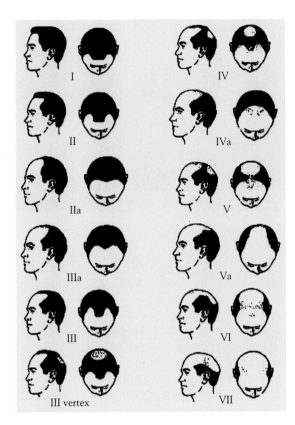

Figure 28.5. *The modified Hamilton–Norwood classification of male androgenetic alopecia.*

and scarring of hair follicles from, for example, trauma, radiation therapy, infection, lupus).

Histopathology

Histological diagnosis is rarely necessary. In cases where diagnosis is equivocal, punch biopsies may be taken. Two 4 mm punch biopsies are taken from the vertex of the scalp, one sectioned horizontally and the other vertically. Horizontal sectioning allows greater number of follicles to be studied and is more useful in diagnosis of AGA.

The main finding is terminal anagen hair being replaced by pseudo-vellus hairs,[48] representing the process of follicular miniaturization. The presence of arrector pili muscle and angiofibrotic streamers distinguishes the vellus hairs from true terminal anagen hairs. The ratio of terminal to vellus hairs reduces from more than 6:1 to less than 4:1.

The anagen to telogen hair count decreases from 12:1 to 5:1.[49]

Others features that may also be seen include follicular fibrosis and perifollicular inflammation. The fibrosis can be seen in around 10% of cases. However, fibrosis may also be seen in a small number of normal scalp biopsies. The inflammation consists of a mild to moderate peri-infundibular lymphohistiocytic inflammatory infiltrate. It is present in up to two-thirds of biopsies,[48] but it is a non-specific feature that is also found in up to one-third of normal scalp biopsies.[49]

Morbidity of androgenetic alopecia

The psychosocial impact of AGA has long been recognized. Bald men are said to look older and to be less popular and less physically and socially attractive. Most men affected by AGA find this a stressful and unwanted event that diminishes body image satisfaction.[50] In contrast, most unaffected men often trivialize or ignore the negative impact of AGA.[51]

Perception by others often plays an important role in creating the low self-esteem suffered by balding men. A Korean study[52] found that the negative perception of balding men by women and non-balding men was similar to the self-reported negative perception by balding men. Importantly, this view was even more common in women than in non-balding men.

Nevertheless, most men with AGA cope well without much impairment of their psychosocial function. Men who are at greater risk of becoming distressed with AGA are those with extensive hair loss, earlier age of onset, strong reliance on physical appearance as a source of self-esteem, pre-existing poor self-esteem, or a lack of a romantic relationship, and those that deem their balding as progressive (often arising from observing their father).[50]

Apart from the psychosocial impact, the physical disadvantages from balding are a loss of protection of the scalp from sunburn, cold, mechanical injury, and ultraviolet light. Ultraviolet exposure may lead to an increased chance of actinic change and skin cancer development. The area should be protected from ultraviolet damage by covering up or with sunscreen.

Management

Before deciding to start treatment, it is important to explore patients' psychosocial morbidity from AGA and their treatment expectations. Then time should be spent on educating patients on the pathogenesis and highlighting to them how prevalent AGA is in the community. Several treatment options are available: topical treatment, oral treatment, surgery, wigs, and camouflage. Regardless of which option is taken up, long-term follow up and consultation is required.

Medical management

Before starting treatment, systemic medications known to induce hair loss, including androgens, retinoids, cytotoxic agents, and anticoagulants, should be ceased where possible. Associated scalp disorders such as seborrheic dermatitis or psoriasis should be treated so that topical preparation can be more effectively applied.

There are two treatments approved in the USA by the Food and Drug Administration for treatment of AGA: topical minoxidil and oral finasteride. Both treatments are able to partially reverse the process of AGA and therefore full regrowth should never be expected. In addition, treatment should be continued indefinitely to maintain its effectiveness. Clinical benefit is only expected after 6–12 months of treatment. Treatment should therefore be continued up to 1 year before re-evaluating whether to continue treatment.

Monitoring of treatment response may potentially be problematic. Doctors rely heavily on patients' subjective assessment of their hair density, and episodic shedding is sometimes more easily noticeable than subtle improvement of hair density over time. A baseline photograph can be helpful, but is unlikely to detect improvement of hair density of less than 20%, which is the maximum amount of regrowth one would expect after treatment of 12–24 months. An objective tool that is used by the authors is a camera mounted on a stereotactic device; a system that is identical to the set-up used

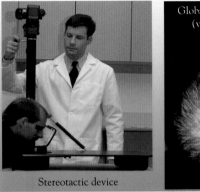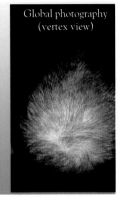

Figure 28.6. *Hair photography using a stereotactic device.*

in the phase III finasteride trials.[53] Six-monthly to yearly photographs are taken of the vertex and frontal hairline for comparison of hair densities at different time points. This set-up is useful in the long-term monitoring of treatment response (Fig. 28.6). Both patient and doctor are able to observe change in hair density. This has proved to be a good motivating factor for patients, and therefore improves patients' compliance with long-term medical treatment. A similar set-up using Polaroid photographs is another alternative.[54]

Topical therapy: minoxidil

Oral minoxidil was originally used as an antihypertensive, with hypertrichosis known to be one if its side effects.[55] Its topical formulation is now widely used as treatment of AGA. The exact mechanism of its action is unknown. It is believed that minoxidil sulfate, the active metabolite, causes the opening of the potassium channel. This in turn increases the negativity of the intracellular potential, and decreases the concentration of intracellular calcium. *In vitro* experiments have shown that epidermal growth factor inhibits hair follicle growth in the presence of calcium. The conversion of minoxidil to minoxidil sulfate is higher in hair follicles than in the surrounding skin and may oppose epidermal growth factor (EGF)-induced inhibition of growth, and thereby delay the onset of catagen phase.[56]

Topical minoxidil is available in two preparations – the 2% and 5% solutions. Both preparations are available over-the-counter in most countries. Minoxidil has been shown in a number of studies to be effective in treatment of AGA.[44,57–61] The preparation of 5% minoxidil has been shown to be superior to 2% minoxidil in promoting hair growth, even after a long period of treatment.[44]

Patients should be educated with the correct expectation of treatment outcome prior to starting therapy. Firstly, a short period of excessive hair shedding is expected in some patients at the start of treatment. This is due to the fact that minoxidil stimulates the induction of anagen phase from resting hair follicles. This in turn causes a short period of previous telogen hair shedding that may last for around 2–8 weeks. This initial period of 'loss of hair' should be seen as an encouraging sign rather than treatment failure.

Secondly, it is also important to advise patients of the importance in long-term therapy, and the financial implications of it. Minoxidil promotes some degree of hair regrowth at the start. Regrowth is more pronounced at the vertex than in the frontal area. Thereafter, patients on treatment (both 5% and 2% minoxidil) will have a continuous deterioration of about 6% per annum decrease in hair weight. The effect of minoxidil only lasts as long as the patient continues to use the preparation. Once treatment is stopped, all minoxidil-dependent hairs will be shed, and any positive effect on hair growth achieved at the start will be lost in 4–6 months. Overall hair density will then return to a point determined by the natural history.[60]

Patients who respond best to minoxidil typically are those who have been recently diagnosed and have a small amount of hair loss. In addition, studies in patients treated with minoxidil have demonstrated that 55% of those with perifollicular micro-inflammation on biopsy had regrowth in response to treatment compared with 77% of patients without inflammation or fibrosis.[61]

Minoxidil should be used twice daily, with one milliliter spread evenly into the entire scalp. The solution should be applied before gels or hairsprays which might reduce absorption. Side effects are uncommon. The 5% preparation has a higher frequency of side effects than the 2% preparation.[62] Skin irritation with itchiness is the most common side effect.[63] Dizziness, tachycardia, and contact allergic dermatitis[64] may also occur infrequently.

Systemic therapy: finasteride

Finasteride is a synthetic azo-steroid that is a potent and highly selective antagonist of type II 5α-reductase. It does not produce generalized anti-androgen effects. It binds irreversibly to the enzyme and inhibits the conversion of testosterone to DHT. Therefore, while the pharmacokinetic half-life is about 8 hours, the biological effect persists for much longer. A daily oral dose of 1 mg reduces scalp DHT by 64% and serum DHT by 68%.[65] A daily oral dose of 5 mg does not produce further decrease in scalp and serum DHT or any further clinical benefit in the treatment of AGA.[66]

The benefits of finasteride on reversing the pathogenesis of AGA have been shown in various studies with convincing evidence.[65–73] Anagen hair count and total hair count increase with treatment, accompanied by an improved anagen–telogen hair ratio.[68] Scalp biopsy study[69] shows an increase in terminal to vellus hair ratio with treatment. This demonstrates the ability of finasteride to stimulate conversion of hair follicles into the anagen phase, and therefore reverse the process of miniaturization.

Maximum benefits of finasteride are achieved with early commencement and long-term maintenance therapy. Approximately two-thirds of men will achieve visible hair re-growth within the first 2 years. Both the vertex and superior frontal scalp region are shown to benefit from treatment, whereas the temporal region and the frontal hairline show minimal benefits.[67,71–73]

In a 5-year multi-center, randomized, placebo-controlled study,[72] 12 months' treatment with finasteride produced an increase of 10% in the mean hair count. Mean hair count declined somewhat thereafter but maintained above baseline after 5 years. On the other hand, the placebo group suffered a progressive decline in hair count at a much faster rate compared with the treatment group, losing about 26% of terminal hairs from baseline after 5 years (Figs. 28.7 and 28.8).

Global photographic assessment (Fig. 28.9) in the same study showed a greater benefit on hair regrowth. Hair thickness was observed to improve

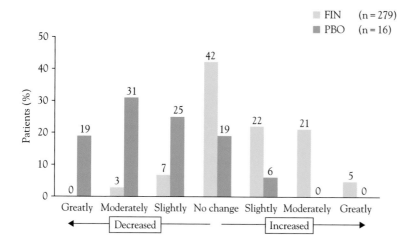

FIN (n = 279)
PBO (n = 16)

Figure 28.7. *Global photographic assessments comparing 5-year finasteride treatment group (FIN) and placebo (PBO) group. Adapted from the Finasteride Male Pattern Hair Loss Study Group.[72] With permission of John Libbey Eurotext.*

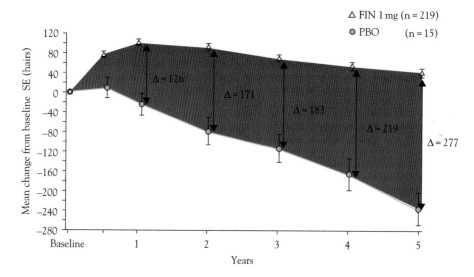

△ FIN 1 mg (n = 219)
⊙ PBO (n = 15)

Figure 28.8. *Hair count mean change from baseline with 5-year treatment of finasteride. FIN, finasteride treatment group; PBO, placebo group; SE, standard error. Adapted from the Finasteride Male Pattern Hair Loss Study Group.[72] With permission of John Libbey Eurotext.*

for up to 24 months of treatment. At 5 years, only 10% of finasteride-treated men had suffered visible deterioration, compared with 75% of placebo-treated men. This longer period of 'regrowth' observed using the global photograph data compared with hair count data is probably due to improvement of hair quality, such as increased growth rate (length) and thickness of hair. This explanation is supported by another study, which demonstrated that finasteride produced a greater benefit in hair weight compared with hair count.[70]

At the end of 12 months, some in the placebo group were randomly crossed over from placebo to treatment with finasteride. These patients, after some loss of hair count in the first 12 months, showed benefit from treatment of finasteride for the remaining 4 years. However, their mean hair count after 4 years of treatment was less than that of the patients who had taken finasteride 'a year earlier' at all comparable time points, with the difference being similar to the amount of hair loss sustained during the year of placebo treatment.

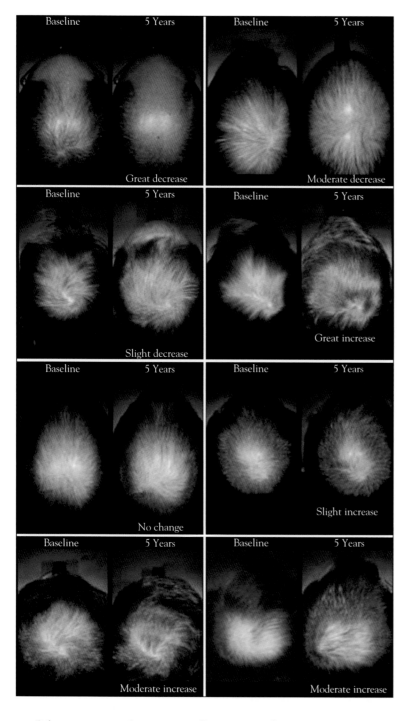

Figure 28.9. *Global photographs showing results of 5 years of treatment with finasteride.*

Other measures of treatment efficacy were also used in the study, which included investigators' clinical assessment of scalp hair and, more importantly, patients' self-administered hair growth questionnaires. Improvements with finasteride were shown in all aspects of assessments.

Finasteride at a dose of 1 mg/day has an excellent safety profile. A low incidence of sexual dysfunction reported after use in the first year include decreased libido (in 1.9%), erectile dysfunction (in 1.4%), and ejaculation disorder (in 1.2%). The rates of occurrence in the placebo groups were 1.3%, 0.6% and 0.5%, respectively. Most of these events resolve on cessation of the drug and, in some cases, with continued treatment. It has been suggested that even these figures overstate the true incidence of sexual dysfunction.[74] With regard to long-term safety data, finasteride has now been in use in urologic patients for over 15 years, with many of them taking a dose of 5 mg/day. There is no effect of long-term use on bone mineral density.[75,76] Reversible painful gynecomastia has been reported[77] and the incidence is thought to be around 0.001%.[78]

Of note, finasteride also causes a moderate reduction in the level of prostate-specific antigen (PSA). This may have implications for patients using PSA as part of screening evaluation of prostate cancer. Previously, it was thought that PSA level should be doubled to correct for effect of finasteride. Recent studies[79] now suggest that finasteride treatment at the 5 mg/day dose affects the serum PSA concentration in a time-dependent manner. The doubling of the PSA value may overestimate the true risk of prostate cancer during the first 6–9 months of finasteride treatment, accurately determine the true PSA value for 1–3 years, and thereafter there may be a possible underestimation of the true PSA value.

Combining finasteride and topical minoxidil

Studies of combination treatment of finasteride and minoxidil were poorly designed. However, animal studies have shown an additive effect when both medications were used concurrently. In order to prevent excessive shedding, patients wishing to switch from one treatment to the other should ensure an overlap period of 3 months before discontinuing the old medication.

Other 5α-reductase inhibitors in development: dutasteride

Dutasteride, a combined type 1 and type 2 5α-reductase, is approved for the treatment of benign prostatic hyperplasia. It has a greater efficacy in reducing DHT levels, and has a serum half-life

of 4 weeks as compared with finasteride (with a half-life of 6–8 hours). As it is known to be teratogenic, patients on dutasteride should avoid donating blood for at least 6 months following cessation of treatment, to prevent the possibility of transfusing a pregnant recepient.[80]

Dutasteride has undergone a recent phase II randomized, placebo-controlled study.[80] At 12 and 24 weeks, dutasteride at a dose of 2.5 mg/day was shown to be superior to finasteride at a dose of 5 mg/day in improving scalp hair growth, as demonstrated both in hair counts and clinical assessment. This is further supported by another randomized, double-blind, placebo-controlled twin study.[81] Dutasteride is well tolerated, and the incidence of the most common sexual side effects is low, tends to decrease over time,[81] and resolves upon drug cessation.

Future drug development: topical anti-androgens

Oral anti-androgens (e.g. spironolactone, cyproterone acetate) are widely used to treat women with AGA. However their use is limited in males owing to systemic anti-androgen effects, affecting libido, male sexual functions, and development of secondary sexual characteristics. A topical anti-androgen, fluridil has recently been rationally developed for use in male AGA. It is designed to be locally metabolized, not systemically resorbable, and degradable into inactive metabolites without anti-androgenic activity.[82] A double-blind, placebo-controlled study shows that patients using topical fluridil had an increase in the anagen–telogen ratio, and the maximum attainable effect is achieved within the first 90 days of daily use. No side effects on libido and sexual performances have been found. Nevertheless, a longer study is required to investigate further its long-term safety and effectiveness in male AGA.

Other drugs

Topical ketoconazole has been reported to be effective for AGA[83] in case reports. However, placebo-controlled trials have not yet been performed. It acts in both an androgen-dependent and androgen-independent manner.

Camouflage and wigs

Camouflage offers a cheap and simple alternative way for patients with mild hair loss. Camouflage treatment works by dyeing the scalp the same color as the hair, and therefore giving the illusion of thicker hair. Sprays of different colors are available. The hair is dried and styled before the dye is sprayed on. Some problems may arise if the hair becomes wet. The spray may dye patients' hands, towels, and pillowcases, although these stains are easily washable. Patients should also be advised to shampoo and remove dye before bedtime every night.

For those with advanced hair loss, good-quality synthetic acrylic or natural-fiber wigs are available. Wigs can be styled and washed, and modern wigs provide excellent coverage that looks natural. Wigs can either be interwoven with existing hair or worn over the top of existing hair. Interwoven wigs requires readjustment every few weeks as hair beneath grows. This is considerably more expensive to maintain. Few patients opt for the options of wigs, since the only wigs people notice are the bad ones. Advice on wigs is usually easily obtainable from the alopecia support groups.

Scalp surgery

The options of scalp surgery in treatment of AGA include transplantation, scalp flaps, and excision of bald scalp, with or without tissue expansion. Young men below the age of 25 should not be considered for scalp surgery, since it is difficult to predict the pattern and degree of hair loss that will occur with age.

Autograft transplantation is the most popular scalp surgery performed these days. The use of artificial fibers has gone out of fashion owing to problems of infection and reaction to foreign bodies. A typical donor site is the occipital scalp region, since occipital hair follicles are resistant to the development of AGA (see the section on pathogenesis, above). A strip of full-thickness occipital scalp is harvested and, under the aid of a dissecting microscope, cut down to small subunits. Minigrafts containing a cluster of hairs are transplanted into slits made with a small scalpel blade. A modified technique uses 'follicular units' containing between one and four hair follicles, which are inserted into smaller needle holes. Both techniques can achieve good results, but follicular unit transplantations have the advantage of being able to achieve much greater hair densities.

The ideal surgical candidate is someone with frontal or mid-frontal hair loss as opposed to hair loss at the vertex. A donor hair density of more than 40 follicular units/cm^2 and with better hair quality (hair thickness) are preferred. Transplanted hairs seem to go into a telogen resting phase after insertion to recipient site. Thus surgical results can only be adequately assessed no less than 3 months after surgery. Concurrent treatment with finasteride, started from 4 weeks prior to transplantation and continued indefinitely, has been shown to improve the density and quality of transplanted hairs.[84]

Major disadvantages of hair transplants include cost, time, and graft results. The number of transplantation sessions required would depend on the size of area to be transplanted, with up to 3000 units transplanted per 'megasession'. There is always a risk of graft failure. This may occur for various reasons, including the skill of the surgeon, careless handling and preparation of the graft units, the density of graft placement, and desiccation of the grafts whilst awaiting insertion.[85]

Scalp reductions result in a more unnatural look with excision scars tending to be more noticeable over time. In addition, the inability to predict further hair loss over time in each patient has meant that the procedures are now uncommonly performed.

Conclusion

AGA is a very common disorder in the community. Although most men with AGA cope well, its negative impact on self-perception is largely neglected by the community. There are a number of treatment options available, all of which require long-term maintenance and follow-up. Careful explanation on pathogenesis and treatment outcome, together with supporting patients' self-esteem, form a huge part management of AGA. Novel treatments for treatment of AGA are under investigation. This, together with the biological structures and changes of hair follicles, has stimulated a great amount of research from stem cell scientists, geneticists, developmental biologists, and immunologists. Hair biology has become an increasingly fruitful field of scientific endeavor.

References

1. Kligman AM. The human hair cycle. J Invest Dermatol 1959; 33: 307–16.
2. Curtois M, Loussouarn G, Horseau C. Hair cycle and alopecia. Skin Pharmacol 1994; 7: 84–9.
3. Van Scott EJ, Ekel TM. Geometric relationships between the matrix of the hair bulb and its dermal papilla in normal and alopecic scalp. J Invest Dermatol 1958; 31: 281–7.
4. Jahoda CA. Cellular and developmental aspects of androgenetic alopecia. Exp Dermatol 1998; 7: 235–48.
5. Obana NJ, Uno H. Dermal papilla cells in macaque alopecia trigger a testosterone-dependent inhibition of follicular cell proliferation. In: van Neste D, Randall VA, eds. Hair Research in the Next Millennium. Elsevier: Amsterdam 1996: 307–10.
6. Randall VA. The use of dermal papilla cells in studies of normal and abnormal hair follicle biology. Dermatol Clin 1996; 14: 585–94.
7. Oliver RF, Jahoda CAB. The dermal papilla and the maintenance of hair growth. In: Rogers GA, ed. The Biology of Wool and Hair. London: Chapman and Hall 1989: 51–67.
8. Whiting DA. Possible mechanisms of miniaturization during androgenetic alopecia or pattern hair loss. J Am Acad Dermatol 2001; 45: S81–6.
9. Sinclair R. Male pattern androgenetic alopecia. BMJ 1998; 317: 865–9.
10. Whiting DA. Scalp biopsy as a diagnostic and prognostic tool in androgenetic alopecia. Dermatol Ther 1998; 8: 24–33.
11. Ellis JA, Sinclair R, Harrap SB. Androgenetic alopecia: pathogenesis and potential for therapy. Expert Rev Mol Med 2002; 2002: 1–11.
12. Setty LR. Hair patterns of scalp of white and Negro males. Am J Phys Anthropol 1970; 33: 49–55.
13. Kuster W, Happle R. The inheritance of common baldness: two B or not two B? J Am Acad Dermatol 1984; 11: 921–6.
14. Ellis JA, Stebbing M, Harrap SB. Polymorphism of the androgen receptor gene is associated with male pattern baldness. J Invest Dermatol 2001; 116: 452–5.
15. Sinclair RD, Greenland K, van Egmond S et al. Men with Kennedy's disease have a reduced risk of androgenetic alopecia. Br J Dermatol 2007; 157: 290–4.
16. Ellis JA, Stebbing M, Harrap SB. Insulin gene polymorphism and premature male pattern baldness in the general population. Clin Sci (Lond) 1999; 96: 659–62.
17. Kaufman KD. Androgen metabolism as it affects hair growth in androgenetic alopecia. Dermatol Clin 1996; 14: 697–711.
18. Hamilton JB. Effect of castration in adolescent and young adult males upon further changes in the proportion of bare and hairy scalp. J Clin Endocrinol Metabol 1960; 20: 1309–18.
19. Griffin JE, Wilson JD. The resistance syndromes: 5α reductase deficiency, testicular feminization and related disorders. In: Baudet AL, Sly WS, Valle D, eds. The Metabolic Basis of Inherited Disease. New York: McGraw Hill, 1989: 1919–44.
20. Imperato-McGinley J, Guerrero L, Gautier T et al. Steroid 5alpha-reductase deficiency in man: an inherited form of male pseudohermaphroditism. Science 1974; 186: 1213–15.
21. Jones LN, Sinclair RD, Rivett DE. Androgen metabolism and human hair growth. Chem Aust 1997; 64: 12–13.
22. Burton JL, Halim MM, Meyrick G et al. Male-pattern alopecia and masculinity. Br J Dermatol 1979; 100: 567–71.
23. Demark-Wahnefried W, Lesko SM, Conaway MR et al. Serum androgens: associations with prostate cancer risk and hair patterning. J Androl 1997; 18: 495–500.
24. Sreekumar GP, Pardinas J, Wong CQ et al. Serum androgens and genetic linkage analysis in early onset androgenetic alopecia. J Invest Dermatol 1999; 113: 277–9.
25. Itami S, Kurata S, Sonoda T et al. Interaction between dermal papilla cells and follicular epithelial cells in vitro: effect of androgen. Br J Dermatol 1995; 132: 527–32.
26. Thornton MJ, Hamada K, Messenger AG et al. Androgen-dependent beard dermal papilla cells secrete autocrine growth factor(s) in response to testosterone unlike scalp cells. J Invest Dermatol 1998; 111: 727–32.
27. Uno H, Adachi K, Montagna W. Morphological and biochemical studies of hair follicle in common baldness of stump-tailed macaque (Macaca speciosa). In: Montagna W, Dobson RL, eds. Hair Growth, Advances in Biology of Skin. Oxford: Pergamon Press 1969: 221–45.

28. Sawaya ME, Price VH. Different levels of 5alpha-reductase type I and II, aromatase, and androgen receptor in hair follicles of women and men with androgenetic alopecia. J Invest Dermatol 1997; 109: 296–300.

29. Randall VA, Thornton MJ, Messenger AG. Cultured dermal papilla cells from androgen-dependent human hair follicles (e.g. beard) contain more androgen receptors than those from non-balding areas of scalp. J Endocrinol 1992; 133: 141–7.

30. Thornton MJ, Laing I, Hamada K et al. Differences in testosterone metabolism by beard and scalp hair follicle dermal papilla cells. Clin Endocrinol (Oxf) 1993; 39: 633–9.

31. Itami S, Kurata S, Takayasu S. 5alpha-reductase activity in cultured human dermal papilla cells from beard compared with reticular dermal fibroblasts. J Invest Dermatol 1990; 94: 150–2.

32. Gan DCC, Sinclair R. Prevalence of male and female pattern hair loss in Maryborough. J Investig Dermatol Symp Proc 2005; 10: 184–9.

33. Norwood OT. Male pattern baldness: classification and incidence. South Med J 1975; 68: 1359–65.

34. Olsen EA, Messenger AG, Shapiro J et al. Evaluation and treatment of male and female pattern hair loss. J Am Acad Dermatol 2005; 52: 301–11.

35. Chen W, Yang CC, Chen GY et al. Patients with a large prostate show a higher prevalence of androgenetic alopecia. Arch Dermatol Res 2004; 296: 245–9.

36. Oh BR, Kim SJ, Moon JD et al. Association of benign prostatic hyperplasia with male pattern baldness. Urol 1998; 51: 744–8.

37. Hawk E, Brewslow RA, Graubard BI. Male pattern baldness and clinical prostate cancer in the epidemiologic follow-up of the first National Health and Nutrition Examination Survey. Cancer Epidemiol Biomarkers Prev 2000; 9: 523–7.

38. Giles GG, Severi G, Sinclair R et al. Androgenetic alopecia and prostate cancer: findings from an Australian case-control study. Cancer Epidemiol Biomarkers Prev 2002; 11: 549–3.

39. Herrera CR, D Agostino RB, Gerstman BB et al. Baldness and coronary heart disease rates in men from the Framingham Study. Am J Epidemiol 1995; 142: 828–33.

40. Ford ES, Freedman DS, Byers T. Baldness and ischemic heart disease in a national sample of men. Am J Epidemiol 1996; 143: 651–7.

41. Lesko SM, Rosenberg L, Shapiro S. A case-control study of baldness in relation to myocardial infarction in men. JAMA 1993; 269: 998–1003.

42. Schnohr P, Lange P, Nyboe J et al. Gray hair, baldness, and wrinkles in relation to myocardial infarction: the Copenhagen City Heart Study. Am Heart J 1995; 130: 1003–10.

43. Lotufo PA, Chae CU, Ajani UA et al. Male pattern baldness and coronary heart disease: the Physicians' Health Study. Arch Intern Med 2000; 160: 165–71.

44. Ahouansou S, Le Toumelin P, Crickx B et al. Association of androgenetic alopecia and hypertension. Eur J Dermatol 2007; 17: 220–2.

45. Ellis JA, Stebbing M, Harrap SB. Male pattern baldness is not associated with established cardiovascular risk factors in the general population. Clin Sci (Lond) 2001; 100: 401–4.

46. Denmark-Wahnefried W, Schildkraut JM, Thompson D et al. Early onset baldness and prostate cancer risk. Cancer Epidemiol Biomarkers Prev 2000; 9: 325–8.

47. Hamilton JB. Patterned hair loss in man: types and incidence. Ann N Y Acad Sci 1951; 53: 708–28.

48. Kligman AM. The comparative histopathology of male pattern baldness and senescent baldness. Clin Dermatol 1986; 6: 108–18.

49. Pinkus H. Differential patterns of elastic fibers in scarring and non-scarring alopecias. J Cutan Pathol 1978; 5: 93–104.

50. Cash TF. The psychological effects of androgenetic alopecia in men. J Am Acad Dermatol 1992; 26: 926–31.

51. Passchier J. Quality of life issues in male pattern hair loss. Dermatol 1998; 197: 217–18.

52. Lee HJ, Ha SJ, Kim D et al. Perception of men with androgenetic alopecia by women and nonbalding men in Korea: how the nonbald regard the bald. Int J Dermatol 2002; 41: 867–9.

53. Sinclair RD, Dawber RP. Androgenetic alopecia in men and women. Clin Dermatol 2001; 19: 167–78.

54. Trueb RM, Itin P. [Photographic documentation of the effectiveness of 1 mg oral finasteride in treatment of androgenic alopecia in the man in routine general practice in Switzerland.] Schweiz Rundsch Med Prax 2001; 90: 2087–93. [in German]

55. Devine BL, Fife R, Trust PM. Minoxidil for severe hypertension after failure of other hypotensive drugs. Br Med J 1977; 2: 667–9.

56. Li M, Marubayashi A, Nakaya Y et al. Minoxidil-induced hair growth is mediated by adenosine in cultured dermal papilla cells: possible involvement of sulfonylurea receptor 2B as a target of minoxidil. J Invest Dermatol 2001; 117: 1594–600.

57. Katz HI, Hien NT, Prawer SE et al. Long-term efficacy of topical minoxidil in male pattern baldness. J Am Acad Dermatol 1987; 16: 711–18.

58. Rietschel RL, Duncan SH. Safety and efficacy of topical minoxidil in the management of androgenetic alopecia. J Am Acad Dermatol 1987; 16: 677–85.

59. Price VH, Menefee E, Strauss PC. Changes in hair weight and hair count in men with androgenetic alopecia, after application of 5% and 2% topical minoxidil, placebo, or no treatment. J Am Acad Dermatol 1999; 41: 717–21.

60. Olsen EA, Weiner MS, Amara IA et al. Five-year follow-up of men with androgenetic alopecia treated with topical minoxidil. J Am Acad Dermatol 1990; 22: 643–6.

61. Whiting DA. Diagnostic and predictive value of horizontal sections of scalp biopsy. J Am Acad Dermatol 1993; 28: 755–63.

62. Olsen SA, Dunlap FE, Funicella T et al. A randomized clinical trial of 5% topical minoxidil versus 2% topical minoxidil and placebo in the treatment of androgenetic alopecia in men. J Am Acad Dermatol 2002; 47: 377–85.

63. Shapiro J, Price VH. Hair regrowth: Therapeutic agents. Dermatol Clin 1998; 16: 341–56.

64. Wilson C, Walkden V, Powell S et al. Contact dermatitis in reaction to 2% topical minoxidil solution. J Am Acad Dermatol 1991; 24: 661–2.

65. Drake L, Hordinsky M, Fiedler V et al. The effects of finasteride on scalp skin and serum androgen levels in men with androgenetic alopecia. J Am Acad Dermatol 1999; 41: 550–4.

66. Roberts JL, Fiedler V, Imperato-McGinley J et al. Clinical dose ranging studies with finasteride, a type2. 5alpha-reductase inhibitor, in men with male pattern hair loss. J Am Acad Dermatol 1999; 41: 555–63.

67. Kaufman KD, Olsen EA, Whiting D et al. Finasteride in the treatment of men with androgenetic alopecia. Finasteride male pattern hair loss study group. J Am Acad Dermatol 1998; 39: 578–89.

68. Van Neste D, Fuh V, Sanchez-Pedreno P et al. Finasteride increases anagen hair in men with androgenetic alopecia. Br J Dermatol 2000; 143: 804–10.

69. Whiting DA, Waldstreicher J, Sanchez M et al. Measuring reversal of hair miniaturization in androgenetic alopecia by follicular counts in horizontal sections of serial scalp biopsies: results of finasteride 1 mg treatment of men and postmenopausal women. J Investig Dermatol Symp Proc 1999; 4: 282–4.

70. Price VH, Menefee E, Sanchez M et al. Changes in hair weight in men with androgenetic alopecia after treatment with finasterdie (1 mg daily): Three- and 4-year results. J Am Acad Dermatol 2006; 55: 71–4.

71. Leyden J, Dunlap F, Miller B et al. Finasteride in the treatment of men with frontal male pattern hair loss. J Am Acad Dermatol 1999; 40: 930–7.

72. The Finasteride Male Pattern Hair Loss Study Group. Long-term (5-year) multinational experience with finasteride 1 mg in the treatment of men with androgenetic alopecia. Eur J Dermatol 2002; 12: 38–49.

73. Stough DB, Rao NA, Kaufman KD et al. Finasteride improves male pattern hair loss in a randomized study in identical twins. Eur J Dermatol 2002; 12: 32–7.

74. Tosti A, Piraccini BM, Soli M. Evaluation of sexual function in subjects taking finasteride for the treatment of androgenetic alopecia. J Eur Acad Dermatol Venereol 2001; 15: 418–21.

75. Tollin SR, Rosen HN, Zurowski K et al. Finasteride therapy does not alter bone turnover in men with benign prostatic hyperplasia—a clinical research center study. J Clin Endocrinol Metab 1996; 81: 1031–4.

76. Matsumoto AM, Tenover L, McClung M et al. The long-term effect of specific type II 5alpha-reductase inhibition with finasteride on bone mineral density in men: results of a 4-year placebo controlled trial. J Urol 2002; 167: 2105–8.

77. Wade MS, Sinclair RD. Reversible painful gynaecomastia induced by low dose finasteride (1 mg/day). Australas J Dermatol 2000; 41: 55.

78. Ferrando J, Grimalt R, Alsina M et al. Unilateral gynecomastia induced by treatment with 1 mg of oral finasteride. Arch Dermatol 2002; 138: 543–4.

79. Marks LS, Andriole GL, Fitzpatrick JM et al. The interpretation of serum prostate specific antigen in men receiving 5alpha-reductase inhibitors: a review and clinical recommendations. J Urol 2006; 176: 868–74.

80. Olsen EA, Hordinsky M, Whiting D et al. The importance of dual 5alpha-reductase inhibition in the treatment of male pattern hair loss: results of a randomized placebo-controlled study of dutasteride versus finasteride. J Am Acad Dermatol 2006; 55: 1014–23.

81. Debruyne F, Barkin J, van Erps P et al. Efficacy and safety of long-term treatment with the dual 5alpha-reductase inhibitor dutasteride in men with symptomatic benign prostatic hyperplasia. Eur Urol 2004; 46: 488–94.

82. Sovak M, Seligson AL, Kucerova R et al. Fluridil, a rationally designed topical agent for androgenetic alopecia: first clinical experience. Dermatol Surg 2002; 28: 678–85.

83. Inui S, Itami S. Reversal of androgenetic alopecia by topical ketoconzole: relevance of anti-androgenic activity. J Dermatol Sci 2007; 45: 66–8.

84. Leavitt M, Perez-Meza D, Rao NA et al. Effects of finasteride (1 mg) on hair transplant. Dermatol Surg 2005; 31: 1268–76.

85. Shiell RC. Modern hair restoration surgery. Clin Dermatol 2001; 19: 179–87.

CHAPTER 29

Diabetes mellitus: focus on type 2 diabetes

D John Betteridge

Introduction

The threat to public health and to men's health from the rapidly increasing prevalence of type 2 diabetes fueled by the epidemic of obesity is enormous. This phenomenon is likely to bring with it an explosion of vascular complications resulting in premature morbidity and mortality from atherosclerosis-related disease – coronary heart disease, stroke, and peripheral vascular disease, in addition to the specific small-vessel or micovascular complications contributing to retinopathy, nephropathy, and neuropathy.

This chapter describes the epidemiology of type 2 diabetes and reviews pre-diabetes and the metabolic syndrome and the preventative measures that have been shown to reduce progression to diabetes. Clearly it is beyond the scope of this chapter to discuss in detail all facets of diabetes management; rather, the focus will be on the management of the increased vascular risk in this population together with the prevention of renal disease: major challenges in men's health.

What is type 2 diabetes?

Diabetes mellitus has been defined by the American Diabetes Association (ADA) as 'a group of metabolic disease characterized by hyperglycemia resulting from defects in insulin secretion, action or both. The chronic hyperglycemia is associated with long-term damage, dysfunction and failure of various organs, especially the eyes, kidney, nerves, heart and blood vessels.' The diagnostic criteria are shown in Table 29.1, together with definitions of impaired glucose tolerance (IGT) and impaired fasting glucose (IFG), which represent intermediate states between normal glucose metabolism and diabetes. As IGT requires an oral glucose tolerance test to make the diagnosis, the ADA introduced a new concept of IFG, orginally set at 6.1 mmol/L and subsequently revised down to 5.6 mmol/L. However the level is still debated.

Type 2 diabetes accounts for the vast majority (>90%) of adult cases of diabetes and represents a heterogeneous disorder characterized by resistance to the action of insulin and β-cell failure. There are strong genetic factors involved in the pathogenesis of type 2 diabetes, as evidenced by the high concordance rate (approximately 90%) in monozygotic twins. Although genetic defects have been identified in rare subgroups of patients, genes explaining the bulk of diabetes remain to be determined. Insulin resistance is a fundamental in the etiology and is also closely linked to a clustering of risk factors: hypertension, raised triglycerides, low levels of high-density lipoprotein (HDL) cholesterol, and obesity (particularly central obesity as measured by waist circumference), in addition to IGT or frank diabetes, often referred to as the metabolic syndrome. As discussed below, this cluster of metabolic risk factors for heart disease as well as diabetes is referred to as the metabolic syndrome, although this concept

Table 29.1. *Criteria for classification of glucose tolerance status according to World Health Organization and the American Diabetes Association criteria*

Glucose tolerance status	Definition	Classification criteria (mmol/L)
Normal glucose tolerance (NGT)	WHO (1999)	FPG <6.1 and 2 h PG <7.8
	ADA (1997)	FPG <6.1
	ADA (2003)	FPG <5.6
Impaired fasting glucose (IFG)	WHO (1999)	FPG ≥6.1 and <7.0 and 2 h PG <7.8
	ADA (1997)	FPG ≥6.1 and <7.0
	ADA (2003)	FPG ≥5.6 and <7.0
Impaired glucose tolerance (IGT)	WHO (1999)	FPG <7.0 and 2 h PG ≥7.8 and <11.1
Diabetes mellitus (DM)	WHO (1999)	FPG ≥7.0 and 2 h PG ≥11.1
	ADA (1997)	FPG ≥7.0
	ADA (2003)	FPG ≥7.0

DM, diabetes mellitus; IFG, impaired fasting glucose; IGT, impaired glucose tolerance; NGT, normal glucose tolerance.
From Goldstein BJ, Müller-Wieland D, Eds. Type 2 diabetes: principles and practice. 2nd edn. New York: Informa Healthcare, 2008.

has been criticized. Diabetes develops when pancreatic islet β-cell production cannot maintain insulin levels – first manifesting itself as lack of first-phase insulin release – to overcome insulin resistance, and blood glucose rises.

Epidemiology of type 2 diabetes

The enormousness of the potential burden of diabetes and its increasing prevalence has been recognized by the United Nations (UN).[1] In an important resolution that encourages member states to 'develop national policies for the prevention, treatment and care of diabetes in line with the sustainable development of their healthcare systems.' Along with this the UN has called for a World Diabetes Day 'to raise public awareness of diabetes and related complications, as well as its prevention and care including through education and the mass media.'

The current global estimate of the number of people with diabetes (mostly type 2) by the International Diabetes Federation (IDF) is 246 million, which amounts to approximately 6% of the world's adult population.[2] This number is estimated to increase by 7 million each year. Diabetes prevalence does vary by region but it is increasing in all regions; it is highest in parts of the western Pacific, the Middle East, the eastern Mediterranean, and North America.[3] Important and worrying trends are the increasing prevalence in the developing world[3] and the escalation of cases in younger people such that children and adolescents are developing a disease that was very much a condition of the middle-aged and elderly and are therefore at increased vascular risk at an earlier age.[4] In the UK, 2.2 million people have a diagnosis of diabetes, mainly type 2, about 4% of the total population. In addition it is estimated that up to 750 000 people have diabetes but are not aware of it. These numbers represent an 11-fold increase since 1940.

Type 2 diabetes is associated with important complications leading to significant morbidity and premature mortality. According to the IDF, diabetes is now the fourth leading cause of death, with 3.8 million deaths annually attributable to the disease.[2] Life expectancy is significantly reduced with affected people losing 5–10 years compared with those without diabetes. This reduction is due mostly to cardiovascular disease (CVD), which accounts for over two-thirds of deaths. In addition to this CVD burden, diabetes is the most important cause of chronic kidney disease requiring renal replacement therapy[5] and the IDF estimates that renal failure accounts for 10–20% of the deaths. Diabetic retinopathy is the major cause of blindness in developed countries and over half of lower limb amputations are attributable to diabetes.

It has been estimated that up to 50% of all people with diabetes are undiagnosed since the condition may remain asymptomatic for many years. Mass screening for asymptomatic disease is not currently recommended because there is as yet no evidence that the prognosis of such cases will be improved by early detection and treatment.[6] However, the possibilities for the prevention of CVD and other complications suggest that screening might be beneficial.[7] In addition, identifying those at risk of developing diabetes should enable effective preventative measures for delaying progression to diabetes.

Those at high risk of type 2 diabetes

There is no doubt that the increasing prevalence of type 2 diabetes closely parallels the increasing prevalence of obesity. Traditionally obesity is defined by the body mass index (BMI) calculated as weight (in kilograms) divided by height (in meters) squared.[8] Many studies have pointed to the increased incidence of diabetes with increasing BMI.[9] The US National Institutes of Health (NIH) has recommended standardized cut-off points for BMI of $\geq 25 \, kg/m^2$ for overweight and $\geq 30 \, kg/m^2$ for obesity. However, there is increasing evidence that it is central or visceral obesity, otherwise known as android or male-type obesity, first referred to by Vague in 1947,[10] that best predicts diabetes and the metabolic syndrome. A good indication of visceral obesity is waist circumference.[11] Ohlson et al. reported that the incidence of diabetes over 13.5 years was low in relation to increasing tertiles of BMI. However, even with BMI in the lowest tertile, waist–hip ratio (WHR) in the upper tertile was associated with a six-fold increased risk of diabetes: this rose to 30-fold in those with BMI and WHR in

the highest tertile.[12] In addition to diabetes, abdominal obesity predicts the clustering of risk factors referred to as the metabolic syndrome. In an 8-year prospective study, the incidence of metabolic syndrome in those with BMI $\geq 30 \, kg/m^2$ was 20%, compared with 10% in those with a BMI $<30 \, kg/m^2$. However, in those with BMI $\geq 30 \, kg/m^2$ and increased waist circumference ($\geq 102 \, cm$ in men and $\geq 88 \, cm$ in women), 33% developed metabolic syndrome.[13] The prevalence of abdominal obesity as defined by waist circumference is reaching epidemic proportions in the USA (36.9% of men and 55.1% of women)[14] and in the UK (29% of men and 26% of women), as it is in many other developed countries.

Central or visceral obesity can be imaged by computed tomography and correlates with waist circumference.[15,16] Visceral obesity is associated with numerous metabolic abnormalities, including insulin resistance, IGT, and type 2 diabetes, dyslipidemia, and hypertension.[17] It has become clear that adipose tissue and particularly visceral adipose tissue is far more than simply a storage organ for triglyceride, in addition, it is an important endocrine and paracrine organ producing hormones involved in energy homeostasis such as leptin but also important inflammatory mediators and factors related to thrombosis [plasminogen activator inhibitor (PAI)-1] and hypertension (the angiotensin system).[18,19] In terms of the relationship between visceral adipose tissue and IGT and type 2 diabetes mellitus, it is important to understand the role of non-esterified fatty acids (NEFA) and a very important adipokine, namely adiponectin. Increasing visceral fat mass is associated with increased delivery of NEFA to the liver,[20] resulting in increased hepatic NEFA oxidation and increased gluconeogenesis: in addition, increased NEFA flux to skeletal muscle results in increased NEFA oxidation and decreased glucose utilization. Both these processes will tend to lead to insulin resistance and hyperinsulinemia and eventually to type 2 diabetes, if there is pancreatic β-cell failure. An associated phenomenon is ectopic fat deposition in muscle and liver, an important feature of insulin resistance and metabolic syndrome.

Adiponectin is the most abundant adipose-specific protein and is a key adipokine related to the metabolic syndrome. This 244-amino-acid protein is encoded by the gene AMP1 on chromosome 3q27. It has a collagen-like fibrous domain and a C1q-like globular domain. Of particular interest is the fact that adiponectin is present in plasma in varying forms produced by multimerization; the high molecular form appears to be most active. There are two receptors: adipoR1 is abundantly expressed in skeletal muscle and adipoR2 is mainly expressed in liver. Importantly, adiponectin secretion and circulating levels are inversely proportional to body fat content.[21–23] Low levels of adiponectin are associated with obesity and particularly visceral fat accumulation, both in animal models and humans. Concentrations are low in insulin resistance and type 2 diabetes and low levels predict diabetes in various populations. Adiponectin concentrations are related to the typical dyslipidemia associated with type 2 diabetes and metabolic syndrome; it is inversely related to triglyceride, apoprotein B and low-density lipoprotein (LDL) and positively to HDL. As the number of components of the metabolic syndrome increase in an individual, a progressive decrease is observed in adiponectin. In some but not all cross-sectional and prospective studies, adiponectin has been shown to be a CVD risk factor independent of traditional risk factors.[21] It has been called the protective adipokine since, experimentally, it can protect the artery against the adverse effects of high levels of adipose-derived factors such as tumor necrosis factor-α, interleukin-6, PAI-1, angiotensinogen, leptin, and resistin.[22,24] In terms of IGT and type 2 diabetes, adiponectin can reduce NEFA flux to the liver and skeletal muscle and reduce insulin resistance and hyperinsulinemia.

From the above discussion it is clear why the IDF in their consensus definition made central obesity as defined by waist circumference a *sine qua non* for the identification of metabolic syndrome, an important predictor of both type 2 diabetes and CVD.

Several studies have shown that it is possible to reduce the progression of IGT to type 2 diabetes. Although pharmacological agents have an impact it is clear that nutrition and lifestyle measures are the way forward in most situations. It has been known for many years that weight reduction in obese subjects will improve insulin sensitivity and carbohydrate and lipid metabolism.[25] Subsequently, several well-conducted trials have demonstrated that these beneficial effects translate into reduced progression to type 2 diabetes.[26–29] In a Swedish study, increased physical activity and weight reduction in people with IGT over a 6-year period halved progression to diabetes compared with a control group.[26] Similar findings have been reported from China.[27] A total of 577 subjects with IGT were randomized to one of four groups; a control group, a diet group, an exercise group, and a diet plus exercise group. After a follow-up period of 6 years there was a 68% incidence of diabetes in the control group. However in the three intervention groups incidence was reduced to 41% in the exercise group and 44% in the diet group. There did not appear to be any additional benefit in the diet and exercise group with an incidence of 46%.[27]

In the Finnish Diabetes Prevention Study, 522 obese men and women with IGT (mean BMI 31 kg/m², mean age 55 years) were randomized to receive individual counseling to reduce weight and total fat intake and to increase fiber intake and physical activity. This group was compared with a control group, which received general oral and written advice. The intervention group achieved a 4.7% weight reduction compared with 0.9% in the control group. This was associated with a 58% reduction in progression to diabetes.[28] In the US Diabetes Prevention Program, overweight people with IGT were advised on lifestyle measures designed to reduce weight by around 7% and physical activity of moderate intensity to at least 150 minutes each week.[29] These measures were associated with a 58% reduction in progression to diabetes compared with a control group (cumulative incidence 4.8 compared with 11 cases per 100 person-years).[29]

Pharmacological interventions in people with IGT using metformin, acarbose, and thiazolidinediones have also been shown to reduce progression to diabetes, but currently these drugs are not licensed for this indication.

Based on the above discussion it is clear that weight reduction and increased physical activity will reduce the development of diabetes in addition to their other important health benefits.

These interventions are highly effective, with numbers needed to treat to prevent one case of diabetes ranging from 21 to 28. Recognizing the importance of these findings the ADA has recommended screening for glucose abnormalities in people aged 45 years and over with BMI $\geq$25 kg/m^2.[30]

Cardiovascular disease in type 2 diabetes

It is beyond the scope of this chapter to discuss the myriad complications of diabetes, and the focus here is on CVD, the largest cause of morbidity and mortality and end-stage renal disease.

Type 2 diabetes is associated with a markedly increased risk of CVD secondary to premature and extensive atherosclerotic vascular disease.[31] The increased risk is present at the time of diagnosis, which is unsurprising given that the majority of people with diabetes have for many years preceding the diagnosis the features of metabolic syndrome. CVD in diabetes has been highlighted in a recent publication from Diabetes UK[32] pointing out that 80% of people with diabetes will die of CVD. In most studies there is a two- to three-fold increased risk of myocardial infarction (MI). Indeed in some but not all studies people with diabetes were found to be at a similar MI risk to people with a previous MI. Importantly, prognosis after MI is worse in diabetes, which argues strongly for primary prevention. A recent report from EMMACE (Evaluation of Methods and Management of Acute Coronary Events) points to the fact that despite advances in management of acute MI, mortality at 18 months in patients with diabetes has remained unchanged between 1995 and 2003.[33]

So far the increased MI risk in known diabetes has been discussed. What about approaching this from the other angle? What is the prevalence of diabetes amongst those with symptomatic coronary disease? An oral glucose tolerance (OGTT) was performed in 181 patients with acute MI not previously diagnosed with diabetes, and IGT or newly detected diabetes was found in 67%; these abnormalities persisted in longer term follow-up.[34] These findings were largely confirmed in a survey of the prevalence of abnormal glucose regulation in 4196 patients with coronary artery disease across Europe involving 110 centers in 25 countries.[35]

Cerebrovascular disease morbidity and mortality is increased two- to six-fold in diabetes and is related to poor glycemic control.[32,36,37] Prognosis post-event is worse in diabets, with increased recurrence, stroke-related dementia, and stroke mortality, arguing (as with MI) for primary prevention. Diabetes is a risk factor for stroke in younger people, as demonstrated in the Copenhagen Stroke Study.[38] A 10-fold risk increase was observed in a study of risk factors for stroke caused by cerebral infarction in younger adults (<55 years).[39]

A further devastating complication of diabetic vascular disease is peripheral vascular disease (PVD), which may lead to gangrene and amputation. Importantly, PVD in diabetes affects smaller arteries, involving infra-popliteal arteries, and it is more commonly associated with vascular calcification,[40] thus making reconstruction more difficult. In a study from the Netherlands, the rates of PVD among groups of patients ranging from normal glucose tolerance to diabetes requiring multiple medications were analyzed. In those with normal glucose tolerance, there was a 7% prevalence of abnormal ankle–brachial pressure indices compared with 21% in those with long-standing diabetes.[41] Patients with diabetes are more likely to have symptomatic disease and amputation.[42] In the Framingham study the risk of claudication in diabetes was 3.5-fold increased in men and 8.6-fold increased in women.[43]

The etiology of atherosclerosis in diabetes is multi-factorial and relates to diabetes-related factors such as hyperglycemia and insulin resistance as well as the major conventional risk factors of cigarette smoking, hypertension, and hypercholesterolemia.[44,45] The major conventional risk factors are important in diabetes but do not explain fully increased CVD disease in diabetes. In the large database of the men (n=347 978) screened to take part in the Multiple Risk Factor Intervention Trial (MRFIT), 5163 reported taking medication for diabetes.[46] Absolute risk of CVD death at the 12-year follow-up was highly significantly greater for diabetic men (approximately three-fold; $p<0.0001$) after adjustment for age, ethnicity, income, cholesterol, systolic blood pressure, and cigarette smoking. As would be expected, the three major risk factors were significant predictors of CVD mortality but at each level of risk in relation to conventional factors, risk in diabetic men was three-fold higher. In men with diabetes, absolute risk of CVD increased more strongly with higher levels of each risk factor and their combination. The authors emphasized 'rigorous, sustained intervention in people with diabetes to control blood pressure, lower serum cholesterol and abolish cigarette smoking and the importance of considering nutritional–hygenic approaches on a mass scale to prevent diabetes'.[46] In the United Kingdom Prospective Diabetes Study (UKPDS), baseline risk factors were analyzed in relation to subsequent risk of MI in newly diagnosed patients with type 2 diabetes.[47] The findings from UKPDS re-enforce and extend those from MRFIT in that the major cholesterol-carrying lipoproteins, LDL and HDL were assessed together with glycosylated hemoglobin. After adjustment for confounding factors, significant associations were identified in order of significance for LDL cholesterol, HDL cholesterol (inverse relationship), glycosylated hemoglobin, systolic blood pressure, and smoking.[47] These findings argue again for a multi-factorial approach to prevention of vascular disease. It is important to note the numerous other factors that may contribute to atherogenesis in type 2 diabetes, including platelet and coagulation abnormalities, activation of the renin–aldosterone system, arterial endothelial damage or dysfunction, and abnormalities of vascular extracellular matrix turnover, amongst others. Discussion of these factors is beyond the scope of this chapter and the reader is referred to comprehensive reviews.[48,49]

Primary and secondary prevention of vascular disease in diabetes

The approach to the primary and secondary prevention of vascular disease needs to be multi-factorial, with attention to all the major risk factors. This is a serious challenge to physician and patient. One of the most important aspects and one that is little researched is the concordance with multiple drug therapy on top of lifestyle measures. However, this should be possible and the potential for considerable benefit has been demonstrated in the Steno

2 study.[50] In this study, multiple risk factor interventions were applied to a group of high-risk patients with type 2 diabetes by targeting hyperglycemia, (goal: glycosylated hemoglobin 5%), hypertension (goal: systolic blood pressure <130 mmHg), cholesterol (goal: <4.5 mmol/L), triglyceride (goal: <1.7 mmol/L), with the addition of aspirin. These interventions produced a reduction in major CVD events of >50% ($p=0.008$) compared with usual care. Despite this intensive approach, achievement of goals was not fully met, the most difficult being glycemic control.[50]

It goes without saying that diet and lifestyle issues are the cornerstone of therapy and for this to be successful a team approach is crucial, involving dieticians, educators, and specialist nurses as well as the physician. The reader is referred to helpful reviews of these issues.[51–53]

Glycemia

There is no doubt that glucose is toxic to the heart and arteries, as well as the microvasculature. There are several possible mechanisms of glucose toxicity including over-activity of the polyol pathway, the hexosamine pathway, the protein kinase C pathway, and advanced glycation end-products, discussed in an authoritative review by Brownlee.[54] In an analysis from UKPDS, glycosylated hemoglobin during the years of follow-up was associated with increasing risk of MI but the relationship was not as strong as that with microvascular end-points.[55] These findings have been confirmed in a meta-analysis of other studies.[56] However, the evidence from randomized controlled trials that reducing glycemia will reduce CVD events is suggestive but not clear-cut. For instance, in UKPDS, more intensive glycemic therapy with either sulfonylurea or insulin was associated with a highly significant reduction in microvascular end-points ($p=0.0099$). However, the impact on MI was of borderline significance ($p=0.052$) with no impact on stroke.[57] It is important to point out that it would be expected from the UKPDS epidemiology data that a 1% reduction in glycosylated hemoglobin would be associated with a 14% reduction in MI, and the actual reduction within the study of 0.9% produced roughly similar effects.

It is clear from epidemiology data that the relationship between glycemia and CVD extends below the level taken for the diagnosis of diabetes. For instance, in a large prospective study (n=10 232) of men and woman aged 45–79 years from Norfolk, UK, those with glycosylated hemoglobin <5% had the lowest CVD rates and mortality. For an increase of glycosylated hemoglobin of 1%, the relative risk of death was 1.24 ($p<0.001$) in men and 1.32 ($p<0.001$) in women. These relationships were independent of other risk factors and persisted when people with diabetes were excluded.[58] Similar findings have been reported from other populations.[59,60] Given these observations it is likely that intervention to control glycemia will need to achieve glycosylated hemoglobin levels near to or in the normal range to demonstrate benefit in terms of CVD. An ongoing study in the USA called ACCORD will, it is hoped, shed further light in this area. However, given the epidemiology evidence confirmed by meta-analysis[56] and a meta-analysis of glycemic intervention, albeit including data from studies in type 1 diabetes,[61] efforts should be directed to achieve best possible glycemic control, which will often necessitate combination drug therapy and eventually in some cases the addition of insulin. A detailed consensus on the management of hyperglycemia from US and European societies has been published detailing available therapeutic options and algorithms.[62] Along with other guidelines, the Joint British Society Guidelines (JBS-2) suggests that the glycosylated hemoglobin target should be <6.5%.[63]

Diabetic dyslipidemia

The changes in plasma lipids seen in metabolic syndrome and type 2 diabetes involve both quantitative and qualitative changes. Importantly, it is present at the time of diagnosis and in the prediabetic period and persists despite treatment of glycemia and requires management in its own right. It is characterized by moderately raised triglycerides, low HDL cholesterol, and the accumulation of cholesterol-rich remnant particles. Total and LDL cholesterol are generally similar to the background population but there are important qualitative changes

in LDL particles, which are smaller and denser. These changes are associated with increased atherogenicity of the particles. In addition, for a given LDL cholesterol the number of particles will be higher if LDL is small. Although LDL cholesterol is generally not increased in type 2 diabetes, it is the most important risk factor for CVD. In addition, the low HDL and raised triglycerides also contribute to vascular risk.[64,65]

There is now considerable information from randomized controlled trials to guide therapy. For secondary prevention of CVD events there have been no trials performed in specific diabetic populations, but sufficient numbers of people with diabetes were included in the major statin trials to allow subgroup analysis, some pre-specified.

The first major statin trial was the Scandinavian Simvastatin Survival Study (4S), which demonstrated that simvastatin 20–40 mg/day significantly reduced overall mortality by 30% together with CVD events in patients with established coronary disease.[66] Two *post hoc* analyses of 4S have been performed to examine effects in diabetic patients. There were 202 known diabetic patients included in 4S. This is a small number and probably represents somewhat atypical patients in that patients were selected on the basis of hypercholesterolemia, and baseline triglyceride exclusion was relatively low. The effects of simvastatin on plasma lipids in diabetic patients were similar to those seen in the overall study with an approximate 35% reduction in LDL cholesterol.

This analysis demonstrated the high risk of diabetic patients post-MI since approximately one-half of those on placebo suffered an event during the follow-up period of 5.4 years.[66] In those on simvastatin, there was a 55% reduction in CVD events ($p=0.002$).[67]

Numbers were much too small to assess effects on overall mortality, although there was a nonstatistically significant 47% reduction. A subsequent analysis identified additional patients (n=483) based on fasting glucose concentrations. In addition, 678 patients were identified with IFT, and glucose levels of 6.1–6.9 mmol/L. There was a significant 42% reduction in major coronary events ($p<0.001$). In the IFG group there was a 43% significant reduction in the primary end-point of overall mortality ($p<0.02$).[68] Results from 4S have been confirmed in subgroup analyses from the other major secondary prevention trials.[69] The Heart Protection Study (HPS) included a large diabetes subgroup, and its analysis was pre-specified.[70]

What is clear from these results is that diabetic patients with established coronary disease benefit from statin therapy in a similar way to those without diabetes. However, there remains a high residual risk. For instance, in HPS the residual risk of a major CVD event in diabetic patients with coronary disease receiving simvastatin 40 mg/day remained higher than in non-diabetic patients with coronary disease on placebo.[70]

It appeared from the 14 randomized controlled trials of statin therapy analyzed by the Cholesterol Treatment Trialists' Collaborators that the greater the LDL reduction the greater the reduction in events.[71] The question arising from this analysis is whether more intensive LDL lowering would achieve more benefit, and this appears to be the case. A recent meta-analysis of the four trials that have examined this question either with different doses of statin or by comparing a less effective statin with a more effective one has shown that more intensive therapy leads to a further 16% reduction in coronary events.[72] In the Treat to New Targets (TNT) trial, more intensive therapy with atorvastatin 80 mg/day was compared with atorvastatin 10 mg/day in 10001 patients with stable coronary disease.[73] Intensive therapy, which achieved an LDL cholesterol of 2 mmol/L, was associated with a 22% risk reduction in the primary end-point (coronary death, non-fatal MI, resuscitated cardiac arrest, and stroke) compared with standard therapy (mean LDL 2.6 mmol/L over a median follow-up of 4.9 years). In the 1501 diabetic patients included in this trial, more intensive therapy was associated with a significant 25% risk reduction ($p=0.026$). Significant differences between the groups in favor of more intensive therapy were also observed for cerebrovascular events (0.69; $p=0.037$) and any cardiovascular event (0.85; $p=0.044$).

On the basis of these new trials the American Heart Association suggested a revision of LDL cholesterol treatment goals to <70 mg/dL (1.8 mmol/L) in those at highest risk, such as those with diabetes and established coronary heart disease.[74]

Given the higher case fatality in diabetic patients with the first vascular event, primary prevention of CVD events is an important consideration in the management of diabetes. The early statin primary prevention trials did not include sufficient diabetic patients to establish significant benefit. The first trial to demonstrate conclusive benefit in diabetic patients was HPS, which included 2912 diabetic patients (aged 40–80 years) and a non-fasting total cholesterol >3.5 mmol/L without symptomatic CVD.[70] In this pre-specified subgroup, the composite primary end-point was coronary death, non-fatal MI, revascularization, and stroke. Patients were randomly allocated to simvastatin 40 mg/day or placebo. Simvastatin therapy was associated with a reduction of LDL cholesterol of 0.9 mmol/L. There was a highly significant 33% reduction in CVD risk in the simvastatin group ($p=0.0003$). This effect was independent of baseline lipids, diabetes duration, diabetic control, and age. The authors calculated that simvastatin therapy over 5 years should prevent first events in approximately 45 people per 1000 people treated. They concluded that statin therapy should be considered routinely in all diabetic patients at sufficiently high risk of major vascular events independent of initial cholesterol levels.[70]

Support for the findings of HPS came from the first end-point trial to be performed specifically in a diabetic population. The Collaborative Atorvastatin Diabetes Study (CARDS) recruited type 2 diabetic patients without previous history of CVD but at least one other risk factor for CVD, namely retinopathy, hypertension, albuminuria, or current cigarette smoking.[75] Baseline LDL cholesterol concentration had to be <4.14 mmol/L and fasting triglyceride concentration <6.78 mmol/L. A total of 2838 patients aged 40–75 years were randomly allocated to atorvastatin 10 mg/day or placebo.

CARDS was designed to have 90% power to detect a reduction of one-third in the primary end-point in the atorvastatin group at a significance level of $p<0.05$. To achieve the specified statistical power, assuming a cumulative annual incidence of 2.35% for the primary end-point in the placebo group, a total of 304 primary end-points needed to accrue. The primary end-point was a composite of time to first occurrence of acute CHD events, coronary revascularization, or stroke. The trial was terminated 2 years earlier than expected because the pre-specified early stopping rule for efficacy had been met. Atorvastatin therapy was associated with a 40% reduction in LDL cholesterol, the median LDL cholesterol during the study being 2.0 mmol/L representing an absolute LDL reduction of 1.2 mmol/L. Allocation to atorvastatin therapy was associated with a 37% reduction in incidence of major CVD events (p=0.001). There was a 36% reduction in acute coronary events, a 31% reduction in revascularizations, and a 48% reduction in stroke. Although not powered for overall mortality there was a 27% reduction in mortality (p=0.059). There was no heterogeneity of effect in respect of baseline lipids, age, duration of diabetes, glycosylated hemoglobin, systolic blood pressure, smoking, or albuminuria.

The authors concluded that atrovastatin was safe and effective in reducing the risk of first CVD events in patients without high LDL cholesterol (mean baseline LDL 3 mmol/L). On the basis of this trial and HPS there seems to be no justification for a particular threshold level of LDL to determine which patients should receive statin therapy. The debate about whether all patients with type 2 diabetes should receive statins should now focus on whether any patients are at sufficiently low risk for statins to be withheld.

The subgroup with diabetes from the Anglo-Scandinavian Cardiac Outcomes Trial Lipid Lowering Arm (ASCOT-LLA) showed a similar trend in reduction of vascular events.[76] This trial is particularly interesting in that the benefits of statin therapy (atorvastatin 10 mg/day) were seen in well-treated hypertensive patients. A total of 2532 diabetic patients were included in ASCOT-LLA, and tests for heterogeneity of effect did not reveal a significant difference in response in this subgroup, although the observed reduction (16%) in the primary endpoint (fatal coronary artery disease and non-fatal MI) did not reach statistical significance. This probably relates to the fact that there were only 84 primary end-points in the diabetes subgroup and greater add-in therapy. Using an expanded composite end-point, analysis of the statin benefits was statistically significant. As with CARDS, this trial was stopped early because the results overall

(36% risk reduction, mean follow-up 3.3 years) passed the pre-specified stopping rule.

What is clear from reviewing all the major trials is that the benefits of statin therapy extend to reduction in stroke as well as CHD. This came as somewhat of a surprise since the epidemiology of cholesterol as a predictor of stroke was unclear.[70,77] Meta-analysis of the statin trials points to a 21% risk reduction for every 1 mmo/L decrease in LDL cholesterol.[37,38] In CARDS, a reduction in stroke of 48% was observed, which suggests a greater benefit than what would be predicted from the 1.2 mmol/L decrease in LDL. However, the confidence intervals of this reduction do include a 25% effect.[75]

Recent guidelines have reflected this new information on the benefits of statin therapy and the fact that the benefits are independent of baseline lipids. The ADA recommends that in diabetic patients aged 40 years or over with total cholesterol >3.5 mmol/L, statin therapy should be given to achieve an LDL reduction of 30–40% regardless of baseline LDL levels and without risk calculation.[78] Similarly, the British Joint Societies guidelines advise that all people with diabetes aged 40 years or over with either type 1 or type 2 diabetes should receive statin therapy with a goal of therapy for total cholesterol <4 mmol/L and an LDL cholesterol <2 mmol/L. For people aged 18–39 years with either type 1 or type 2 diabetes, statins should be given in those with retinopathy, nephropathy, poor glycemic control defined as glycosylated hemoglobin >9%, elevated blood pressure requiring drug therapy, total cholesterol >6 mmol/L, features of the metabolic syndrome, or a family history of diabetes.[63]

Lipid lowering with fibrates

There is much less information available from major CVD end-point clinical trials of fibrate drugs to guide clinical practice. In the Helsinki Heart Study, a primary prevention trial in 4082 men with non-HDL cholesterol >5.2 mmol/L, gemfibrozil therapy reduced coronary heart disease events by 35%.[78] This reduction is greater than would have been expected from the cholesterol reduction observed. In a *post hoc* analysis the benefits of gemfibrozil were found to occur principally in patients with a ratio of total to HDL cholesterol ratio of >5 who were also hypertriglyceridemic. In this subgroup, there was a 71% risk reduction. In the small subgroup of diabetic patients (n=135) included, the incidence of coronary death and MI was significantly higher (7.4% vs 3.3%), but the 68% risk reduction in the diabetic patients with gemfibrozil did not reach statistical significance possibly because of the small numbers.[79]

Bezafibrate was also used in a large secondary prevention trial conducted in Israel – the Bezafibrate Infarct Prevention (BIP) trial. The overall result did not reach statistical significance[80] but in a *post hoc* analysis of those with evidence of the metabolic syndrome there was a significant risk reduction.

In the Veterans Administration HDL Trial (VAHIT), gemfibrozil 1200 mg/day was compared with placebo in 2531 men with stable coronary artery disease and low HDL cholesterol (baseline HDL 0.8 mmo/L, LDL 2.8 mmol/L). Gemfibrozil therapy was associated with a 22% risk reduction in coronary death and non-fatal MI ($p=0.006$) after a mean follow-up of 5.1 years.[81] In a subgroup of 309 diabetic patients, a composite end-point of coronary death, stroke, and MI was reduced by 32%. In VAHIT there was no effect on LDL cholesterol but HDL increased by 5–6% and triglycerides fell by 31%, suggesting benefit beyond LDL lowering.

In the recent Fenofibrate Intervention and Event Lowering in Diabetes (FIELD) study, fenofibrate was compared with placebo in 9795 diabetic patients (aged 50–75 years) with type 2 diabetes and not taking a statin at study entry.[47] The diabetic population consisted of patients with previous CVD (n=2131) but the majority had no previous disease (n=7764). The primary end-point was coronary death and non-fatal MI. After a median follow-up of 5 years, 288 patients on placebo and 256 on fenofibrate had a first coronary event, a relative risk reduction of 11% (0.89, 95% CI 0.75–1.05; $p=0.16$) was observed in the fenofibrate group. This was associated with a statistically significant 24% reduction in non-fatal MI but a statistically non-significant increase in coronary mortality. Total mortality was 6.6% in the placebo group and 7.3% in the fenofibrate group. Clearly this result is disappointing and there was no effect in those with established disease. Fenofibrate effects on HDL were small and there was more add-in statin therapy in the placebo group. In addition,

fenofibrate increased homocysteine concentrations, which may have an adverse effect on vascular risk.

Whatever the explanation for the outcome of this large trial, the guidelines for therapy in diabetes should remain unaltered, with statins the first-line therapy in the overwhelming majority of patients.[82]

Future trends in lipid therapy

Statins have dramatically improved outcome in patients with diabetes, and the priority now is to transfer this knowledge into clinical practice. There is a perception amongst physicians that diabetic patients without CVD should not be treated to the same goals of therapy as those with known CVD.[83] However, despite statin therapy there remains a significant residual risk particularly in those with established disease. This is exemplified by the results of HPS. In those people with diabetes and CVD the residual risk in those treated with simvastatin 40 mg/day remained higher than in those patients in the placebo group without diabetes but with symptomatic CVD.[26] Clearly, more recent trials have shown the benefits of more intensive therapy but an additional approach may be to target the next important lipid parameter, namely HDL, in addition to intensive LDL lowering.

As discussed earlier, increasing HDL may protect against atherogenesis in several different ways but what is missing is clinical trial data such as exist for LDL lowering. HDL can be increased by diet and lifestyle measures and various drugs. The statins in most patients have a relatively small impact on HDL. The fibrates are traditionally used to increase HDL but the data from the major trials show that their effect is small. In addition, the only fibrate with good evidence from randomized controlled trials is gemfibrozil, and this agent should not be combined with statins because of a serious drug interaction. Nicotinic acid derivatives have a larger effect on HDL, and studies with these agents do suggest benefit on CVD, mainly from surrogate end-point studies. In the diabetic patient, smaller doses of nicotinic acid and its derivatives, particularly prolonged-release preparations, which significantly increase HDL, are likely to have less adverse effects on diabetic control than the higher doses used in the past.[84]

However, newer approaches are clearly required. These new approaches may involve the PPAR gamma agonist, pioglitazone. For example, in the PROactive study, a study of secondary prevention in diabetes, the increase in HDL was 9% and it is likely that some of the benefit in reducing vascular events observed in this study was related to this effect.[85] Another development is the endocannabinoid receptor blocker, rimonabant, which produces similar effects on HDL.[86] It is of interest that both peroxisome proliferator activated receptor (PPAR) gamma agonist and rimonabant increase adiponectin levels in diabetic patients, which may explain the impact on HDL. The first cholesterol ester transfer protein inhibitor, torcetrapib, which increased HDL by approximately 50%, turned out to be toxic and has been withdrawn.[87]

Until there is more evidence from randomized controlled trials to guide combination therapy, the author's approach in patients where LDL is the goal but triglycerides remain raised or HDL is low is to use a secondary goal of therapy, namely non-HDL cholesterol set at 0.8 mmol/L above the LDL goal. To achieve this secondary goal, statin dosage should be increased or a more effective statin (such as atorvastatin or rosuvastatin) substituted. Addition of the specific cholesterol absorption inhibitor, ezetimibe, is very helpful in reducing LDL by a further 20–25% when added to maximum tolerated statin.

Hypertension

The benefits of effective management of hypertension are well established[63] and do not need to be reviewed here. Rather, the focus is on the particular benefits to be achieved in the high-risk population of those with type 2 diabetes. In addition to the benefits in reducing stroke, congestive heart failure, and coronary events, the potential benefit in preventing and delaying progression of retinopathy and nephropathy is huge.

Many hypertension studies over recent years have included representative numbers of people with diabetes, and in several studies specific diabetic populations have been targeted – some of these

trials are discussed here. The epidemiology from UKPDS was clear: increasing blood pressure was associated with MI but also with microvascular events.[88] This finding predicts the outcome of the UKPDS hypertension sub-study performed in 1148 hypertensive patients (mean blood pressure 160/94 mmHg). Patients were randomly allocated to 'tight' control (blood pressure goal <150/85 mmHg) with captopril or atenelol as main treatment, or less 'tight' control (blood pressure goal <180/105 mmHg). The pre-defined clinical end-points were time to occurrence of first clinical end-point related to diabetes (sudden death, death from hyperglycemia or hypoglycemia, fatal or non-fatal MI, angina, heart failure, amputation, vitreous hemorrhage, retinal photocoagulation, blindness in one eye, or cataract extraction); death related to diabetes; or death from all causes. In the 'tight' control group (mean blood pressure 144/82 mmHg) there was a 24% reduction in diabetes-related end-points (95% CI 8–38%; $p=0.0046$) compared with the less 'tight' group (mean blood pressure 154/87 mmHg). Deaths related to diabetes were reduced by 32% (6–51%; $p=0.019$). All cause mortality was not significantly reduced. Tighter blood pressure control also reduced development and progression of diabetes.

This is an important study and provides clear evidence for the benefit of lowering blood pressure; hypertension affects about 40% of patients at the age of 45 years, increasing to 60% at 75 years. An important practice point is that in the 'tight' control group, 29% of patients required three or more anti-hypertensive agents to achieve the target pressure.[89]

The Hypertension Optimal Treatment (HOT) study included 1501 diabetic hypertensive patients out of a total of 18 790.[90] In the group randomized to a target diastolic pressure ≤80 mmHg (mean achieved 81 mmHg), the risk of major CVD events was halved ($p=0.005$) in comparison with the group (targeted to ≤90 mmHg). Baseline therapy in this study was the calcium-channel blocker, felodipine.

A subgroup analysis of the Systolic Hypertension in the Elderly Programme (SHEP), which used a low-dose diuretic-based anti-hypertensive regimen, demonstrated benefits in older diabetic patients with isolated systolic hypertension. Out of

4736 hypertensives aged >60 years and with systolic pressure ≥160 mmHg and diastolic pressure <90 mmHg, 583 had diabetes. The baseline regimen consisted of low dose chlorthalidone with step up to atenelol or reserpine. In the diabetic group, the 5-year major CVD end-points were reduced by 34%, which was similar to that observed in non-diabetics, but the absolute risk reduction was twice as great for those with diabetes, reflecting their higher risk.[91]

In a further study focusing on systolic hypertension, the Systolic Hypertension in Europe trial (Syst-Eur), very favorable results were observed in the diabetes subgroup (n=492; total population, 4695) with systolic blood pressure 160–219 mmHg and diastolic blood pressure <95 mmHg. Baseline active treatment in this trial was the calcium-channel blocker, nitrendipine. After a relatively short median follow-up of 2 years, CVD mortality fell significantly by 76% and overall mortality by 55%, a considerably greater benefit than seen in those without diabetes.[92]

A large group of diabetic patients (the micro-HOPE study) were included in the Heart Outcomes Prevention Evaluation study (HOPE).[93] A total of 3577 high-risk diabetic patients, mean age 65 years and mean diabetes duration 11.6 years on usual care, were randomly allocated to the angiotensin converting enzyme (ACE) inhibitor, ramipril 10 mg/day. In addition to important effects in reducing MI (22%), stroke (33%), CVD death (37%), and overall mortality (24%), ramipril therapy reduced a composite of microvascular end-points (nephropathy, dialysis, or laser therapy for retinopathy) by 16%. These effects were observed irrespective of the presence of left ventricular dysfunction, microalbuminuria, or hypertension at baseline. Indeed, blood pressure was generally already well controlled in those diabetic patients with hypertension, and approximately 40% of patients at baseline were not classified as hypertensive.[93] A question remains as to how much of the benefit in micro-HOPE was conferred by the small additional effects on blood pressure and how much was conferred by other effects of the ACE inhibitor.

In the Losartan Intervention for Endpoint Reduction in Hypertension (LIFE) study 9153 hypertensive patients with left ventricular hypertrophy were randomly allocated to an angiotensin 2 receptor blocker, losartan, or an atenelol-based regimen.[94,95] The large diabetes subgroup (n=1195) had a mean age of 67 years and a mean blood pressure of 177/96 mmHg. During the 4-year study, blood pressure reduction was roughly similar in the losartan (17/11 mmHg) and the atenelol (19/11 mmHg) groups. The composite primary end-point (CVD death, MI, or stroke) occurred in 103 patients in the losartan group compared with 139 in the atenelol group (0.76; 95%CI 0.5–0.98; p=0.031). Of interest, diabetes is independently related to left ventricular hypertrophy, which is magnified in the presence of hypertension; in the LIFE study, losartan was more effective in reversing left ventricular hypertrophy, which is likely to be related to the improved CVD outcomes. An interesting finding to emerge from the non-diabetic population in the LIFE study was that significantly fewer patients developed new-onset diabetes in those treated with the angiotensin 2 receptor blocker.

From the above discussion, it is clear that the diabetic population benefits considerably from effective management of hypertension, with important effects not only on CVD events but also on microvascular end-points. Indeed, in UKPDS, blood pressure management was more effective in reducing vascular events than glucose management. However, this observation should not detract from the need for the best possible glycemic control, as observed by Mogensen in his editorial, in which he refers to the double jeopardy of high blood pressure and high glucose in type 2 diabetes.[96] Indeed, the additive effects of glycemia and blood pressure on both microvascular events and on MI have been well demonstrated in UKPDS,[97] and patients who underwent 'intensive' glucose management and 'tight' blood pressure control had fewer diabetes-related end-points than those on either policy or neither (p for trend, 0.024).

From the above it should be clear that intensive management of hypertension is a very important aspect of risk management in type 2 diabetes. Along with other national and international guidelines, JBS-2 suggests a target of <130/80 mmHg. To achieve this target combination therapy is generally required.

Hypertension and prevention of kidney disease

Longstanding diabetes is the major contributor to the global burden of chronic kidney disease (CKD) requiring replacement therapy.[5,98,99] Importantly, the clinical course of nephropathy from microalbuminuria to clinical proteinuria to kidney failure can be modified substantially. In addition, an intriguing association exists between proteinuria and increased CVD risk such that many patients die from CVD before reaching end-stage kidney disease.[100,101] This relationship is not fully explained but may represent generalized endothelial dysfunction. It is likely that efforts to reverse proteinuria and reduce nephropathy will translate into CVD reduction as well as a reduction in end-stage kidney disease and the need for renal replacement.

A seminal observation by Mogensen in 1976 has led to major benefit to the diabetic population. He demonstrated that decline in glomerular filtration rate (GFR) was correlated with blood pressure in longstanding diabetic patients with proteinuria, and that lowering of pressure could plateau the decline.[102] Since that initial observation it has become clear from many studies that hypertension is a major determinant of progression of nephropathy and that anti-hypertensive therapy helps to preserve the GFR and to reduce mortality.[103]

There has been considerable debate as to whether drugs that target the renin–angiotensin system (RAS), such as ACE inhibitors or angiotensin 2 receptor blockers, have effects on reno-protection beyond what would be expected from the blood pressure reduction. These drugs produce the greatest reductions in urinary albumin excretion rate. In the RENAAL study (Reduction of Endpoints in Non-Insulin Dependent Diabetes Mellitus with the Angiotensin II Antagonist, Losartan), losartan 50–100 mg/day was compared with placebo in 1513 hypertensive patients with proteinuria.[104] Conventional therapy, including diuretics, β-adrenergic blockers, α-blockers, and calcium-channel blockers, were used in both groups and other angiotensin 2 receptor blockers and ACE inhibitors were excluded. The primary end-point was a composite of doubling in serum creatinine, end-stage renal disease, or death. The study was discontinued early because of

publication of the HOPE study, which showed that ACE inhibition reduced CVD outcomes in a similar population group.[93] Over the 4-year study, there was a 16% risk reduction in the primary end-point ($p=0.02$), with a 25% reduction in the doubling of serum creatinine, a 28% reduction in end-stage renal disease, and a 20% reduction in end-stage renal disease or death.

The Irbesartan Diabetic Nephropathy Trial (IDNT) also employed an angiotensin 2 receptor blocker. It recruited 1715 patients with hypertension and nephropathy, serum creatinine levels of 89–266 μmol/L in women and 106–266 μmol/L in men, and a protein excretion rate of at least 900 mg/day.[105] Patients were randomized to daily treatment with irbesartan 300 mg/day, amlodipine 10 mg/day, or placebo. Target blood pressure control for all three groups was <135/85 mmHg. The primary composite end-point was a doubling of baseline serum creatinine, end-stage renal disease, or all-cause mortality.[105] The mean follow-up ranged from 2.5 to 2.6 years between the treatment arms. Irbesartan therapy was associated with a reduction of 20% in the primary end-point compared with the placebo group ($p=0.024$) and a 23% reduction compared with the amlodipine group ($p=0.006$). Proteinuria was significantly reduced in the irbesartan group but not in the placebo group or the amlodipine group.

The impact of irbesartan has also been studied in the Irbesartan Micoalbuminuria Type 2 Trial (IRMA-II). A total of 590 hypertensive patients with microalbuminuria were randomized to placebo, irbesartan 150 mg/day, or irbesartan 300 mg/day. The primary end-point was time to onset of clinical proteinuria and the follow-up period was 2 years. Compared with patients who did not take the angiotensin 2 receptor blocker, there was a 70% relative risk reduction ($p=0.0004$) in the progression to clinical proteinuria.[106]

The effect of the angiotensin 2 receptor blocker, valsartan, was compared with the calcium-channel blocker, amlodipine, on the urinary albumin excretion rate (UAER) in the Micoalbuminuria Reduction with Valsartan (MARVAL) study. For the same degree of blood pressure control, UAER was significantly reduced with the angiotension 2 receptor blocker, certainly suggesting an effect independent of blood pressure.[107]

From the above discussion it would appear that inhibition of the RAS has reno-protective effects; however, this concept has been challenged. For instance in a *post hoc* analysis of the Antihypertensive and Lipid-Lowering Treatment to Prevent Heart Attack Trial (ALLHAT), which compared ACE inhibitor, calcium-channel blocker, and a diuretic on CVD outcomes, no difference in the incidence of end-stage renal disease or a ≥50% GFR reduction was seen between the ACE inhibitor, lisinopril, compared with the chlorthalidone group in those with diabetes at baseline and in the whole group.[108] However, ALLHAT was not designed as a renal study in that there were no measures of albuminuria and the ACE inhibitor dose was low. A meta-analysis has also challenged a specific reno-protective effect of ACE inhibitor or angiotensin 2 receptor blockers, concluding that the benefits of RAS inhibition are probably the result of an effect on blood pressure.[109]

How can the approach to reno-protection be summarized? It is clear that effective blood pressure lowering with any intervention is reno-protective. Reduction of proteinuria with inhibitors or angiotension 2 receptor blockers appears to be independent of blood pressure, and the controversy relates to whether this translates into hard renal end-points independent of blood pressure lowering. However, several recent analyses have pointed to the relationship between reduction of proteinuria and renal and CVD outcomes.[110,111]

The debate with regard to ACE inhibitors and angiotensin 2 receptor blockers is largely academic in terms of routine management of hypertension in the diabetic patient, since the requirement for multiple drug therapy is the norm for optimal blood pressure control and the great majority of physicians will include an ACE inhibitor or an angiotensin 2 receptor blocker in their approach to drug therapy.

Summary

The almost exponential increase in the prevalence of type 2 diabetes presents major challenges for men's health, given that it brings with it important morbidity and mortality from vascular complications.

In this chapter I have detailed the size of the problem and reviewed how progression from pre-diabetes to clinical diabetes can be delayed. The importance of CVD has been described and the evidence base for preventive measures reviewed. The opportunities for preventive medicine are enormous and should translate into huge benefit for patients.

References

1. United Nations. UN Resolution in Diabetes, UN Resolution 61/225 [available at: http://www.unitefordiabetes.org/campaign/resolution.html].
2. International Diabetes Federation. Facts and Figures: Did You Know? [available at: http://www.idf.org/home/index].
3. International Diabetes Federation. Diabetes Atlas, 3rd edn. Brussels, Belgium: International Diabetes Federation, 2006 [available at:http://www.eatlas.idf.org/media].
4. Pinhas-Hamiel O, Zeitler P. Acute and chronic complications of type 2 diabetes mellitus in children and adolescents. Lancet 2007; 369: 1823–31.
5. Molitch ME, De Fronzo RA, Franz MJ et al. Nephropathy in diabetes. Diabetes Care 2004; 27(Suppl 1): S79–83.
6. Engelgau MM, Narayan KM, Herman WH. Sceening for type 2 diabetes. Diabetes Care 2000; 23: 1563–80.
7. Engelgau MM, Colagiuri S, Ramchandran A et al. Prevention of type 2 diabetes: issues and strategies for identifying persons for interventions. Diabetes Technol Ther 2004; 6: 874–82.
8. Keys A, Fidanza C, Karvonen MJ et al. Indices of relative weight and obesity. J Chronic Dis 1972; 25: 329–43.
9. National Institutes of Health, National Heart, Lung and Blood Institute. Clinical guidelines on the identification, evaluation and treatment of overweight and obesity in adults – the evidence report. Bethesda, MD: National Institutes of Health, 1998.
10. Vague J. La differenciation sexuelle, facteur déterminant des formes de l'obésité. Presse Med 1947; 30: 339–40.
11. Lean ME, Han TS, Morrison CE. Waist circumference as a measure for indicating need for weight management. BMJ 1995; 311: 158–61.

12. Ohlson LO, Larsson B, Svadsudd K et al. The influence of body fat distribution on the incidence of diabetes mellitus. 13.5 years of follow-up of the participants in the study of men born in 1913. Diabetes 1985; 34: 1055–8.

13. Han TS, Williams K, Sattar N et al. Analysis of obesity and hyperinsulinaemia in the development of metabolic syndrome: San Antonio Heart Study. Obes Res 2002; 10: 923–31.

14. Ford ES, Mokdad AH, Giles WH. Trends in wiast circumference among US adults. Obes Res 2003; 11: 1223–3.

15. Miyazaki Y, Glass L, Triplitt C et al. Abdominal fat distribution and peripheral and hepatic insulin resistance in type 2 diabetes mellitus. Am J Physiol Endocrinol Metab 2002; 282: E1135–43.

16. Pouliot MC, Despres JP, Lemieux S et al. Waist circumference and abdominal sagittal diameter: best simple anthropometric indexes of abdominal visceral adipose tissue accumulation and related cardiovascular risk in men and women. Am J Cardiol 1994; 73: 460–8.

17. Eckel RH, Grundy SM, Zimmet PZ. The metabolic syndrome. Lancet 2005; 365: 1415–28.

18. Lyon CJ, Law RE, Hsueh WA. Minireview, adiposity, inflammation and atherogenesis. Epidemiol 2003; 144: 2195–200.

19. Trayhurn P, Wood IS. Adipokines, inflammation and the pleiotropic role of white adipose tissue. Br J Nutr 2004; 92: 347–55.

20. Nielsen S, ZengKui Guo C, Johnson M et al. Splanchnic lipolysis in human obesity. J Clin Invest 2004; 113: 1582–8.

21. Matsuzawa Y. Therapy insight: adipocytokines in metabolic syndrome and related cardiovascular disease. Natl Clin Pract Cardiovasc Med 2006; 3: 35–42.

22. Whitehead JP, Richards AA, Hickman IJ et al. Adiponectin, a key adipokine in the metabolic syndrome. Diabetes Obes Metab 2006; 8: 264–80.

23. Lara-Castro C, Fu Y, Hong Chung B, Garvey WT. Adiponectin and the metabolic syndrome: mechanisms mediating risk for metabolic and cardiovascular disease. Curr Opin Lipidol 2007; 18: 263–70.

24. Hopkins TA, Ouchi O, Shibata R, Walsh K. Adiponectin actions in the cardiovascular system. Cardiovasc Res 2007; 74: 11–18.

25. Olefsky JM, Reaven GM, Farquhar JW. Effects of weight reduction on obesity: studies of carbohydrate and lipid metabolism. J Clin Invest 1974; 53: 64–76.

26. Eriksson KF, Lindgarde F. Prevention of type 2 diabetes mellitus by diet and physical exercise. The 6-year Malmo feasibility study. Diabetologia 1991; 31: 891–8.

27. Pan X-R, Li G-W, Wang J-X et al. Effects of diet and exercise in preventing NIDDM in people with impaired glucose tolerance. The Da Qing IGT and Diabetes Study. Diabetes Care 1997; 20: 537–44.

28. Tuomilehto J, Lindstrom J, Eriksson JG et al. Prevention of type 2 diabetes mellitus by changes in lifestyle among subjects with impaired glucose tolerance. N Engl J Med 2001; 344: 1343–50.

29. Knowler WC, Barrett-Connor E, Fowler SE et al. Reduction in the incidence of type 2 diabetes with lifestyle intervention or metformin. N Engl J Med 2002; 346: 393–403.

30. American Diabetes Association. The prevention or delay of type 2 diabetes. Diabetes Care 2002; 25: 742–9.

31. Zimmet PZ, Alberti KGMM. The changing face of macrovascular disease in non-insulin-dependent diabetes mellitus: an epidemic in progress. Lancet 1997; 350: 1–4.

32. Diabetes UK. Diabetes heartache. The hard reality of cardiovascular care for people in diabetes. Diabetes UK, 2007.

33. Cubbon RM, Wheatcroft SB, Grant PJ et al. on behalf of the EMMACE (Evaluation of Methods and Management of Acute Coronary Events) Investigators. Temporal trends in mortality of patients with diabetes mellitus suffering acute myocardial infarction: a comparison of over 3000 patients between 1995 and 2003. Europ Heart J 2007; 28: 540–5.

34. Norhammar A, Tenerz A, Nisson G et al. Glucose metabolism in patients with acute myocardial infarction and no previous diagnosis of diabetes mellitus: a prospective study. Lancet 2002; 359: 2140–4.

35. Bartnik M, Ryden L, Ferrari R et al. ON behalf of the Euro Heart Survey investigators. Eur Heart J 2004; 25: 1880–90.

36. Barrett-Connor E Khaw KT. Diabetes mellitus: an independent risk factor for stroke? Am J Epidemiol 1988; 128: 116–23.

37. Stegmayr B, Asplund K. Diabetes is a risk factor for stroke: a population perspective. Diabetologia 1995; 38: 1061–8.

38. Morgensen H, Nakayama H, Raaschon HO, Olhsen TS. Stroke in patients with diabetes: the Copenhagen Stroke Study. Stroke 1994; 25: 1977–84.

39. You RX, McNeil JJ, O'Malley HM et al. Risk factors for stroke due to cerebral infarction in young adults. Stroke 1997; 28: 1913–18.

40. Jade EB, Oyibo SO, Chalmers N, Boulton AJ. Peripheral arterial disease in diabetic and non diabetic patients. Diabetes Care 2001; 24: 1433–7.

41. Beks PJ, Mackaay AJ, de Neeling JN et al. Peripheral arterial disease in relation to glycaemic level in an elderly Caucasian population: the Hoorn Study. Diabetologia 1995; 38: 86–96.

42. Uusitupa MI, Niskanen Lk, Siitonen O et al. 5-year incidence of atherosclerotic vascular disease in relation to general risk factors, insulin level and abnormalities in lipoprotein composition in non insulin dependent diabetic and non diabetic subjects. Circulation 1990; 82: 27–36.

43. Kannel WB, McGee DL. Update on some epidemiologic features of intermittent claudication: the Framingham Study. J Am Geriatr Soc 1985; 33: 13–18.

44. Laakso M, Lehto S. Epidemiology of macrovascular disease in diabetes. Diabetes Rev 1997; 5: 294–315.

45. Falk E. Pathogenesis of atherosclerosis. J Am Coll Cardiol 2006; 47: C7–12.

46. Stamler J, Vaccaro O, Neaton JD, Wentworth D for the Multiple Risk Factor Intervention Trial Research Group. Diabetes, other risk factors and 12-year cardiovascular mortality for men screened in the Multiple Risk Factor Intervention Trial. Diabetes Care 1993; 16: 434–44.

47. Turner RC, Millns H, Neil HAW. For the United Kingdom Prospective Diabetes Study Group. Risk factors for coronary artery disease in non insulin dependent diabetes mellitus: United Kingdom Prospective Diabetes Study (UKPDS: 23). BMJ 1998; 316: 823–8.

48. Varughese GI, Tomson J, Lip GYH. Type 2 diabetes mellitus: a cardiovascular perspective. Int J Clin Pract 2005; 59: 798–816.

49. Beckman JA, Creager MA, Libby P. Diabetes and atherosclerosis. Epidemiology, pathophysiology and management. JAMA 2002; 287: 2570–81.

50. Gade P, Vedel P, Larsen N et al. Multifactorial intervention and cardiovascular disease in patients with type 2 diabetes. N Engl J Med 2003; 348: 383–93.

51. Franz MJ, Bantle JP, Beebe CA et al. Evidence-based nutrition principles and recommendations for the treatment and prevention of diabetes and related complications. Diabetes Care 2002; 25: 148–298.

52. Sigal RJ, Kenny GP, Wasserman DH et al. Physical activity/exercise and type 2 diabetes. Diabetes Care 2004; 27: 2518–39.

53. Mensing CR, Boucher J, Cypress M et al. Nutritional standards for diabetes self-management education. Diabetes Care 2000; 23: 682–9.

54. Brownlee M. The pathobiology of diabetic complications. Diabetes 2005; 54: 1615–25.

55. Statton IM, Adler AI, Neil HAW et al. Association of glycaemia with macrovascular and microvascular complications of type 2 diabetes (UKPDS: 35): prospective observational study. BMJ 2000; 321: 405–12.

56. Selvin E, Marinopoulos S, Berkenblit G et al. Meta analysis: glycosylated haemoglobin and cardiovascular disease in diabetes mellitus. Ann Intern Med 2004; 141: 421–31.

57. United Kingdom Prospective Diabetes Study Group. Intensive blood-glucose control with sulphonylureas or insulin compared with conventional treatment and risk of complications in patients with type 2 diabetes (UKPDS 33). Lancet 1998; 352: 837–53.

58. Khaw K-T, Wareham N, Bingham S et al. Association of haemoglobin A1c with cardiovascular disease and mortality in adults: the European Prospective Investigation into Cancer in Norfolk. Ann Intern Med 2004; 141: 413–20.

59. Blake GJ, Pradhan AD, Manson JE et al. Relationship between haemoglobin A1c level and future cardiovascular events among women. Arch Intern Med 2004; 164: 757–61.

60. Selvin E, Coresh J, Golden SH et al. Glycaemic control and coronary heart disease in persons with or without diabetes: the Atherosclerosis Risk in Communities study. Arch Intern Med 2005; 165: 1910–16.

61. Stettler C Allemann S, Juni P et al. Glycaemic control and macrovascular disease in types 1 and 2 diabetes mellitus: Mea-analysis of randomized trials. Am Heart J 2006; 152: 27–38.

62. Nathan DM, Buse JB, Davidson MB et al. Management of hyperglycaemia in type 2 diabetes; a consensus algo-rhythm for the initiation and adjustment of therapy. A consensus statement from the American Diabetes Association and the European Association for the Study of Diabetes. Diabetologia 2006; 49: 1711–21.

63. JBS 2. Joint British Societies guidelines on prevention of cardiovascular disease in clinical practice. Heart 2005; 91(Suppl V): V1–52.

64. Taskinen MR. Diabetic dyslipidaemia: from basic research to clinical practice. Diabetologia 2003; 46: 733–49.

65. Betteridge DJ. Dyslipidaemia and diabetes. Pract Diabetes Int 2001; 18: 201–8.

66. Scandinavian Simvastatin Survival Study Group (4S). Randomised trial of cholesterol lowering in 4444 patients with coronary heart disease: the Scandinavian Simvastatin Survival Study. Lancet 1994; 344: 1383–9.

67. Pyorala K, Pedersen TR, Kjekshus J et al. Cholesterol lowering with simvastatin improves prognosis of diabetic patients with coronary heart disease. A subgroup analysis of the Scandinavian Simvastatin Survival Study (4S). Diabetes Care 1997; 20: 614–20.

68. Haffner SM, Alexander CM, Cook TJ et al. Reduced coronary events in simvastatin-treated patients with coronary heart disease and diabetes or impaired fasting glucose levels. Subgroup analysis in the Scandinavian Simvastatin Survival Study. Arch Intern Med 1999; 159: 2661–7.

69. Ryden L, Standl E, Bartnik M et al. The task force on diabetes and cardiovascular diseases of the European Society of Cardiology (ESC) and of the European Association for the Study of Diabetes (EASD). Guidelines on diabetes, pre-diabetes and cardiovascular diseases: executive summary. Eur Heart J 2007; 28: 88–136.

70. Heart Protection Study Collaborative Group. MRC/BHF Heart Protection Study of cholesterol lowering with simvastatin in 5963 people with diabetes: a randomized placebo-controlled trial. Lancet 2003; 361: 2005–16.

71. Cholesterol Treatment Trialists' (CTT) Collaborators. Efficacy and safety of cholesterol-lowering treatment: prospective meta-analysis of data from 90,056 participants in 14 randomised trials of statins. Lancet 2005; 366: 1267–78.

72. Cannon CP, Steinberg BA, Murphy SA et al. Meta-analysis of cardiovascular outcomes trials comparing intensive versus moderate statin therapy. J Am Coll Cardiol 2006; 48: 438–55.

73. Shepherd J, Barter P, Carmena R et al. Effect of lowering LDL cholesterol substantially below recommended levels in patients with coronary heart disease: the Treating to New Targets (TNT) Study. Diabetes Care 2006; 29: 1220–6.

74. Grundy SM, Cleeman JI, Merz CNB et al. For the Coordinating Committee of the National Cholesterol Education Program. Implications of recent clinical trials for the National Cholesterol Education Program Adult Treatment Panel III guidelines. Circulation 2004; 110: 227–39.

75. Colhoun HM, Betteridge DJ, Durrington PN et al. on behalf of the CARDS investigators. Primary prevention of cardiovascular disease in type 2 diabetes in the Collaborative Atorvastatin Diabetes Study (CARDS): multicentre randomized placebo-controlled trial. Lancet 2004; 364: 685–96.

76. Sever PS, Dahlof B, Poylter NR et al. Prevention of coronary and strokes events with atorvastatin in hypertensive patients who have average or lower than average cholesterol concentrations in the Anglo-Scandinavian Cardiac Outcomes Trial-Lipid Lowering Arm (ASCOT-LLA): a multicentre randomized controlled study. Lancet 2003; 361: 1149–58.

77. Amarenco P, Labreuche J, Lavallée P, Touboul PJ. Statins in stroke prevention and carotid atherosclerosis: systematic review and up-to-date meta-analysis. Stroke 2004; 35: 2902–9.

78. Frick MH, Elo O, Haapa K et al. The Helsinki Heart Study: primary prevention trial with gemfibrozil in middle-aged men with dyslipidaemia. Safety of treatment changes in risk factors and incidence of coronary heart disease. N Engl J Med 1987; 317: 1237–45.

79. Koskinen P, Mantarri M, Manninen V et al. Coronary heart disease in NIDDM patients in the Helsinki heart study. Diabetes Care 1992; 15: 820–5.

80. Bezafibrate Infarction Prevention Study Group. Secondary prevention by raising HDL cholesterol and reducing triglycerides in patients with coronary artery disease: the Bezafibrate Infarction Prevention (BIP) study. Circulation 2000; 102: 21–7.

81. Rubins HB, Robins SJ, Collins D et al. for the Veterans Affairs HDL Intervention Trial (VAHIT). Gemfibrozil for the secondary prevention of coronary heart disease in men with low levels of high density lipoprotein cholesterol. N Engl J Med 1999; 241: 410–18.

82. The FIELD Study Investigators. Effects of long-term fenofibrate therapy on cardiovascular events in 9795 people with type 2 diabetes mellitus (the FIELD study): randomized, controlled trial. Lancet 2005; 366: 1849–61.

83. Leiter LA, Betteridge DJ, Chacra AR et al. on behalf of the AUDIT Study Steering Committee. AUDIT study. Evidence of global undertreatment of dyslipidaemia in patients with type 2 diabetes. Br J Diabetes Vasc Dis 2006; 6: 31–41.

84. Van Gaal LF, Peiffer F, Ballaux D. Reducing cardiovascular disease in patients with type 2 diabetes: the potential contribution of nicotinic acid. Diabetes Vasc Risk 2002; 5: 344–51.

85. Dormandy JA, Charbonnel B, Eckland DJA et al. Secondary prevention of macrovascular events in patients with type 2 diabetes in the PROactive Study (PROspective pioglitAzone Clinical Trial. In macroVascular Events): a randomized controlled trial. Lancet 2005; 366: 1279–88.

86. Despres JP, Golay A, Sjostrom L for the Rimonabant in Obesity-Lipids Study Group. Effects of rimonanbant on metabolic risk factors in overweight patients with dyslipidaemia. N Engl J Med 2005; 353: 2121–34.

87. Barter PJ, Caulfield M, Eriksson M et al. for the ILLUMINATE Investigators. Effects of torcetrapib in patients at high risk for coronary events. N Engl J Med 2007; 357: 2109–22.

88. Adler AI, Stratton MK, Neil HAW et al on behalf of the UK Prospective Diabetes Study group. Association of systolic blood pressure with macrovascular complications of type 2 diabetes. (UKPDS 36): prospective observational study. BMJ 2000; 321: 412–19.

89. UK Prospective Diabetes Study (UKPDS) Group. Tight blood pressure control and risk of macrovascular and microvascular complications in type 2 diabetes. (UKPDS 38). BMJ 1998; 317: 703–13.

90. Hansson L, Zanchetti A, Carruthers SG et al. Effect of intensive blood-pressure lowering and low dose aspirin in patients with hypertension: principle results of the Hypertension Optimal Treatment (HOT) randomized trial. Lancet 1998; 351: 1755–62.

91. Curb JD, Pressel SL, Cutler JA et al. Systolic hypertension in the elderly cooperative research group. Effect of diuretic-based antihypertensive treatment on cardiovascular disease risk in older diabetic patients with isolated systolic hypertension. JAMA 1996; 273: 1886–92.

92. Tuomilehto J, Rastenyte D, Berkenhager WH et al. For the Systolic Hypertension in Europe Trial Investigators. Effects of calcium channel blockade in older patients with diabetes and systolic hypertension. N Engl J Med 199; 340: 677–84.

93. Heart Outcomes Prrevention Evaluation (HOPE) Study Investigators. Effects of ramipril on cardiovascular and microvascular outcomes in people with diabetes mellitus: results of the HOPE study and MICRO-HOPE substudy. Lancet 2000; 355: 253–9.

94. Dahlof B, Devereux RB, Kjeldsen SE et al. Cardiovascular morbidity and mortality in the Losartan Intervention for Endpoint Reduction in Hypertension study (LIFE): a randomized trial against atenelol. Lancet 2002; 359: 1004–10.

95. Lindholm LH, Ihsen H, Dahlof B et al. for the LIFE Study Group. Cardiovascular morbidity and mortality in patients with diabetes in the Losartan intervention for endpoint reduction in hypertension Study (LIFE): a randomized trial against atenelol. Lancet 2002; 359: 1004–10.

96. Mogensen CE. Combined high blood pressure and glucose in type 2 diabetes: double jeopardy. British trials show clear benefit of treatment, especially blood pressure reduction. BMJ 1998; 317: 693–4.

97. Stratton IM, Cull CA, Adler AI et al. Additive effects of glycaemia and blood pressure on risk of complications in type 2 diabetes; a prospective observational study. (UKPDS 75). Diabetologia 2006; 49: 1761–9.

98. Atkins RC. The changing patterns of chronic kidney disease: the need to develop strategies for prevention relevant to different regions and countries. Kidney Int 2005; 98(Suppl): S83–5.

99. Roderick P, Davies R, Jones C et al. Simulation model of renal replacement therapy: predicting future demand in England. Nephrol Dial Transplant 2004; 19: 692–701.

100. Mogensen CE, Cooper ME. Diabetic renal disease: from recent studies to improved clinical practice. Diabetic Med 2004; 21: 4–17.

101. Curtis BM, Levin A, Parfrey PS. Multiple risk factor intervention in chronic kidney disease: management of cardiac disease in chronic kidney disease patients. Med Clin North Am 2005; 89: 511–23.

102. Mogensen CE. Progression of nephropathy in long term diabetics with proteinuria and effect of initial anti-hypertensive treatment. Scand J Clin Lab Invest 1976; 36: 383–8.

103. Grossman E, Messerli FH, Goldbourt U. High blood pressure and diabetes mellitus: are all hypertensive drugs created equal? Arch Intern Med 2000; 160: 2447–52.

104. Brenner BM, Cooper ME, de Zieuw D et al. Effects of losartan on renal and cardiovascular outcomes in patients with type 2 diabetes and nephropathy. N Engl J Med 2001; 345: 861–9.

105. Lewis EJ, Hunsicker LG, Clarke WR et al. for the Collaborative Study Group. Renoprotective effect of the angiotensin-receptor antagonist irbesartan

in patients with nephropathy due to type 2 diabetes. N Engl J Med 2001; 345: 851–60.

106. Parving HH, Lehnert H, Brochner-Mortensen J et al. for the Irbesartan in Patients with microalbuminuria Study Group. The effect of irbesartan on the development of diabetic nephropathy in patients with type 2 diabetes. N Engl J Med 2001; 345: 870–8.

107. Viberti G, Wheeldon NM for the Micoalbumin Reduction with Valsartan (MARVAL) Sudy Investigators. Micoalbuminuria with type 2 diabetes mellitus: a blood pressure-independent effect. Circulation 2002; 106: 672–8.

108. Rahman M, Pressel S, Davis BR et al. Renal outcomes in high-risk hypertensive patients treated with an angiotensin-converting enzyme inhibitor or a calcium channel blocker vs diuretic: a report from the Antihypertensive and Lipid-Lowering treatment to prevent Heart Attack Trial (ALLHAT). Arch Intern Med 2005; 165: 936–46.

109. Casas JP, Chua W, Loukogeorgakis S et al. Effect of inhibitors of the renin-angiotensin system and other anti-hypertensive drugs on renal outcomes: systematic review and meta-analysis. Lancet 2005; 366: 2026–33.

110. Hovind P, Tarnow L, Rossing P et al. Improved survival in patients obtaining remission of nephrotic range albuminuria in diabetic nephropathy. Kidney Int 2004; 66: 1180–6.

111. Ibsen H, Olsen MH, Wachtell K et al. Does albuminuria predict cardiovascular outcomes on treatment with losartan versus atenelol in patients with diabetes, hypertension and left ventricular hypertrophy? The LIFE study. Diabetes Care 2006; 29: 595–600.

Men and the gastro-intestinal system

CHAPTER 30

Esophagitis and peptic ulcer disease

Adam Humphries, Sean Preston

Introduction

Complications secondary to gastric acid are the most common cause of upper gastrointestinal symptoms that result in patients presenting to either primary or secondary care. In the 1980s Warren and Marshall established the role of *Helicobacter pylori* in the formation of peptic ulceration, which, in addition to the advent of acid suppression by proton pump inhibitors (PPIs), has dramatically altered the clinical landscape with regard to diagnosis and treatment of this condition. This chapter discusses the etiology, epidemiology, pathology, clinical presentation, investigation, current management, and complications of both esophagitis and peptic ulcer disease (PUD).

Esophagitis

Reflux esophagitis

Gastro-esophageal reflux disease (GERD) is the major cause of esophagitis, and is defined as the reflux of stomach contents into the esophagus causing symptoms sufficient to impair quality of life. In the Western world 10–20% of the population suffer heartburn more that once weekly, but this figure falls to less than 5% in Asia,[1] with dietary and lifestyle factors being likely explanations for the geographical difference.

The esophagus is protected from free reflux of gastric contents by various mechanisms. Although its epithelial lining contains a few bicarbonate-secreting submucosal glands, it is the tight epithelial junctions of the surface esophageal squamous cells that provide the greatest barrier against damage. In addition to this, the diaphragm in combination with the lower esophageal sphincter (LOS) – a 3–4cm length of contracted smooth muscle – acts as the main physiological protective mechanism.

The pathophysiology of GERD is multi-factorial, but transient lower esophageal sphincter relaxations (TLOSRs) are thought to be the most important mechanism, particularly in mild disease.[2-4] TLOSRs are the reduction in lower esophageal sphincter (LOS) pressure not associated with swallowing, and these have been likened to the lower esophageal equivalent of burping, allowing gastric contents to reflux back into the esophagus. They are not, however, thought to play a major role in the more severe end of the GERD spectrum, where permanently low LOS pressures and anatomical disruption of the gastroesophageal junction predominate. Various foodstuffs (fat, chocolate, caffeine), as well as alcohol, smoking, and medications (anticholingerics, calcium-channel blockers, β-blockers, and nitrates), all decrease the LOS pressure (Fig. 30.1), therefore predisposing to gastric reflux, which can be exacerbated by delayed gastric emptying and poor esophageal clearance.

Hiatus hernia

A hiatus hernia involves a portion of the upper stomach protruding through the diaphragmatic

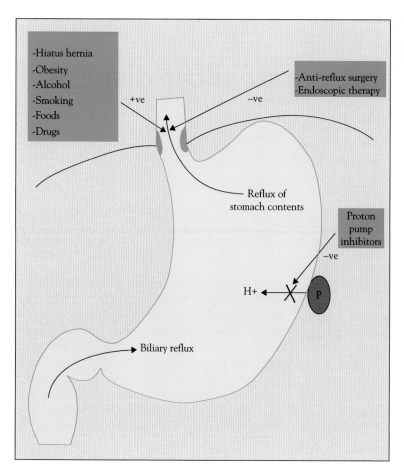

Figure 30.1. *Different physiological mechanisms in gastroesophageal reflux disease. P, parietal cell.*

hiatus into the thoracic cavity. In addition to the LOS, the crural diaphragm also acts to maintain the integrity of the gastroesophageal barrier. In patients with a sliding hernia the contribution of the diaphragm is lost, mainly at times of low LOS pressure and during deep inspiration and straining, therefore predisposing to reflux. Hiatus hernia is seen in significantly more patients with esophagitis than those without, and is associated with prolonged acid exposure and poor esophageal clearance.[5,6] Hiatus hernia size has also been shown to correlate with the severity of esophagitis.[7]

Obesity

The worldwide prevalence of obesity continues to increase rapidly, and being overweight (defined as a body mass index >25 kg/kg^2) increases the risk of GERD by 50% and doubles the risk of esophageal adenocarcinoma.[8] Increased waist circumference has also been shown to be associated with an increased risk of Barrett's esophagus and a greater severity of GERD symptoms.[9] The exact mechanisms are unclear, but TLOSRs have been shown to be longer and to be associated with more frequent reflux episodes in obese patients.[10,11] Obesity also predisposes to the disruption of the esophagogastric junction leading to hiatus hernia and increased intragastric pressure.[10,12] The role of weight loss and obesity surgery in the reversal of these pathophysiological changes is still unclear.

Clinical presentation

The classical symptoms of GERD are heartburn or acid regurgitation (or both), but they can also include nausea or occasionally dysphagia and vomiting. Heartburn usually occurs during and after meals, while recumbent, or on bending forward and is often exacerbated by alcohol, caffeine, and certain foods. Patients with GERD can also present with other extra-esophageal symptoms such as chest pain, abdominal pain, sleep disturbance, laryngitis, cough, and dental erosions.[13,14] Dysphagia cannot simply be attributed to GERD, particularly in the context of weight loss, and an esophageal malignancy must be excluded on an urgent basis.

Clinical examination is especially important in the elderly, where an upper gastrointestinal cancer needs to be considered.

Investigations

The choice of investigations is dependent upon both age and history. Blood tests should include a complete blood count to detect anemia. An endoscopy or a barium swallow should be performed in those patients with any alarm features such as dysphagia, vomiting, unintentional weight loss, anorexia, or iron-deficient anemia to exclude an underlying cancer. There is no current evidence to support screening endoscopy to detect esophageal adenocarcinoma in patients with chronic heartburn.[15] For all other patients, upper gastrointestinal endoscopy is not warranted unless there is sufficient doubt about the cause of symptoms, or they are not responding to appropriate medical management.

Various endoscopic classification systems exist for reflux esophagitis, of which the Los Angeles classification system is the most widely used (Table 30.1).

A barium swallow should be considered in patients who complain of significant dysphagia for which no cause is found at endoscopy. For those patients who have a normal endoscopy and barium swallow and who are not responding to anti-secretory therapy, 24-hour esophageal pH studies and manometry are useful for objective assessment of acid reflux in order to guide further management.

Management
Conservative measures

Lifestyle advice focusing on weight loss, smoking cessation, and the avoidance of dietary precipitants is very important and must be emphasized. Other simple measures such as elevation of the head while sleeping by putting bricks under the head of the bed, eating small regular meals during the day, and not

Table 30.1. *Los Angeles classification for endoscopic assessment of reflux esophagitis*

Grade A	One or more mucosal breaks no longer than 5 mm, none of which extends between the tops of the mucosal folds
Grade B	One or more mucosal breaks more than 5 mm long, none of which extends between the tops of two mucosal folds
Grade C	Mucosal breaks that extend between the tops of two or more mucosal folds, but that involve less than 75% of the esophageal circumference
Grade D	Mucosal breaks that involve at least 75% of the esophageal circumference

eating late at night can also be beneficial. Many patients with mild symptoms can be managed successfully with lifestyle measures and on-demand simple antacids and alginates.

Medical therapy

For those with more severe symptoms in whom conservative measures are not sufficient, PPIs are the most effective form of treatment and are the mainstay of medical treatment for most patients. They have been shown to be superior to both H2 receptor antagonist (H2RA) and placebo both in the healing of esophagitis and in preventing relapse of symptoms with maintenance treatment.[16,17] There have been many studies comparing the efficacy of the various PPIs and there are only marginal differences between different preparations. Esomeprazole 40 mg may be superior in severe esophagitis,[18] and it has been shown to demonstrate higher healing rates in reflux esophagitis than standard-dose PPIs (lansoprazole 30 mg, omeprazole 20 mg, pantoprazole 40 mg, or rabeprazole 20 mg).[19] A simple management strategy is to give a high-dose PPI for 4–8 weeks in order to heal the esophagitis and then step down to either on-demand therapy (PPI, H2RA, or alginate) or long-term maintenance treatment at a low dose as symptoms dictate. There is a lack of evidence to support prokinetic therapy being superior to placebo.[16]

For those patients who have no endoscopic evidence of acid reflux and do not respond to medical management, further investigation with esophageal pH studies can be useful to determine objective evidence of acid reflux. Patients can then be categorized into two groups, as having:

- Non-erosive reflux diseases (NERD)
- Functional heartburn.

The NERD group includes patients with positive documentation of abnormal acid reflux and those with normal pH testing but a positive correlation between symptoms and reflux events.[20] This is the most common presentation of GERD, and various mechanisms have been proposed, including mucosal hypersensitivity, intra-esophageal distention by gas and reflux of non-acid gastric contents.[21] There may be some response to antacid treatment.

The Rome III criteria[20] define functional heartburn as symptoms that have been present for at least 6 months prior to diagnosis and have been currently active for 3 months, for which there is absence of pathologic gastroesophageal reflux, achalasia, or other motility disorders with a recognized pathologic basis. Functional heartburn does not respond to PPIs and management can be very difficult. In patients who are also experiencing dyspepsia, treatment of H. pylori, if present, may be of benefit. Antidepressives are widely used but are of uncertain benefit; psychological therapies have been shown to help.

Long-term PPI therapy results in chronic hypo- or achlorhydria and secondary hypergastrinemia. In H. pylori-infected patients this results in a corpus-dominant gastritis as opposed to antral gastritis, leading on to atrophic gastritis and thus potentially gastric cancer,[22] although there is no current evidence to support a higher incidence of gastric cancer in H. pylori-positive patients taking long-term PPI therapy, and clinical trials have shown long-term PPI use to be safe and effective.[23] However, in those patients on long-term PPI medication then treating for H. pylori, if present, reverses this process[24] and is therefore advised. Other potential complications of longstanding hypochlorhydria include iron and vitamin B12 deficiency and an increased susceptibility to gastrointestinal infections and Clostridium difficile.[25] There is no evidence to support directly the theory that H. pylori eradication increases or worsens GERD.[23,24,26,27]

Endoscopic therapies

Over recent years several endoscopic therapies have been developed for the treatment of GERD, with the aim of providing a minimally invasive alternative to long-term medication or surgery.[28] There are currently no definitive indications for endoscopic therapy, and evidence is lacking to support its routine use.[29]

Surgery

There is no consensus regarding which patients should be referred for surgery. Several randomized controlled trials comparing anti-reflux surgery versus PPI therapy have shown better or similar outcomes.[30–33] Anti-reflux surgery does, however, carry a significant risk of complications such as dysphagia, pneumothorax, esophageal perforation, and vascular injury and it is not recommended for patients whose symptoms are well controlled on medical therapy.[34] For a small group of carefully selected patients with ongoing severe symptoms despite maximal medical therapy and objective evidence of acid reflux that correlates with symptoms, then surgery (a laparoscopic Nissen fundoplication) should be considered. Surgery may also benefit those patients with large sliding hiatus hernias who do not respond completely to PPI therapy.

Complications
Benign esophageal strictures

Peptic strictures can form as a result of prolonged acid reflux. A combination of high-dose PPI therapy and endoscopic dilatation can be employed successfully in most cases. Other therapeutic options include endoscopic steroid injection with triamcinolone.

Barrett's esophagus

Barrett's esophagus is a premalignant condition that can be defined pathologically as the metaplastic replacement of squamous esophageal epithelium by columnar epithelium in the distal esophagus,[35] and it is thought to result as a complication

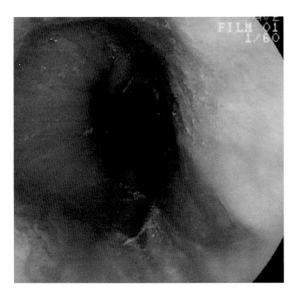

Figure 30.2. *A tongue of Barrett's esophagus (at the 5 o'clock position).*

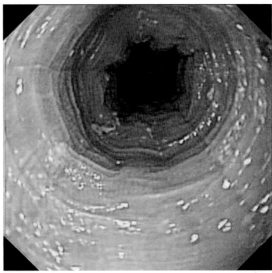

Figure 30.3. *Rings of eosinophilic esophagitis.*

of GERD. Barrett's esophagus is recognized at endoscopy (Fig. 30.2) on the basis of macroscopic changes, and is then confirmed histologically on biopsy. Patients have a 2–25% risk of developing mild to severe dysplasia, and a 2–5% risk of esophageal adenocarcinoma.[36] Current guidelines from the British Society of Gastroenterology recommend that all patients should be on high-dose PPI treatment and undergo second-yearly endoscopic screening if they are considered fit for treatment.[15] Although symptoms are usually well controlled in Barrett's esophagitis patients on PPI therapy, there is no clinical evidence that this treatment prevents or reverses progression to dysplasia and adenocarcinoma.

Surgery (esophagectomy) currently remains the gold-standard treatment for high-grade dysplasia and adenocarcinoma, although the risks are high with an operative mortality of 1.6–9.4% and an overall morbidity of 30–35%.[36–38] Because of this there has been focus on developing local endoscopic treatments for high-grade dysplasia or early esophageal adenocarcinoma. The current three main modalities are photodynamic treatment, thermal therapy, and endoscopic mucosal resection; all are minimally invasive and have shown promising results in clinical trials.[36] Although these techniques are not yet widely available, they offer the possibility

of potential curative treatment, particularly in elderly, frail patients, and this will have further implications for future screening criteria.

The Aspirin Esomeprazole Chemoprevention Trial (AspECT) is an on-going, large, randomized, controlled study involving more than 5000 patients with Barrett's esophagus, evaluating the benefit if PPI therapy with or without low-dose aspirin.

Eosinophilic esophagitis

Eosinophilic esophagitis (Fig. 30.3) is being increasingly recognized, especially amongst children and young adults. Patients often present with symptoms of esophageal dysfunction and GERD but are unresponsive to PPIs. At endoscopy atypical mucosal findings, such as edema or white exudates, may be seen and esophageal biopsies showing >15 eosinophils per high-power field are required to confirm the diagnosis.[39] Treatment options include removal of potential food allergens, and topical and oral corticosteroids, with biological therapies currently being evaluated.

Infectious esophagitis and systemic disease

Various infectious agents can also cause esophageal inflammation. These include herpes simplex virus,

Table 30.2. *Etiology of peptic ulcer disease*

Helicobacter pylori

Non-steroidal anti-inflammatory drugs and aspirin

Malignancy

Zollinger–Ellison syndrome

Severe systemic stress or illness

Smoking and alcohol

candidiasis, and cytomegalovirus in immunocompromised patients or those receiving antibiotics. In addition the esophagus may be involved in certain systemic diseases such as Crohn's disease, Churg–Strauss syndrome, pemphigoid, and other autoimmune diseases.

Peptic ulcer disease

Peptic ulceration occurs when there is a breach in the gastric or duodenal mucosa extending through the muscularis mucosa into the submucosa or deeper. Most PUD is caused either by *H. pylori* or NSAIDs, and developments over the past 30 years in our understanding of its pathophysiology have greatly improved both prevention and treatment. The lifetime prevalence of PUD is approximately 500–1000 per 10 000 of the population in developed countries, with a sex ratio of 1 : 1, and there has been a significant decline over the past 10 years.[40] The main causes of PUD are summarized in Table 30.2.

Peptic ulcers are formed when there is an imbalance between the gastroduodenal mucosal defenses and the damaging effects of gastric juices and *H. pylori* infection. Food stimulates the release of acetylcholine from vagal afferents and gastrin from G cells located in the gastric antrum. Gastrin then stimulates enterochromaffin-like cells in the gastric body to produce histamine that acts directly, along with gastrin, to stimulate acid production from the parietal cell located in the upper body and fundus. Acetylcholine also directly stimulates the parietal cell acid pump via the muscarinic receptor.

Endocrine cells present in the gastric antrum, known as D cells, produce somatostatin and are stimulated by acid secretion; this suppresses gastrin production and parietal cell acid production via a negative feedback loop (Fig. 30.4).

Mucosal protection is achieved by a number of mechanisms. Goblet cells produce and maintain a layer of protective mucus, and bicarbonate secretion by epithelial cells acts to sustain a neutral pH environment immediately surrounding the epithelial surface. Prostaglandin production by mucus cells acts directly on the parietal cell to decrease acid production, promote mucosal blood flow, and stimulate production of both mucus and bicarbonate.

Helicobacter pylori

H. pylori is a Gram-negative microaerophilic bacillus and is the main cause of gastroduodenitis and PUD in addition to being the leading cause of gastric cancer worldwide,[41] having been classified by the WHO as a class 1 carcinogen. The prevalence of *H. pylori* is estimated at 50% worldwide, although there is wide geographical variation, with much higher prevalence in developing countries.[42] Humans are the main reservoir and the infection is typically acquired in early childhood, predominantly via direct human–human contact in developed countries and via the feco-oral route in developing countries, with increased socio-economic development being associated with a decreased prevalence.[42–44]

The location and distribution of *H. pylori* in the stomach and complex interactions between bacterium and host, together with bacterial virulence factors all determine the clinical outcome of infection. Determinants of the host response to infection have been focused on gene polymorphisms related to the innate and acquired immune system.[45] Certain *H. pylori* strains are more pathogenic than others and several important virulence factors have been identified: cytotoxin vacuolating toxin A; CagA, a product of the gene cluster *cag pathogenicity island* (*cagPAI*), which contains many genes that appear to be related to *H. pylori* pathogenicity; and BabA$_2$, an outer-membrane-bound adhesin protein, which *H. pylori* uses to adhere to gastric epithelial cells.[46,47] Persistent *H. pylori* infection causes continuous gastric inflammation in virtually all infected

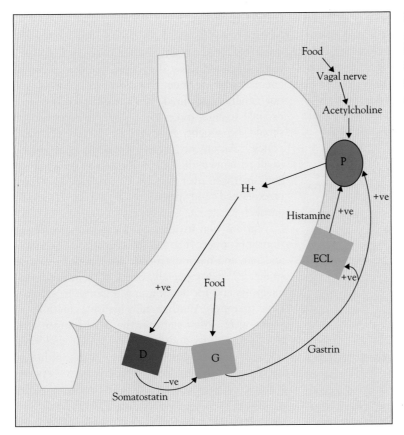

Figure 30.4. *Autoregulation of acid secretion; P, parietal cell; ECL, enterochromaffin-like cell; G, gastrin-producing cells; D, somatostatin-producing endocrine cells.*

persons,[48] but only 10–20% of carriers develop significant gastric disease.[46]

Duodenal ulcers

Duodenal ulceration (Fig. 30.5) is associated with an antral-predominant *H. pylori* gastritis. This results in acid hypersecretion caused by suppression of somatostatin cells with resulting increased gastrin production by antral G cells. The increased acid production directly damages the duodenal mucosa, and also allows *H. pylori* to colonize areas of gastric metaplasia in the duodenum, causing further mucosal inflammation.[47,49]

Gastric ulceration

Most benign gastric ulcers are associated with a corpus-predominant chronic *H. pylori* gastritis; if *H. pylori* is not present then NSAIDs are usually the cause. Patients with gastric ulceration tend to have normal rates of acid secretion or acid hyposecretion, however, acid suppression helps healing.[49]

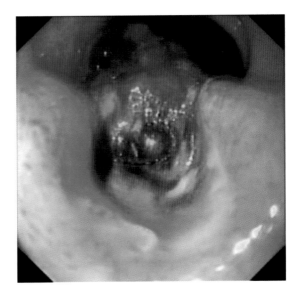

Figure 30.5. *A duodenal ulcer with a central visible vessel.*

395

Both direct and indirect consequences of *H. pylori* infection are likely to contribute to mucosal inflammation and ulceration, via toxin release and the secondary effects of the vigorous host inflammatory response, respectively. All gastric ulcers need to be biopsied at endoscopy, with follow-up endosopy 8–12 weeks later to exclude an underlying gastric malignancy.

Gastric cancer

H. pylori infection predisposes to distal, non-cardia gastric cancer, causing chronic gastritis and initiating the pre-cancerous sequence of chronic active non-atrophic gastritis, multifocal atrophy, and intestinal metaplasia that can subsequently develop into dysplasia and invasive carcinoma.[41,45,49,50] Patients have reduced acid secretion, owing to a corpus-dominant gastritis that reduces parietal cell acid secretion. *H. pylori* is also the most important risk factor for gastric mucosa-associated lymphoid tissue (MALT) lymphomas.

Non-steroidal anti-inflammatory drugs

Between 30% and 35% of hospital admissions for bleeding gastric and duodenal ulcers are caused by NSAIDs or aspirin;[51] users have a three- to five-fold increased risk of upper gastrointestinal complications.[52] NSAIDs promote gastroduodenal mucosal injury through direct toxic effects and the inhibition of the cyclo-oxygenase-1 pathway, with subsequent reduction of prostaglandin synthesis; the imbalance results in the development of erosions and ulceration.

Clinical presentation

Most patients present with symptoms of dyspepsia, classically defined as burning upper abdominal or epigastric pain or discomfort after meals, which may be relieved by food or antacids. Dyspepsia is often polysymptomatic and patients may have associated heartburn, nausea, or vomiting. Occasionally patients have an upper gastrointestinal bleed as their first presentation of PUD. The history should focus on risk factors such as NSAID or aspirin use, previous peptic ulcers, and *H. pylori* infection.

In older patients examination is, again, focused on detecting signs of upper gastrointestinal cancer such as an abdominal or epigastric mass or cervical lymphadenopathy.

Investigations

In patients with no alarm features (i.e. no gastrointestinal bleeding, unintentional weight loss, vomiting, epigastric mass, dysphagia, or iron-deficiency anemia) who are under 55 years of age, endoscopy is not generally required. Blood should be tested to exclude anemia, and evidence for *H. pylori* infection should be sought, followed by a 'test-and-treat' policy.[50] An urgent gastroscopy should be requested in all patients with alarm features, and on a routine basis in those over the age of 55 years who have unexplained and persistent dyspepsia of recent onset.[53]

Various non-invasive tests exist for the detection of *H. pylori*. The ^{13}C-urea breath test is simple and safe and has a diagnostic accuracy of <95% in studies.[50,54] It is especially useful both in the initial diagnosis and for determining response to eradication therapy. Another non-invasive method of assessing *H. pylori* status is the stool antigen test, with a sensitivity and specificity of 91% and 93%, respectively.[55] *H. pylori* serology testing, although inexpensive, is unable to differentiate between current and previous infection and accuracy varies according to the antibody used. There are a few occasions where serology does have advantages over breath testing – results of serology are not affected by PPI therapy or antibiotics, and it can be recommended for assessing *H. pylori* infection in patients with bleeding ulcers and other conditions associated with a low bacterial density (i.e. gastric atrophy and MALT lymphoma).

At endoscopy presence of *H. pylori* infection can be confirmed either with rapid urease testing via antral biopsy or with histological biopsy. The rapid urease test has a sensitivity of >98%,[56] although false-negative results do occur with PPI therapy, and in those patients a biopsy from the gastric body should also be taken.

Management

Advice should be given regarding lifestyle factors that might be contributing to symptoms (e.g. smoking and excessive alcohol intake), in addition to the discontinuation of any medication that has gastric toxicity. A 4–8-week course of PPI therapy should be prescribed to heal any inflammation, but treating *H. pylori* with appropriate eradication therapy is key. Recommended first-line eradication consists of triple therapy using a PPI with clarithromycin and amoxicillin given twice daily.[50] Where there are high rates of clarithromycin resistance, metronidazole may be used instead.[50,57] A recent large European multi-center, double-blind, randomized study showed no significant difference in terms of efficacy, safety, and patient compliance between durations of one or two weeks of therapy.[58] Owing to increasing antibiotic resistance to both clarithromycin and metronidazole, eradication rates have been decreasing – eradication rates on an intention-to-treat basis are currently around 80% for first-line therapy.[58,59] Treatment failures are due to either antibiotic resistance or poor patient compliance. If symptoms persist then *H. pylori* eradication should be confirmed with breath testing. If the patient is still positive for *H. pylori* then further eradication using second-line antibiotics should be administered.[59] These include bismuth-based quadruple therapy[50] and other combinations containing levofloxacin, rifabutin, or furazolidone.[50,60–62] *H. pylori* can be cultured from gastric biopsies and the antibiotic regimen determined from sensitivities.

For patients with PUD in whom the prescription of aspirin or NSAIDs cannot be stopped, *H. pylori* should be tested for and eradicated if present.[53] Co-prescription of a protective drug such as a PPI should be considered, or a less gastro-toxic alternative, such as a selective cyclo-oxygenase-2 inhibitor, substituted for the NSAID.

Non-ulcer dyspepsia

There has been much debate over the issue of *H. pylori* eradication in patients who have dyspepsia but no endoscopic evidence of inflammation or ulceration. The current evidence supports eradication therapy since it has a small but significant effect on symptoms in these patients and economic modeling suggests that this modest benefit may be cost effective.[63]

Conclusions

GERD and PUD represent the two most common upper gastrointestinal disorders encountered in general clinical practice, and account for significant morbidity and mortality. Owing to the recent advances in our knowledge of the underlying pathophysiology and the advent of PPIs, most patients can be successfully managed in primary care without the need for referral and invasive investigations. With regard to PUD, the importance of ensuring that *H. pylori* has been successfully eradicated is key, along with the rationalization of NSAID use.

References

1. Dent J, El-Serag HB, Wallander MA, Johansson S. Epidemiology of gastro-oesophageal reflux disease: a systematic review. Gut 2005; 54: 710–17.

2. Dent J, Holloway RH, Toouli J, Dodds WJ. Mechanisms of lower oesophageal sphincter incompetence in patients with symptomatic gastrooesophageal reflux. Gut 1988; 29: 1020–8.

3. Dodds WJ, Dent J, Hogan WJ et al. Mechanisms of gastroesophageal reflux in patients with reflux esophagitis. N Engl J Med 1982; 307: 1547–52.

4. Mittal RK, McCallum RW. Characteristics and frequency of transient relaxations of the lower esophageal sphincter in patients with reflux esophagitis. Gastroenterology 1988; 95: 593–9.

5. Emerenziani S, Habib FI, Ribolsi M et al. Effect of hiatal hernia on proximal oesophageal acid clearance in gastro-oesophageal reflux disease patients. Aliment Pharmacol Ther 2006; 23: 751–7.

6. Sontag SJ, Schnell TG, Miller TQ et al. The importance of hiatal hernia in reflux esophagitis compared with lower esophageal sphincter pressure or smoking. J Clin Gastroenterol 1991; 13: 628–43.

7. Jones MP, Sloan SS, Rabine JC et al. Hiatal hernia size is the dominant determinant of esophagitis presence and severity in gastroesophageal reflux disease. Am J Gastroenterol 2001; 96: 1711–17.

8. Hampel H, Abraham NS, El-Serag HB. Meta-analysis: obesity and the risk for gastroesophageal reflux disease and its complications. Ann Intern Med 2005; 143: 199–211.

9. Corley DA, Kubo A, Levin TR et al. Abdominal obesity and body mass index as risk factors for Barrett's esophagus. Gastroenterology 2007; 133: 34–41.

10. Wu JC, Mui LM, Cheung CM, Chan Y, Sung JJ. Obesity is associated with increased transient lower esophageal sphincter relaxation. Gastroenterology 2007; 132: 883–9.

11. El-Serag HB, Ergun GA, Pandolfino J et al. Obesity increases oesophageal acid exposure. Gut 2007; 56: 749–55.

12. Pandolfino JE, El-Serag HB, Zhang Q et al. Obesity: a challenge to esophagogastric junction integrity. Gastroenterology 2006; 130: 639–49.

13. Fry LC, Monkemuller K, Malfertheiner P. Functional heartburn, nonerosive reflux disease, and reflux esophagitis are all distinct conditions—a debate. Con Curr Treat Options Gastroenterol 2007; 10: 305–11.

14. Farrokhi F, Vaezi MF. Extra-esophageal manifestations of gastroesophageal reflux. Oral Dis 2007; 13: 349–59.

15. British Society of Gastroenterology. Guidelines for the management of Barrett's columnar lined epithelium [available from: http://www.nsg.org.ukSG].

16. Khan M, Santana J, Donnellan C, Preston C, Moayyedi P. Medical treatments in the short term management of reflux oesophagitis. Cochrane Database Syst Rev 2007; CD003244.

17. Donnellan C, Sharma N, Preston C, Moayyedi P. Medical treatments for the maintenance therapy of reflux oesophagitis and endoscopic negative reflux disease. Cochrane Database Syst Rev 2005; CD003245.

18. Coron E, Hatlebakk, JG, Galmiche JP. Medical therapy of gastroesophageal reflux disease. Curr Opin Gastroenterol 2007; 23: 434–9.

19. Edwards SJ, Lind T, Lundell L. Systematic review: proton pump inhibitors (PPIs) for the healing of reflux oesophagitis – a comparison of esomeprazole with other PPIs. Aliment Pharmacol Ther 2006; 24: 743–50.

20. Drossman DA. The functional gastrointestinal disorders and the Rome III process. Gastroenterology 2006; 130: 1377–90.

21. Savarino V, Savarino E, Parodi A, Dulbecco P. Functional heartburn and non-erosive reflux disease. Dig Dis 2007; 25: 172–4.

22. Schenk BE, Kuipers EJ, Nelis GF et al. Effect of Helicobacter pylori eradication on chronic gastritis during omeprazole therapy. Gut 2000; 46: 615–21.

23. Klinkenberg-Knol EC, Nelis F, Dent J et al. Long-term omeprazole treatment in resistant gastroesophageal reflux disease: efficacy, safety, and influence on gastric mucosa. Gastroenterology 2000; 118: 661–9.

24. Kuipers EJ, Nelis GF, Klinkenberg-Knol EC et al. Cure of Helicobacter pylori infection in patients with reflux oesophagitis treated with long term omepra-zole reverses gastritis without exacerbation of reflux disease: results of a randomised controlled trial. Gut 2004; 53: 12–20.

25. Louw JA. Peptic ulcer disease. Curr Opin Gastroenterol 2006; 22: 607–11.

26. McColl KE, Dickson A, El-Nujumi A, El-Omar E, Kelman A. Symptomatic benefit 1–3 years after H. pylori eradication in ulcer patients: impact of gastroesophageal reflux disease. Am J Gastroenterol 2000; 95: 101–5.

27. Malfertheiner P, Dent J, Zeijlon L et al. Impact of Helicobacter pylori eradication on heartburn in patients with gastric or duodenal ulcer disease — results from a randomized trial programme. Aliment Pharmacol Ther 2002; 16: 1431–42.

28. Rothstein R, Filipi C, Caca K et al. Endoscopic full-thickness plication for the treatment of gastroesophageal reflux disease: a randomized, sham-controlled trial. Gastroenterology 2006; 131: 704–12.

29. Pace F, Costamagna G, Penagini R, Repici A, Annese V. Review article: endoscopic anti-reflux procedures – an unfulfilled promise? Aliment Pharmacol Ther 2008; 27: 375–84.

30. Anvari M, Allen C, Marshall J et al. A randomized controlled trial of laparoscopic nissen fundoplication versus proton pump inhibitors for treatment of patients with chronic gastroesophageal reflux disease: one-year follow-up. Surg Innov 2006; 13: 238–49.

31. Mahon D, Rhodes M, Decadt B et al. Randomized clinical trial of laparoscopic nissen fundoplication compared with proton-pump inhibitors for treatment of chronic gastro-oesophageal reflux. Br J Surg 2005; 92: 695–9.

32. Mehta S, Bennett J, Mahon D, Rhodes M. Prospective trial of laparoscopic nissen fundoplication versus proton pump inhibitor therapy for gastroesophageal reflux disease: seven-year follow-up. J Gastrointest Surg 2006; 10: 1312–16; discussion 1316–17.

33. Lundell L, Miettinen P, Myrvold HE et al. Continued (5-year) followup of a randomized clinical study comparing antireflux surgery and omeprazole in gastroesophageal reflux disease. J Am Coll Surg 2001; 192: 172–9; discussion 179–81.

34. Vakil N. Review article: the role of surgery in gastro-oesophageal reflux disease. Aliment Pharmacol Ther 2007; 25: 1365–72.

35. Flejou JF. Barrett's oesophagus: from metaplasia to dysplasia and cancer. Gut 2005; 54: 16–12.

36. Deviere J. Barrett's oesophagus: the new endoscopic modalities have a future. Gut 2005; 54: i33–7.

37. Sauvanet A, Mariette C, Thomas P et al. Mortality and morbidity after resection for adenocarcinoma of the gastroesophageal junction: predictive factors. J Am Coll Surg 2005; 201: 253–62.

38. Zaninotto G, Parenti AR, Ruol A et al. Oesophageal resection for high-grade dysplasia in Barrett's oesophagus. Br J Surg 2000; 87: 1102–5.

39. Furuta GT, Liacouras CA, Collins MH et al. Eosinophilic esophagitis in children and adults: a systematic review and consensus recommendations for diagnosis and treatment. Gastroenterology 2007; 133: 1342–63.

40. Ehlin AG, Montgomery SM, Ekbom A, Pounder RE, Wakefield AJ. Prevalence of gastrointestinal diseases in two British national birth cohorts. Gut 2003; 52: 1117–21.

41. Correa P, Houghton J. Carcinogenesis of Helicobacter pylori. Gastroenterology 2007; 133: 659–72.

42. Brown LM. Helicobacter pylori: epidemiology and routes of transmission. Epidemiol Rev 2000; 22: 283–97.

43. Magalhaes Queiroz, DM, Luzza F. Epidemiology of Helicobacter pylori infection. Helicobacter 2006; 11: 1–5.

44. Lehours P, Yilmaz, O. Epidemiology of Helicobacter pylori infection. Helicobacter 2007; 12: 1–3.

45. Moss SF, Malfertheiner P. Helicobacter and gastric malignancies. Helicobacter 2007; 1: 23–30.

46. Hocker M, Hohenberger P. Helicobacter pylori virulence factors—one part of a big picture. Lancet 2003; 362: 1231–3.

47. Suerbaum S, Michetti P. Helicobacter pylori infection. N Engl J Med 2002; 347: 1175–86.

48. Dooley CP, Cohen H, Fitzgibbons PL et al. Prevalence of Helicobacter pylori infection and histologic gastritis in asymptomatic persons. N Engl J Med 1989; 321: 1562–6.

49. Calam J, Baron JH. ABC of the upper gastrointestinal tract: pathophysiology of duodenal and gastric ulcer and gastric cancer. BMJ 2001; 323: 980–2.

50. Malfertheiner P, Megraud F, O'Morain C et al. Current concepts in the management of Helicobacter pylori infection: the Maastricht III Consensus Report. Gut 2007; 56: 772–81.

51. Langman MJ. Ulcer complications associated with anti-inflammatory drug use. What is the extent of the disease burden? Pharmacoepidemiol Drug Saf 2001; 10: 13–19.

52. Hernandez-Diaz S, Rodriguez LA. Association between nonsteroidal anti-inflammatory drugs and upper gastrointestinal tract bleeding/perforation: an overview of epidemiologic studies published in the 1990s. Arch Intern Med 2000; 160: 2093–9.

53. National Institute for Health & Clinical Excellence (NICE). Managing dyspepsia in adults in primary care (2004). [Available from: www.nice.org.uk].

54. Gisbert JP, Pajares JM. Review article: C-urea breath test in the diagnosis of Helicobacter pylori infection – a critical review. Aliment Pharmacol Ther 2004; 20: 1001–17.

55. Gisbert JP, Pajares JM. Stool antigen test for the diagnosis of Helicobacter pylori infection: a systematic review. Helicobacter 2004; 9: 347–68.

56. Yousfi MM, El-Zimaity HM, Cole RA, Genta RM, Graham DY. Comparison of agar gel (CLOtest) or reagent strip (PyloriTek) rapid urease tests for detection of Helicobacter pylori infection. Am J Gastroenterol 1997; 92: 997–9.

57. Ford A, Moayyedi P. How can the current strategies for Helicobacter pylori eradication therapy be improved? Can J Gastroenterol B 2003; 17: 36B–40B.

58. Zagari RM, Bianchi-Porro G, Fiocca R et al. Comparison of 1 and 2 weeks of omeprazole, amoxicillin and clarithromycin treatment for Helicobacter pylori eradication: the HYPER Study. Gut 2007; 56: 475–9.

59. Di Mario F, Cavallaro LG, Scarpignato C. 'Rescue' therapies for the management of Helicobacter pylori infection. Dig Dis 2006; 24: 113–30.

60. Gisbert JP, Morena F. Systematic review and meta-analysis: levofloxacin-based rescue regimens after Helicobacter pylori treatment failure. Aliment Pharmacol Ther 2006; 23: 35–44.

61. Saad RJ, Schoenfeld P, Kim HM, Chey WD. Levofloxacin-based triple therapy versus bismuth-based quadruple therapy for persistent Helicobacter pylori infection: a meta-analysis. Am J Gastroenterol 2006; 101: 488–96.

62. Vakil N, Megraud F. Eradication therapy for Helicobacter pylori. Gastroenterology 2007; 133: 985–1001.

63. Moayyedi P, Axon AT. Review article: gastro-oesophageal reflux disease—the extent of the problem. Aliment Pharmacol Ther 2005; 22: 11–19.

Men and mental/emotional health and trauma

CHAPTER 31

Men and mental health

Alan Pringle

Introduction

Taylor and Field suggest that we all think we know what mental health is but that actually it is very difficult to clearly define.[1] Mental health can be defined negatively, as the absence of disease, or functionally as what a person is able to do, and in attempts to define mental health commentators frequently wrestle with the presence or absence of the features versus functionality debate. It is perhaps significant, then, that although in their 'Health of the Nation' document[2] the UK government set a target to 'improve significantly the health and social functioning of mentally ill people' there was no attempt to define what mental illness actually was.

The World Health Organization (WHO) has a functional view of mental health, defining it as 'A state of well being in which the individual realizes his or her own abilities, can cope with the normal stresses of life, and is able to make a contribution to the community.'[3] WHO claims that all people should be healthy enough to participate actively in a social life and that health should have importance given to esthetic and social factors.[4] WHO definitions have been criticized, despite being admirable, for being utopian and unrealistic, with Banyard[5] going so far as to suggest that if this definition is correct, then he has never had a good day's health in his life.

Whilst some believe that mental health problems are primarily biological in nature and constitute a definite disease process, others dispute the existence of mental illness *per se*, claiming that, since there is

no change in structure or function in any part of the body when mental illness is diagnosed, then the phenomenon experienced is not a disease. Despite continued debate around defining mental health, the impact that poor mental health has on the patient, his or her family, and society as a whole is devastating. It is the strength of this impact that Kirby et al.[6] suggest has driven the huge changes in policy and practice around mental health care in recent years, primarily in response to the sheer number of people who present with mental health difficulties.

Pringle and Sayers[7] suggest that although men, as a distinct group, have not always been identified as a definite subgroup in writings on mental health in the way that women have, the particular problems experienced by men are now starting to be acknowledged in psychology and sociology literature and are beginning to feature in mainstream mental health research. One of the main reasons for this may be the fact that, statistically, men's mental health, especially younger men's, is showing marked changes in presentation.

Prior and Hayes[8] observe that the beginning of the new century has seen an increase in the male population of mental health inpatient facilities so that men now outnumber women as inpatients in the UK. Another example of this rise in presentation can be seen in the number of men formally admitted to National Health Service hospitals in England and Wales under sections 2, 3, and 4 of the Mental Health Act. In recent years, formal admissions of men in England has risen from

403

8673 per year in 1990 to 13400 in 2003–2004.[9] There has also been a rise in young men entering the psychiatric system for substance misuse problems and for personality disorder.

History of avoidance

Men have a long and well-documented history of avoidant behavior in response to illness. Newland[10] suggests men are more likely to 'tough' out illness, give priority to work commitments over treatment and rest, feel that illness equals weakness, to fear the consequences of illness and disease, and to be less likely than women to discuss their health. When men do discuss health, Pack[11] comments that their attitudes to their own health is encapsulated in behaviors that include demonstrating a 'macho' approach, making jokes, ignoring symptoms, and working through pain. Stoicism and suppression of emotion are values often associated with masculine role socialization.[12]

In mental health these behaviors of avoidance are also found. Steward and Harmon[13] suggest that men will often measure their mental health by the presence of such concepts as stoicism, self-reliance, strength, work, status, and aggression and show 'traditional' strength by denying any vulnerability and exhibiting restricted emotionality. Rees et al.[14] whilst acknowledging some movement away from this view within the male population, suggest that there are still many who cling to the sex stereotypes.

This acknowledged avoidance behavior makes it difficult to be sure about the figures and trends in the mental health of men in general. For example, the UK Office of National Statistics[15] suggests that although women are more likely to have been treated for a mental health problem than men (29% compared with 17%), this could be because, when asked, women are more likely to report symptoms of common mental health problems.

Precursors to mental health problems in men

Wilkins[16] suggests that precursors for the development of mental health difficulties in men can be

examined by focusing on distinct area of men's lives. These, he suggests, include the influences of family, finances, and employment as well as the communities within which those with mental health problems live.

Family

The role of a stable family life in helping children to develop positive attitudes and strategies that contribute towards good mental health is well documented. Lamb[17] suggests that, for many years, research on children's development and wellbeing generally focused on the dynamics between mothers and their children but that some research has begun to focus on the importance of quality time that takes place between fathers and children. For example, a study by Flouri and Buchannan[18] was based on 17000 children who were born in the UK in 1958 and who were followed up at ages 7, 11, 16, 23, and 33 years. This study found that good father–child relationships are associated with an absence of emotional and behavioral difficulties in adolescence and greater academic motivation. It also found that boys who had involved fathers were less likely to be in trouble with the police as they grew older. This echoed Amato,[19] Gould et al.,[20] and McCann,[21] whose studies found that in families in which there was little or no involvement with a father there was a marked increase in behavioral disorders, psychiatric diagnosis, and suicide. It appears then that as the UK government's 1998 consultation paper 'Supporting Families' says: 'Fathers have a crucial role to play in their children's upbringing.'[22]

The impact of family breakdown can be profound on men and boys caught up in the process. MIND[23] proposes that in the UK when a relationship breaks down, it is men who may lose touch with their children as well as their partner and who are more likely to have to find a new home since courts award custody of children to mothers in 91% of cases. Family situation also appears to be an important factor in the rates of suicide for men. The UK Office for National Statistics[24] showed that the suicide rate for widowed and divorced men was more than double the rate for married men and that the suicide rate for single men is markedly greater than that for married men.

Flouri and Buchannan[18] also confirmed a link between the level of involvement by the father and a boy being in trouble with the police, with a significantly higher proportion of boys with little or no involvement with their father offending compared with boys with a highly involved father. From a mental health perspective this is significant because of the relationship between custodial experience and mental health difficulties. Men make up approximately 96% of the prison population in the UK, and the Office for National Statistics found that a large proportion of prisoners have mental health problems. Fifty-eight percent of male remand prisoners, for example, were assessed as having significant neurotic symptoms and over 20% of male prisoners stated that they had made a serious attempt at suicide at some point in their lives.

Finances and employment

Having the financial wherewithal to meet the daily necessities of life is an important precursor of mental wellbeing. Bonner et al.[25] draw what they call the explicit link between poverty, social exclusion, and mental illness and they felt that poverty is the cornerstone on which social exclusion is built. The inability to provide financially for themselves and their family is seen by many men as a testament to their failure as a person.

Unemployment is high amongst those labeled as mentally ill, and a diagnosis can in some cases make people feel almost unemployable. Experiencing satisfaction at work is an important predisposing factor for positive mental health in men, with one of the reasons for this being the importance of 'breadwinning' as a cultural indicator of the 'male role'. Over the past 40 years there have been dramatic changes in patterns of employment in the UK. Mining, steel manufacturing, ship-building and other heavy industries, which traditionally employed men, have closed, while the newly created jobs have tended to be in the service sector, often seen in the traditional view as 'women's work'.

Community and family

The feeling of acceptance by and belonging to a community has a profound effect on a person's belief about whether he or she is included or excluded socially. Bertram and Stickley[26] suggest that the

relationship between social exclusion and mental health problems is complex, with many of the elements of exclusion being, in different circumstances, both causal factors and consequences of mental ill health. This is echoed by Repper and Perkins,[27] who claim that people actually diagnosed with a mental illness are among the most 'excluded' in society and that this exclusion only adds to the cycle in which the exclusion has a negative impact on the symptoms and the symptoms increase the chances of being excluded.

Mental health conditions in men

The most commonly presenting clinical conditions men are likely to be diagnosed with are depression, psychosis, and personality disorder.

Depression

Alexander[28] describes how depressed men may not be diagnosed as severely mentally ill and, as such, approximately twice as many women as men are reported to suffer from depression. Despite this, three times as many men take their own lives. According to Real[29] these types of statistics highlight the presence of what is known as 'hidden' or 'covert' depression. Real goes on to claim that depression may also be a factor behind several of the problems we think of as being typically male, such as alcohol and drug abuse, domestic violence, and failures in intimacy. Emslie et al.[30] propose that men and women actually experience depression in a similar way, but have different ways of manifesting and expressing their distress. They go on to describe the findings of Brownhill et al.[31] who found that, although both men and women tried to avoid emotional distress by attempting to block out negative thoughts, men were more likely to be overwhelmed after a longer period of time and release the emotion in the form of anger or violence, while women were more prepared to release emotions early by crying and seeking help. Wilhelm et al.[32] suggest, however, that once a diagnosis is made and men are actively treated, there are few sex differences in severity or course of established episodes of major depression.

The effective range of treatments available for depression, ranging from talking treatments through pharmacological interventions and electro-convulsive therapy, appear to have as much efficacy in men as in women. As Elmslie et al.[30] point out, however, the actual symptoms of depression (e.g. lack of confidence and assertiveness, low self-worth, and feelings of lack of entitlement to physician time and resources) also contribute to problems in accessing help. Perhaps the most worrying thing for those involved with mental healthcare is the outcome for those who do actively avoid treatment for depression. The statistics for men, especially young men, and suicide make for poignant reading.

Suicide

In response to concern around suicide, a specified target in the UK government's White Paper, 'Our Healthier Nation'[33] was a reduction in suicides by at least 20% by 2010 from the 1999 baseline. This was followed in 2002 by the National Suicide Prevention strategy. Key measures in the strategy included reducing the suicide risk of men aged under 35 years, who are most likely to take their own lives, for example by improving the treatment of alcohol and drug misuse among young men who self-harm.

The result has been a drop in the rate of young male suicide in the period from 1998 to 2005. A progress report published by the National Institute for Mental Health in England acknowledges that good progress is being made towards meeting the government target to reduce suicide by 20% by 2010. Despite this welcome development, suicide remains the major cause of death of men aged 25–34 according to Davidson and Lloyd,[34] with young men almost four times more likely to take their life through suicide than women.[7]

The method chosen to attempt suicide has a definite sex influence, with men predominantly choosing hanging and firearms as a method over the female preference of self-poisoning.[35] Among firearm suicides, shotguns are used in over three-quarters of cases,[36] with handguns and other firearms making up the rest. Sport and occupational use were the main reasons for gun ownership.

When statistics for men and self-poisoning were reviewed, it was found that 40% of people who had overdosed were aged 55 years and over and nearly half had a previous history of self-harm. Alcohol was involved in more than half of the

incidents. In considering the whole question of suicide in men in the UK, Gunnell et al.[37] draw the conclusion that the increases in young male suicide in England and Wales in the past 30 years have paralleled rises in a number of risk factors for suicide in this age group, namely unemployment, divorce, alcohol and drug abuse, and declines in marriage.

Psychosis

Psychoses are relatively low prevalence disorders that have a disproportionately negative impact on individuals and society. This is often because the features of psychosis can have a dramatic impact on a range of aspects of a person's life, including perception, cognition, mood, personality, behavior, and movement. Women and men are approximately equally affected by psychotic conditions. In young adults the disease begins in males on the average a few years earlier than in women, whilst in contrast it affects more women when the psychosis first becomes manifest at older ages.

Schizophrenia is by far the most commonly diagnosed of the psychoses, and the National Institute for Mental Health in England suggests that recovery from the condition is possible.[38] The most usual course of the disorder, however, generally involves numerous active phases of illness with residual phases of impairment between episodes. While full remissions from schizophrenia do occur, most people have at least some residual symptoms of varying severity. Generally, 25% of people experience a complete recovery, 40% experience recurrent episodes of psychosis with some degree of social disability and periods of unemployment, while 35% may remain chronically disabled.

Stefan et al.[39] describe how schizophrenia in the past was often thought of as 'a disease of unknown etiology' but suggest that a combination of factors increase predisposition to the condition. These include genetic factors, the presence of obstetric complications, prenatal infection, reaction to adverse life events, and the inability to deal effectively with stress. It appears that no one event but rather a combination of a range of risk factors interact to propel the person over a threshold for the development of the condition. One statistic that has been of note in this area is the high numbers of people of Afro-Caribbean origin to be given a diagnosis of psychosis. Robinson,[40] amongst others, however, urges caution with this trend, suggesting that diagnosis that is made from a monocultural perspective has the possibility of 'viewing behaviors, values and lifestyles that differ from the Euro-American norm' as abnormal.

In recent years there has been a growing literature both in academic fields and in the media generally about the possible links between cannabis and the development of psychosis. Whilst Kemp[41] proposes that substance abuse is a significant problem in the treatment of young people with their first psychosis owing to its potentially distorting impact on presenting symptoms, being able to find what Moore et al.[42] feel is *conclusive proof* that cannabis can cause psychotic or affective symptoms that persist beyond transient intoxication is difficult. Amar and Potvin[43] and Moore et al.[42] do, however, conclude that there is now sufficient evidence to warn young people that using cannabis *could* increase their risk of developing a psychotic illness later in life.

Although pharmacological interventions remain the main initial method for intervening in active presentations of psychosis, Sayer et al.[44] suggest that cognitive behavioral techniques are increasingly used as adjuncts to medication in the treatment of psychosis. This is possible, they feel, because there is now a growing workforce of nurses and other professionals trained in the use of cognitive behavioral interventions for psychosis.

Personality disorder

Health professionals have not always agreed about how best to identify personality disorders. Manning[45] claims that personality disorder is the subject of considerable psychiatric controversy and that its classification, diagnosis, and treatment are disputed not only within psychiatry, but also within the closely related fields of forensic and psychological work. The fourth edition of the *Diagnostic and Statistical Manual of Mental Disorders* (DSM-IV) lists 10 distinct subtypes of personality disorder, with each one linked to a different set of attitudes, emotions, and behaviors. In their document 'Personality disorder – no longer a diagnosis of exclusion' the Department of Health suggests that personality disorder in adults has its origins in childhood

disturbance.[46] Men are more likely than women to be diagnosed with antisocial, paranoid, and schizoid or schizotypal personality disorders, with antisocial personality disorder the most common diagnosis.

Adults who present with antisocial personality disorder have often been subjected to severe neglect and abuse and are likely to have a parent or caregiver who has had a psychiatric disorder and has difficulties in parenting. Key factors in the development of antisocial personality disorder include the early onset of conduct problems, persistent antisocial behavior, and the presence of attention-deficit–hyperactivity disorder. There is currently no reliable method of identifying adolescents who are at high risk for developing antisocial personality disorder in adult life. The mental health charity MIND claims that this group is hugely over-represented in the prison population in the UK, among whom antisocial personality disorder is found in 63% of male remand prisoners and 49% of sentenced male prisoners.

Some clinicians are sceptical about the effectiveness of treatment interventions for personality disorder and, as such, can be reluctant to accept people with a primary diagnosis of personality disorder for treatment. A range of treatment interventions are, however, available for personality disorder, including psychological treatments and drug therapy, and there is a growing body of literature available on the efficacy of treatment approaches such as psychosocial interventions and cognitive behavioral therapy. Bateman and Tyrer[47] conclude that whilst more research is needed, there are real grounds for optimism that therapeutic interventions can work for personality disorders.

Other conditions

The huge number of potential diagnoses offered by ICD-10 and DSM-IV reflect the complexity of mental health problems and treatment, and men have the potential to develop almost every one of the conditions included in the texts. Men are prone to the development of all the symptoms of anxiety, obsessive–compulsive disorder, and eating disorders that the public often primarily associate with women.

One specific area in which men present prominently is post-traumatic stress disorder (PTSD) related to occupation. People at high risk of developing PTSD include combat veterans, fire-fighters, and victims of violence, groups in which men are likely to be over-represented. Studies of groups of at-risk people show that they are at least three times more likely to have PTSD than the general population. PTSD is a condition that appears to be increasing in its prevalence.[48]

Musruck and Pringle[49] describe how PTSD sufferers show the development of characteristic symptoms following exposure to an extreme trau-matic, including avoidance of reminders of the trauma, symptoms of hyperarousal including hyper-vigilance for threat, exaggerated startle responses, irritability, difficulty in concentrating, and sleep problems. PTSD sufferers also describe symptoms of emotional numbing. These include inability to have any feelings, feeling detached from other people, giving up previously significant activities, and amnesia for significant parts of the event. Many PTSD sufferers experience other associated symp-toms, including depression, generalized anxiety, shame, guilt, and reduced libido, which contribute to their distress and affect their functioning.

The role of alcohol and drugs

The co-occurrence of substance misuse and psychi-atric disorders (dual diagnosis) has been, according to Lowe and Abou-Saleh[50] increasingly recognized in the UK, where clinical studies of patients with severe mental disorders can show high rates of substance misuse with poor clinical and social out-come. Coombes and Wratten[51] suggest common examples of dual diagnosis include depression with cocaine use, alcohol addiction with panic reactions, and personality disorder with episodic drug use. These patients often fall 'between the cracks' of the separate general psychiatric and addiction services, and this comorbidity is associated with increased levels of violence and suicide and with worse out-comes, including frequent and prolonged inpatient episodes.

The National Service Framework for Mental Health, whilst emphasizing the importance of tack-ling dual diagnosis, failed to provide standards and service models to address the challenges, but a Dual Diagnosis Good Practice Guide has been published

in the UK by the Department of Health.[52] This document suggested that substance misuse among people with mental health problems is not uncom-mon and that the relationship between the two problems is complex. In recognition of this, the guidelines suggest that it is important that all people presenting to general psychiatric services (and not just addiction services) be screened to detect sub-stance misuse. This it is felt has helped bring about the development of dedicated dual diagnosis teams in community settings.

Addressing the problem

In the Western world, the health of men in general is poorer than that of women. Mortality rates are higher for men and they use health services less often than women, even when reproductive services have been accounted for.[53] Despite this situation, specific services aimed at men have been slow to develop. Well woman clinics have mushroomed to cater for various needs but, perhaps with the exception of assessing cardiovascular disease risk, little has been done specifically for men.[54]

Clearly some thought has to continue to be given to help create services that address the differ-ing needs of men and women in mental health care. Services should acknowledge that men may seek 'masculine' solutions to problems of emotional distress whereas approaches to improving mental health often rely on messages perceived as 'feminine', for example, preparedness to 'open up' or admitting to vulnerability.[16] The failure of men to access services has resulted in men often being blamed for being poor consumers of health services, and so being seen to be victims of their own behavior.[55] Addressing the challenges of improving men's uptake of services may involve service providers focusing on the areas of education, attitudes, and environment.

Men are seen as having a poor uptake of educa-tional material around health but it may well be that men simply have a different approach to seeking information. Tudiver and Talbot[56] suggest that the initial approach by men seeking help for health-related issues tends to be indirect and that men tend to view their partners and friends as their initial resource for help in mental health. Cotton et al.[57] note that males show significantly lower recognition of symptoms associated with mental illness and are more likely to endorse the use of alcohol to deal with mental health problems.

Initiatives are needed to raise the awareness of the prevalence of depression, combined with a better understanding of the illness and promotion of good mental health. McKenzie[58] emphasizes the importance of educating men about the symptoms of psychiatric disorders, reducing the stigma of mental ill health, making services more accessible to working men, and utilizing language and approaches that are relevant and comprehensible.

White and Cash[59] suggest that personal and professional attributes of the individual healthcare workers were an essential factor affecting the success of interventions with men. These key attributes included being non-judgmental, being non-threatening, being male-focused, being creative, being willing to go to the men, being able to see beyond the showing off of the lads, being able to use humor appropriately, and being willing to wait for success, since some initiatives can take months (if not years) to be accepted.

Emslie et al.[30] claim that while both men and women valued good communication skills in health professionals, men tended to value skills that helped them to talk, while women valued listening skills. Good and Wood[60] suggest that one way to increase men's use of counseling services would be to focus less on emotional expressiveness and more on instrumental changes and control. When considering the environment, Newland[10] describes a report from the Men's Health Forum in which men stated that they often felt unwelcome in 'feminized' premises in terms of decor and display material, and perceived a sex bias in the provision of some services.

Examples of progress

Men remain a difficult group to engage but examples using the ideas outlined above can be found in both interventions and in health promotional work. The Brother to Brother (B2B) project in London, for example, used drama workshops and creative exercise with black youth workers and young men to foster discussions on issues such as masculinity, fatherhood, attitudes and beliefs about sex, and emotional wellbeing. There are other examples of successful initiatives for men's health, including outreach health clinics, slimming and lifestyle clubs, and health promotion in unconventional venues.

Some football clubs in the UK have been involved in health promotional activities with their local health authorities. An example is the Alive and Kicking project in Coventry, which encouraged multi-disciplinary working with young men to help develop more healthy lifestyles. Although this project focused mostly on physical aspects of health, such as diet, fitness, smoking, sexual behavior, and cancer awareness, it showed that work that was associated closely with a recognized team, in this case Coventry City, could help to engage men in health promotional activities.

Using this male-dominated world of football, a range of initiatives to tackle mental health issues can also be found. The Derwent Valley Rovers project uses involvement in playing football as the method of having an impact on the mental health of participants. Similar initiatives are found with the Positive Mental Attitude League in London and the Care Services Improvement Partnership league in Manchester, which, every 5 weeks during the football season, brings together over 200 service users to the JJB Soccer Dome in Trafford Park, Manchester.

Another example of using football in health promotion is the 'It's a Goal!' project, which was launched in 2004 at Macclesfield Town Football Club, a side who play in the second Division of the English football league and which is now run at Manchester United's Old Trafford stadium and at Plymouth Argyle Football Club. Pringle and Sayers[7,61] describe how this project bases a Community Mental Health Nurse in the stadium and uses group-working techniques that utilize the language and metaphor of football to engage with men around mental health issues.

Other innovative ideas for mental health interventions with men include the development of mental health service user-led support groups; groups in arts, drama, and writing; and support for men who have experienced childhood sexual abuse.

Conclusions

Despite the difficulties in defining what mental health actually is, promoting mental health has become a major component of the government's overall health strategy. Reflecting this, the National Service Framework For Mental Health[2] put an emphasis on mental health promotion and outlined standards for mental health care, focusing on the mental health needs of working-age adults up to the age of 65. The document outlines seven district standards that each care provider has to meet. The standards focus on health promotion, access to services, working with carers, and the prevention of suicide. Each standard is evidence-based and felt to be achievable.

If these goals are to be achieved for men with mental health issues, then services and initiatives must recognize the specific needs of men as a distinct group. Robbins[62] proposes that men must be given the time, study, and respect that they need to function in an ever more complicated world and environment. This, according to Baker,[54] highlights the need for men's health to be included when policies are made, and for health services to be tailored and made more accessible for men.

Banks[63] optimistically suggests that developing services that genuinely address these issues may be helped in the UK by the 2007 'Gender Equality Duty Act', which, for the first time, makes it a legal requirement to deliver all services in the public sector on a sex-equitable basis by outcome rather than process. In other words, the National Health Service will have to demonstrate not only that it is addressing sex health issues but that the results are as near as possible the same for both sexes.

Although there is much that health services can do to target and improve men's health, White[64] feels that to be effective in this area we must realize that men's health is not a medical issue but a societal one and that as such a much broader approach needs to be taken when addressing the issue. This means that co-operative working between not just health and social agencies but also community facilities, support groups, retail and food outlets, health facilities, and even football clubs holds out hope for a more integrated approach that can help to address issues to do with men's health.

References

1. Taylor S, Field D. Sociology of Health and Health Care, 4th edn. Oxford: Blackwell Science, 2007.
2. Department of Health. Saving Lives; Our Healthier Nation. London: The Stationary Office, 2002.
3. World Health Organization. Mental Health Fact Sheet N130. Geneva: World Health Organization, 1999.
4. World Health Organization. Global Strategy of Health for All by the Year 2000. Geneva: World Health Organization, 2000.
5. Banyard P. Applying Psychology to Health. London: Hodder and Stoughton, 1996.
6. Kirby S, Mitchell G, Cross D et al. Mental Health Nursing Competencies for Practice. London: Palgrave Macmillan, 2004.
7. Pringle A, Sayers P. It's a goal: basing a community psychiatric nursing service in a local football stadium. J R Soc Promot Health 2004; 124: 234–8.
8. Prior B, Hayes C. Changing places: men replace women in mental health beds in Britain. Soc Policy Adm 2001; 35: 397–410.
9. Department of Health. Statistics on Formal Admission Under the Mental Health Act. London: The Stationary Office, 2004.
10. Newland J. Not going for checkups: is it a guy thing? Nurse Pract 2006; 31: 6.
11. Pack S. It only hurts when I laugh. Prof Nurse 2005; 20: 56.
12. Lee C, Owens G. The Psychology of Men's Health. Buckingham: Open University Press, 2002.
13. Stewart D, Harmon K. Mental health services responding to men and their anger. Int J Mental Health Nurs 2004; 13: 249–54.
14. Rees C, Jones M, Scott T. Exploring men's health in a men-only group. Nurs Stand 2005; 9: 38–40.
15. Office of National Statistics. Better or Worse: A Longitudinal Study of the Mental Health of Adults in Great Britain, London: Office of National Statistics, 2003.
16. Wilkins D. Policy-makers must ask: will it make us happier? Available at http://www.menshealthforum.org.uk/userpage1.cfm?item_id=1962.
17. Lamb ME. The Role of the Father in Child Development, 3rd edn. New York: John Wiley Sons, 1997.
18. Flouri E. Buchanan A. What predicts good relationships with parents in adolescence and partners in adult life; findings from the 1958 British Birth Cohort. J Fam Psychol 2002; 16: 186–98.

19. Amato PR. Father–child relations, mother–child relations, and offspring psychological well-being in early adulthood. J Marriage Fam 1994; 56: 1031–42.

20. Gould MS, Shaffer D, Fisher P, Garfinkel R. Separation/divorce and child and adolescent completed suicide. J Am Acad Child Adolesc Psychiatry 1997; 37: 155–62.

21. McCann R. On Their Own; Boys Growing Up Unfathered. Sydney: Finch, 2000.

22. Department of Health. Supporting Families; a Consultative Document. London: The Stationary Office, 1998.

23. MIND. Men's Mental Health. Available at: http://www.mind.org.uk/Information/Factsheets/Men, 2007.

24. Office of National Statistics. Social Focus on Men. London: Office of National Statistics, 2001.

25. Bonner L, Barr W, Hoskins A. Using primary care-based mental health registers to reduce social exclusion in patients with severe mental illness. J Psychiatr Mental Health Nurs 2002; 9: 585–93.

26. Bertram G, Stickley T. Mental health nurses, promoters of inclusion or perpetuators of exclusion? J Psychiatr Mental Health Nurs 2005; 12: 387–95.

27. Repper J, Perkins R. Social Inclusion and Recovery, a Model for Mental Health Practice. London: Baillière Tindall, 2003.

28. Alexander J. Depressed men: an exploratory study of close relationships. J Psychiatr Mental Health Nurs 2001; 8: 67–75.

29. Real T. I Don't Want to Talk About It: Overcoming the Secret Legacy of Male Depression. New York: Fireside Simon and Schuster, 1997.

30. Emslie C, Ridge D, Zieblands S and Hunt K. Exploring men's and women's experiences of depression and engagement with health professionals: more similarities than differences? A qualitative interview study Fam Pract 2007; 8: 827–38.

31. Brownhill S, Wilhelm K, Barclay L, Schmied V. 'Big build': hidden depression in men. Aust N Z J Psychiatry 2005; 39: 921–31.

32. Wilhelm , Roy K, Mitchell P, Brownhill S, Parker G. Gender differences in depression risk and coping factors in a clinical sample. Acta Psychiatr Scand 2002; 106: 45–53.

33. Department of Health. Saving Lives: Our Healthier Nation. London: The Stationary Office, 1999.

34. Department of Health. Supporting Families: a Consultative Document. London: The Stationary Office, 1998.

35. Bennewith O, Gunnell D, Kapur N et al. Suicide by hanging: a multicentre study based on coroners' records in England. Br J Psychiatry 2005; 186: 260–1.

36. Haw C, Sutton L, Simkin S et al. Suicide by gunshot in the United Kingdom: a review of the literature. Med Sci Law 2004; 44: 295–310.

37. Gunnell D, Middleton N, Whitley E, Dorling D, Frankel S. Why are suicide rates rising in young men but falling in the elderly – a time-series analysis of trends in England and Wales 1950–1998. Soc Sci Med 2003; 57: 595–611.

38. NIMHE. Guiding Statement on Recovery. London: The Stationary Office, 2004.

39. Stefan M, Travis M Murray RM. An Atlas of Schizophrenia. London: Parthenon, 2002.

40. Robinson L. Race, Communication and the Caring Professions. Buckingham: Open University Press, 1998.

41. Kemp M. Promoting the health and wellbeing of young black men using community-based drama. Health Educ 2006; 106: 186–200.

42. Moore THM, Zammit S, Lingford-Hughes A et al. Cannabis use and risk of psychotic or affective mental health outcomes: a systematic review. Lancet 2007; 370: 319–28.

43. Amar MB Potvin S. Cannabis and psychosis: what is the link? J Psychoactive Drugs 2007; 39: 31–42.

44. Sayer J, Ritter S, Gournay K. Beliefs about voices and their effects on coping strategies. J Adv Nurs 2000; 31: 1199–205.

45. Manning N. Psychiatric diagnosis under conditions of uncertainty: personality disorder, science and professional legitimacy. Sociol Health Illn 2000; 22: 621–39.

46. Department of Health. Personality Disorder: No Longer a Diagnosis of Exclusion – Policy Implementation Guidance for the Development of Services for People with Personality Disorder. London: The Stationary Office, 2003.

47. Bateman AW, Tyrer P. Psychological treatment for personality disorders. Advances Psychiatr Treat 2004; 10: 378–88.

48. O'Brien M, Nutt D. Loss of consciousness and post-traumatic stress disorder: A clue to aetiology and treatment. Br J Psychiatry 1998: 102–4.

49. Musruck D, Pringle A. The treatment of Post Traumatic Stress Disorder in a Korean War veteran using Scripted Exposure and EMDR. Ment Health Nurs 2003; 23: 4–9.

50. Lowe AL, Abou-Saleh MT. The British experience of dual diagnosis in the National Health Service. Acta Neuropsychiatr 2004; 16: 41–6.

51. Coombes L, Wratten A. The lived experience of community mental health nurses working with people who have dual diagnosis: a phenomenological study. J Psychiatr Ment Health Nurs 2007; 14: 382–92.

52. Department of Health. Mental Health Policy Implementation Guide. Dual Diagnosis Good Practice Guide. London: The Stationary Office, 2002.

53. Lee C, Owens G. The Psychology of Men's Health. Buckingham: Open University Press, 2002.

54. Baker P. Men's health policy. J R Soc Promot Health 2004; 124: 205–6.

55. Courtenay W. Behavioural factors associated with disease, injury, and death among men: evidence and implications of prevention. J Mens Stud 2000; 9: 81–142.

56. Tudiver F Talbot Y. Why don't men seek help? Family physicians' perspectives on help-seeking behaviour in men. J Fam Pract 2000; 48: 47–52.

57. Cotton SM, Wright A, Harris MG et al. Influence of gender on mental health literacy in young Australians. Austr N Z J Psychiatry 2006; 40: 790–6.

58. McKenzie S. The strong silent type. Public Health News 2006; 5: 14–15.

59. White AK, Cash K. Report on the First Phase of the Study on Men's Usage of the Bradford Health of Men Services. Leeds: Leeds Metropolitan University, 2005.

60. Good GE, Wood PK. Male gender role conflict, depression, and help. Seeking: do college men face double jeopardy? J Counse Dev 1995; 74: 70–5.

61. Pringle A, Sayers P. It's a goal! The half time score. Men Health Nurs 2006; 26: 14–17.

62. Robbins A. Introduction to men's mental health. J Mens Health Gend 2004; 1: 359–64.

63. Banks I. The Vienna declaration: just one more thing? J Mens Health Gend 2007; 4: 220–1.

64. White AK. Report on the Scoping Study on Men's Health. London: Department of Health, 2001.

CHAPTER 32

Trauma in male health

Tatum Tarin, Simon Kimm, Jack McAninch, Daniel Rosenstein

Introduction

Trauma to the external genitalia is an uncommon event. Because of the relatively protected position of the penis and testicles between the thighs and pubic bone, these organs are usually able to avoid direct injury from blunt or penetrating forces. Nonetheless, the external genitalia may be severely injured by direct trauma or be secondarily injured in association with more extensive injuries such as burns. The primary care physician may encounter these patients in the urgent care setting, and must be prepared to diagnose and treat genital injuries expeditiously. Mismanagement of these injuries may result in significant physical and psychological consequences, which are often difficult to foresee at the time of injury. Fortunately, treatment protocols for genital injuries have been well defined and confirmed by multi-center experience in the urologic literature. This chapter reviews the management of the most common types of trauma to the penis, urethra, testes, and scrotum.

Anatomy and physiology

The penis is composed of paired corpora cavernosa and the corpus spongiosum. The two corpora cavernosa are the bodies primarily responsible for erectile function. They contain delicate vascular erectile tissue, and are enclosed in a thick fibrous sheath known as the tunica albuginea. Superficial to this is Buck's fascia, which encloses all three corporal structures. A loose elastic layer known as dartos fascia runs deep to the skin of the penis and scrotum (Fig. 32.1). The arterial blood supply to the penis is via the deep internal pudendal arteries. The principal vascular structures of the penis run longitudinally along its dorsal (upper) aspect as the dorsal neurovascular bundles. These consist of paired dorsal arteries and a deep dorsal vein running between them, along with sensory nerves from the glans. A central (cavernosal) artery runs through the center of each corporal body. The skin of the penis and scrotum receives its blood supply from the superficial external pudendal artery, which arborizes into a fine vascular plexus running through the dartos fascia. The corpus spongiosum and urethra are supplied by the bulbourethral arteries, which course forward to anastomose with the dorsal circulation within the glans of the penis (Fig. 32.2).

The urethra is an epithelial-lined conduit for urine and semen which has an elastic submucosa surrounded by the vascular tissue of the corpus spongiosum. When discussing trauma and reconstruction, it is meaningful to subdivide the urethra into five segments. The most proximal portion of the urethra begins at the bladder outlet, and courses through the prostate – this is referred to as the prostatic urethra. The membranous urethra passes through the perineal membrane, and is surrounded only by the striated urethral sphincter (Fig. 32.3). The prostatic and membranous urethras are also collectively referred to as the posterior urethra.

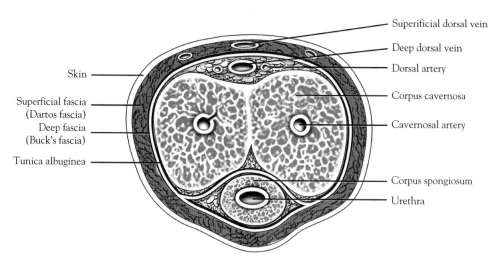

Figure 32.1. *Cross-section of the penis illustrating the relationship of the neurovascular structures to the corporal bodies and urethra. Note the relationship of the superficial fascia (dartos fascia) to the deep fascia (Buck's fascia).*

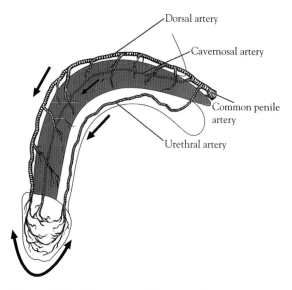

Figure 32.2. *Illustration of the arterial supply of the deep structures of the penis. The common penile artery is the terminal branch of the internal pudendal artery. Note the anastomosis of the dorsal and the bulbourethral arteries at the level of the glans penis.*

The membranous urethra is the location where the urethra reaches its widest caliber. The anterior urethra is surrounded by the corpus spongiosum and glans penis. It is subdivided from proximal to distal into the bulbar urethra, the pendulous urethra, and the fossa navicularis. The fossa navicularis is the location where the urethra reaches its narrowest caliber.

The scrotum consists of a sac of corrugated skin surrounding a sheet of dartos muscle. The testis resides within three fascial layers referred to as the outer, middle (or cremasteric), and inner spermatic fascia. The testis is immediately surrounded by visceral and parietal layers of tunica albuginea. The testis is closely attached posterolaterally to the epididymis. The principal blood supply to the testis is the testicular (or internal spermatic) artery, which originates from the aorta anterior and medial to the renal arteries (Fig. 32.4). It also receives collateral blood flow from the deferential artery, which runs parallel to the vas deferens. The spermatic cord contains the vas deferens, the pampiniform plexus (divisions of the spermatic vein), the internal and external spermatic arteries, and various lymphatics and nerves. The cord runs from the testis through the inguinal canal.

Injuries to the penis

Penile fracture
A fractured penis implies disruption of the tunica albuginea surrounding the corpora cavernosa. This injury typically occurs during vigorous intercourse,

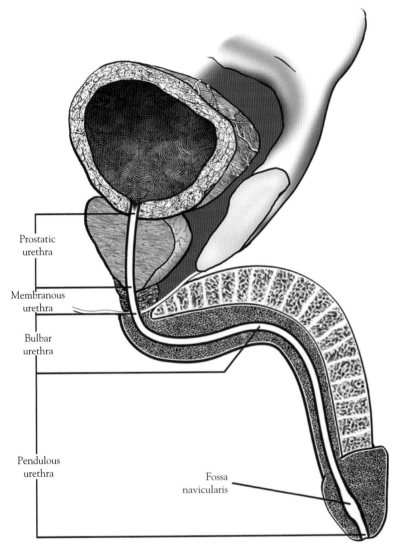

Figure 32.3. *The anatomy of the urethra is divided into the anterior and the posterior segments. The posterior segment comprises the prostatic urethra and the membranous urethra. The anterior segment comprises the bulbous urethra, the pendulous urethra, and the fossa navicularis.*

Prostatic urethra

Membranous urethra

Bulbar urethra

Pendulous urethra

Fossa navicularis

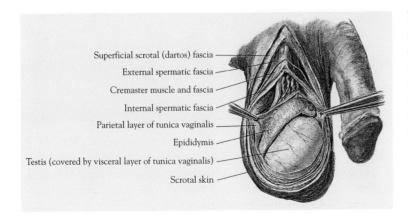

Superficial scrotal (dartos) fascia

External spermatic fascia

Cremaster muscle and fascia

Internal spermatic fascia

Parietal layer of tunica vaginalis

Epididymis

Testis (covered by visceral layer of tunica vaginalis)

Scrotal skin

Figure 32.4. *Fascial layers of the scrotum. Superficial (left) and deeper (right) layers. Note that the vascular supply of the testis runs within the deepest fascial layers, and thus is usually spared in superficial (skin loss) injuries of the scrotum. From reference 1.*

when the rigid penis is misdirected against the partner's pubic bone resulting in buckling trauma. This injury may also be self-inflicted by abrupt bending of the erect penis during masturbation. The classic history involves the scenario described above, with patients usually reporting a popping sound as the tunica tears, followed by pain, penile swelling, and rapid detumescence. The laceration is classically found on the pendulous part of the penis, but more proximal tears have been reported. There is frequently a delay in presentation to hospital, presumably secondary to patient embarrassment.

Physical examination typically reveals a swollen, ecchymotic penis (Fig. 32.5). The fracture line in the tunica is often palpable. There is often a clot lying over or near the fracture site, which corresponds to the cavernosal rupture site. Urethral injury is associated with penile fracture in up to one-third of cases. Retrograde urethrography should be performed to rule out suspected urethral injury – particularly in the presence of gross hematuria, inability to void, or blood at the urethral meatus. Adjunctive imaging studies in penile fracture are usually unnecessary, since the clinical picture is frequently adequate to expedite therapy. Ultrasound and magnetic resonance imaging have both been used occasionally to visualize the fracture site on the

corporal bodies, but are rarely indicated. Cavernosography is an invasive but sensitive test to detect cavernosal fracture, but it is mostly used to exclude cavernosal rupture in an unusually ambiguous presentation.

We recommend immediate exploration and surgical repair of penile fracture. When compared to non-operative management, this approach results in a faster recovery, less morbidity, less erectile dysfunction, and less long-term penile curvature. The penis is explored via a circumcising incision, and the entire length of the corporal bodies and urethra are inspected. The corporal laceration is closed with absorbable sutures (Fig. 32.6). If an associated urethral injury is present, it is repaired in a spatulated fashion over a catheter. Patients who undergo this type of expedient repair have a low complication rate and usually avoid disabling and disfiguring penile curvature in the postoperative period.

Penile amputation

Penile amputation is a very rare entity, arising largely from self-mutilation in the hands of a psychotic patient. Most psychotic patients respond well to psychiatric rehabilitation, and the vast majority will not attempt to repeat amputation. It may also be caused by violent assault or as a devastating

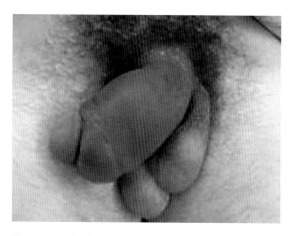

Figure 32.5. *Gross appearance of the fractured penis. Note the massive edema along the shaft. This clinical picture has been characterized as the 'eggplant deformity.'*

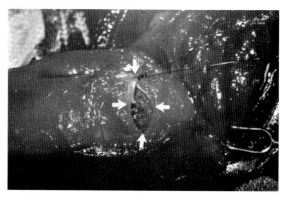

Figure 32.6. *Intraoperative photograph of the fractured penis revealing the site of the tear in the tunica albuginea of the corpus cavernosum. This is repaired in a watertight fashion with an absorbable suture. From reference 2.*

complication of circumcision. The largest published series of penile amputations comes from Thailand where, historically, this was considered acceptable retribution for philandering husbands. Expeditious penile replantation is the treatment of choice. Replantation is best accomplished using microvascular techniques, if available.

The penis is remarkably resistant to cold ischemia, and successful replantation has been accomplished up to 24 hours after amputation. The penis should be preserved in a saline-soaked gauze and placed within a sterile plastic bag. This bag is then immersed in ice slush, which increases ischemic tolerance of the amputated segment (Fig. 32.7).

Microsurgical replantation of the amputated penis involves two-layer closure of the urethra over a catheter in order to stabilize the remainder of the repair. The tunica albuguinea of the corporal bodies are re-approximated in a watertight fashion. At least one dorsal artery and the dorsal vein should be re-approximated. Dorsal nerve repair through the epineureum is also warranted, if possible (Fig. 32.8). Urinary drainage from the bladder should be diverted with a suprapubic catheter. If microsurgical techniques are not available, the penis may be replanted using macroscopic techniques, whereby only the urethra and the corporal bodies are re-approximated. The incidence of skin loss and urethral stricture is significantly higher using the latter technique. Remarkably, return of partial or complete erectile function has been reported in many cases in the months following replantation.

If the amputated segment if not available, the corpora should be debrided and closed, with a urethrostomy formed. The patient may then consider less optimal choices, such as phallic construction or advancement of penile stump.

Gunshots and penetrating penile injury

Penile gunshot and penetrating injuries are uncommon outside wartime settings. Eighty percent of these patients will have injuries to adjacent organs, which require evaluation. The urethra is injured in approximately 50% of cases, and thus retrograde urethrography should be performed prior to exploration, if possible. Most of these injuries may be debrided and repaired primarily with a good functional outcome. The exception is in the case of a close-range shotgun injury, where massive and diffuse tissue destruction is present. The damaged tissues should be debrided and allowed to declare themselves in terms of the extent of injury. They may then be repaired in a staged fashion.

Corporal injuries should be closed with buried absorbable suture. Associated urethral injury should be closed primarily in a watertight fashion over a Foley catheter. A more superficial laceration that is superficial to Buck's fascia may be debrided and closed primarily.

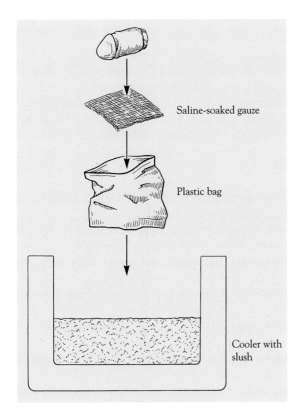

Figure 32.7. *The 'bag within a bag' technique of preservation of the amputated penis for transport reduces warm ischemic time. From reference 3.*

Saline-soaked gauze

Plastic bag

Cooler with slush

Injuries to the urethra

Posterior (membranous) urethral injuries

The vast majority of membranous urethral injuries occur in association with a pelvic fracture, and more

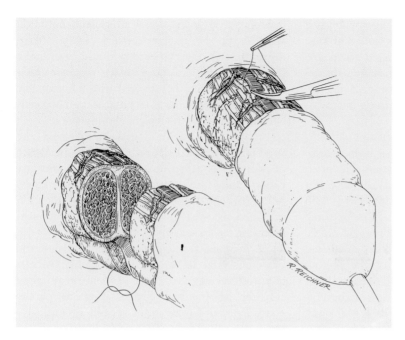

Figure 32.8. *Microsurgical replantation of the amputated penis. Note that initial urethral and corporal reanastomosis stabilizes the penis for subsequent microanastomosis of the dorsal neurovascular structures. From reference 3.*

specifically in association with bilateral pubic rami fractures (Fig. 32.9). The prostate is anchored behind the pubic rami via the puboprostatic (pubourethral) ligaments. When a deforming force fractures the pubic ramus and distracts the bony fragment superiorly and posteriorly, the resulting displacement will tear through the membranous urethra – typically at the point of departure of the bulbous urethra. The membranous urethra may rarely be injured by bullets or other projectiles. Thus, the physician encountering patients with pelvic trauma must maintain a high index of suspicion for urethral injury.

Appropriate early recognition and treatment of prostatomembranous urethral disruption significantly reduces long-term morbidity. Although these patients have often suffered critical orthopedic, vascular, and visceral injuries, it is often the sequelae of the urethral injury (incontinence and erectile dysfunction) that cause the most morbidity after all the other injuries have healed.

Clinically, these patients present with blood at the meatus, inability to void, and a palpably full bladder. The prostate has been described as 'high-riding', but this sign is unreliable, since a normal (non-displaced) prostate may be impalpable

secondary to the surrounding pelvic hematoma. A perineal hematoma may or may not be present. Finding any of these signs warrants a retrograde urethrogram. An attempt at catheter placement in this setting prior to urethrography may have serious consequences if the urethra has been disrupted.

The findings on retrograde urethrography dictate subsequent management steps. It is important to highlight that oblique and lateral decubitus views are necessary in order to visualize the bulbous and membranous urethra adequately. A normal retrograde urethrogram rules out significant urethral injury, and a Foley catheter may then be placed for urinary drainage. Placement of the catheter in the setting or pelvic fracture with hematuria should be immediately followed by a cystogram in order to rule out an associated bladder or bladder neck laceration.

If the retrograde urethrogram demonstrates extravasation of contrast at the level of the membranous urethra with or without bladder filling, a prostatomembranous urethral disruption is present (Fig. 32.10). Initial and early management of these injuries remains a controversial and widely debated topic in traumatic and reconstructive urology. Current treatment options include suprapubic catheter

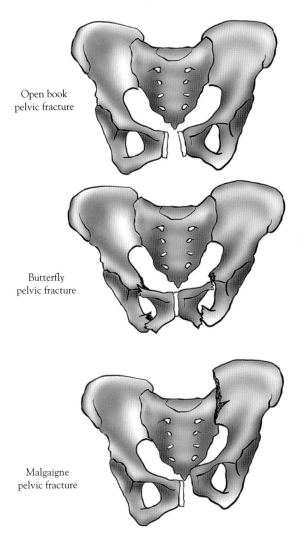

Open book
pelvic fracture

Butterfly
pelvic fracture

Malgaigne
pelvic fracture

Figure 32.9. *Diagram of different pelvic fractures associated with prostatomembranous urethral disruption.*

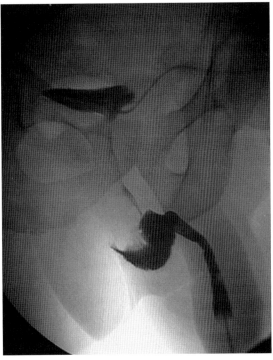

Figure 32.10. *Retrograde urethrogram documenting prostatomembranous urethral disruption. Note the extravasation of radiographic contrast with no bladder filling. From reference 4.*

placement alone followed by delayed reconstruction 3–12 months later; suprapubic catheter placement followed by endoscopic placement of an aligning catheter (to bring the severed ends of the urethra into alignment); and urethral reconstruction in the early post-injury period. Regardless of the initial management chosen for critically injured patients with pelvic trauma, the urologist's main priority is to achieve urinary drainage – typically with a suprapubic catheter. If the patient is stable and

the urologist has adequate expertise and equipment, an attempt to place an aligning catheter may follow. Endoscopic realignment does not appear to increase complications if properly performed, and may simplify a later posterior urethral reconstruction by bringing the urethral ends into alignment. It appears that while most patients managed with aligning catheters will heal with urethral stricture, many will heal with strictures mild enough to be managed by a direct vision internal urethrotomy.

Delayed primary sutured coaptation of the urethra (typically within a few days of the initial injury) is rarely employed in the USA, but this approach has gained enthusiasm in parts of Europe. This approach involves exploration of a maturing pelvic hematoma and placement of sutures into the prostatic apex and severed urethral margins.

419

The long-term results have yet been reported, but rates of incontinence, erectile dysfunction, and recurrent strictures appear higher with this approach.

Open placement of a suprapubic catheter is indicated in a setting where bladder inspection and repair is planned (e.g. in the case of a bladder neck laceration). A suprapubic catheter may also be placed at the time of concomitant orthopedic plating of the anterior pubic arch. Another absolute indication for open suprapubic catheter placement in the case of simultaneous rectal or vascular injury. In these complicated cases, irrigation and drain placement are warranted, but no attempt to expose or repair the urethral disruption should be made at the time of the acute injury.

Delayed reconstruction may be undertaken at 3–12 months, depending on the rate of healing of the other injuries. It is beyond the scope of this chapter to outline technical aspects of posterior urethral reconstruction, but certain key points deserve mention. The vast majority of prostatomembranous urethral disruptions may be successfully repaired via a perineal approach in a single stage. Following excision of all the scar tissue separating the two urethral ends, the urethra is adequately mobilized to allow a tension-free anastomosis (Fig. 32.11). Endoscopic techniques that attempt reconstruction by coring through the scar to bridge the defect ('cut-to the light' procedures) between the two ends have unacceptably high failure rates. Because of the complexity of this type of reconstructive surgery and the relative paucity of patients requiring it, it is best undertaken in referreal centers where urologists have developed special expertise in this area.

Anterior urethral injuries

Anterior urethral injuries are distinctly rare, encompassing at most 10% of urethral injuries. These injuries are most commonly caused by a blunt straddle type injury, where the bulbar urethra is crushed up against the pubic rami. Penetrating trauma to this region (stab or gunshot injury) is rarely encountered. Patients may present with blood at the meatus, inability to void, or an expanding scrotal hematoma which may contain extravasated urine. Retrograde urethrography is mandatory to diagnose this injury.

Because of the rarity of these injuries, management algorithms have been based upon small series.

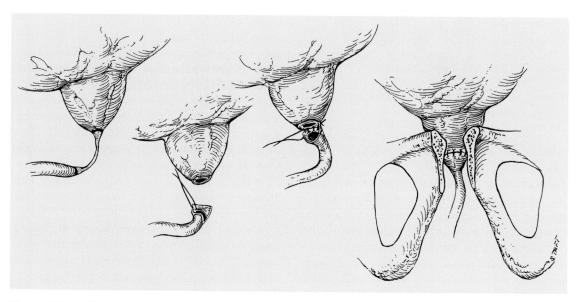

Figure 32.11. *Prostatomembranous urethral stricture: successful repair demands total stricture excision followed by spatulation and tension-free anastomosis of the bulbar urethra to the prostatic apex.*

The management options for the treatment of anterior urethral injuries includes primary catheter realignment followed by delayed repair or suprapubic urinary diversion followed by delayed repair. In a retrospective review of 78 cases of anterior urethral injury (81% managed initially with suprapubic tube diversion and delayed repair, and 19% managed with primary catheter realignment), Park and McAninch reported that the majority of these patients would require surgical intervention.[5] However, those who had been initially managed with a primary realignment required complex flap or graft urethroplasty more often than those managed with a suprapubic tube and delayed treatment. After transperineal urethroplasty, their success rate was 95% with a mean follow-up of 25 months. Initial management with suprapubic urinary diversion and delayed repair may also lead to the best outcomes in the setting of shotgun blasts or high-velocity projectiles.

Scrotal and testicular injuries

Traumatic injuries to the testes and scrotum may result from either blunt or penetrating insults. The relative mobility of the testes usually allows them to swing away from crushing forces. The fibrous tunica albuginea usually protects the delicate seminiferous tubules within from further trauma. However, a significant deforming force may cause rupture of the tunica – clinically known as testicular fracture. Scrotal contusions that do not rupture the tunica but nonetheless produce significant hematomas within the wall of the scrotum may be clinically difficult to distinguish from a fractured testicle.

Although once believed to be rare, the risk of testicular rupture following major blunt scrotal trauma may be as high as 50%. The most common etiologies are assault and sports-related injuries, but testicular trauma may be self-inflicted in the unusual trans-sexual patient. Penetrating trauma secondary to gunshot wounds is uncommon, but may occasionally be self-inflicted from a loaded firearm misplaced in a pocket. Penetrating injury is more likely to require testicular exploration.

Clinical findings are often non-specific, but usually include significant pain and a swollen, ecchymotic scrotum. Because of rapid expansion of the scrotal hematoma, it is often difficult to appreciate the testicular contour on physical examination. A history of forceful trauma should raise suspicion of testicular rupture. In penetrating trauma, associated injuries to the penis, perineum, and femoral vessels should be considered and ruled out.

While scrotal imaging may serve as a useful adjunct to physical examination in suspected testis trauma, the definitive diagnosis of testis rupture is made surgically. It is thus most appropriate to explore a grossly abnormal scrotum without ultrasonography when the index of suspicion is high. However, ultrasound may be useful in equivocal cases. In a recent review of the San Francisco General Hospital experience, testicular ultrasound – using the single radiographic finding of heterogeneous echo pattern of the testicular parenchyma with a loss of contour definition – was found to have a 93.5% specificity and a 100% sensitivity in detecting testis rupture.[6] Other radiographic findings, including continuity of the tunica albuginea and hematocele, have been evaluated in predicting testis rupture but have been found to have lower sensitivity and specificity.

Early scrotal exploration and repair of testicular rupture results in the highest testis salvage rate. Observation of the traumatized testis results in higher orchiectomy rates, and also significantly increases the patient's disability period. Non-operative management is usually complicated by infection, testicular atrophy, or necrosis.

The operative approach via a midline scrotal incision permits full exposure of both testes and spermatic cords, as needed. Large scrotal hematomas are then evacuated. All necrotic testicular parenchyma is debrided, and the tear in the tunica albuginea is closed. Penetrating injury through the spermatic cord is more likely to result in orchiectomy at the time of exploration. Typically, a Penrose drain may be left in place if hemostasis is in question. Testicular salvage is possible in most cases, and spermatogenesis and endocrine (testosterone production) function is thus preserved.

Testicular amputation injuries are fortunately uncommon, and are usually self-inflicted by a psychotic patient. Unlike the penis, the testes do

421

not tolerate prolonged periods of warm ischemia. Testicular replantation is thus reserved for cases of bilateral amputation or amputation of a solitary testis. This involves microsurgical re-anastomosis of the testicular artery, vasovasostomy, and re-approximation of two or three of the spermatic veins. The overlying amputated skin is not vascularized by the deep structures, and thus is usually not replantable. The ideal coverage of the replanted testis is via primary scrotal closure with remaining scrotal skin.

Genital skin loss

Historically, genital skin avulsion resulted from accidental entanglement of clothing and underlying skin in farm or rotary machinery. Currently these injuries arise more commonly secondary to motorcycle or bicycle deceleration trauma whereby the genital skin is avulsed as the rider is thrown forward. The most common overall cause of genital skin loss is in the setting of necrotizing genital gangrene (Fournier's gangrene), in which necrotic genital skin is debrided acutely.

Genital skin usually avulses along a loose, avascular plane, which usually spares the deeper structures. On the penis, it will dissect superficial to Buck's fascia, while the scrotal skin usually dissects superficially to the external spermatic fascia. The testes, cords, urethra, and corporal bodies are thus usually left intact.

Because of the tremendous elasticity of genital skin, the scrotum may usually be closed primarily when as much as 60% of the skin surface area has been lost. If primary closure is not possible, the testes and cords are left exposed and dressed during the perioperative period with moist saline gauze dressings. The wound itself may be continuously debrided with wet-to-dry dressing changes three to four times daily. More recently, vacuum-assisted closure of perineal wounds has been reported to accelerate wound healing after surgical debridement has been completed. If the wound is clean and fit for reconstruction at this point, split thickness skin grafts (STSGs) may be applied. If the wounds are contaminated, the testes are placed in subcutaneous thigh pouches for delayed scrotal reconstruction

with STSGs or local thigh flaps. Thigh pouches protect the testes well and ease subsequent reconstructive efforts. Testes that are left exposed for a prolonged period develop a thick fibrous peel which impedes graft take. In contrast, thigh pouches prevent the formation of this fibrous covering.

Scrotal reconstruction with meshed STSGs taken from the thigh or buttock usually provides an esthetically pleasing outcome. The grafts ultimately assume a dependent, rugated appearance which mimics the native scrotum. The donor site usually re-epithelializes with minimal complication. Local thigh flaps may also be used, but this may be more labor-intensive and the ultimate cosmetic outcome is not optimal compared to STSGs.

In the case of avulsed penile shaft skin, STSG reconstruction also provides an excellent result. Meshed grafts should be avoided on the penis because of their tendency towards contracture. It is important to excise any remaining subcoronal skin prior to grafting, since this residual skin may have impaired lymphatic drainage and lead to circumferential lymphedema.

Genital burn injuries

Genital burn injuries may be caused by thermal, electrical, or chemical energy sources. Thermal burns of the genitalia are usually associated with more extensive burns of adjacent tissues. These burns are treated by complete arrest of the burning process (usually by removal of burning clothing). Initial treatment should include aggressive fluid resuscitation and evaluation of depth and extent of the burn. A Foley catheter should be placed early in the resuscitation period unless the urethra is obviously involved in the burn. In this case, suprapubic catheter placement is advised.

Most genital thermal burns are first- or second-degree, and will usually heal with local wound care and rarely require debridement. Conversely, third-degree genital burns of the penis or scrotum require prompt debridement of non-viable tissue, followed by STSG reconstruction as previously described. This approach may decrease infection rates and ultimately obviate formation of a genital burn scar, which usually results when third-degree burns are managed conservatively. Chemical burns are managed with initial flushing of burned surfaces with copious amounts of sterile water. The injury is the managed as outlined for thermal burns.

Electrical burns to the genitalia may be particularly devastating because tissue destruction is often far deeper and more extensive than the visible surface burn indicates. Evaluation should thus include cystoscopy and sigmoidoscopy in order to rule out associated pelvic organ damage. Electrical burns may cause extensive muscle necrosis and consequent myoglobinuria and hemoglobinuria, both of which lead to renal insufficiency. Electrical burns may require repeat debridement before skin graft or myocutaneous flap reconstruction may be undertaken.

Conclusion

Trauma to the male genitalia may range from a tiny superficial laceration to a devastating complete avulsion of the penis and testicles. The physician treating the traumatized patient has to recognize and treat some or all of the injuries outlined in this chapter. The treatment plans described herein provide a basic framework for up-to-date management of the most common genital injuries seen in clinical practice.

References

1. Netter FH. Atlas of Human Anatomy. West Caldwell, NJ: Ciba-Geigy, 1989; 365.
2. Miller KS, McAninch JW. Penile fracture and soft tissue injury, initial management and reconstruction of male genital amputation injuries. In: McAninch JW, ed. Traumatic and Reconstructive Urology. Philadelphia, PA: WB Saunders, 1996: 693–8.
3. Jordan GH. Lower Genitourinary Tract Trauma and Male External Genital Trauma. AUA Updates Series vol. 19, 2000; Lessons 10–12.
4. Dixon CD. Diagnosis and acute management of posterior urethral disruptions. In: McAninch J, ed. Traumatic and Reconstructive Urology. Philadelphia, PA: WB Saunders, 1996: 347–55.
5. Park S, McAninch J. Straddle injuries to the bulbar urethra: management and outcomes in 78 patients. J Urol 2004; 171: 722–5.
6. Buckley JC, McAninch JW. Use of ultrasonography for the diagnosis of testicular injuries in blunt scrotal trauma. J Urol 2006; 175: 175–8.

Suggested reading

Bhanganada K, Chayavatana T, Pongnumkul C et al. Surgical management of an epidemic of penile amputations in Siam. Am J Surg 1983; 146: 376–82.

Bourree M, Kozianka J. 6 years VAC in general surgery: clinical data from 128 patients. Zentralbl Chir 2006; 131(Suppl 1): S100–4.

Brandes SB, McAninch JW. External genital trauma: amputation, degloving and burns. Atlas Urol Clin North Am 1998; 6: 127–42.

Corrales JG, Corbel L, Cipolla B et al. Accuracy of ultrasound diagnosis after blunt testicular trauma. J Urol 1993; 150: 1834–6.

Jordan GH. Initial management and reconstruction of male genital amputation injuries. In: McAninch JW, ed. Traumatic and Reconstructive Urology. Philadelphia, PA: WB Saunders, 1996: 673–81.

Koraitim M. Pelvic fracture urethral injuries: the unresolved controversy. J Urol 1999; 161: 1433–41.

McAninch JW, Santucci RA. Genitourinary trauma. In: Walsh PC et al., eds. Campbell's Urology. 8th edn. Philadelphia, PA: WB Saunders, 2002: 3707–44.

Morey AF, Hernandez J, McAninch JW. Reconstructive surgery for trauma of the lower urinary tract. Urol Clin North Am 1999; 26: 49–60.

Morey AF, McAninch JW. Genital skin loss and scrotal reconstruction. In: Ehrlich RM, Alter GJ, eds. Reconstructive and Plastic Surgery of the External Genitalia. Philadelphia, PA: WB Saunders, 1999: 414–22.

Mouraviev V, Coburn M, Santucci R. The treatment of posterior urethral disruption associated with pelvic fractures: comparative experience of early realignment versus delayed urethroplasty. J Urol 2005; 173: 873–6.

Mydlo J. Surgeon experience with penile fracture. J Urol 2001; 166: 526–9.

Nudell DM, Morey AF, McAninch JW. Penile trauma. In: Graham S, ed. Glenn's Urologic Surgery. Philadelphia, PA: Lippincott, Williams and Wilkins, 1998: 599–608.

Tiguert R, Harb J, Hurley P et al. Management of shotgun injuries to the pelvis and lower genitourinary system. Urol 2000; 55: 193–7.

CHAPTER 33

Men and suicide: assessment and management in a primary care setting

Nick Hervey, Dominique LeTouze

Background

Suicide, the act of deliberately killing oneself, is often under-reported. It is one of the three leading causes of death globally among people aged 15–44 years. In 2000, around a million people died from suicide, a worldwide mortality rate of 16 per 100 000, or one death every 40 seconds. The World Health Organization estimates that more people die each year from suicide than in all the world's armed conflicts.[1]

Across the world, men are almost three times as likely to take their own life as women.[2] Male suicides have increased more rapidly than female suicides since 1950.[1]

Suicide rates vary internationally. Some countries in South America and in the Middle East report suicide rates of 1 per 100 000 or below. The highest rates are in Eastern European and the former Soviet Union, with Russia and Belarus both reporting suicide rates over 60 per 100 000.[1] The UK had a mid-range male suicide rate of 17.5 per 100 000 in 2005.[3] In England, unlike the global picture, suicide rates have fallen across the whole population in recent years.[4] However, English men are still more likely to commit suicide than English women.

All national rates hide wide internal variability. In the UK suicides are highest in Wales, the north-east and the north-west.[5] Caution should therefore be exercised when comparing global suicide rates. Definitions of suicide or accidental death differ markedly, affecting the number of suicides reported.

It is also possible that the stigma associated with suicide may influence reporting, with some suicides being recorded as accidents to avoid distress to relatives.

Which men commit suicide?

Figure 33.1 shows that those most at risk of suicide are young and elderly men. Elderly men commit suicide two to three times more often than younger age groups.[2] However, rates have increased among young men, and in England, suicide is the leading cause of death among men aged under 35 years.[6] As younger men are less likely to die from other causes, suicide represents a greater mortality burden in that age group than in elderly men.

Elderly men

Elderly men experiencing painful physical illness and disability are more prone to suicide than others. Poor physical health is often accompanied by coexistent depressive illness.[7] Social isolation and loneliness among older men who survive their peers and partner may also cause depression and often act as risk factors for suicide.

Young men

Like older men, young men who commit suicide often have mental health problems. Unlike older men, though, young men are thought to be more vulnerable to unemployment, family breakdown, and substance misuse.[8] Other influential factors are thought to be HIV diagnosis and media coverage (e.g. of a celebrity taking his own life).[9] Rutter and

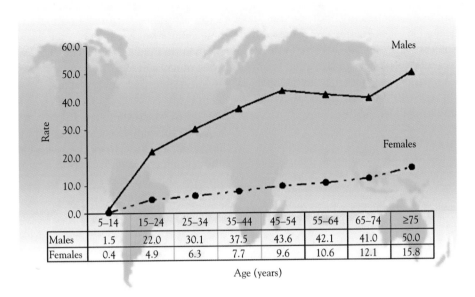

	5–14	15–24	25–34	35–44	45–54	55–64	65–74	≥75
Males	1.5	22.0	30.1	37.5	43.6	42.1	41.0	50.0
Females	0.4	4.9	6.3	7.7	9.6	10.6	12.1	15.8

Age (years)

Figure 33.1. *Global suicide rates per 100 000 (2000), with distribution by sex and age.*

Behrendt[10] have suggested that a sense of hopelessness, hostility, negative self-concept, and isolation appear to be common to many cases of adolescent suicide.

Why men?

Violent methods

It is well recorded that women make more suicide attempts than men, but men tend to choose more violent methods and are therefore more likely to succeed. Among men in England, hanging and suffocation are the most common methods, accounting for half of all such deaths.[2] Perhaps owing to the fact that suicide can be impulsive, ease of access to all lethal methods increases the likelihood of taking one's life. For example, access to a firearm increases risk,[11] with guns responsible for three times as many suicides as any other method in the USA.[12] Measures to limit access to suicide methods, for example by reducing toxicity of domestic gas, making car emissions safer, erecting barriers at common suicide sites, and limiting the packet size or prescriptions of some drugs, have all helped to reduce suicide rates.[2,13]

Mental illness

A history of mental health problems is the most common predictor of suicide in both men and women, associated with 90% of events.[1] Suicide is the most common cause of death in schizophrenic patients, with data from the UK indicating that 20% of suicide victims during the period 1996–1998 had a diagnosis of schizophrenia.[14] The likelihood of suicide in diagnosed alcoholics has been estimated to be between 60 and 120 times that for the rest of the population.[15]

Loss

Social or emotional loss, of loved ones and social networks, can leave men isolated and lonely, and bereavement through suicide creates a particular risk of future suicide in relatives. For men, loss of employment status or economic security, for example through redundancy or retirement, also heightens risk. Lewis and Sloggett[16] found a strong association between suicide and unemployment, with those who were unemployed being over one and a half times more likely to commit suicide than employed people. For many people, work represents status, a valuable contribution to society, and economic

425

stability, the loss of which can be devastating. Durkheim suggested that feelings of alienation and isolation from one's community increase suicide rates.[17] Associated with alienation are issues that themselves increase risk such as poor self-esteem, impoverished social contacts, and mental health problems. In England and Wales men living in the most deprived areas are twice as likely to commit suicide as those in the least deprived areas.[18]

Psychosocial factors

Other factors are more difficult to measure. Some authors have suggested that suicide is more acceptable to men than women, and more acceptable in certain cultures. As such, men may be more likely to see it as a final solution to their troubles.

Despite many people presenting to primary care prior to a suicide attempt, men, especially young men, may find it harder to express their distress fully. In recent research, this was one of a number of barriers that prevented men from seeking assistance from mental health services. Another was that men felt that health professionals often failed to recognize or treat these problems.[19]

Importance of primary care in preventing suicide

Over 80% of successful suicide victims visit a general practitioner in the 6-month period before their death, and 50% of them within a month. Primary care practitioners have the ability to reduce suicide rates substantially if they are equipped with the knowledge and skills to assess and manage suicide ideation successfully. It is impossible to know how many suicides are already prevented each year in this way.

A distinction is sometimes made between those who express suicidal ideation and those who attempt suicide – the latter often termed parasuicides. However, research has shown that many people who attempt suicide later go on to take their own life. When looking at suicide from a prevention perspective it is important to view each case of suicidal ideation as an indicator of risk, falling on a spectrum of suicidality along which people move depending on circumstance.

Assessment of suicide risk

Although there are many demographic and clinical factors associated with risk (Table 33.1) of suicide, these cannot be relied upon when assessing suicide risk in an individual person. Suicide can also occur in the absence of these factors, and they are probably most effective in predicting long-term risk. Suicide can be characterized as an existential life position in which there is a balance of possibilities in a person's mind, some of which it would be difficult for a partner, friend, or professional to recognize, but which leave the person a rational choice. However this minimizes the very real disturbance that characterizes many suicides.

The evidence suggests that right up until the final stages, those who go on to kill themselves agonize as to whether or not suicide should be carried out. This means that for a clinician it is crucial to reach out to a person presenting as hopeless and to offer hope, which initially should be done by listening in a non-judgmental way. However, some

Table 33.1. *Risk factors for suicide*

Major indicators	Accompanying factors
Previous suicide attempts	Social isolation
Family history of suicide	No employment
	Abuse of alcohol or drugs
Existence of a well-formed plan	No close personal relationship
Access to the means	Tidying up of personal affairs
Presence of active thinking about suicide and the means	History of mental health problems
Inability to see anything positive about the future	Legal problems, conflict with law
	Experience of child abuse
Presence of psychosis	
Presence of depression	Loss, including physical health, bereavement
Presence of a recently made will	

people act on sudden impulse, and where a clinician is aware of suicidal ideation it is vital to explore likely triggers for suicidal feelings and to share techniques for buying time and pre-empting crises. Identifying possible lifelines and support systems can defuse episodes of acute risk. It is important to prevent the narrowing of conceptual thinking to a dichotomy – a form of Hobson's choice: death or an unbearable life. People do still have a choice, and healthcare professionals can help by widening the options that a person feels are available.

The final evaluation of risk must depend on individual clinical judgment, with a differential weighting of the risk factors in each person. The full evaluation of risk can only be completed with a detailed clinical assessment containing a comprehensive review of the history, the present risk, the current mental state, and the diagnosis, where possible. Despite the low sensitivity of risk factors, they are still a vital element of any clinical assessment. They can also be a useful check indicating caution, if they are present in numbers when the general view is one of low risk.

The process of interviewing a suicidal person

Given that many people are ambivalent about killing themselves, it is essential that the environment and atmosphere that you create are conducive to the person talking about what is going on in his inner world. Someone may be indifferent, excited, or appalled by what he is contemplating, and it is important for a clinician to reduce the levels of expressed emotion whilst being able to gain the person's confidence. In many cases, however, doctors remain unaware of their patients' suicidal ideation because they have not directly assessed this. Research findings suggest suicide rates can be reduced by as much as 30% if primary care providers are trained in risk identification. Interview technique is therefore a major factor in determining whether someone shares his thinking with a clinician. Table 33.2 gives some guidance for interviewing a suicidal person.

Your interview may be one of the last opportunities to bridge the gap created by a person's

Table 33.2. *Guidance for interviewing a suicidal person*

- Ensure that you have a quiet space that the person feels comfortable in, and minimize the risk of interruptions
- Offer something to drink
- Allow time for an unhurried assessment
- Start the interview with non-directive, open-ended questions, allowing the patient to talk about what is important to him
- Use language that is appropriate for the person, taking account of possible cultural and faith beliefs
- Avoid using judgmental and challenging statements
- Listen to what the person is saying, and watch for non-verbal cues
- Go over recent events and take note of particular values that the person puts on different statements or behaviors
- Complete a mental state examination
- Directly address suicidal motivation

mistrust with the world around him and the loss of hope that his situation could ever change for the better. Ignoring basic clinical practice or being abrupt, dismissive, or unsympathetic may confirm suicidal despair.

It is important to lead into the whole topic of suicide gradually, thus offering sensitivity to the person's predicament, giving him the confidence to share his thoughts with you. Direct questions about suicidal ideas are important, but there is other circumstantial evidence (see Table 33.1) that is also important and that may emerge when gathering background data. Wherever possible you should, with the patient's agreement, take the opportunity to talk to relatives, who often have important background information, which you can cross-check with what the patient has told you. The patient may have omitted key information, either inadvertently or in an attempt to undermine the efficacy of your assessment. Family members may be in possession of information about small changes in behavior, which themselves do not indicate suicidal intention but when assembled present a worrying picture.

Sequence of questions

Some practitioners are concerned that asking about suicide might raise an option that someone might not otherwise have considered. There is no research evidence to suggest this is the case and in fact patients have often reported that it is a relief when someone finally raises the subject with them. Although asking a direct question about suicidal thinking may seem counterintuitive, it is no different from many other major questions that seem taboo, the airing of which in fact brings relief and a chance for resolution. It is essential, though, to take a graduated approach, starting with factors that might indicate that the person has resources to combat his feelings of despair and negativity, and leading into an exploration of the depth of the misery. Table 33.3 gives a suggested sequence of questions for assessing risk.

Once suicidal ideation has been elicited it is vital that a further series of questions are asked to determine how strongly the ideas are held: will they persist and worsen without help?; are they likely to be acted upon?; and can the person give any reassurances about his safety until the next time he is seen? Can the person say anything else that indicates that he envisages being around at a future point in time? It is also important to evaluate any factors that might worsen the situation (e.g. the presence of a spouse with whom he is at breaking point) and establish what help is available.

The questions in Table 33.3 are not intended to be exclusive or adopted in a rigid way. Although some are clearly 'leading' they can be asked in an open-ended way, offering them as one choice amongst several. The key challenge though is to avoid any aggressive or coercive questioning at all costs. Empathic listening and sharing will allow the person to open up to the interviewer. Some patients, in particular those with personality disorder or depression accompanied by morbid thinking, may well be placed at risk by aggressive interviewing.

In gathering information from relatives and other sources, it is important to remember that suicidal intent can fluctuate wildly, often from one hour or day to the next, and therefore it is helpful to reassess at intervals whenever possible to get a more longitudinal view.

Table 33.3. *Sequential questions for assessing risk*

- Ask a series of questions designed to find out if a person has any hope, gets any pleasure out of his life, feels able to cope with the day ahead, or sees a point to life
- This should be followed by questions that assess if the person ever despairs about things, feels he can't face another day, that life is a burden, that he wishes it would all end
- Ask if the person, feels that he is responsible for things that are happening around him
- Check if the person knows why he feels this way
- Then ask specifically if the person has thought of ending his life, and if so how often currently
- Has the person thought about specific methods or means of doing so
- Has the person ever acted on any suicidal intentions before
- Ask if the person feels able to resist any suicidal thoughts or has any thoughts about what they could do to make these thoughts go away

Developing a care plan

It is helpful to identify positive and supportive factors. Emphasizing the ways that people can help themselves can empower them to realize suicide is not the only way to take control of the situation. It is important whenever possible to get their agreement to share the plan with other family members and agencies to increase the support network. The factors in Table 33.4 may have protective value that can be emphasized and used in a care plan. Ensuring that the plan is followed up is vital to its success and will encourage a suicidal person to re-visit health services.

Post-suicide

It is essential in the wake of a suicide to consider the needs of both staff and family members. Whenever

Table 33.4. *Protective factors*
▪ Good physical and mental health
▪ Strong social networks and social integration (including family, school, faith community)
▪ Responsibility for dependants
▪ Strong religious or spiritual faith, or a sense of meaning and purpose to life
▪ Limited access to suicide methods
▪ Early identification and appropriate treatment of mental health problems
▪ Economic security in older age
▪ Belief that suicide is wrong

possible there should be a debrief for staff to learn from the event and to ensure that family members are supported. Sometimes staff are tempted to withdraw from a family, fearful of recriminations and litigation, but this is a mistake. It is crucial that relatives are offered an opportunity to grieve and helped with the bereavement process. There are a number of information leaflets[20] and packs available to help with this. Evidence suggests that the death of a family member by suicide is itself a significant risk factor for suicide, so help offered at this time could be crucial to the wellbeing of relatives.

Training

There are several training schemes available nationally in the UK, some targeted at frontline staff who need specific expertise in assessing and working with suicide risk, and others aimed at staff in a range of organizations who may need to be able to identify emerging risk. The STORM package[21] (Skills-based Training On Risk Management) is flexible and adaptable to meet the needs of different organizations. It is evidence-based, has been formally evaluated, and has the advantage of being based on a cascade model of delivery. Once trained, STORM facilitators from the organization can deliver training to their colleagues. Similarly, the ASIST[22] (Applied Suicide Intervention Skills Training) course consists of 2 days of training with an emphasis on suicide first aid and helping a person to stay safe and seek

further help. It is important for staff to receive training because insensitive and ill-informed approaches carry a high risk.

Health promotion to reduce suicide risk

In the UK, there are a number of issues for Mental Health Commissioners to consider in relation to suicide. Under Standard One of the National Service Framework for Mental Health, local implementation teams are tasked with producing a Mental Health Promotion Strategy. This should include consideration of wider initiatives to reduce suicide. Clearly many of the demographic factors that affect suicide rates are likely to be affected only by wider regeneration and neighborhood renewal schemes, but there are intervention models that can address individual needs for support in a crisis. These are predicated upon the notion that a range of supports will reduce the possibility of someone reaching crisis point. In particular they may be aimed at risk groups such as young men, people dependent on drugs and alcohol, and the elderly with physical health problems.

The key elements of such interventions are the provision of information, education, and support. A good example of such a model is CALM[23] (Campaign Against Living Miserably), a scheme in Merseyside in north-west England based on a 24-hour help-line and a website specifically designed to appeal to young people. Its approach is to encourage young men to open up and discuss their problems, rather than to think it is 'macho' to cope on their own. Using the medium of wider health promotion helps to reduce the centrality of suicidal fears for a person by offering a range of support on other health worries, including smoking, testicular cancer, obesity, sensible drinking, and diabetes. This can encourage people to talk more generally about their concerns, including those relating to interpersonal relationships, which are often at the root of suicidal feelings.

Strengthening communication between young men, their peers, family, advice services, general practitioners, and other professionals has been shown to reduce risk,[11] and the same principle can apply to elderly people. Good referral and communication between agencies to ensure that a person is supported in all aspects of his life will reduce risk factors and highlight issues of concern in a timely manner, and so prevent unnecessary deaths.

Acknowledgments

The authors would like to thank Rosie MacQueen and Wanda Garcia for their comments and assistance in drafting this article.

References

1. World Health Organization Suicide Prevention (SUPRE), 2007. Available at: http://www.who.int/mental_health/prevention/suicide/suicideprevent/en [Accessed 7 October, 2007].
2. Diekstra RF, Gulbinat W. The epidemiology of suicidal behaviour: a review of three continents. World Health Stat Q 1993; 46: 52–68.
3. Office of National Statistics. Suicide, 2007. Available at: http://www.statistics.gov.uk/CCI/nugget.asp?ID=1092&Pos=6&ColRank=2&Rank=1000 [Accessed 13 October, 2007].
4. National Institute of Mental Health in England. National Suicide Prevention Strategy for England: Annual Report on Progress 2006. Leeds, UK: Department of Health, 2007.
5. National Statistics. News Release: Suicides Reach 30 Year Low in 2003, 2005. Available at: http://www.statistics.gov.uk/pdfdir/suicide0305.pdf [Accessed 13 October 2007].
6. Men's Health Forum. Soldier it! Young Men and Suicide, 2002. Available at: http://www.menshealthforum.org.uk/uploaded_files/mhfsuicideauditfinal.pdf [Accessed 10 October, 2007].
7. Cattell H. Suicide in the elderly. Adv Psychiat Treat 2000; 6: 102–8.
8. EPPI-Centre. A Scoping Exercise for a Review of the Effectiveness of Health Promotion Interventions of Relevance to Suicide Prevention in Young Men (19–34). London: EPPI-Centre, Institute of Education, 2002.
9. Hawton K. Why has suicide increased in young males? Crisis 1998; 19: 119–24.
10. Rutter PA, Behrendt AE. Adolescent suicide risk: four psychosocial factors. Adolescence 2004; 39: 295–302.
11. Romero M, Wintermute GJ. The epidemiology of firearm suicide in the United States. J Urban Health 2002; 79: 39–48.
12. Streib EW, Hackworth J, Hayward TZ et al. Firearm suicide: use of firearm injury and death surveillance system. J Trauma 2007; 62: 730–34.
13. Shah R, Uren Z, Baker A et al. Trends in suicide from drug overdose in the elderly in England and Wales, 1993–1999. Int J Geriatr Psychiatry 2002; 17: 416–21.
14. Appleby L, Shaw J, Amost T et al. Safer Services. Report of the National Confidential Inquiry into Suicide and Homicide by People with Mental Illness. London: The Stationery Office, 1999.
15. McIntosh C, Ritson B. Treating depression complicated by substance misuse. Adv Psychiatr Treat 2001; 7: 357–64.
16. Lewis G, Sloggett A. Suicide, deprivation and unemployment: record linkage study. BMJ 1998; 317: 1283–6.
17. Durkheim E. Le suicide. Paris: F Alcan, 1897.
18. Office for National Statistics. Health Statistics Q 2006; 31: 6–22.
19. Strike C, Rhodes AE, Bergmans Y et al. Fragmented pathways to care: the experiences of suicidal men. Crisis 2006; 27: 31–8. Cited in: Centre for Suicide Prevention. Men and Suicide: Part 1 – Risk Factors. Available at: http://www.suicideinfo.ca/csp/assets/alert65.pdf [Accessed 17 October, 2007].
20. Department of Health. Help is at Hand: a Resource for People Bereaved by Suicide and Other Sudden Traumatic Death. London: Central Office of Information, 2006.
21. STORM Training, available at: http://www.medicine.manchester.ac.uk/storm/TheSTORMPackage/
22. ASIST Training, available at: http://www.asist.org.uk/attend.html
23. The CALM Zone website, available at: http://www.thecalmzone.net

CHAPTER 34

Alcohol

Brian Wells

Introduction

A wide historical literature on the subject of alcohol can be traced back over many centuries. Recent developments and a selection of 'classic' papers are listed in the Further Reading section of this chapter. Ethyl alcohol is a sedative drug rapidly absorbed in the upper gastrointestinal tract. Use leads to dose-related altered inhibitions, inebriation, loss of consciousness, coma, diminished reflexes, and eventual death by respiratory depression (the traditional phases of general anesthesia). The neurobiological mechanisms involved are complex.

The four basic types of drinking

Experimental drinking

Alcohol is sampled in a variety of socio-cultural settings. An 'altered state' may be experienced – the effect of the drug ethyl alcohol. Some enjoy it, others remain indifferent. Despite initial nausea and vomiting that may occur, a significant number (who may progress to dependence) will vividly remember that first experience. It is unlikely that they will remember the first time they tasted chocolate.

Parents, friends, religion, culture and sub-culture are highly influential, so that alcohol (and other drugs) may or may not be part of child, adolescent and early adult development.

Drinking patterns vary according to what is available, acceptable, in fashion, and advertised locally. Drunkenness is rarely seen in Italy (although this is changing among young people), while neighboring France maintains a seven times greater prevalence of alcoholic liver cirrhosis. Younger men in the UK and USA currently tend to drink beer; perhaps cold lager directly from the can or bottle, warm ale (from straight glasses) is drunk more in northern Great Britain and Ireland; while Australian men are renowned beer drinkers despite their global surplus of wines. Tastes alter, income varies, friends and drinking patterns change. A wine cellar may become the gourmet equivalent of a collection of art or vintage cars.

In some cultures drinking may be illegal, shameful (especially among women), a source of derision or a reason for imprisonment and even execution. With international variations in law, advertising and government policy, the World Health Organization estimates that there are at least 2 billion regular users of alcohol worldwide. Most of these people have moved from experimental drinking to recreational drinking.

Recreational drinking

Recreational drinking is a sociable, pleasurable part of normal life in most cultures. Recreational drinkers are responsible and enjoy modest amounts of their chosen beverages, causing no harm to themselves or others. Drinking may be light, moderate, or 'heavy'. Those who drink two units daily may live longer than teetotallers, owing to the antioxidant properties of ethanol (the beverage itself being irrelevant).

A generalization is that recreational drinkers can 'take it or leave it'. They may choose to get drunk at times or use alcohol to celebrate, for 'Dutch courage', or for solace after a difficult day. They do not self-medicate with alcohol on a regular basis and tend to enjoy the taste as well as the effect. Usually they sip their drinks and a pattern of 'social' drinking is established, which may vary over time.

Hazardous and harmful (problem) drinking

Alcohol is second only to tobacco as the world's biggest 'drug problem'. Because most cultures include alcohol consumption as part of normal life, attempts to reduce excessive drinking have been fraught with debate, controversy, and lack of efficacy. There is much current interest in 'sensible' drinking. In the UK a number of policy documents have recently been published, with particular emphasis on curbing the sub-cultural phenomenon of binge drinking in young people. Paradoxically and controversially, licensing hours have been extended so that alcohol is more widely available. Problems relating to consumption of cannabis, heroin, cocaine, club-drugs, and other 'pharmaceuticals' are minor compared with the public health concerns caused by the use and misuse of tobacco and alcohol. This is a global phenomenon, with a long and complex history.

Men drink more than women: 38% of men in England (but 16% of women) have an 'alcohol use disorder' (hazardous, harmful or dependent drinking). Men suffer more consequences although this is changing. Crime, violence, morbid jealousy, murder, spread of HIV, self-harm, accidents, depression, suicide, attendance for medical or surgical care, child abuse, and imprisonment are all strongly correlated with excessive use of alcohol. Family life is seriously affected. Billions of dollars are lost each year resulting from absenteeism, underperformance, and crime as a direct result of problematic drinking.

Harmful drinkers tend to drink more (certainly than the recommended guidelines) and experience problems on a regular basis as a direct result of alcohol consumption. Physical and psychological health may be seriously affected, as well as socio-economic

Box 34.1.

Hazardous drinking

Has the potential to become harmful and may cause tissue damage

It may be seen in:

- anyone consuming more than the recommended limits
- binge-drinkers (drinking 8 units over 24 hours for men, 6 units for women)

Recommended limits

No more than 3–4 units a day (for men)

No more than 2–3 units a day (for women)

0 units (for pregnant women)

Note: 1 unit is one small glass of wine; half a pint (284 ml) of normal-strength lager, cider, or beer, or one measure of spirits (8–10 g of alcohol).

function. Harmful drinkers suffer a variety of adverse consequences, as does society as a whole. The features of hazardous drinking are outlined in Box 34.1, as are some recommendations for safe drinking levels.

A significant number of problem drinkers will move on to dependent drinking.

Dependent drinking (alcoholism)

The hallmark of dependent drinking is that alcohol becomes important to the person who is becoming dependent. Dependent drinkers seek out people and situations that involve the consumption of alcohol, perhaps finding employment in industries where alcohol is available or acceptable. Over time, they begin to display features that include a strong desire or compulsion to drink and an altered tolerance, with regular withdrawal symptoms that are relieved by alcohol, consumption of which persists despite clear evidence of harm and neglect of socio-economic function.

Alcohol dependence can be spectacular and obvious (sometimes at an early age). More commonly, it is an insidious process and only gradually do those around (family, employers, friends) become aware. The person who is becoming dependent is often genuinely unaware or has only partial insight (denial). This can lead to arguments and stigmatization of 'the alcoholic', who tends to break promises, causing mistrust and other problems.

Alcohol dependence may be moderate or severe. To complicate matters, patterns of dependent drinking can vary from a gradual increase in regular 'top-up' drinking over decades, to long periods of abstinence or moderate drinking that may suddenly lead to a chaotic binge that can last for several days or weeks.

Severe alcohol dependence is easy to diagnose. Mild-to-moderate dependence is where time, skill, collateral 'evidence' and experience are required. The distinction between heavy recreational, problematic, and dependent drinking is important. After years of research, controversy, debate, and the development of operational definitions (ICD10, DSM-1V), it is now generally agreed (in some cases argued) that dependent drinkers are unlikely to be able to return to 'normal drinking' and are in danger of progressing into severe dependence with all associated consequences.

On a population basis, alcohol dependence subtracts an average of 4.2 disability-adjusted life-years (DALYs) per person. For comparison, tobacco use subtracts 4.1 DALYs, AIDS 6.0 DALYs, 'illicit' drug use 0.8 DALYs, and type 1 diabetes 0.1 DALYs.

It is estimated that between 60% and 80% of worldwide alcohol dependence occurs in men (although the 'hidden' population of women is rising) and that 6–9% of regular male drinkers in the UK and USA drink in a dependent manner. In recent years attention has been given to the adverse effects of alcohol dependence upon the 'family system' and the children of alcoholics, which, combined with genetic processes that require further clarification, leads to ongoing trans-generational complications.

Alcohol dependence may mimic a host of physical and psychological disorders. It is frequently the **cause** (rather than result) of mood disorders, anxiety-related conditions, and apparent disorders of personality. It is frequently missed as a treatable diagnosis. The physical complications of excessive drinking are listed in Box 34.2.

Management of problem drinking

Government and workplace policies, national laws, religious and cultural beliefs, and family values may

---

Box 34.2. *Physical complications of excessive drinking*

These may be direct or indirect (e.g. malnutrition due to pancreatitis or liver disease). Note also that 85% of dependent drinkers smoke.

Direct consequences

- Acute intoxication, coma, and death from overdosage (often young men rapidly drinking a bottle of spirits)
- Aspiration (of vomit with loss of reflexes)
- Accidents

Gastroenterological disorders

- Alcoholic liver disease – fatty liver, alcoholic hepatitis, alcoholic cirrhosis (rates of which have doubled in the UK over the past decade)
- Acute and chronic pancreatitis
- Gastritis and peptic ulceration
- Mallory–Weiss syndrome (due to vomiting)

Musculoskeletal disorders

- Gout
- Osteoporosis
- Myopathy

Endocrine disorders

- Pseudo-Cushing's syndrome
- Male hypogonadism (low testosterone levels and erectile dysfunction)

Cancers – increased risk for certain cancers

- Oropharynx
- Esophagus
- Liver (following alcoholic cirrhosis)
- Possibly breast cancer in women

Cardiovascular disease

- Alcohol-related arrythmias
- Hypertension (especially in binge drinkers)
- Cerebrovascular disease or stroke
- Coronary heart disease
- Alcoholic cardiomyopathy

(Continued)

Box 34.2. *(Continued)*

Respiratory disease

- Pneumonia
- Tuberculosis
- Carcinoma of the lung (associated with smoking)

Metabolic disorders

- Hypoglycemia
- Hypothermia
- Alcoholic ketoacidosis (rare)
- Hyperlipidemia

Hematological effects

- Anemia
- Macrocytosis
- Iron deficiency
- Neutropenia and thrombocytopenia

Disorders of the central and peripheral nervous system

- Seizures (often resulting from alcohol withdrawal)
- Alcoholic cerebellar degeneration
- Alcohol amblyopia
- Wernicke–Korsakoff syndrome
- Alcoholic pellagra encephalopathy
- Alcoholic 'dementia'
- Central pontine myelinolysis
- Marchiafava–Bignami disease
- Hepatic encephalopathy
- Peripheral neuropathy
- Fetal alcohol syndrome

Skin disease

- Psoriasis
- Discoid eczema
- Fungal infections

Immune deficiency

Increased cross-tolerance to anesthetic agents

variably influence the harm caused by excessive drinking. The years of Prohibition in the USA are often viewed as an era of hedonistic illicit behavior controlled by corrupt politicians and mobsters. There were, at that time, a minimal number of alcohol-related problems in that country (in other words, Prohibition was in fact a huge, albeit unpopular, success as a harm-reduction strategy).

The availability of alcohol and other drugs, however controlled (e.g. by price, law, age-restriction) remains the one constant factor in all data so far gathered in attempts to prevent, reduce, or control the harm caused by excessive use of alcohol and other drugs. Such attempts include pricing initiatives in certain Scandinavian cities, where alcoholic beverages are so expensive that, come the weekend, people stay at home to drink until late at night, when they then go out to dance venues, leading to the extraordinary sight of drunken people from all ages and socio-economic groups stumbling in and out of taxis at 2.00 or 3.00 a.m. This cultural phenomenon results in high levels of cirrhosis as a result of weekend 'binge' drinking, in mainly non-dependent people.

Clinical awareness

Excessive and dependent use of alcohol and other drugs are often missed or undeclared or are too infrequently at the forefront of the clinician's mind. In a busy primary care setting, the patient's relationship with alcohol may be minimized or ignored.

In emergency departments, inebriated patients are seen commonly (as are their families), and it can be difficult to do anything other than deal with the presenting complaints. Drunken people do not respond well to what they may view as a judgmental, accusatory or pejorative stance taken by others. They can, however, respond well to empathic suggestions that may lead to action taken at some point in the future.

It is strongly recommended that the subject of alcohol and other drug use should be raised in a non-judgmental manner as routine 'healthcare' practice in all clinical settings. Validated screening instruments can be easily and rapidly completed during assessment, the FAST (20 seconds) and AUDIT (2 minutes) questionnaires having been extensively researched and translated into many languages. Hematological and biochemical investigations (mean corpuscular volume, γ-glutamyl transferase, carbohydrate deficient transferrin, and blood or breath alcohol levels) may be useful indicators of excessive alcohol consumption, although these can be unremarkable in even severely dependent drinkers. Sometimes a family member may mention alcohol or drugs or resultant behavior as a problem.

If there is the hint or more obvious evidence of a drinking problem or dependence, it is prudent either to spend more time on a brief intervention or to refer the patient for a specialist assessment.

Brief interventions

Time-consuming, detailed assessment is required in only those cases of dependence that are 'difficult'. Brief interventions consisting of a few minutes of informed advice by any healthcare professional can alter the course of hazardous drinking. This may be extended to a 20–30-minute session using basic motivational interviewing skills, aimed at changing the behavior of problematic drinkers, by workers trained in such techniques. Such interventions have been shown to have a sustainable effect upon those who are able to modify their drinking. However, those who have moved into moderate dependence are best advised to seek further assessment and help.

Specialist assessment

Men and women becoming dependent on alcohol and other drugs are always in adverse circumstances by the time they present for assessment (which may be under duress from family or employer). The process should initiate a useful treatment 'direction', as opposed to the mere accumulation of information that fails to inspire someone who is probably in a difficult situation.

Trust needs to be established, insight gained, and motivation enhanced as part of the assessment process – ideally in collaboration with 'significant others' who are able to contribute in a productive, rather than an antagonistic or confrontational, manner. Low self-esteem (usually present) leads to

evasive and deflective responses in people who feel threatened. The objective of a detailed assessment is to facilitate the taking of positive steps forward with a condition that remains highly stigmatized.

Several sessions may be required. Motivational interviewing techniques are often used, in a process that should 'bring to life' the evolution of an addictive disorder that needs to be understood and recognized by the index patient. Differing therapeutic styles may be used to elicit a mutual understanding. Each situation is different, so it may be appropriate to cover the ground in an order or manner that is engaging, to avoid awkwardness and defensive 'minimization'. The traditional psychiatric assessment (Box 34.3) may need to become atypical and flexible, while investigations, including urine and hair testing (for drugs), can be used to positive and constructive effect.

The key questions that require understanding and formulation are:

- Is the index patient **dependent** upon alcohol or drugs?
- If so, what is the **degree** of dependence?
- Is anyone at **risk** of harm (family members, the public, motorists, etc)?
- Is urgent action or treatment required?
- How can the clinician work with the patient and family to facilitate positive change?

Treatment

Treatment is essentially the mutual agreement of realistic goals that should be directed towards the best interests of everyone involved. While true for medicine as a whole, treatment for substance misuse may include the protection of children as a priority. Families may have endured years of failed treatment attempts. 'Addiction' can be chronic, and relapse is common; smoking as the most glaring example, with some attempts at 'treatment' actually making matters worse, the index patient perhaps becoming more secretive and difficult to live with.

Cutting down on consumption may be a realistic goal where the patient is not dependent. Many heavy and problematic drinkers will either abstain, or reduce their intake to safe levels following a 'brief

Box 34.3. *Traditional psychiatric assessment*

Demographic details

The current situation (often some form of crisis)

A picture of the recent history that has led to the meeting

Previous help-seeking for this type of problem

Personal history (birth, childhood, schooling, siblings, family atmosphere, achievements)

Family history

Occupational history (with problems relating to alcohol and drugs being quietly noted)

Relationship and sexual history (including HIV risk behaviors)

Past medical, surgical, and 'psychiatric' episodes (including accidents, treatment for 'depression')

Trauma (physical and emotional)

Current and past relationship with the criminal justice system

Risk behaviors (driving, child-care, etc.)

Current personal and domestic circumstances

Relationship with other drugs (illicit and prescribed)

A detailed typical drinking day or week (preferably recent, at a time of heavy drinking)

Mental state examination (including cognitive function)

Physical examination (often ignored or neglected)

intervention' as described previously. In cases of dependence, unless the patient becomes abstinent, problems are likely to worsen for everyone involved. A small number of dependent patients simply stop their use of alcohol and drugs (spontaneous remission). The majority will relapse at some point and require a form of supportive treatment. The more severely dependent will rapidly revert into 'dependent' use.

Abstinence-based treatments

Abstinence-based treatments may be 'drop-in', outpatient, day-care, or intensively residential in format. A plethora of techniques aimed towards abstention, some of which are evidence-based, many of which hinge upon the beliefs of the therapist or institution, are available. Usually, a process of motivation and negotiation takes place enabling the patient and family to undergo a cognitive–perceptual shift with the aid of community reinforcement and support. Such negotiations are commonly met with initial resistance, and careful 'reading' of the situation is required in order to proceed in a productive manner.

Historically in the UK, the thrust of treatment has been led by psychologists with an orientation based upon learning theory. Alcohol dependence has been viewed as a learned behavior, which can be modified by techniques such as cognitive behavioral therapy (CBT), with attempts at controlled drinking having been the norm until the recent past. There has been much (sometimes volatile) professional debate, most of which has now subsided as a result of 'landmark' re-evaluations of dependent drinkers who were initially claimed to have resumed satisfactory drinking patterns. Further scrutiny of these cohorts revealed that most subjects had either died or reinstated into dependent drinking.

In the USA, where alcohol dependence has been viewed as a 'disease' by the American Medical Association, thousands of residential 28-day programs were set up during the 1950s, 1960s, and 1970s. These were usually covered by health insurance (hence the 28 days) allowing patients and families to undergo an experiential process consisting of group therapy, one-to-one counseling, and personal assignments, during which they 'internalized' the understanding of 'alcoholism' being a progressive illness for which there is no cure. Recovery, however, is deemed possible; based on a framework of total abstention from alcohol (and from other mood-altering drugs) with vigorous participation in a process of recovery as suggested by the 'Twelve-Step Movement' (exemplified by Alcoholics Anonymous and other twelve-step organizations).

However, in the 1990s a system of managed care was introduced, causing the majority of these residential centers to close. Those that survived either became 'licensed psychiatric facilities' or specialist (often not-for-profit) units that weathered the financial storm. Meanwhile variations of this model had gradually been transported to the UK, Scandinavia, Australia, and South Africa, and more recently to the Middle East and India, where they are becoming generally accepted as the most efficacious form of treatment ('rehab') in these countries. Some units offer specialist facilities for families, professionals (doctors, lawyers, and pilots), and those with eating disorders and other 'co-morbid' conditions. There remain many professional sceptics who do not accept the 'disease model' or what they view as the religious element of the twelve-step ideology. While other mutual self-help groups and organizations exist, few have stood the test of time. Some workers continue with non-evidence-based techniques (e.g. hypnosis, cathartic experience, psychodrama). Most psychodynamic practitioners will not entertain the treatment of an alcohol-dependent client until the client has achieved sufficient abstinence and ego-strength to benefit from such work.

The controversial extreme is an orchestrated intervention. The dependent person attends what he or she believes will be a work-related meeting, only to find the room full of relatives, employers and, poignantly, even the children. Letters may be read aloud, tears may be shed, while the index patient is told that while he or she is loved and appreciated, the following steps (usually the immediate admission to a residential facility) will be required to avoid serious consequences such as job loss, divorce and family fragmentation. If the patient agrees to the terms put forward, he or she is offered support and re-employment after the therapy, subject to agreement to a process of 'recovery' and monitoring for the presence of alcohol and drugs, and also subject to behavior being acceptable.

Such 'ambush' types of intervention must be carefully crafted by the interventionist, taking full account of available 'leverage' (sticks and carrots), and having rehearsed the process with all persons present, who must be 'on board' no matter how painful it may be. This must include consideration of the process back-firing. The patient may walk out, self-harm, or live with resentment.

While remaining controversial and viewed as a 'high-risk', ethically dubious strategy by critics, there are many people who have been successfully coerced into treatment with excellent results.

Many US physicians with substance use disorders have been subjected to orchestrated interventions and given 'offers they cannot refuse'. Recent data show impressive results for those who complete the 90 day residential program at the Betty Ford Unit for Professionals (and other similar institutions) that include a residential 'family week', followed by regular and consistent post-treatment monitoring (urine and hair testing). During the 'monitoring period', 81% had negative urine test results. Most doctors (95%) who completed monitoring were still licensed and working as physicians at five years post-treatment. These (astounding) results cannot be ignored, and the principles of post-treatment monitoring are now being applied to 'non-professional' patients with early outcome measures that appear highly promising (personal communication from the recently formed Betty Ford Institute).

Orchestrated and brief interventions are the two extremes. More commonly, a middle road is found that will nudge the dependent patient into abstinence over a variable period of time, with or without a formal treatment experience. A useful tactic when meeting resistance may be to encourage patients to sip and enjoy 3 units of alcohol daily (2 for women) for the next 6–12 months. If they can achieve this, the likelihood is that they are not dependent. If they cannot, they may be able to 'see for themselves', and internalize the need and motivation for abstinence.

Highly confrontational methods aimed at 'breaking the denial' are old-fashioned and ineffective. Far more effective are those that are empathic and that facilitate a productive experience for patients and their families.

CBT is a well-researched, evidence-based technique that aims to modify maladaptive or 'erroneous' beliefs, as well as to provide coping strategies, problem-solving and social skills. It may be effectively used in combination with other modes of treatment in assisting dependent drinkers towards abstinence, and it is a fundamental tool in the prevention of relapse.

Motivational enhancement therapy (MET) is a style of treatment that is covertly directive.

The traditional style – taking a detailed history followed by overt directive advice – is replaced by strategies that 'roll with resistance', utilizing open-ended questions and structured reflective feedback that effectively mobilize the patient's own resources to gain insight and motivation to take action.

Project Match, a landmark outpatient study (costing some US$37 million), demonstrated that MET, cognitive behavioral coping skills therapy and twelve-step facilitation are all powerful treatments. At 1-year follow-up they all had equal efficacy. The 15-year follow-up shows that dependent patients who attend support groups such as Alcoholics Anonymous are more likely to have remained abstinent (personal communication).

Residential treatment is expensive and has not yet been formally validated as superior to outpatient or day-care except in severe dependence, 'complicated' cases, or in cases where the situation at home is untenable. It therefore exists largely in the private sector and for those with means or healthcare insurance.

Provision in the public sector is variable. Funding for effective alcohol services in the UK is complex and has been inadequate, despite the rhetoric, compared with that available for 'drug' services. There are long waiting times that lose the opportunity to capitalize on 'the crisis' that initiates contact (the teachable moment). Treatment generally comprises an assisted withdrawal combined with 'counseling' of variable quality, usually with an MET or CBT orientation. Therapists require adequate training. There remain a number of 'counselors' in both the public and private sectors who have little training other than their own experiences of 'recovery'. This is changing as funding sources increasingly require demonstrable accreditation, follow-up reports, and the application of evidence-based techniques.

Pharmacological treatments

A medically assisted withdrawal from alcohol (detoxification) may or may not be required, bearing in mind that this is simply the initiation of abstinence and not an effective psychosocial treatment in itself. Most patients can remain ambulant or be treated on an outpatient basis.

Drugs with a cross-tolerance to alcohol, usually benzodiazepines (oxazepam, diazepam, chlordiazepoxide) are administered until sufficient dosage over 24 hours minimizes or removes alcohol withdrawal symptoms (tremor, sweating, nausea). If there is a history of epilepsy or convulsions on previous attempts at withdrawal, additional anticonvulsant cover may be advisable. The dosage is then tapered over an appropriate time period (usually 3–10 days) allowing comfortable and safe withdrawal. B vitamins are often administered as routine and must be given (as parenteral thiamine) if Wernicke–Korsakoff syndrome is suspected. *Post mortem* studies suggest that 80% of such cases remain undiagnosed.

Delerium tremens is not in itself a characteristic of alcohol withdrawal and can usually be avoided with adequate assisted withdrawal. Should it manifest (usually 24–150 hours after cessation of alcohol) it must be regarded as a life-threatening emergency, and is best treated by a medical team in hospital.

Upon achieving abstinence, the use of disulfiram may be helpful, either in chronic recidivism or for enhancement of confidence. The dangers of drinking on top of disulfiram must be carefully explained, recorded, and understood by the patient, many of whom claim to have 'drunk on top of Antabuse' to no ill effect.

Naltrexone and acamprosate may be helpful in initial stages. It is claimed that both drugs reduce the desire to drink, and that if a lapse or relapse occurs it is relatively short lived. Studies show naltrexone to be superior, although in the UK it remains unlicensed for alcohol dependence.

The results of genomic and other 'biological' research that is under way are awaited with interest. It may be that biological markers will allow future prediction of tendencies towards dependence upon alcohol and other drugs. At the present time it is known that 'alcoholism runs in families'. There are genetic factors involved (based on evidence from twin studies, etc.), and if the 'addiction' is not to alcohol, it may manifest itself with other extreme and compulsive behaviors (related to drugs, food, gambling, sex, work, and other forms of 'instant gratification').

Post-treatment 'cross-addiction' to other drugs and behaviors is well documented, and often leads to a process of relapse. Success requires a vigilant, interesting and balanced form of recovery.

The family needs to become part of the process and sometimes requires more attention than the index patient. Family members are often 'damaged' as a result of living with alcohol dependence for many years. It takes time for trust to be re-established and in circumstances where only the index patient embraces recovery, subsequent family fragmentation is extremely common ('I'm no longer with the person that I married'). Recovery involves change. Family members who 'send the patient to treatment' are often surprised when, on return, he or she is spending time at support groups, resuming responsibilities previously neglected, and visibly re-prioritizing. Unless the family is also 'in recovery', problems occur, values become different, and post-treatment divorce rates are high (in excess of 50%).

Modern treatments for alcohol dependence are extremely effective. Patients in active recovery for longer than 3–5 years have a good prognosis, tend to be good employees, and describe an enjoyable 'journey', based upon abstinence, personal growth, development of new interests, and enhanced self-esteem.

Patients who are difficult to treat

- Despite all attempts at treatment (including liver transplants) some dependent patients will continue to drink until their premature death.
- Adolescents and young adults.
- The elderly (often widowed).
- Colleagues and members of one's own family.
- VIPs, celebrities, and the very wealthy (and their children).
- Those with co-morbid psychiatric conditions (e.g. bipolar illness, severe personality disorders).
- Severe, long-term poly-substance users.
- Those in chronic pain and with various other 'physical' conditions.

- Those suffering certain types of brain damage or trauma.

Useful attitudes to adopt

- There is no such thing as a 'hopeless case'.
- Always leave the door open.
- One day, something may 'click'.
- Work as part of a team.
- Be open to different strategies and treatment models.
- Know when to refer elsewhere.
- Enjoy continued professional development.

Conclusions

Alcohol enhances the health, pleasure, and quality of life in more than one-third of the global population, and the alcohol industry is a highly significant factor in world economics. For socio-biological reasons, many people drink to excess and develop alcohol use disorders, which account for and contribute to the premature deaths of predominantly men, while having an impact upon families and societies. Those who choose to misuse alcohol contribute to the stigma assigned to men and women who are in need of help.

Alcohol use disorders are preventable and highly treatable. Despite their prevalence and media profile, international policies remain muddled while effective treatments are unavailable to many in need. This can be partly attributed to history, stigma, lack of awareness, and real difficulties in the delivery of convincing research, both epidemiological and clinical, into this aspect of human behavior.

Acknowledgments

I am honored to be asked to contribute this chapter in the 3rd edition of so important a book. While not an award ceremony, I must thank my mentors, Dr Garrett O'Connor MD, Professors Griffith Edwards and Herbert D Kleber, as well as close friends and colleagues, Drs William Shanahan,

Gillian Tober, Duncan Raistrick, Anne Geller and Nicholas F Colangelo, for their wisdom, inspiration, dedication and humor.

Suggested reading

Abel EL, Sokol RJ. A revised conservative estimate of the incidence of foetal alcohol syndrome and its economic impact. Alcohol Clin Exp Res 1991; 15: 514–24.

American Psychiatric Association. Diagnostic and Statistical Manual of Mental Disorders, 4th edn. (DSM-IV). Washington DC: American Psychiatric Association, 1994.

Babor TF. Tackling alcohol misuse in the UK. BMJ 2008; 336: 455.

Babor TF, Hofmann M, Del Boca FK et al. Types of alcoholics, I: evidence for an empirically derived typology based on indicators of vulnerability and severity. Arch Gen Psychiatry 1992; 49: 599–608.

Ball DM, Murray RM. Genetics of alcohol misuse. Br Med Bull 1994; 50: 18–35.

British Medical Association. Alcohol misuse: tackling the UK epidemic. British Medical Association Board of Science, 2008.

Chapman WD, Hingson RW, Merrigan DM et al. A randomized trial of treatment options for alcohol-abusing workers. N Engl J Med 1991; 325: 775–82.

Chiauzzi EJ, Liljegren S. Taboo topics in addiction treatment. J Subst Abuse Treat 1993; 10: 303.

Chick J. Delirium tremens. BMJ 1989; 298: 3–4.

Cook CCH. Aetiology of alcohol misuse. In: Chick J, Cantwell R, eds. Seminars in psychiatry: alcohol and drug misuse, London: Royal College of Psychiatrists, 1994: 94–125.

Davidson KM. Diagnosis of depression in alcohol dependence: changes in prevalence with drinking status. Br J Psychiatry 1995; 166: 199–204.

Davies DL. Normal drinking by recovered alcohol addicts. Q J Stud Alcohol 1962; 23: 194–204.

Dawson SA, Grant BF, Stinson FS et al. Recovery from DSM-IV alcohol dependence: United States, 2001–2002. Addict 2005; 100: 281–92.

Department of Health. Models of care for alcohol misusers. London: Stationery Office, 2006.

Department of Health, Safe, Sensible, Social. The next steps in the national alcohol strategy – a summary. London: Stationery Office, 2007.

Edwards G, Marshall EJ, Cook CCH. The Treatment of Drinking Problems: a Guide for the Helping Professions, 4th edn. Cambridge: Cambridge University Press, 2003.

Edwards G, Anderson P, Babor TF et al. Alcohol Policy and the Public Good. Oxford: Oxford University Press, 1994.

Edwards G, Davies DL. 'Normal drinking in recovered alcohol addicts': the genesis of a paper. Drug Alcohol Dep 1994; 35: 249–59.

Edwards G, Gross MM. Alcohol dependence: provisional description of a clinical syndrome. BMJ 1976; 1: 1058–61.

Heather N, Robertson I. Controlled drinking. London: Methuen, 1981.

Goldman D, Oroszi G, Ducci F. The genetics of addictions: uncovering the genes. Laboratory of Neurogenetics, National Institute on Alcohol Abuse and Alcoholism, USA, 2005.

Hemström O, Leifman H, Ramstedt M. The ECAS survey on drinking patterns and alcohol-related problems. In: Norström T, ed. Alcohol in Postwar Europe: Consumption, Drinking Patterns, Consequences and Policy Responses in 15 European Countries. Stockholm: Almqvist and Wiksell, 2002: 115–36.

Hodgson R, Alwyn T, John B, Thom B, Smith A. The FAST alcohol screening test. Alcohol Alcoholism 2002; 37: 61–6.

Humphreys K. Circles of recovery: self-help organisations for addictions. Cambridge: Cambridge University Press, 2004.

Jellinek EM. The Disease Concept of Alcoholism. New Brunswick: Hillhouse Press, 1960.

Johnson VE. I'll Quit Tomorrow. New York: Harper and Row, 1980.

Jones S, Casswell S, Zhang J-F. The economic costs of alcohol-related absenteeism and reduced productivity in the working population of New Zealand. Addict 1995; 90: 1453–62.

King DE, Mainous AG, Geesey ME. Adopting moderate alcohol consumption in middle age: subsequent cardiovascular events. Am J Med 2008; 121: 201–6.

Lingford-Hughes A, Welch S, Nutt D. Evidence based guidelines for the pharmacological management of substance misuse, addiction and co-morbidity: recommendations from the British Association for Psychopharmacology. J Psychopharmacol 2004; 18: 293–335.

Marlatt G, Gordon J. Relapse prevention. New York: Guilford Press, 1985.

McLellan AT, Skipper GS, Campbell M, DuPont RL. Five year outcomes in a cohort study of physicians treated for substance use disorders in the United States. BMJ 2008; 337: a2038.

Miller W, Rollnick S. Motivational interviewing: preparing people to change addictive behaviour. New York: Guilford Press, 1991.

Miller WR, Heather N, Hall W. Calculating standard drink units: international comparisons. Br J Addict 1991; 86: 43–7.

National Institute on Alcohol Abuse and Alcoholism. Drinking and driving. Alcohol Alert 31. Rookville, MD: 1996; 1–3.

Parker AJR, Marshall EJ, Ball DM. Diagnosis and management of alcohol use disorders. BMJ 2008; 336: 496–501.

Pendery ML, Maltzman IM, West LJ. Controlled drinking by alcoholics? New findings and a re-evaluation of a major affirmative study. Science 1982; 217: 169–75.

Project MATCH Research Group. Matching alcoholism treatment to client heterogeneity: Project MATCH post-treatment drinking outcomes. J Stud Alcohol 1997; 58: 7–29.

Raistrick D, Heather N, Godfrey C. Review of the Effectiveness of Treatment for Alcohol Problems. London: National Treatment Agency for Substance Misuse, 2006.

Room R, Babor TF, Rehm J. Alcohol and public health. Lancet 2005; 365: 519–30.

Savola O, Niemela O, Hillbom M. Blood alcohol is the best indicator of hazardous alcohol drinking in young adults and working-age patients with trauma. Alcohol Alcoholism 2004; 39: 340–5.

Shepherd J. Violent crime: the role of alcohol and new approaches to the prevention of injury. Alcohol Alcoholism 1994; 29: 5–10.

Sher KJ. Children of alcoholics. Chicago: University of Chicago Press, 1991.

Sobell MB, Sobell LC. Second-year treatment outcome of alcoholics treated by individualised behaviour therapy: results. Behav Res Ther 1976; 14: 195–215.

Thomson AD, Marshall EJ. The natural history and pathophysiology of Wernicke's encephalopathy and Korsakoff's psychosis. Alcohol Alcoholism 2006; 41: 151–8.

Timko C, DeBenedetti A, Billow R. Intensive referral to 12-step self-help groups and 6-month substance use disorder outcomes. Addict 2006; 101: 678–88.

Tober G, Raistrick D. Motivational dialogue preparing addiction professionals for motivational interviewing practice. London: Routledge, 2007.

UKATT Research Team. Effectiveness of treatment for alcohol problems: findings of the randomised UK alcohol treatment trial (UKATT). BMJ 2005; 311: 541–4.

Vaillant GE. The Natural History of Alcoholism. Cambridge: Harvard University Press, 1983.

World Health Organization. AUDIT – The Alcohol Use Disorders Identification test: Guidelines for Use in Primary Care, 2nd edn. Geneva: World Health Organization, 2001.

World Health Organization. Brief Intervention for Hazardous and Harmful Drinking: a Manual for Use in Primary Care. Geneva: World Health Organization, 2001.

World Health Organization. Global status report on alcohol. Geneva: World Health Organization, 2004.

World Health Organization. The ICD-10 Classification of Mental and Behavioral Disorders: Clinical Descriptions and Diagnostic Guidelines. Geneva: World Health Organization, 1992.

Men and their lifestyle

CHAPTER 35

Exercise and health

Roy J Shephard

Introduction

A growing number of men now view regular exercise as important to their health.[1] There are substantial difficulties in ascertaining population levels of physical activity from available questionnaire data,[2-4] and estimates vary substantially from one report to another (Fig. 35.1). Nevertheless, at least 25% of US men report engaging in no physical activity during the preceding month,[5,6] and only a minority of men in most developed countries take the amount of exercise that US and Canadian agencies currently recommend for the maintenance of good health.[7] After considering briefly some definitions of physical activity and prevention,[8] this chapter looks at a number of chronic health problems in which exercise has proven benefit.[9,10] It explores what is known about appropriate patterns of exercise for maximizing these benefits,[11,12] and it considers methods of avoiding hazards associated with an excessive volume and intensity of physical activity (particularly musculoskeletal injuries and heart attacks).

Definitions

Types of physical activity
The term 'exercise' implies that physical activity is being undertaken deliberately, either individually or as a group, with the objective of enhancing health or improving physical condition.[9] But for any given pattern and intensity of energy expenditure, most of the health benefits that are associated with a formal exercise program can also be realized through participation in other forms of physical activity, including sport and such instrumental activities as physically demanding occupations, do-it-yourself tasks, household chores, care of dependants, and walking or cycling to and from work. In recent years, the emphasis of those concerned with population health has shifted away from recommending participation in centrally located exercise classes and sport teams (where much of a person's potential exercise time may be lost in travel to the sports facility); instead, the focus has been on increasing the activity content of the normal day (the so-called active living approach).[13]

Types of prevention
The preventive value of an increase in physical activity may be realized at any one of four points in the natural history of disease, termed primary, secondary, tertiary, and quaternary prevention.[14]

Primary prevention
A primary preventative program acts before any abnormalities of health can be detected even by sophisticated laboratory testing. For example, a man who adopts an adequate amount of physical activity may be able to keep his serum lipids within the recommended normal range throughout his lifespan.

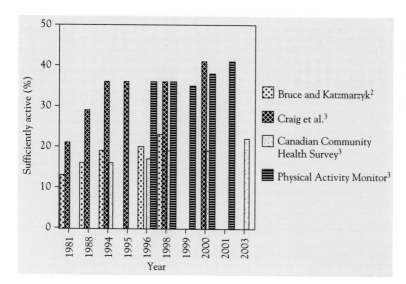

Figure 35.1. *Estimates of the percentage of the Canadian adult population taking adequate amounts of physical activity (i.e. 12.5 kJ/kg per day, or 3 MET hours per day).*

Secondary prevention

Secondary prevention is instituted when the scores for laboratory tests have become abnormal but there is still no clinical evidence of disease. For example, a program for the secondary prevention of ischemic heart disease would be strongly recommended if a man had an increase of serum cholesterol or other abnormalities of serum lipids.

Tertiary prevention

Many rehabilitation programs offer tertiary prevention. For example, 'post-coronary' exercise classes are designed to maximize the recovery of cardiac function and reduce the likelihood of a recurrence following a clinical episode of myocardial infarction.

Quaternary prevention

Quaternary exercise programs seek to minimize symptoms and enhance the quality of life when there is little possibility of restoring full health. For example, moderate physical activity may be recommended to reduce muscle wasting in a person who has established AIDS, cancer, or muscular dystrophy.

Conditions in which regular physical activity has proven benefit

There are some immediate benefits of exercise, such as the relief of anxiety or depression, the

Table 35.1. *Aspects of health that are enhanced by regular physical activity*

Mood state

Obesity

Diabetes mellitus

Lipid disorders

Hypertension

Cardiovascular disease

Congestive heart failure

Some forms of cancer

Osteoporosis

Smoking withdrawal

Chronic obstructive pulmonary disease

Immune function

Loss of functional capacity with aging

management of stress, and better patterns of sleeping, but most of the health dividends of regular physical activity are long-term in nature (Table 35.1).[9,10] Evidence of the long-term benefits comes mainly from epidemiological research, which shows linkages between good health and either a high level of physical activity or the adoption of an active lifestyle. Such data can never provide categorical evidence of causality. Nevertheless, application of Bradford Hill's criteria (Table 35.2) allows a strong case to be made for the existence of a cause-and-effect relationship between regular physical activity and the prevention of chronic medical conditions, particularly if the data have been statistically adjusted to allow for potential intervening factors such as socioeconomic class and smoking habits.[15]

Obesity

Obesity develops in most men during middle age, largely because of an imbalance between the amount of energy consumed as food and drink, and the quantity of energy expended over a typical day. Physicians sometimes look for a gross imbalance, but obesity more commonly occurs because a hard to perceive (0.5–1.0%) discrepancy between the intake and output of energy is repeated on a daily basis. For example, a man may have begun using his car instead of walking or cycling to the corner drug store.

The prevalence of obesity has increased in many populations over the past 30 years (Fig. 35.2),[16] to the point that there is talk of a worldwide epidemic of obesity.[17,18] The most probable explanation of

Table 35.2. *Bradford Hill's criteria, used in testing the inference of a causal association between regular physical activity and a given manifestation of health. From reference 15*

Strength of the association
The association must be a strong one; thus, the risk of a particular form of ill health must be low if a man is active, but high if he is inactive (this is commonly expressed as a risk ratio, setting the risk at 1.0 for the person who is totally inactive)

Consistency
The association must be reported consistently by investigators across differing types of population in many countries, preferably also using different methods to assess physical activity

Specificity
The association between physical activity and health must be specific, with a minimum of confounding factors that could also influence health. In fact, active people tend to be non-smokers, and are distinguished by a higher average level of education and socioeconomic status; however, multivariate techniques permit adjustment for these confounding influences

Temporality
There should be an appropriate time relationship between physical activity and health; thus, benefit is generally not observed unless physical activity is maintained

Biological gradient
There should be a gradation of health benefit, depending on the dose of physical activity received

Plausibility
There should be a plausible biological mechanism to explain how an increase in physical activity could enhance health

Coherence
The hypothesis that is advanced should provide a coherent explanation of available data

Experimental verification
It should be possible to obtain experimental verification of the proposed benefits if humans or animals participate in a randomized controlled trial of exercise; it is difficult to persuade humans to enter a lengthy trial of primary prevention, but experimental verification has been possible in some areas of secondary and tertiary prevention

Analogy
If a basis is proposed for the health benefits of exercise (e.g. a decrease in body fat), then similar benefit should be seen if body fat is reduced by some other mechanism

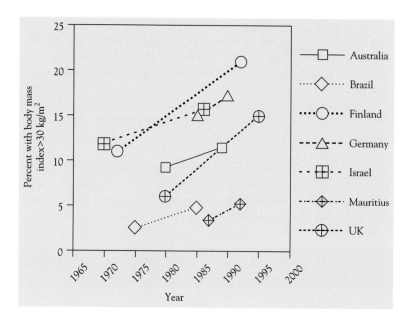

Figure 35.2. *Trends of obesity (body mass index >30 kg/m²) among adult men in various countries, based on data accumulated by Flegal.[16]*

this phenomenon is a progressive decrease in daily energy expenditure, as cars have been used for personal transportation, work has become ever more closely tied to computer screens, and power tools have minimized energy expenditures around the home. If this is indeed the case, then the problem should be corrected by an increase in daily energy expenditure[19] provided that this is maintained on a regular basis and is not matched by an increased intake of food.

Many physicians have monitored obesity in terms of the body mass index. This criterion is useful in assessing population trends. If a person is known to have gained mass over the past 10 years, this is also likely to be due to an accumulation of fat. On the other hand, if the body fat content is reduced by an increase in physical activity, there is not necessarily a corresponding decrease in body mass. As a man becomes more active, his weight is augmented by an increase of blood volume, muscle growth, and a strengthening of bones. Thus, to assess the extent of fat loss during an exercise program, it is necessary to make more direct measurements of body fat content, using such methods as skinfold calipers or underwater weighing.

In general, 1 g of body fat is metabolized to compensate for every 29 kJ (7 kcal) of negative energy balance. However, if a drastic energy deficit is imposed, this may cause a 10–15% reduction in resting metabolism (around 500 kJ/day), adding to the difficulty in reducing body fat content. The problem of a decrease in resting metabolism is greatest if obesity is addressed by dieting, and there is some evidence that regular bouts of exercise help to limit the decrease in average resting energy expenditure, because a stimulation of metabolism persists long after the exercise bout has ceased.[20] Nevertheless, the volume of activity needed either to prevent or to reverse obesity seems larger than currently recommended for health – possibly as much as 90 minutes per day.[21]

Diabetes mellitus

Exercise is recommended for people with type 1 diabetes mellitus, mainly to realize general health benefits and to reduce the risk of late complications such as microvascular and atherosclerotic disease. The need for insulin is generally decreased by exercise, and if a patient has recently begun a regular exercise program it is wise to re-evaluate his or her insulin dosage. It is also important for the affected person to carry a source of readily assimilated carbohydrate, in case hypoglycemia develops during or immediately following exercise.

Prospective studies suggest that the risk of developing maturity-onset (type 2) diabetes mellitus is inversely related to the person's level of habitual physical activity.[22,23] Moreover, regular exercise has a positive impact upon the control of blood glucose in those people in whom the disease is already established.[22] A regular exercise program can reduce the patient's need for insulin, and diminish the likelihood of complications. The prescribed exercise must consider the patient's increased risk of a cardiovascular incident; if there is evidence of diabetic neuritis, particular care must be taken to avoid skin injuries or infections, and if there is a diabetic retinitis, it is important to avoid activities that could precipitate intra-ocular hemorrhage and retinal detachment.[24]

Lipid disorders

Although dietitians make much of the virtues of adopting a low-cholesterol diet, a large fraction of the body's cholesterol is synthesized in the liver; thus, physical inactivity and a positive energy balance (over-eating) play important roles in the genesis of hypercholesterolemia. Conversely, an increase in daily energy expenditure and the development of a negative energy balance will augment serum high-density lipoprotein cholesterol levels, with less consistent reductions in total cholesterol, low-density lipoprotein cholesterol and triglyceride concentrations.[25] There is insufficient information to establish a clear dose–response curve, but some evidence suggests that a substantial weekly volume of activity (for example, walking or jogging 15 km per week) is needed to enhance the body's lipid profile.

Hypertension

Regular physical activity induces a small but therapeutically useful reduction in both systolic and diastolic pressures.[26,27] In the normotensive person, the change may be no more than 3–4/2 mmHg, but in those with established hypertension, a larger average reduction of 7/6 mmHg is observed. Such responses are perhaps less than could be achieved in the rare person who is totally compliant with powerful hypotensive drugs but, on the other hand, they are clinically significant, and benefit is realized without the various complications of pharmaco-

therapeutic options such as physical and mental fatigue – indeed, unlike drug treatment, regular exercise is likely to yield important dividends in other, unrelated areas of health.

Cardiovascular disease

The value of vigorous exercise in the prevention and treatment of ischemic heart disease is now widely accepted;[28–30] there is also growing evidence for the prevention of at least certain types of stroke, but this is less conclusive.[30,31] Epidemiological studies of both occupational activity and leisure pursuits have documented the effectiveness of physical activity in the primary and secondary prevention of myocardial infarction and sudden death; the risk of a clinical incident is at least two or three times greater in those with a sedentary lifestyle than in those who engage regularly in recommended levels of physical activity.[32]

Following a cardiac incident, the successful adoption of an exercise program is more likely in men than in women. Meta-analyses suggest that there is a small (20–30%) reduction in the risk of a fatal recurrence among those who adhere to a prescribed exercise regimen.[33–35] An exercise program also strengthens residual myocardial function, allowing an earlier return to work and an enhancement of the patient's quality of life. A further advantage of attending formal exercise sessions regularly is that the patient then receives regular advice on other aspects of lifestyle such as smoking withdrawal, diet, weight control, and a resumption of marital relations.

Congestive heart failure

There is growing recognition that a progressive exercise regimen has value in the tertiary treatment of patients with stable congestive heart failure. Much of the limitation of function seen in those with congestive heart failure reflects difficulty in perfusing weakened skeletal muscles, and an exercise prescription that combines aerobic activity with a muscle-strengthening regimen can thus do much to reduce symptoms and enhance the patient's quality of life.[36,37]

Cancer

Epidemiological research has shown significant associations between regular occupational or leisure activity and a reduced risk of both all-cause and certain specific types of cancer,[38–40] The main benefit is a reduced likelihood of tumors in the descending colon, although the mechanism of protection remains uncertain.[41] Some studies have also suggested a reduced risk of prostate cancers.[38]

In those with established tumors, regular exercise helps to elevate mood and reduce muscle wasting. If leukocyte counts have been depressed by irradiation, it is important to ensure that this trend is not exacerbated by over-intensive exercise.[42] If prostate cancer has been treated by antigonadotrophic hormones, this weakens both muscles and bones, and here again exercise can play a restorative role.

Osteoporosis

Osteoporosis is often considered a condition of post-menopausal women, but it can also affect older men, particularly if they have a prostatic carcinoma and are being treated by androgen inhibitors. Regular exercise stimulates bone formation through a piezo-electric effect. Benefit is seen only if the activity involves weight-bearing (e.g. running) or takes the form of resisted muscle contractions.[43,44] Recent animal studies suggest that mechanical impulses are most effective in stimulating osteogenesis if they are separated by intervals as long as 30 seconds, and there may be a finite limit to the number of beneficial impulses per exercise session.[45]

Cigarette withdrawal

The proportion of cigarette smokers is substantially smaller among men who are physically active, particularly those involved in endurance sports. Such people tend to be a sub-sample of the population who have adopted a healthy overall lifestyle, although there is also some evidence that regular endurance activity increases the likelihood of successful cigarette withdrawal.[46]

Chronic obstructive pulmonary disease

A number of centers now offer tertiary rehabilitation programs for people who have developed chronic obstructive pulmonary disease. Severe breathlessness makes class participation less easy than it is following a heart attack. Even successful exercisers are unlikely to restore damaged pulmonary tissue, and the scores on pulmonary function tests usually remain unchanged as a program progresses. Nevertheless, many participants note an increase in subjective wellbeing.[47] This could partly reflect an enhanced mood state, and a further contributing factor is a strengthening of skeletal muscles weakened by prolonged physical inactivity.[48]

Immune function

Occasional reports suggest that both single bouts of very prolonged activity (such as an ultramarathon run) and periods of peak training for Olympic competition have a negative effect on certain aspects of immune function (for instance, the number or activity of circulating natural killer cells decreases, and the mucosal concentration of immunoglobulins diminishes). Moreover, these changes are associated with a short-term increase in susceptibility to infections of the respiratory tract.[49] On the other hand, regular moderate training seems to have a positive effect on immune function, and it may also help to counter the progressive loss of immune function that is associated with aging.[50]

Loss of functional capacity with aging

Perhaps the strongest argument for engaging in a regular program of physical activity is the potential to limit the deterioration of function that is a usual concomitant of aging. Both maximal aerobic power and peak muscle force typically decrease by some 10% with each decade of adult life.[51] Such changes can restrict the employment potential of men in physically demanding jobs. Perhaps even more importantly, if functional deterioration continues unchecked, at some age between 80 and 85 years the person becomes unable to undertake even the activities of normal daily living without help. Independence is then lost, and there is a corresponding deterioration in the quality of life.[52,53]

The rate of loss of cardiac and muscular function is relatively similar for an active and an inactive person, but at any given age training augments the functional capacity of the inactive person by as much as 20%. Such training in effect turns back the biological clock by as much as 20 years, with a corresponding enhancement of the functional capacity and quality of life.[51]

Appropriate patterns of exercise prescription

Some patients are impressed and motivated if they are given a detailed 'exercise prescription'.[54] Unfortunately, attempts to offer them precise advice are hampered by uncertainties regarding the optimal setting, characteristics, and dose (volume, intensity, frequency, and duration) of physical activity needed for good health.[12] Moreover, failure to comply with a detailed prescription can become a source of guilt or anxiety. For many people, the best advice may be to begin by taking a little more exercise than they are currently attempting, and (provided that there are no untoward symptoms) to increase this amount on a weekly basis until the currently recommended minimal level is reached or personal goals are met.

Setting

Debate continues on the relative merits of group versus home exercise programs. Depending on personality and levels of occupational stress, some men prefer the bonhomie of a sports team or group classes and the associated social interactions, but others prefer to take their exercise individually, in the quiet of the country or their garden.

In high-risk people, potential advantages of the group setting are regular consultation with well-trained professionals and access to any equipment that might be needed for cardiac resuscitation. Against such benefits must be set the need to exercise at a fixed time of day, the direct costs of facilities and equipment, and the substantial but less direct 'opportunity cost' involved in driving to an exercise class in a large city. Perhaps the optimal solution, particularly for high-risk patients, is to begin a program with one supervised exercise session per week, supplementing this by a home prescription to be performed four or five times per week; the frequency of supervised sessions can be reduced subsequently, as the exerciser becomes familiar with an appropriate pattern of physical activity and learns any symptoms warning of a

need to moderate the volume or intensity of activity sessions.

Characteristics

Traditionally, exercise programs have focused on aerobic activities, with a view to enhancing cardiovascular function. However, there is now growing appreciation of the need to provide an adequate training stimulus to each of the major muscle groups at least twice per week, to take all of the joints of the body through their full range of motion on a regular basis, and to enhance bone formation by suitable weight-bearing or resisted exercise.[54]

Volume, intensity, frequency, and duration

Many professional bodies and international conferences have attempted to reach a consensus on the minimum volume and intensity of exercise needed to maintain health.[12] Unfortunately, a succession of differing recommendations[56,57] has reduced the credibility of the exercise scientists and left patients uncertain as to what is appropriate.

Plainly, the necessary duration and intensity of exercise are inversely related; the duration of effort can be reduced if the intensity is higher. Furthermore, a given absolute intensity of activity provides a stronger relative training stimulus as a person becomes older.[8] Many middle-aged men are interested only in the minimal amount of activity that will maintain their health, but highly competitive 'type A' people may have a dangerous desire to out-perform their friends, reasoning that if a little activity is good, more will be even better for them. From the viewpoint of health, there seems little to be gained from an intensity of effort that surpasses the person's normal aerobic training zone (60–70% of maximal oxygen intake). Most people perceive this intensity of exercise as 'moderately hard'; it is at a level where breathing is perceptible, but the exerciser can still maintain a normal conversation.

In terms of aerobic activity, a common current recommendation is to take at least 30 minutes of moderate intensity activity (>50% of maximal oxygen intake) on most days of the week;[55,56] however, if the person's initial fitness does not permit a

451

30-minute exercise session, there is some suggestion that the 30 minutes of activity can be accumulated as several 10–15-minute bouts.[58] The World Health Organization has warned that this is less than the minimum volume needed to control body mass,[21] and Canadian authorities have therefore argued that if the chosen activity is of only moderate intensity, then its duration should be at least 60 minutes per day (Table 35.3).[13,59]

In part because there are many health objectives, there is little consensus on an optimal regimen.[11,59] Possibly, some of the health benefits of exercise such as the control of obesity are obtained if exercisers expend a critical total volume of energy, whereas other needs, such as cardiovascular conditioning, are only obtained if the intensity of effort reaches the aerobic training zone.

Perhaps the answer is to focus on the problem that is most likely to reduce a person's quality-adjusted life expectancy; this factor is probably a loss of independence in old age, and a regimen designed to enhance cardiovascular fitness seems best suited to preventing such an outcome.[60] In the absence of better information, another alternative is to adopt an anthropological approach, recommending the pattern of physical activity to which humans have adapted over countless millennia – prolonged bouts of moderate intensity exercise;[61] incidentally, this should serve the goal of maintaining cardio-respiratory function.

Avoiding the hazards of exercise

The potential hazards faced by those who engage in excessive exercise include catastrophic cardiovascular incidents, musculoskeletal injury, and immunosuppression. However, the average man is likely to take too little rather than too much exercise, so that care should be taken to avoid

---

Table 35.3. *Pattern of physical activity recommended to maintain and enhance health*

Aerobic activity
Large muscle activity such as walking, jogging, cycling or cross-country skiing at an intensity between 50 and 85% of the person's maximal oxygen intake (60–90% of the age-predicted maximal heart rate), performed for 20–60 minutes per session on most days of the week; the activity should be sufficient to produce some sweating and shortness of breath

Unfit people should begin at the lower end of the intensity range, and should attempt to continue exercising for 60 minutes, using split sessions if necessary

Fit people can exercise at the higher end of the intensity range, with a corresponding reduction in exercise duration

Muscular activity
Strength training should be sufficient to maintain the person's fat-free body mass. At least twice per week, exercisers should make between eight and 12 repetitions of eight to 12 different exercises, each at 60% of one-repetition maximal force, and involving the main muscle groups of the body

Flexibility
Each of the major joints in the body should be taken through their full range of motion on a regular basis; flexibility can be enhanced by making gentle stretching movements at the end of the range of motion

Bone strength
The strength of the major bones should be enhanced by ensuring a combination of adequate calcium intake and weight-bearing or resisted activity

Body fat
The body fat content should be brought below 20% through a combination of an increased daily energy expenditure and a modest reduction of food intake

Table 35.4. *The Canadian Physical Activity Readiness Questionnaire (PAR-Q), a self-administered instrument for adults aged 15–69 years*

Physical Activity Readiness
Questionnaire - PAR-Q
(revised 2002)

PAR-Q & YOU

(A Questionnaire for People Aged 15 to 69)

Regular physical activity is fun and healthy, and increasingly more people are starting to become more active every day. Being more active is very safe for most people. However, some people should check with their doctor before they start becoming much more physically active.

If you are planning to become much more physically active than you are now, start by answering the seven questions in the box below. If you are between the ages of 15 and 69, the PAR-Q will tell you if you should check with your doctor before you start. If you are over 69 years of age, and you are not used to being very active, check with your doctor.

Common sense is your best guide when you answer these questions. Please read the questions carefully and answer each one honestly: check YES or NO.

YES	NO		
☐	☐	1.	Has your doctor ever said that you have a heart condition <u>and</u> that you should only do physical activity recommended by a doctor?
☐	☐	2.	Do you feel pain in your chest when you do physical activity?
☐	☐	3.	In the past month, have you had chest pain when you were not doing physical activity?
☐	☐	4.	Do you lose your balance because of dizziness or do you ever lose consciousness?
☐	☐	5.	Do you have a bone or joint problem (for example, back, knee or hip) that could be made worse by a change in your physical activity?
☐	☐	6.	Is your doctor currently prescribing drugs (for example, water pills) for your blood pressure or heart condition?
☐	☐	7.	Do you know of <u>any other reason</u> why you should not do physical activity?

If

you

answered

YES to one or more questions

Talk with your doctor by phone or in person BEFORE you start becoming much more physically active or BEFORE you have a fitness appraisal. Tell your doctor about the PAR-Q and which questions you answered YES.

• You may be able to do any activity you want — as long as you start slowly and build up gradually. Or, you may need to restrict your activities to those which are safe for you. Talk with your doctor about the kinds of activities you wish to participate in and follow his/her advice.

• Find out which community programs are safe and helpful for you.

NO to all questions

If you answered NO honestly to all PAR-Q questions, you can be reasonably sure that you can:
• start becoming much more physically active – begin slowly and build up gradually. This is the safest and easiest way to go.
• take part in a fitness appraisal – this is an excellent way to determine your basic fitness so that you can plan the best way for you to live actively. It is also highly recommended that you have your blood pressure evaluated. If your reading is over 144/94, talk with your doctor before you start becoming much more physically active.

→ **DELAY BECOMING MUCH MORE ACTIVE:**
• if you are not feeling well because of a temporary illness such as a cold or a fever – wait until you feel better; or
• if you are or may be pregnant – talk to your doctor before you start becoming more active.

PLEASE NOTE: If your health changes so that you then answer YES to any of the above questions, tell your fitness or health professional. Ask whether you should change your physical activity plan.

Informed Use of the PAR-Q: The Canadian Society for Exercise Physiology, Health Canada, and their agents assume no liability for persons who undertake physical activity, and if in doubt after completing this questionnaire, consult your doctor prior to physical activity.

> **No changes permitted. You are encouraged to photocopy the PAR-Q but only if you use the entire form.**

NOTE: If the PAR-Q is being given to a person before he or she participates in a physical activity program or a fitness appraisal, this section may be used for legal or administrative purposes.

"I have read, understood and completed this questionnaire. Any questions I had were answered to my full satisfaction."

NAME _____

SIGNATURE _____   DATE_____

SIGNATURE OF PARENT _____   WITNESS _____
or GUARDIAN (for participants under the age of majority)

> **Note:** This physical activity clearance is valid for a maximum of 12 months from the date it is completed and becomes invalid if your condition changes so that you would answer YES to any of the seven questions.

CSEP
SCPE © Canadian Society for Exercise Physiology   Supported by: [■+■] Health Santé
Canada Canada   continued on other side...

(Continued)

Table 35.4. (*Continued*)

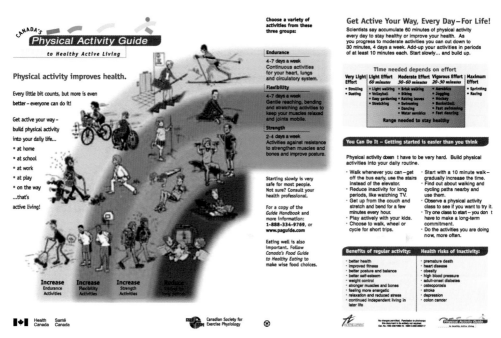

PAR-Q & YOU

...continued from other side

Physical Activity Readiness
Questionnaire - PAR-Q
(revised 2002)

Source: Canada's Physical Activity Guide to Healthy Active Living, Health Canada, 1998 http://www.hc-sc.gc.ca/hppb/paguide/pdf/guideEng.pdf
© Reproduced with permission from the Minister of Public Works and Government Services Canada, 2002.

FITNESS AND HEALTH PROFESSIONALS MAY BE INTERESTED IN THE INFORMATION BELOW:

The following companion forms are available for doctors' use by contacting the Canadian Society for Exercise Physiology (address below):

The **Physical Activity Readiness Medical Examination (PARmed-X)** – to be used by doctors with people who answer YES to one or more questions on the PAR-Q.

The **Physical Activity Readiness Medical Examination for Pregnancy (PARmed-X for Pregnancy)** – to be used by doctors with pregnant patients who wish to become more active.

References:
Arraix, G.A., Wigle, D.T., Mao, Y. (1992). Risk Assessment of Physical Activity and Physical Fitness in the Canada Health Survey
    Follow-Up Study. **J. Clin. Epidemiol.** 45:4 419-428.
Mottola, M., Wolfe, L.A. (1994). Active Living and Pregnancy, In: A. Quinney, L. Gauvin, T. Wall (eds.), **Toward Active Living: Proceedings of the International
    Conference on Physical Activity, Fitness and Health**. Champaign, IL: Human Kinetics.
PAR-Q Validation Report, British Columbia Ministry of Health, 1978.
Thomas, S., Reading, J., Shephard, R.J. (1992). Revision of the Physical Activity Readiness Questionnaire (PAR-Q). **Can. J. Spt. Sci.** 17:4 338-345.

For more information, please contact the:

Canadian Society for Exercise Physiology
202-185 Somerset Street West
Ottawa, ON K2P 0J2
Tel. 1-877-651-3755 • FAX (613) 234-3565

Online: www.csep.ca

The original PAR-Q was developed by the British Columbia Ministry of Health. It has been revised by an Expert Advisory Committee of the Canadian Society for Exercise Physiology chaired by Dr. N. Gledhill (2002).

Disponible en français sous le titre «Questionnaire sur l'aptitude à l'activité physique - Q-AAP (revisé 2002)».

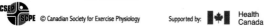 © Canadian Society for Exercise Physiology

Supported by: Health Canada Santé Canada

Table 35.5. *The Canadian Physical Activity Readiness Medical Examination (PARmed-X)*

Physical Activity Readiness
Medical Examination
(revised 2002)

PARmed-X
PHYSICAL ACTIVITY READINESS
MEDICAL EXAMINATION

The PARmed-X is a physical activity-specific checklist to be used by a physician with patients who have had positive responses to the Physical Activity Readiness Questionnaire (PAR-Q). In addition, the Conveyance/Referral Form in the PARmed-X can be used to convey clearance for physical activity participation, or to make a referral to a medically-supervised exercise program.

Regular physical activity is fun and healthy, and increasingly more people are starting to become more active every day. Being more active is very safe for most people. The PAR-Q by itself provides adequate screening for the majority of people. However, some individuals may require a medical evaluation and specific advice (exercise prescription) due to one or more positive responses to the PAR-Q.

Following the participant's evaluation by a physician, a physical activity plan should be devised in consultation with a physical activity professional (CSEP-Professional Fitness & Lifestyle Consultant or CSEP-Exercise Therapist™). To assist in this, the following instructions are provided:

PAGE 1: • Sections A, B, C, and D should be completed by the participant BEFORE the examination by the physician. The bottom section is to be completed by the examining physician.

PAGES 2 & 3: • A checklist of medical conditions requiring special consideration and management.

PAGE 4: • Physical Activity & Lifestyle Advice for people who do not require specific instructions or prescribed exercise.

• Physical Activity Readiness Conveyance/Referral Form - an optional tear-off tab for the physician to convey clearance for physical activity participation, or to make a referral to a medically-supervised exercise program.

This section to be completed by the participant

A PERSONAL INFORMATION:

NAME _____

ADDRESS _____

_____

_____

TELEPHONE _____

BIRTHDATE _____ GENDER _____

MEDICAL No. _____

B PAR-Q: Please indicate the PAR-Q questions to which you answered YES

- ❏ Q 1 Heart condition
- ❏ Q 2 Chest pain during activity
- ❏ Q 3 Chest pain at rest
- ❏ Q 4 Loss of balance, dizziness
- ❏ Q 5 Bone or joint problem
- ❏ Q 6 Blood pressure or heart drugs
- ❏ Q 7 Other reason:

C RISK FACTORS FOR CARDIOVASCULAR DISEASE:
Check all that apply

- ❏ Less than 30 minutes of moderate physical activity most days of the week.
- ❏ Currently smoker (tobacco smoking 1 or more times per week).
- ❏ High blood pressure reported by physician after repeated measurements.
- ❏ High cholesterol level reported by physician.
- ❏ Excessive accumulation of fat around waist.
- ❏ Family history of heart disease.

Please note: Many of these risk factors are modifiable. Please refer to page 4 and discuss with your physician.

D PHYSICAL ACTIVITY INTENTIONS:

What physical activity do you intend to do?

_____

_____

_____

_____

This section to be completed by the examining physician

Physical Exam:

Ht	Wt	BP i)	/
		BP ii)	/

Conditions limiting physical activity:

- ❏ Cardiovascular
- ❏ Musculoskeletal
- ❏ Respiratory
- ❏ Abdominal
- ❏ Other

Tests required:

- ❏ ECG
- ❏ Blood
- ❏ Exercise Test
- ❏ Urinalysis
- ❏ X-Ray
- ❏ Other

Physical Activity Readiness Conveyance/Referral:

Based upon a current review of health status, I recommend:

Further Information:
- ❏ Attached
- ❏ To be forwarded
- ❏ Available on request

- ❏ No physical activity
- ❏ Only a medically-supervised exercise program until further medical clearance
- ❏ Progressive physical activity:
  - ❏ with avoidance of: _____
  - ❏ with inclusion of: _____
  - ❏ under the supervision of a CSEP-Professional Fitness & Lifestyle Consultant or CSEP-Exercise Therapist™
- ❏ Unrestricted physical activity–start slowly and build up gradually

CSEP / SCPE © Canadian Society for Exercise Physiology

Supported by: Health Canada Santé Canada

1

(Continued)

Table 35.5. *(Continued)*

PARmed-X   PHYSICAL ACTIVITY READINESS MEDICAL EXAMINATION

Following is a checklist of medical conditions for which a degree of precaution and/or special advice should be considered for those who answered "YES" to one or more questions on the PAR-Q, and people over the age of 69. Conditions are grouped by system. Three categories of precautions are provided. Comments under Advice are general, since details and alternatives require clinical judgement in each individual instance.

	Absolute Contraindications	Relative Contraindications	Special Prescriptive Conditions	
	Permanent restriction or temporary restriction until condition is treated, stable, and/or past acute phase.	Highly variable. Value of exercise testing and/or program may exceed risk. Activity may be restricted. Desirable to maximize control of condition. Direct or indirect medical supervision of exercise program may be desirable.	Individualized prescriptive advice generally appropriate: • limitations imposed; and/or • special exercises prescribed. May require medical monitoring and/or initial supervision in exercise program.	**ADVICE**
Cardiovascular	❑ aortic aneurysm (dissecting) ❑ aortic stenosis (severe) ❑ congestive heart failure ❑ crescendo angina ❑ myocardial infarction (acute) ❑ myocarditis (active or recent) ❑ pulmonary or systemic embolism—acute ❑ thrombophlebitis ❑ ventricular tachycardia and other dangerous dysrhythmias (e.g., multi-focal ventricular activity)	❑ aortic stenosis (moderate) ❑ subaortic stenosis (severe) ❑ marked cardiac enlargement ❑ supraventricular dysrhythmias (uncontrolled or high rate) ❑ ventricular ectopic activity (repetitive or frequent) ❑ ventricular aneurysm ❑ hypertension—untreated or uncontrolled severe (systemic or pulmonary) ❑ hypertrophic cardiomyopathy ❑ compensated congestive heart failure	❑ aortic (or pulmonary) stenosis—mild angina pectoris and other manifestations of coronary insufficiency (e.g., post-acute infarct) ❑ cyanotic heart disease ❑ shunts (intermittent or fixed) ❑ conduction disturbances • complete AV block • left BBB • Wolff-Parkinson-White syndrome ❑ dysrhythmias—controlled ❑ fixed rate pacemakers	• clinical exercise test may be warranted in selected cases, for specific determination of functional capacity and limitations and precautions (if any). • slow progression of exercise to levels based on test performance and individual tolerance. • consider individual need for initial conditioning program under medical supervision (indirect or direct).
			❑ intermittent claudication	progressive exercise to tolerance
			❑ hypertension: systolic 160-180; diastolic 105+	progressive exercise; care with medications (serum electrolytes; post-exercise syncope; etc.)
Infections	❑ acute infectious disease (regardless of etiology)	❑ subacute/chronic/recurrent infectious diseases (e.g., malaria, others)	❑ chronic infections ❑ HIV	variable as to condition
Metabolic		❑ uncontrolled metabolic disorders (diabetes mellitus, thyrotoxicosis, myxedema)	❑ renal, hepatic & other metabolic insufficiency	variable as to status
			❑ obesity ❑ single kidney	dietary moderation, and initial light exercises with slow progression (walking, swimming, cycling)
Pregnancy		❑ complicated pregnancy (e.g., toxemia, hemorrhage, incompetent cervix, etc.)	❑ advanced pregnancy (late 3rd trimester)	refer to the "PARmed-X for PREGNANCY"

References:

Arraix, G.A., Wigle, D.T., Mao, Y. (1992). Risk Assessment of Physical Activity and Physical Fitness in the Canada Health Survey Follow-Up Study. **J. Clin. Epidemiol.** 45:4 419-428.

Mottola, M., Wolfe, L.A. (1994). Active Living and Pregnancy, In: A. Quinney, L. Gauvin, T. Wall (eds.), **Toward Active Living: Proceedings of the International Conference on Physical Activity, Fitness and Health.** Champaign, IL: Human Kinetics.

PAR-Q Validation Report, British Columbia Ministry of Health, 1978.

Thomas, S., Reading, J., Shephard, R.J. (1992). Revision of the Physical Activity Readiness Questionnaire (PAR-Q). **Can. J. Spt. Sci.** 17: 4 338-345.

The PAR-Q and PARmed-X were developed by the British Columbia Ministry of Health. They have been revised by an Expert Advisory Committee of the Canadian Society for Exercise Physiology chaired by Dr. N. Gledhill (2002).

No changes permitted. You are encouraged to photocopy the PARmed-X, but only if you use the entire form.

Disponible en français sous le titre «Évaluation médicale de l'aptitude à l'activité physique (X-AAP)»

Continued on page 3...

2

(Continued)

Table 35.5. (*Continued*)

Physical Activity Readiness
Medical Examination
(revised 2002)

	Special Prescriptive Conditions	**ADVICE**
Lung	❑ chronic pulmonary disorders	special relaxation and breathing exercises
	❑ obstructive lung disease	breath control during endurance exercises to tolerance; avoid polluted air
	❑ asthma	
	❑ exercise-induced bronchospasm	avoid hyperventilation during exercise; avoid extremely cold conditions; warm up adequately; utilize appropriate medication.
Musculoskeletal	❑ low back conditions (pathological, functional)	avoid or minimize exercise that precipitates or exasperates e.g., forced extreme flexion, extension, and violent twisting; correct posture, proper back exercises
	❑ arthritis—acute (infective, rheumatoid; gout)	treatment, plus judicious blend of rest, splinting and gentle movement
	❑ arthritis—subacute	progressive increase of active exercise therapy
	❑ arthritis—chronic (osteoarthritis and above conditions)	maintenance of mobility and strength; non-weightbearing exercises to minimize joint trauma (e.g., cycling, aquatic activity, etc.)
	❑ orthopaedic	highly variable and individualized
	❑ hernia	minimize straining and isometrics; stregthen abdominal muscles
	❑ osteoporosis or low bone density	avoid exercise with high risk for fracture such as push-ups, curl-ups, vertical jump and trunk forward flexion; engage in low-impact weight-bearing activities and resistance training
CNS	❑ convulsive disorder not completely controlled by medication	minimize or avoid exercise in hazardous environments and/or exercising alone (e.g., swimming, mountainclimbing, etc.)
	❑ recent concussion	thorough examination if history of two concussions; review for discontinuation of contact sport if three concussions, depending on duration of unconsciousness, retrograde amnesia, persistent headaches, and other objective evidence of cerebral damage
Blood	❑ anemia—severe (< 10 Gm/dl) ❑ electrolyte disturbances	control preferred; exercise as tolerated
Medications	❑ antianginal ❑ antiarrhythmic ❑ antihypertensive ❑ anticonvulsant ❑ beta-blockers ❑ digitalis preparations ❑ diuretics ❑ ganglionic blockers ❑ others	NOTE: consider underlying condition. Potential for: exertional syncope, electrolyte imbalance, bradycardia, dysrhythmias, impaired coordination and reaction time, heat intolerance. May alter resting and exercise ECG's and exercise test performance.
Other	❑ post-exercise syncope	moderate program
	❑ heat intolerance	prolong cool-down with light activities; avoid exercise in extreme heat
	❑ temporary minor illness	postpone until recovered
	❑ cancer	if potential metastases, test by cycle ergometry, consider non-weight bearing exercises; exercise at lower end of prescriptive range (40-65% of heart rate reserve), depending on condition and recent treatment (radiation, chemotherapy); monitor hemoglobin and lymphocyte counts; add dynamic lifting exercise to strengthen muscles, using machines rather than weights.

*Refer to special publications for elaboration as required

The following companion forms are available online: http://www.csep.ca/forms.asp

The **Physical Activity Readiness Questionnaire (PAR-Q)** - a questionnaire for people aged 15-69 to complete before becoming much more physically active.

The **Physical Activity Readiness Medical Examination for Pregnancy (PARmed-X for PREGNANCY)** - to be used by physicians with pregnant patients who wish to become more physically active.

For more information, please contact the:

Canadian Society for Exercise Physiology
202 - 185 Somerset St. West
Ottawa, ON K2P 0J2
Tel. 1-877-651-3755 • FAX (613) 234-3565 • Online: www.csep.ca

Note to physical activity professionals...
It is a prudent practice to retain the completed Physical Activity Readiness Conveyance/Referral Form in the participant's file.

 © Canadian Society for Exercise Physiology

Supported by: Health
Canada   Santé
Canada

Continued on page 4...

3

(*Continued*)

Table 35.5. (*Continued*)

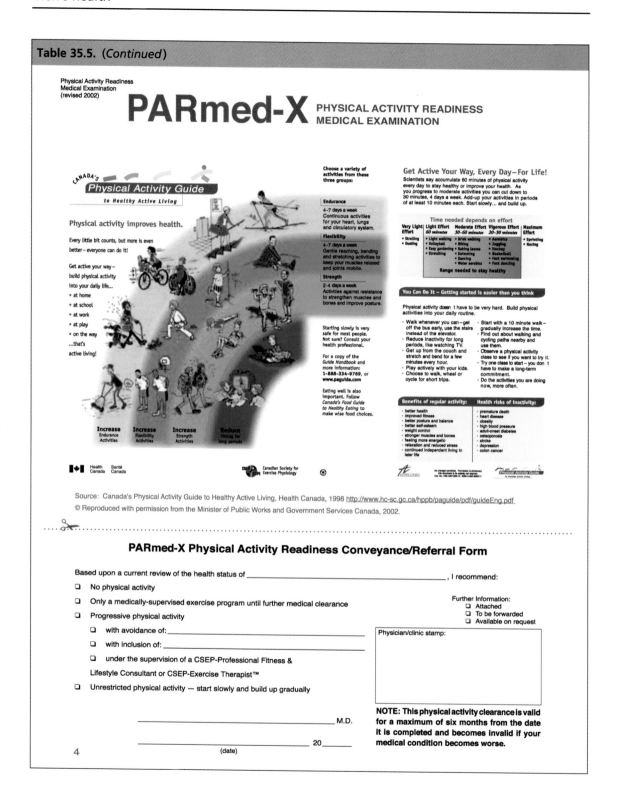

Source: Canada's Physical Activity Guide to Healthy Active Living, Health Canada, 1998 http://www.hc-sc.gc.ca/hppb/paguide/pdf/guideEng.pdf
© Reproduced with permission from the Minister of Public Works and Government Services Canada, 2002.

PARmed-X Physical Activity Readiness Conveyance/Referral Form

Based upon a current review of the health status of _____ , I recommend:

❑ No physical activity

❑ Only a medically-supervised exercise program until further medical clearance

❑ Progressive physical activity

    ❑ with avoidance of: _____

    ❑ with inclusion of: _____

    ❑ under the supervision of a CSEP-Professional Fitness &

Lifestyle Consultant or CSEP-Exercise Therapist™

❑ Unrestricted physical activity — start slowly and build up gradually

Further Information:
❑ Attached
❑ To be forwarded
❑ Available on request

Physician/clinic stamp:

_____ M.D.

_____ 20_____
(date)

NOTE: This physical activity clearance is valid for a maximum of six months from the date it is completed and becomes invalid if your medical condition becomes worse.

4

the deterrent effect of excessive warnings and precautions.

Cardiovascular incidents

The risk of a cardiovascular incident is increased 5–50-fold during exercise, depending on its intensity.[62,63] In young adults, danger may come from rupture of an aneurysm, a congenital abnormality of the coronary vasculature, or a familial cardiomyopathy, but in older men the problem usually reflects latent or known ischemic heart disease.

The hazard associated with the exercise bout is more than offset by a reduced risk of cardiovascular incidents during subsequent rest; in consequence, the overall risk is two to three times greater for an inactive than for an active person.[63,64] The danger of exercise is greatest if the intensity of exercise is high, and if there is associated emotional stress. Risks also seem to be greater in the morning than later during the day. Simple precautions include asking potential exercisers about cardiac risk factors and completing a simple self-administered clearance questionnaire such as the Canadian Physical Activity Readiness Questionnaire (PAR-Q) (Table 35.4);[13,54] if the answers to any of the questions on this simple, self-administered instrument are positive, a physician should be consulted before any drastic increase in physical activity. The physician who is undertaking an exercise clearance may find it helpful to complete a more detailed aide-memoire, such as the Canadian Physical Activity Readiness Medical Examination (PARmed-X) (Table 35.5). A thorough clinical history should identify many of the patients with familial cardiomyopathy, and other congenital abnormalities may be revealed by a competent physical examination. There are few other guidelines that can reduce the risk of cardiovascular events. Recommendations to undertake echocardiography and electrocardiography on all potential exercisers seem misplaced; the resulting observations would be difficult to interpret, with many false-positive results and much unnecessary iatrogenic disease.[65,66]

Musculo-skeletal injuries

Musculoskeletal injuries are much more likely than a cardiovascular incident.[67] Individual types of activity show a hierarchy of risk – for example,

alpine skiing and snow-boarding are much more dangerous than fast walking. Particularly in older men if eyesight, hearing and balance are impaired and healing is slow, low-risk activities should be recommended. Some men find motivation from involvement in competitive sports. Such people are particularly vulnerable to injury if excessive competition is provided by younger or stronger opponents, and if the playing area and safety equipment are poorly maintained.

Debate continues on the value of a formal warm-up in the prevention of muscle and tendon injuries, although many recent papers find no advantage from this practice.[68,69] On the other hand, there is no evidence that a gentle start to an exercise program is harmful, and it seems logical to anticipate that if the viscosity of the tissues is reduced by a gradual warming, then the risk of muscle and tendon tears will be reduced.

Conclusions

Regular physical activity makes an important contribution to many areas of men's health, preventing chronic disease, maximizing function after the onset of ill health, and maintaining independence into old age. If practiced wisely, it is a very pleasant form of therapy with few side effects, and it merits wider recommendation by practicing physicians.

References

1. Nolin B, Prud'homme D, Godin G et al. Enquête québécoise sur l'activité physique et la santé 1998. Quebec: Institut National de la Santé du Québec, 2002.
2. Bruce MJ, Katzmarzyk PT. Canadian population trends in leisure-time physical activity levels, 1981–1998. Can J Appl Physiol 2002; 27: 681–90.
3. Craig CL, Russell SJ, Cameron C et al. Twenty-year trends in physical activity among Canadian adults. Can J Pub Health 2004; 95: 59–63.
4. Katzmarzyk PT, Tremblay MS. Limitations of Canada's physical activity data: implications for monitoring trends. Appl Physiol Nutr Metab 2007; 32: S185–94.

5. Macera CA, Powell KE. Population attributable risk: implications of physical activity dose. Med Sci Sports Exerc 2001; 33(Suppl 6): S635–39.

6. Hughes E, McCracken M, Roberts H et al. Surveillance for certain health behaviors among states and selected local areas – behavioral risk factor surveillance system, United States, 2004. MMWR Morb Mortal Wkly Rep 2006; 55: 1–24.

7. Canadian Fitness and Lifestyle Research. Meeting Guidelines. Ottawa, ON: Canadian Fitness and Lifestyle Research Institute, 1998: Bulletin 31.

8. Bouchard C, Shephard RJ. Physical activity, fitness, and health: the model and key concepts. In: Bouchard C, Shephard RJ, Stephens T, eds. Physical Activity, Fitness and Health. Champaign, IL: Human Kinetics Publishers, 1994: 77–88.

9. Bouchard C, Shephard RJ, Stephens T. Physical Activity, Fitness and Health. Champaign, Illinois: Human Kinetics Publishers, 1994.

10. Bouchard C, Blair SN, Haskell W. Physical Activity and Health. Champaign, IL: Human Kinetics Publishers, 2007.

11. Kesaniemi YA, Danforth E, Jensen MD et al. Dose–response issues concerning physical activity and health: an evidence-based symposium. Med Sci Sports Exerc 2001; 33(Suppl 6): S351–8.

12. Warburton DER, Katzmarzyk PT, Rhodes RE et al. Evidence-informed physical activity guidelines for Canadian adults. Appl Physiol Nutr Metab 2007; 32(Suppl 2E): S16–S68.

13. Canadian Society of Exercise Physiology. The Canadian Physical Activity, Fitness and Lifestyle Appraisal. CSEP'S Plan for Healthy Active Living. Ottawa, ON: Canadian Society for Exercise Physiology, 1996.

14. Shephard RJ. Aerobic Fitness and Health. Champaign, IL: Human Kinetics Publishers, 1994.

15. Hill AB. Principles of Medical Statistics. Oxford: Oxford University Press, 1971.

16. Flegal KM. The obesity epidemic in children and adults: current evidence and research issues. Med Sci Sports Exerc 1999; 31(Suppl 11): S509–14.

17. Katzmarzyk PT, Ardern CI. Overweight and obesity mortality trends in Canada 1985–2000. Can J Publ Health 2004; 95: 16–20.

18. Shephard RJ. Can sports physicians play a role in controlling the obesity epidemic? In: Shephard RJ, ed. Year Book of Sports Medicine, 2006. Philadelphia: Elsevier Mosby, 2007, xix–xxv.

19. Ross R, Janssen I. Physical activity, total and regional obesity: dose–response considerations. Med Sci Sports Exerc 2001; 33: S521–7.

20. Tremblay A, Fontaine E, Poehlman ET et al. The effect of exercise training on resting metabolic rate in lean and moderately obese individuals. Int J Obes 1986; 10: 511–17.

21. World Health Organization. Obesity: Preventing and Managing the Global Epidemic. Report of a WHO Consultation. Geneva: World Health Organization, 1998.

22. Kelley DE, Goodpaster BH. Effects of exercise on glucose homeostasis in type 2 diabetes mellitus. Med Sci Sports Exerc 2001; 33(Suppl 6): S495–501.

23. Williamson DF, Vinicor F, Bowman BA. Primary prevention of type 2 diabetes mellitus by lifestyle intervention; implications for health policy. Ann Intern Med 2004; 140: 951–7.

24. Leon AS. Exercise in the prevention and management of diabetes mellitus and blood lipid disorders. In: Shephard RJ, Miller HS, eds. Exercise and the Heart in Health and Disease. New York: Marcel Dekker, 1999; 355–421.

25. Leon AS, Sanchez OA. Response of blood lipids to exercise training alone or combined with dietary intervention. Med Sci Sports Exerc 2001; 33(Suppl 6): S502–15.

26. Fagard RH. The influence of exercise intensity on the blood pressure response to dynamic physical training. Med Sci Sports Exerc 2001; 33(Suppl 6): 484–92.

27. Pescatello LS, Franklin BA, Fagard R et al. American College of Sports Medicine: Position Stand. Exercise and hypertension. Med Sci Sports Exerc 2004; 36: 533–53.

28. Wannamethee SG, Shaper AG, Alberti KG. Physical activity, metabolic factors and the incidence of coronary heart disease and type 2 diabetes. Arch Intern Med 2000; 160: 2108–16.

29. Emberson JR, Whincup PH, Morris RW et al. Lifestyle and cardiovascular disease in middle-aged British men: the effect of adjusting for within person variation. Eur Heart J 2005; 26: 1774–82.

30. Kohl HW. Physical activity and cardiovascular disease: evidence of a dose response. Med Sci Sports Exerc 2001; 33(Suppl 6): S472–83.

31. Lee CD, Folsom AR, Blair SN. Physical activity and stroke risk: A meta-analysis. Stroke 2003; 34: 2475–81.

32. Powell KE, Thompson PD, Caspersen CJ et al. Physical activity and the incidence of coronary heart disease. Ann Rev Public Health 1987; 8: 253–87.

33. Oldridge NB, Guyatt G, Fischer M et al. Randomized trials of cardiac rehabilitation:

combined experience of randomized clinical trials. JAMA 1988; 260: 945–50.

34. Iestra JA, Kromhout D, van der Schouw YT et al. Effect size estimates of lifestyle and dietary changes on all-cause mortality in coronary artery disease patients: a systematic review. Circulation 2005; 112: 924–34.

35. Taylor RS, Unal B, Critchley JA et al. Mortality reductions in patients receiving exercise-based cardiac rehabilitation: how much can be attributed to cardiovascular risk factor improvements? Eur J Cardiovasc Prev Rehabil 2006; 13: 369–74.

36. Delagardelle C, Feiersen P, Autier P et al. Strength/endurance training versus endurance training in congestive heart failure. Med Sci Sports Exerc 2002; 34: 1868–72.

37. Shephard RJ. Exercise for patients with congestive heart failure. In: Stanek B, ed. Optimising Heart Failure Management. Auckland: Adis Publications, 2000; 71–89.

38. Shephard RJ, Futcher R. Physical activity and cancer: How may protection be maximized? Crit Rev Oncogen 1997; 8: 219–72.

39. Thune I, Furberg A-S. Physical activity and cancer risk: dose–response and cancer, all sites and site specific. Med Sci Sports Exerc 2001; 33(Suppl 6): S530–50.

40. Lee IM. Physical activity and cancer prevention. Data from epidemiological studies. Med Sci Sports Exerc 2003; 35: 1823–7.

41. Shephard RJ, Shek PN. Associations between physical activity and susceptibility to cancer. Possible mechanisms. Sports Med 1998; 26: 293–315.

42. Fairey AS, Courneya KS, Field CJ et al. Physical exercise and immune system function in cancer survivors: a comprehensive review and future directions. Cancer 2002; 94: 539–51.

43. Vuori I. Dose-response of physical activity and low back pain, osteoarthritis, and osteoporosis. Med Sci Sports Exerc 2001; 33(Suppl 6): S551–86.

44. Warburton DE, Gledhill N, Quinney A. Musculoskeletal fitness and health. Can J Appl Physiol 2001; 26: 217–37.

45. Umemura Y, Ishiko T, Yamauchi T et al. Five jumps per day increase bone mass and breaking force in rats. J Bone Min Res 1997; 12: 1480–5.

46. Shephard RJ. Exercise and lifestyle change. Br J Sports Med 1989; 23: 11–22.

47. Carter R, Coast JR, Idell S. Exercise training in patients with chronic obstructive pulmonary disease. Med Sci Sports Exerc 1992; 24: 281–91.

48. Couillard A, Maltais F, Saey D et al. Exercise-induced quadriceps oxidative stress and peripheral muscular dysfunction in patients with chronic obstructive pulmonary disease. Am J Respir Crit Care Med 2003; 167: 1664–9.

49. Nieman DC. Is infection risk linked to exercise workload? Med Sci Sports Exerc 2000; 32(Suppl 7): S406–11.

50. Shinkai S, Konishi M, Shephard RJ. Aging and immune response to exercise. Can J Physiol Pharmacol 1998; 76: 562–72.

51. Shephard RJ. Aging, Physical Activity and Health. Champaign, IL: Human Kinetics Publishers, 1997.

52. Shephard RJ. Quality of life in old age: a key reason for promoting 'sport for all'. In: Simard C, Thibault G, Goulet C et al., eds. Actes du VIIIe Congrès Mondiale du Sport pour Tous. Quebec: Sports Internationaux du Québec, 2001: 529–39.

53. Paterson DH, Covindasamy D, Vidmar M et al. Longitudinal study of determinants of dependence in an elderly population. J Am Geriatr Soc 2004; 52: 1632–8.

54. American College of Sports Medicine. ACSM's Guidelines for Exercise Testing and Prescription, 7th edn. Philadelphia: Lippincott Williams and Wilkins, 2005.

55. Shephard RJ. Relative vs. absolute intensity of exercise in a dose–response context. Med Sci Sports Exerc 2001; 33(Suppl 6): S400–18.

56. Shephard RJ. Whistler. A Health Canada/CDC Conference on 'Communicating physical activity and health messages: Science into practice'. Am J Prev Med 2002; 23: 221–5.

57. Shephard RJ. What is an effective dose of physical activity? In: Shephard RJ, ed. Year Book of Sports Medicine, 2004. Philadelphia: Elsevier Mosby, 2005; xvii–xii.

58. Hardman AE. Issue of fractionalization of exercise (short vs long bouts). Med Sci Sports Exerc 2001; 33(Suppl 6): S421–7.

59. Shephard RJ, ed. Advancing the future of physical activity measurements and guidelines. Appl Physiol Nutr Metab 2007; 32(Suppl 2E): S1–224.

60. Paterson DH, Jones GR, Rice CL. Physical activity guidelines for older adults. Appl Physiol Nutr Metab 2007; 32(Suppl 2E): S69–108.

61. Shephard RJ. Physical activity and aging: some ecological perspectives. In: Siniarski A, Wolanski N, eds. Ecology of Aging. Delhi: Kamla Raj Enterprises, 2000: 93–108.

62. Vuori I. Sudden death and exercise: effects of age and type of activity. Sport Sci Rev 1995; 4: 46–84.

63. Shephard RJ. Exercise and sudden death: An overview. Sport Sci Rev 1995; 4: 1–13.

64. Siscovick DS, Weiss NS, Fletcher RH et al. The incidence of primary cardiac arrest during vigorous exercise. N Engl J Med 1984; 311: 874–7.

65. Shephard RJ. Exercise, hypertrophy, and cardiomyopathy in young and older athletes. In: Shephard RJ, Miller HS, eds. Exercise and the Heart in Health and Disease. New York: Marcel Dekker, 1999; 223–38.

66. Shephard RJ. Preparticipation screening of young athletes: an effective investment? In: Shephard RJ, ed. Year Book of Sports Medicine, 2005. Philadelphia: Elsevier Mosby, 2006; xix–xv.

67. Pate R, Macera CA. Risks of exercising. Musculoskeletal injuries. In: Bouchard C, Shephard RJ, Stephens T, eds. Physical Activity, Fitness, and Health. Champaign, IL: Human Kinetics Publishers, 1994: 1008–18.

68. Shrier I. Stretching before exercise does not reduce the risk of local muscle injury: a critical review of the clinical and basic science literature. Clin J Sports Med 1999; 9: 221–7.

69. Olsen OE, Myklebust G, Engebretsen L et al. Exercises to prevent lower limb injuries in youth sports: Cluster randomized trial. BMJ 2005; 330: 449–52.

CHAPTER 36

Obesity and men's health

David Haslam

History

The 2200-year-old Terracotta Army of Chinese Emperor Qin is known as the eighth wonder of the world, and comprises at least 8000 life-size figures molded from clay, each one unique in size, facial features, hair style, clothing, and posture, and each is sculpted in incredible detail. Buried with the Emperor to ensure his continued high status in the afterlife, most of the characters are military: foot soldiers, archers, cavalry, generals, and so on; others are accountants and administrators. Of all the thousands of statues, only one is obese: the entertainer – included to ensure that the Emperor could still enjoy a good laugh at someone else's expense between battles. The comedic appeal of the obese male has been evident throughout history. Even before a fat man speaks, the audience is already in his thrall, the sight of a rotund abdomen ensuring warmth and mirth. The fact holds true almost universally, throughout the Italian Atellan plays, comedia dell'arte, English mummers plays, and in literature, where roly-poly characters such as Sancho Panza – literally 'Mr Gut' – amuse the reader with their buffoonery. Falstaff was a self-confessed 'goodly portly man, i'faith, and a corpulent, of a cheerful look, a pleasing eye, and a most noble carriage'.

In 1811, Thomas Jameson explained the phenomenon of the funny fat man. He defined the years between age 28 and 58 as the era of male perfection, but neglected to mention that it should also be the era during which men prepare to stay as healthy as possible from 59 onwards: 'Corpulency steals imperceptibly on most men, between the ages of thirty and fifty-seven. In many cases the belly becomes prominent. A moderate degree of obesity is certainly a desirable state of body at all times, as it indicates a healthy condition of the assimilating powers [and] diminishes the irritability of the system, since fat people are remarked for good humour'. Many obese men are indeed characterized by good humor; rotund, plethoric men can be the very embodiment of conviviality, for instance standing at the bar, holding court to the assembly of drinkers.

More recently, the cinema has frequently portrayed fat men in a similar fashion. One of the earliest clips to have survived dates from 1912, entitled 'Fat Man on a Bicycle'. It stars Fred Evans as the amusing character Pimple, teaching an hilariousy incompetent fat friend to ride a bike, resulting in a variety of innocent bystanders and trades people suffering side-splitting slapstick sequelae.[1] John Bunny, Fatty Arbuckle, Oliver Hardy, and more recently actors such as Robert Morley and Richard Griffiths have carried the torch, alongside stand-up comics such as Bernard Manning and Peter Kay.

The 'fat is funny' concept is not universally male in either show business or everyday life; carnivals and circuses of bygone ages were inhabited by female 'fat freaks' with names such as Jolly Ollie and Dolly Dimples – rosy-cheeked Cushie Butterfields populate every soap opera and television drama – but it is a role most often filled by the stout male. When such a character appears on the stage or screen, the audience can tuck into their popcorn safe in the knowledge that an unthreatening corpulent clown will entertain them cleanly and warmly; the actor's girth representing a shop window; a promise of the material in store.

Unfortunately the same shop window represents an entirely different inventory to the medical practitioner. Ever since Hippocrates pronounced that corpulent men die sooner than their lean counterparts, it has been known that obesity is unhealthy; that an expanded abdomen is the outward physical sign of internal metabolic dysfunction. In 1765 the surgeon Joannes Morgagni, better known for lending his name to parts of the testicle, carried out *post mortem* studies on people who had died young or quickly, and described fat deposits within the abdomen and beneath the diaphragm.[2] In 1829, another surgeon William Wadd provided similar evidence, describing one *post mortem* examination: 'The omentum was a thick fat apron.

The whole of the intestinal canal was embedded in fat, as if melted tallow had been poured into the cavity of the abdomen; and the diaphragm and the parietes of the abdomen must have been strained to their very utmost extent, to have sustained the extreme and constant pressure of such a weighty mass. So great was the mechanical obstruction,... that the wonder is, not that he should die, but that he should live'.[3]

Prevalence

Almost a quarter of the male population is now obese, as assessed by body mass index (BMI). Waist circumference is a much more accurate way to assess obesity, as it is directly proportional to the level of a person's cardiometabolic risk: the statistics reveal an alarming obesity rate of almost 30% by this measure.[4]

The UK Government's Foresight report 'Tackling Obesities' reveals the extent of the problem of obesity (Fig. 36.1). Although certain people have a

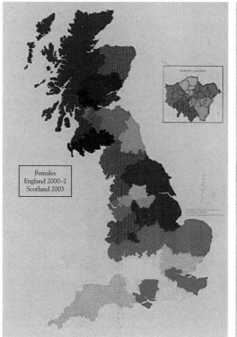
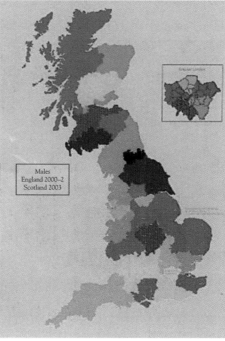
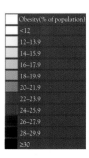

Figure 36.1. *Prevalence of obesity in England and Scotland, by region.*

genetic predisposition to obesity and overweight, public health recognizes the obesogenic or toxic environment as a major cause of obesity. The term 'passive obesity' has been coined to describe the method by which the average man, who lives an ordinary life, using technology as it is intended to be used, and eating the food presented to him, becomes overweight or obese, as if by osmosis. The existence of the term passive obesity implies the parallel existence of 'active obesity'. There is no doubt that in some people, unwise personal choices, and overindulgence in inappropriate foods, and enjoyment of sedentary pursuits – gluttony and sloth – do play a formative role in their condition, but the fact that two-thirds of the population are fat reveals that there is a lot more to the problem than greed and laziness.

Physical activity is rare in most people's work and leisure lives. TVs and DVDs and computer games are more common than ever, and are controlled by remote controls. Emails take away the necessity to deliver messages by hand, even from one room to another. Getting up to answer the phone is an anachronism, since the mobile phone revolution, and even doors respond automatically without being pushed; escalators and elevators take the strain in hotels and public buildings (the stairs are often out of bounds to visitors as a health hazard); and there are more cars per household than ever before. The current generation of adults is the first in history that has never experienced food shortage. Since post-War rationing, food has become plentiful, ubiquitous, cheap, available all day and night, and unhealthier in quality, and it is being served in ever bigger portions. The expression 'optimal default' describes the ideal state, whereby in any given situation, the act that a person is automatically, intrinsically drawn to performing is the healthy option – in other words a default to the optimum healthy behavior. For example, when walking into a hotel, a person might, instead of a battalion of lifts, be confronted with an attractive, sweeping marble staircase, with shallow steps, and a plush carpet, with a series of paintings half way up, which require closer viewing, and this would draw the person into the optimum default of walking. A lift must, of course be available but need not be presented as the only option. On approaching the fizzy drinks section in a supermarket, the obvious choice should be the most healthy one; cheaper, easily reached, and most attractively packaged.

Impact

Unfortunately, the human environment has evolved millions of times more rapidly than the metabolic pathways, and in the 30 years it has taken for the obesity epidemic to become established, we have not had the chance to evolve to protect ourselves, and have no instinct to avoid food and unnecessary activity. Natural selection has turned on us. Those people who once had the capacity to lay down excess food as energy stores in fatty tissue were able to thrive in times of fast and famine, and therefore had superior genetic predisposition and were programmed to survive. Now, however, it is the identical phenotype, which faced with an abundance of food and no innate ability to modify intake, is being selected to die prematurely. In order to avoid the health consequences associated with sedentary behavior and over-efficient energy storage, physical activity must be included within daily life, and food intake must be carefully monitored and adjusted. People must force themselves to move their body from A to B, for fun, necessity, or profit, without the use of external forces, as often as possible, and must fuel the effort with as healthy a food intake as possible, combining low saturated fat with a reduction in refined carbohydrates.

The comic habitus of the obese male is no longer funny. When an obese man enters the physician's office, the response is worry, not comfort; medical concern rather than mirth. Men even have a particular type of obesity named after them. In the 1940s, the French physician Jean Vague reflected the work of Morgagni and Wadd, describing the android or apple shape assumed by obese men, in contrast to female gynoid, pear-shaped obesity. Unfortunately for the male, the central adiposity denoted by the apple is the dangerous variety. There should be no moral or ethical objection to fat from the medical profession, many of whom share the same body morphology; but the simple fact is that being obese is very bad for health, and should be appropriately managed.

Hippocrates took the first step in recognizing risk factors for ill health, correctly observing that obesity was a risk factor for sudden death. It has taken several thousand years for modern science to provide the supportive evidence for his remark, which finally arrived with the Paris Prospective Study, which was set up in 1967, and is still reporting a broad range of evidence based on 23 years of follow-up of over 7000 apparently healthy middle-aged men.[5] The Paris study recently focused on the 118 sudden deaths and 192 fatal myocardial infarctions that occurred amongst this cohort, reporting a massive increase in risk of both conditions conferred upon a person by abdominal obesity (Fig. 36.2).

The increased incidence of sudden death amongst abdominally obese people is highly significant. Data collected recently from male drivers at motorway service stations in the UK compound the sense of alarm, by revealing that:

- 81.4% of the male driving population are overweight or obese, compared with around two-thirds of the general population;
- 34.6% are obese, compared with less than 24% of the general population;
- the average weight of male drivers is 91.6 kg;
- the average driver is obese by both waist circumference and BMI; and
- the average driver has a raised resting pulse rate, another marker of increased cardiovascular risk.

Bearing in mind that the male driving population most at risk includes heavy goods vehicle drivers, taxi drivers, and bus drivers, the at-risk population from a driver's sudden incapacitation at the wheel also involves the general public.

Whereas Hippocrates only had abdominal girth to rely upon to estimate risk, the modern physician has a wealth of prognostic indicators to call upon. Comorbid diseases such as type 2 diabetes, hypertension, and hypercholesterolemia can be picked up by simple screening measures. Predictors of future cardiometabolic illness can be assessed easily and cheaply in the general population, and a risk evaluation score created, based on Framingham, Sheffield, or other risk engines. The renowned French–Canadian physician JP Despres has described the 'triglyceridemic waist' whereby a person with abdominal obesity and a fasting triglyceride level >2 mmol/l can be confidently labeled as being at high risk for cardiovascular disease. However, although medical science has the knowledge to predict and prevent illness, thereby avoiding personal suffering, reducing the workload of healthcare professionals, and saving much money to the wider economy, the knowledge is not being utilized, and the opportunity to reduce the burden of disease is being missed.

Fig. 36.3 demonstrates the increase risk of coronary heart disease with increasing levels of obesity in men, but only as assessed with the inclusion of waist circumference, rather than BMI. The man at

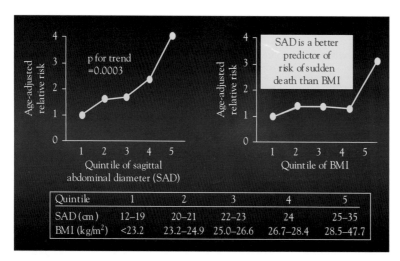

Figure 36.2. *Abdominal obesity predicts adverse outcomes such as sudden death. BMI, body mass index; SAD, sagittal abdominal diameter. From reference 5.*

Quintile	1	2	3	4	5
SAD (cm)	12–19	20–21	22–23	24	25–35
BMI (kg/m²)	<23.2	23.2–24.9	25.0–26.6	26.7–28.4	28.5–47.7

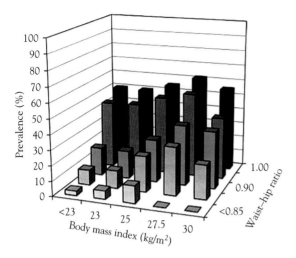

Figure 36.3. *Prevalence (%) of predicted 10 year risk of coronary heart disease ≥15% according to waist–hip ratio and body mass index in men aged 35–74 years. From reference 6.*

the lowest risk in this study appears at the front right. He is officially obese, with a BMI of ≥30 kg/m², but he has a normal waist–hip ratio, and presumably an athletic build.[6] One of the highest risk men, however is shown at the back on the left: he has a normal BMI of <23 kg/m², but a high waist–hip ratio: a skinny man with a pot belly. It is important to include waist circumference in assessing the health of a person otherwise high-risk people such as him slip through the net.

Geoff visited the surgery for the first time at age 47, as his son's tonsillitis coincided with his wife's admission to hospital for a minor operation. His son required, and received antibiotics, but on casual assessment, Geoff appeared significantly abdominally obese. Basic screening revealed a waist circumference of 130 cm, weight of 140 kg, and BMI of 43 kg/m². Second-tier screening recorded a blood pressure of 150/90 mmHg, a fasting total cholesterol of 6.8 mmol/L, and a fasting plasma glucose of 6.9 mmol/L. Geoff therefore failed to fulfil the criteria for diabetes, hypertension, or hypercholesterolemia *per se*, but by dint of his borderline blood pressure and lipid profile and his impaired fasting glucose he had a massively

increased risk score for future cardiovascular disease. In people like Geoff, multiple borderline risk factors multiply up, equating to high risk, and it is not acceptable merely to monitor borderline blood pressure in the presence of a series of other borderline risk factors. Unfortunately there are no implementable guidelines that call for screening of individuals like Geoff, or that highlight the management of the obese individual at high risk for cardiometabolic disease. The likes of Geoff must wait until the almost inevitable heart attack, stroke, or diagnosis of diabetes to occur to be confident of receiving the basic medical management that their level of risk deserves. At the point of diagnosis with a life-threatening illness, Geoff will receive state-of-the-art medical input, and gold standard intervention on his portfolio of risk factors, by which time it will be too late to help him avoid overt disease. Obese individuals should be offered screening for multiple risk factors, and their risk managed accordingly, with specific concern to their underlying obesity.

Sudden death is undoubtedly something all men would wish to avoid. So is erectile dysfunction, another disease linked with obesity. Erectile dysfunction is an important phenomenon in its own right, but it is also an early signal of impending cardiovascular disease. Erectile dysfunction and sudden death are different ends of the spectrum of the same disease, a spectrum that involves obesity and a huge catalog of comorbidities. It is essential that obese people seek medical help to assess their likelihood of serious comorbid disease, and that clinicians act upon that information to modify their patients' risk of illness.

The metabolic syndrome was formally defined in 1988 by Professor Gerald Reaven, to describe and explain scientifically the observed clustering together of illnesses such as diabetes, blood pressure, and heart disease in susceptible people. The most recent criteria for the metabolic syndrome were drawn up by the International Diabetes Federation, and make allowances for different ethnic backgrounds, since, for instance South Asian men are at much higher risk of diabetes at more modest levels of obesity than their 'Europid' counterparts.

It has been estimated that between 20% and 30% of middle-aged people in industrialized countries may already suffer from the metabolic syndrome, and are therefore twice as likely to die from, and three times as likely to suffer, a heart attack or stroke compared with people without the metabolic syndrome. They also have a five-fold greater risk of being diagnosed with type 2 diabetes – the fourth or fifth leading cause of death in the developed world – and adding to the 230 million current cases worldwide. Another estimate suggests that as few as 30% of all adults exhibit none of the major characteristics of the syndrome.

The new International Diabetes Federation definition of the metabolic syndrome states that a person must have central obesity (defined as waist circumference ≥94 cm for Europid men and ≥80 cm for Europid women, with ethnicity-specific values for other groups) plus any two of the following four factors:

- raised triglyceride level [≥150 mg/dL (1.7 mmol/L)], or specific treatment for this lipid abnormality
- reduced high-density lipoprotein (HDL) cholesterol [<40 mg/dL (1.03 mmol/L) in males and <50 mg/dL (1.29 mmol/L) in females] or be on specific treatment for this lipid abnormality
- raised blood pressure (systolic ≥130 mmHg or diastolic ≥85 mmHg) or be on treatment of previously diagnosed hypertension
- raised fasting plasma glucose [≥100 mg/dL (5.6 mmol/L)], or previously diagnosed type 2 diabetes.

The Paris Prospective Study, which had scientifically linked the phenomenon of sudden death with abdominal obesity, went one step further in 2007, broadening the net to assess the effect of metabolic syndrome, rather than isolated obesity, on sudden deaths, and discovered a staggering 68% increase in the prevalence of sudden death in the presence of the metabolic syndrome, underlining the potentially catastrophic dangers many men carry towards morbidity and mortality. The concept of the metabolic syndrome has undoubtedly been successful in providing the link between these conditions with the same etiological pathways, and

in making their management more robust and co-ordinated. However, although diabetes, blood pressure, and cardiovascular disease are the most important strands of the metabolic syndrome, other conditions that are part of the same metabolic dysfunction are potentially overlooked because they fall outside the traditional criteria – conditions such as certain cancers and non-alcoholic steatohepatitis (NASH), which are also all directly linked to intra-abdominal adiposity.

Put simply, fat, especially that situated within the abdomen, is directly associated with a whole catalog of diseases, and must therefore be dealt with in that context, as a disease process. Adipose tissue is not merely an inert yellow mass of padding used to store excess energy, but a dangerous metabolically active bodily organ. Abdominal fat, wrapped within the omentum of the gut, can be considered to be the body's largest endocrine gland in obese people, which, rather than being the source of useful hormones, secretes inflammatory factors known as adipocytokines into the portal circulation, which lead directly to endothelial dysfunction, and plaque formation, and are the precursors of cardiovascular disease.

Another fundamental metabolic flaw in obese people is insulin resistance, which has a number of serious consequences, including the release of atherosclerotic free fatty acids from adipose tissue into the bloodstream. But possibly the best recognized sequel of insulin resistance is type 2 diabetes. When sugar is absorbed from the stomach into the blood stream, insulin is secreted by pancreatic β-cells, which enables skeletal muscle to take up sugar for energy. If a person is resistant to effects of insulin, the level of sugar in the blood will be driven upwards, causing the pancreas to produce extra insulin to compensate: hyperinsulinemia. Eventually the β-cells of the pancreas fail to maintain insulin production, sugar levels are uncontrollable, and impaired glucose control and frank diabetes develop. Insulin resistance, however, occurs only in muscle, liver, and adipose tissue; other organs of the body were described, by Professor Reaven himself, as 'innocent bystanders' of the hyperinsulinemic state, and react in different ways. The toxic state brought about by the combination of high circulating insulin and the presence of adipocytokines such as tumor necrosis factor-α is responsible for the long list of diseases.

The most important casualty of the abnormal metabolism in obese people is the heart and circulation, damage to which leads to cardiovascular disease. The first stage in the onset of cardiovascular disease is inflammation of the walls of the arteries caused by the combination of high insulin and inflammatory toxins produced by adipose tissue. This is exacerbated by the atherogenic cholesterol abnormalities typically found in obesity – low HDL cholesterol levels and low-density lipoprotein (LDL) cholesterol particles, which lead to plaque formation in the arterial wall; the plaques subsequently rupture, causing a thrombus to form, and myocardial infarction or stroke ensue. Furthermore, blood tends to be too viscous in obese people – hypercoagulability is caused by increased plasminogen activator inhibitor 1, making thrombosis even more likely. Over a third of deaths in the UK are caused by cardiovascular disease, and obesity, along with the resultant abnormal metabolism, is the leading factor, along with smoking.

Findings from a major study of over 300 000 adults followed up for almost 7 years reported that for each unit change in BMI a 9% difference in ischemic heart disease events occurred, with a change of 8% in hypertensive deaths and ischemic strokes.[7] Dyslipidemia progressively develops as BMI increases from 21 kg/m^2. There is a very close link between obesity, particularly abdominal obesity, and high blood pressure; up to two-thirds of cases of hypertension are linked with obesity. Obese people have over five times the risk of developing hypertension, and people who are 20% overweight are eight times more likely to develop it.

NASH is being increasingly recognized and is rapidly rising in prevalence. It is one of the leading causes of end-stage liver failure in the developed world owing to the progression from benign nonalcoholic fatty liver disease (NAFLD) to cirrhosis, portal hypertension, and sometimes even hepatocellular carcinoma. The changes in the liver normally associated with alcohol damage are seen in NASH, but the main etiological factor is obesity – patients with NASH are more insulin resistant than those with benign fatty liver alone. The symptoms of NASH can be vague; some people describe tiredness and abdominal discomfort but it is usually asymptomatic, and signs of liver disease are rare. Raised liver function tests may be the only indication of NAFLD, which may lead to the discovery of an abnormal appearance of the liver on ultrasound. NASH occurs in between 2% and 9% of the population, of whom 50% will develop fibrosis, 30% will develop cirrhosis, and 3% will end up with liver failure or transplantation.

Obese drivers are not only at risk of sudden death due to cardiovascular disease, but also put themselves, their passengers, and innocent bystanders at risk because of sleep apnea, which increases the risk of road traffic accidents by up to seven times. Sleep apnea is caused by the compression of the airways by fatty tissue around the neck and is characterized by episodes of disrupted breathing, recurring up to 30 times a night. The patient may be unaware of the problem, but may snore loudly, pause in the normal respiratory pattern for 10 seconds or more, then grunt loudly, before resuming a normal breathing pattern. Sleep apnea affects around 4% of the population and is four times as common in men than women. Although it can lead to pulmonary hypertension, right heart failure, hypertension, stroke, and arrhythmias, the main risk is accidental injury caused by daytime somnolence and falling asleep in inappropriate situations, for instance while driving a vehicle.

Obesity can lead to joint and musculoskeletal problems from childhood onwards, but the problems are not exclusive to weight-bearing joints. Other joints such as the wrist are also affected, implying a metabolic rather than simply a mechanical cause.

Obesity, alongside smoking, is the biggest preventable cause of cancer in the developed world, being linked with around 20 different malignancies, including cancer of the breast, uterus, colon, pancreas, and testes and non-Hodgkins lymphoma. Ten percent of all cancer deaths among non-smokers are estimated to be related to obesity. One study followed 28 000 obese patients for up to 29 years, and reported an increased cancer incidence of 33% compared with the general population.[8]

The ultimate outcome of obesity is death, not just sudden death as demonstrated by the Paris study, but also premature death from a variety of causes. Fig. 36.4 illustrates the premature mortality linked with obesity, demonstrating that, for instance, a man aged 20, with a BMI of 33 kg/m², is likely to lose 4 years of life, and a 30-year-old with the same BMI, 3 years of life, whereas a 20-year-old with a BMI ≥45 can expect to lose 13 years of life.[9]

In the USA, whereas mortality from most diseases is dropping, deaths due to diabetes are increasing, due to the obesity epidemic, and the subsequent diabetes timebomb (Fig. 36.5). The same will happen in the UK unless drastic measures are taken.

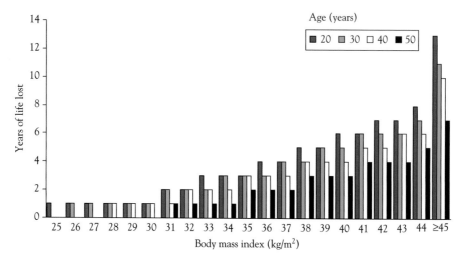

Figure 36.4 *Impact of obesity on mortality and years of life lost.*

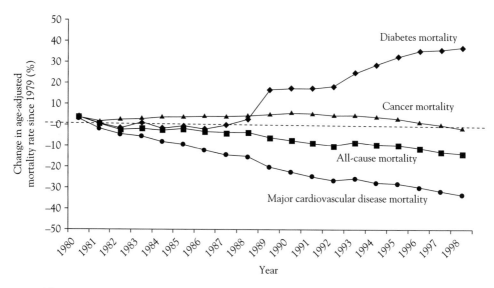

Figure 36.5 *Change in age-adjusted mortality rates since the year 1979 in the USA by cause of mortality (Centers for Disease Control and Prevention Mortality Database).*

Treatment

Weight loss should aim to be gradual, at around 0.5–1 kg (1–2 lb) per week, by sustainable changes and a balanced diet, along with brisk physical activity of 60–90 minutes per day, but in many patients a more pragmatic approach is required.

Some dietary regimens can be maintained better than others, and low-carbohydrate diets such as the Atkins diet have a substantial evidence base. A recent comparison revealed that after 6 months, people on low-carbohydrate diets had lost more weight than those randomized to low-fat diets, although after a year the effects were even.[10] Triglyceride and HDL cholesterol levels changed more favorably in low-carbohydrate diets, but total and LDL cholesterol levels changed more favorably in low-fat dieters. Against the Atkins regimen is the expectation to increase fat intake, and not to worry about butter or fatty meat. A more recent development has been the 'Total Wellbeing Diet' developed by the Commonwealth Scientific and Industrial Research Organisation (CSIRO) in Australia, which recommends high protein and low carbohydrate, with a lower fat intake than Atkins, making it healthier and more balanced.[11] So far a limited amount of evidence suggests that weight loss occurs secondary to a lower calorie intake, assisted by the increased satiety induced by high protein intake.[12]

Interventions such as meal replacements and low calorie diets and very low calorie diets are appropriate for certain people, generally those who have failed on more traditional regimens – and they have an excellent long-term evidence base.

Increased activity is an essential facet of weight management regimens, but activity alone is unlikely to induce significant weight loss, owing to increase in muscle mass, which is denser than fat. Physical activity does, however, have significant health benefits regardless of whether weight loss occurs:

- improved control of type 2 diabetes
- improvement in lipid profile, in particular increase in HDL cholesterol
- improvement in blood pressure
- improved insulin sensitivity
- improved self-esteem, and reduction in symptoms of depression and anxiety
- improved day-to-day functional capacity
- reduced risk of colorectal cancer.

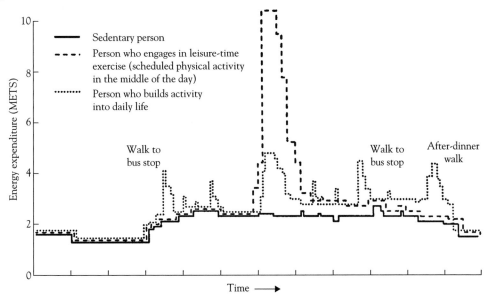

Figure 36.6. *Contrasting patterns of energy expenditure (represented by the area under the curve) of daily activities. The area under the curve is greatest for the person who is constantly engaged in low-intensity activity. From reference 13.*

471

A rough guide to the level of physical activity required is 10 000 steps per day measured by a pedometer, but any increase is hugely beneficial and leads to extremely rapid improvements in health. The best and most sustainable method of increasing activity is to build it into daily life, for example by climbing the stairs instead of using the escalators and walking to work, or at least part of the way (Fig. 36.6).

Diet and physical activity are, and will always be, the first-line treatments for obesity, but second-line remedies including drugs and surgery have an important role to play. The three pharmacological agents currently available are orlistat, sibutramine, and rimonabant, which act in different ways to reduce food intake, absorption, or metabolism by varying degrees and mechanisms. In the past, some of the most toxic chemicals known to man have been used in the management of obesity, including mercury, arsenic, strychnine, and amphetamines, but modern drugs are entirely separate entities: well tolerated and effective in the appropriate circumstances. As well as inducing weight reduction, they also improve other risk factors including glycemic control, lipid profile, and blood pressure. They should be taken under the supervision of a doctor, nurse, or pharmacist, alongside diet and physical activity measures.

The term 'bariatric surgery' applies to surgical techniques specifically intended to induce weight loss, and include procedures that restrict the size of

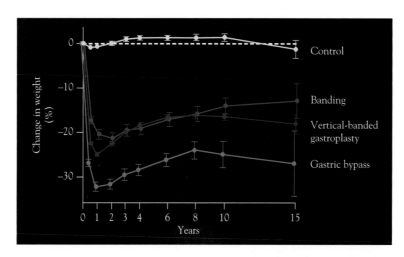

Figure 36.7. *Weight change over time after treatment for obesity by banding, vertical-banded gastroplasty, or gastric bypass. From reference 14.*

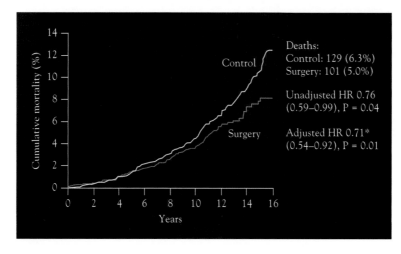

Figure 36.8. *Mortality reduction after weight-reduction surgery. HR, hazard ratio. From reference 14.*

the stomach, or reduce the functional capacity of the stomach and bowel, by bypassing parts of the tract. Such procedures are amongst the most clinically effective and cost-effective techniques in any field of medicine, and have been shown to induce immense, sustained weight loss (Fig. 36.7) and the reversal of comorbidities, including diabetes, in over 90% of cases (Fig. 36.8).

The recently reported outcome data from the large Swedish Obese Subjects study shows scientifically, for the first time ever, what Hippocrates himself already knew over 3000 years ago, and what practicing physicians have been aware of for centuries: that weight reduction significantly improves mortality and prevents premature death.[14]

References

1. http://www.screenonline.org.uk/film/id/730648/index.html
2. 'The Seats and Causes of Diseases Investigated by Anatomy 1765. Joannes Baptista Morgagni, 1765 Epistola anatoma clinica XXI.' De Sedibus et Causis Morborum per Anatomen indagata.
3. Wadd W. Comments on Corpulency, Lineaments on Leanness. London: Ebers, 1829.
4. Ruston D, Hoare J, Henderson L et al. National Diet and Nutrition Survey, vol. 4. London: Office of National Statistics, 2004.
5. Empana JP, Ducimetiere P, Charles MA, Jouven X. Sagittal abdominal diameter and risk of sudden death in asymptomatic middle-aged men: the Paris Prospective Study I. Circulation 2004; 110: 2781–5.
6. Nanchahal K, Morris JN, Sullivan LM, Wilson PW. Coronary heart disease risk in men and the epidemic of overweight and obesity. Int J Obes Relat Metab Disord 2005; 29: 317–23.
7. James WPT, Jackson-Leach R, Ni Mhurchu C et al. Overweight and obesity (high body mass index). In: Ezzati M, Lopez AD, Rodgers A, Murray CJL, eds. Comparative Quantification of Health Risks: Global and Regional Burden of Disease Attributable to Selected Major Risk Factors, Vol. 1. Geneva: World Health Organization, 2004: 497–596.
8. Wolk A, Gridley G, Svensson M et al. A prospective study of obesity and cancer risk (Sweden). Cancer Causes and Control 2001; 12: 1321.
9. Fontaine KR, Redden DT, Wang C et al. Years of life lost due to obesity. JAMA 2003; 289: 187.
10. Nordmann A, Nordmann A, Briel M et al. Effects of low-carbohydrate vs low-fat diets on weight loss and cardiovascular risk factors. A meta-analysis of randomized controlled trials. Arch Intern Med 2006; 166: 285–93.
11. http://www.csiro.au/ [accessed 1 January, 2007].
12. Clifton PM, Noakes M, Keogh J, Foster P. Effect of an energy reduced high protein red meat diet on weight loss and metabolic parameters in obese women. Asia Pac J Clin Nutr 2003; 12: S10.
13. Blair SN, Kohl HW, Gordon NF, Paffenbarger RS Jr. How much physical activity is good for health? Annu Rev Public Health 1992; 13: 99–126.
14. Sjöström L, Narbro K, Sjöström CD et al. Effects of bariatric surgery on mortality in Swedish obese subjects. N Engl J Med 2007; 357: 741–52.

CHAPTER 37

Smoking and lung cancer

Richard Doll

Early evidence

Use of tobacco

The smoking of tobacco was introduced into Europe in the fifteenth century when it was recommended as a therapy for a wide range of conditions. Its use for pleasure was discouraged by church and state and it was not until the end of the sixteenth century that the smoking of tobacco in pipes came to be adopted widely, at first in Britain, whence it spread to the Netherlands and then to the rest of the continent.

Gradually the way in which tobacco was most commonly used changed. By the end of the seventeenth century, its use as nasal snuff had spread from France and largely replaced the smoking of pipes and this form remained common until a century later when it, in turn, began to be replaced by the smoking of cigars, which had long been smoked in a primitive form in Spain and Portugal. By then cigarettes were already being made in South America and their use had spread to Spain, but it was not until after the Crimean War that cigarette smoking began to be adopted widely and by the end of the nineteenth century to have begun to replace cigar smoking. Consumption of cigarettes increased rapidly in the First World War and by the end of the Second World War they had largely replaced all other tobacco products in most developed countries. By this time, smoking had become so much the norm for men that, in Britain, some 80% were regular smokers.

For its impact on health, the important change in the use of tobacco was the swing to cigarettes, which was brought about by two industrial developments. The first was a new method of curing tobacco. With the old method, the smoke that had come from pipes and cigars was alkaline, irritating, and difficult to inhale. The nicotine in it was, however, predominantly in the form of a free base and it could be absorbed across the oral and pharyngeal mucosa. Blood levels of nicotine could consequently be high and addiction was readily produced; but only small amounts of other constituents were absorbed. The new method of flue-curing was introduced in North Carolina in the mid nineteenth century.[1] It exposed the leaf to high temperatures and increased its sugar content, thereby causing the pH of the smoke to be acid. In this environment, the nicotine was predominantly in the form of salts and was dissolved in smoke droplets, which were less irritating than the free base and easier to inhale. With each inhalation there was a rapid rise in the level of nicotine in the blood which was perceived in the brain and was particularly satisfying to addicts, but other constituents of the smoke were unfortunately also absorbed and distributed throughout the body.

The second development was mechanical: namely, the introduction of cigarette making machines. One was patented in 1880 and was eventually adapted to work so efficiently that 120 000 cigarettes of good quality could be produced every 10 hours by one machine, the equivalent of the production of about 100 unassisted workers. As a result the price fell and a mass market became feasible.

Health effects

Until cigarette smoking became common very little evidence of harmful effects was detected – for the good reason that relatively little harm was probably caused. One harmful effect, the production of cancer of the lip, was recognized at the end of the eighteenth century by Sömmering[2] in Germany and to this was added, in the course of the next hundred years, the production of cancers of the tongue and other parts of the mouth on the basis of clinical series in France,[3] Germany[4] and the UK[5] – findings that are now simply explained because we know that these cancers can be produced at least as easily by the smoking of pipes and cigars as by the smoking of cigarettes. Little attention was, however, paid to them by clinicians, who characterized cancer of the lip as the result of smoking clay pipes, which was a custom of agricultural workers, in whom the risk was enhanced by exposure to ultraviolet light. One disease, however, was unequivocally attributed to tobacco, and taught as being so, namely, tobacco amblyopia. It was described by Beer[6] in 1817 and occurred in heavy pipe smokers in combination with malnutrition and was probably caused by the cyanide in smoke not being detoxified because of a deficiency of vitamin B12.[7] The disease is no longer seen, at least in developed countries.

With the advent of the twentieth century, several new diseases began to be associated with smoking: first, intermittent claudication described by Erb in 1904,[8] and second a rare form of peripheral vascular disease affecting relatively young people, now named after Buerger[9] who recognized it in 1908 and called it thrombo-angiitis obliterans. Both diseases were made much more common by smoking, with the latter almost limited to smokers; but neither reached the epidemic proportions that two other relatively new diseases achieved in the next few decades. One was myocardial infarction, which was first described at autopsy in 1876[10] but was not diagnosed in life until 1910.[11] Subsequently

it was reported progressively more often every year for four or five decades. Hoffman, an American statistician, linked the increase with the increasing consumption of cigarettes as early as 1920.[12] Several clinical studies of the relationship with smoking were published, but no substantial evidence was found until 1940, when English et al reported an association in the records of the Mayo Clinic.[13] Their findings led them to conclude that the smoking of tobacco probably had 'a more profound effect on younger individuals owing to the existence of relatively normal cardiovascular systems, influencing perhaps the earlier development of coronary disease'. That cigarette smoking played a part in the increasing incidence of the disease was eventually clearly demonstrated. The association was not close enough for it to have been the only cause of the increase, or even probably the most important, and, unlike the other disease that burst into medical prominence in the first half of the twentieth century, the full explanation of its rapid increase is still a matter for debate.[14]

The other disease was cancer of the lung. A small cluster of cases in tobacco workers in Leipzig[15] had led Rottmann to suggest, in 1898, that it might be caused by the inhalation of tobacco dust, but the first suggestion that it might be due to smoking was not made until 1912 when Adler noted that, although the disease was rare, it appeared to have become somewhat less so.[16] Many people were subsequently struck by the parallel increase in the consumption of cigarettes and the incidence of the disease and by the frequency with which patients with lung cancer described themselves as heavy smokers and several even ventured to suggest that the two were related.[17–21] Experiments were consequently undertaken in the 1920s to see if cancer could be caused in animals by the application of tobacco tars to the skin. These generally failed and the one that did not, carried out by Roffo[22,23] in the Argentine, was dismissed in the UK because he had produced the tar at irrelevantly high temperatures.[24] Two case–control studies in Germany reported a strong association between smoking and lung cancer and led to the conclusion that increased smoking might be the most important cause of the increase in the disease[25,26] but their methodology was weak and the conclusion dubious.

Similar results were, however, also found in a third study in the Netherlands.[27]

Modern knowledge

Origin

Modern knowledge of the effect of smoking dates from the 1950s when the evidence that it caused cancer of the lung became compelling.[28,29] Cohort studies were initiated to check the validity of the conclusions drawn from case–control studies and these soon began to reveal that smoking was quantitatively related to mortality from a wide range of diseases other than lung cancer. Such studies have now been carried out in China,[30] Japan,[31] Norway,[32] Sweden,[33] and Canada[34] as well as in the UK and the USA and have been extended to cover the past two decades, when most smokers in the last two countries have been smoking cigarettes for nearly all their smoking lives.[35,36] The results have all been broadly consistent, though they have differed in detail, depending on differences in past smoking habits and in exposure to other agents with which smoking has interacted.

Altogether, cigarette smoking has been found to be positively associated with nearly 40 diseases or causes of death and negatively associated with eight others. In a few instances the associations are due to confounding with other factors that are the causes of the conditions, but the great majority arise because tobacco smoke is a direct contributory cause. This is not as surprising as might at first appear: for it arises partly because of the complexity of tobacco smoke which contains over 4000 chemicals, and partly because many of the diseases are different clinical manifestations of common underlying pathologies, such as DNA damage, cytotoxicity, vascular occlusion and damage to the small airways.

Harmful effects

The principal harmful effects of prolonged cigarette smoking are illustrated by the results of the American Cancer Society's most recent study of a million people[34] (and personal communication) and of the study of 34 000 male British doctors initiated by the British Medical Research Council.[35] The American cohort was followed for 9 years from 1982, but the first 2 years' observations have been omitted to reduce the 'healthy responder effect': that is, the tendency for healthy people to respond more readily to questionnaires than people who are sick, which biases observed mortality rates downwards. In the subsequent 7 years over 80 000 deaths were recorded. In the British study, the cohort was followed for 40 years from 1951 with changes in smoking habits recorded at intervals of 5–12 years throughout. Over 20 000 deaths were recorded.

Table 37.1 shows the risk of death in continuing cigarette smokers relative to that in lifelong non-smokers from 22 causes of death. In both studies the risks are standardized for age in single years according to the age distribution of the populations at risk and, in the British study, also for year of observation. In a few instances, data are given for only one study, either because the number of deaths in the other was too small to provide reliable results or because the relevant diagnostic code was not used. For each cause of death, a figure is given for the percentage of deaths attributed to it in England and Wales in 1993[37] as an indication of its relative importance.

The relative risks, which vary from 1.3 to 1 to infinity to 1 (because no death occurred in a non-smoker) are all statistically significant ($p < 0.01$) and qualitatively similar in both studies. The exceptionally high relative risk for cancers of the mouth, pharynx, and larynx in the British study, which have been grouped together because of paucity of numbers, had wide confidence limits because only two deaths from this group of cancers were observed in non-smokers.

Table 37.2 shows the corresponding risks in the British study for ex and current cigarette smokers and for light and heavy smokers (that is, for men smoking less than 15 or 25 or more cigarettes a day). With one exception, the risks for ex-smokers are intermediate between those for non-smokers and current smokers and all are higher in heavy smokers than in light. The exception is the mortality from asthma and that is due to the effect of asthma on smoking habits, rather than the reverse, as sufferers from the disease tend to stop smoking or to reduce the amount smoked. The findings for cancer of the lung are outstanding because of the high relative

Table 37.1. *Principal diseases caused in part by smoking: ratios of mortality rates in male cigarette smokers and lifelong non-smokers (References 35, 36 and personal communication)*

Cause of death (% of deaths England and Wales 1993)		Ratio of mortality rates	
		British doctors 1951–91	US population 1984–91
Cancers of mouth, pharynx and larynx	(0.4)	24.0	11.4
Cancer of esophagus	(1.0)	7.5	5.6
Cancer of lung	(5.6)	14.9	23.9
Cancer of pancreas	(1.0)	2.2	2.0
Cancer of bladder	(0.8)	2.3	3.9
Ischemic heart disease	(25.3)	1.6	1.9
Hypertension	(0.5)	1.4	2.4
Myocardial degeneration	(2.0)	2.0	
Pulmonary heart disease*	(0.3)	∞	2.1
Other heart disease	(3.0)	–	
Aortic aneurysm	(1.6)	4.1	6.3
Peripheral vascular disease	(0.1)	–	9.7
Arteriosclerosis	(0.5)	1.8	2.7
Cerebral vascular disease	(10.6)	1.5	1.9
Chronic bronchitis and emphysema	(4.5)	12.7	17.6
Pulmonary tuberculosis	(0.1)	2.8	–
Asthma[†]	(0.3)	2.2	1.3
Pneumonia	(9.4)	1.9	2.5
Other respiratory disease	(1.4)	1.6	
Peptic ulcer	(0.7)	3.0	4.6
All causes		1.8	2.5

*No death was reported in non-smoking doctors.
†Smokers include ex-smokers, as asthma may itself cause cessation of smoking.

risk from smoking and the frequency with which the disease occurs in the population.

Other harmful effects caused in part by smoking are listed in Box 37.1. For these, evidence has often had to be obtained from case–control studies: for cancers of the pelvis and body of the kidney, because they are seldom identified separately in the certified causes of death used in most cohort studies; for cancers of the stomach, liver and cervix and for myeloid leukemia because they are only weakly related to smoking, so that large numbers and evidence to exclude confounding have been needed; for cancers of the lip and nose and for Crohn's disease because they are too uncommon for substantial numbers of deaths to be observed in even the largest cohort studies. Five of the other

Table 37.2. *Principal diseases in men caused in part by smoking: ratios of mortality rates in ex-cigarette smokers and in cigarette smokers of different amounts and rates in lifelong non-smokers[35]*

Cause of death	Ratio of mortality rates			
	Ex-cigarette smokers	Current cigarette smokers, smoking per day		
		Any number	1–14	25 or more
Cancer of mouth, pharynx and larynx	3.0	24.0	12.0	48.0
Cancer of esophagus	4.8	7.5	4.3	11.3
Cancer of lung	4.1	14.9	7.5	25.4
Cancer of pancreas	1.4	2.2	1.9	3.1
Cancer of bladder	1.6	2.3	2.2	2.8
Ischemic heart disease	1.2	1.6	1.4	1.8
Hypertension	1.03	1.4	0.9	1.9
Myocardial degeneration	1.4	2.0	2.0	2.8
Pulmonary heart disease*	(7)	(10)	(5)	(21)
Aortic aneurysm	2.2	4.1	2.5	5.4
Arteriosclerosis	0.8	1.8	1.4	3.1
Cerebral vascular disease	1.1	1.5	1.4	1.7
Chronic bronchitis and emphysema	5.7	12.7	8.6	22.5
Pulmonary tuberculosis	2.0	2.8	1.8	5.0
Asthma	2.8	1.8	1.5	1.6
Pneumonia	1.3	1.9	1.6	2.4
Other respiratory disease	1.5	1.6	1.4	1.7
Peptic ulcer	1.5	3.0	1.4	4.5
All causes	1.2	1.8	1.5	2.3

*For pulmonary heart disease mortality rates are given in place of mortality ratios as the rate in non-smokers was zero.

six conditions are seldom or never fatal and evidence has principally been obtained in case–control studies or surveys and only occasionally in cohort studies in which special enquiries have been made about the condition of interest.

Evidence that all these effects can be caused by smoking varies in strength. It includes, in nearly all cases, increases in risk with the amount smoked, decreases in risk since smoking stopped, qualitatively similar findings in different populations in which cigarette smoking has been prolonged, and biologically plausible mechanisms by which the risk of developing the disease could be affected. For some the evidence is very strong. For chronic obstructive pulmonary disease it includes observations on a cohort of workers in whom the rate of deterioration

Box 37.1. Other harmful effects caused in part by smoking

Cancer of lip[38,39]

   nose[38,39]

   stomach[38,39]

   pelvis of kidney[38–40]

   body of kidney[38,39]

   liver[38,39]

   cervix uteri[38,39]

Myeloid leukemia[38,39]

Crohn's disease[41]

Osteoporosis[42]

Periodontitis[43]

Tobacco amblyopia[44]

Age-related macular degeneration[45–47]

Reduced fecundity[48]

Reduced growth of fetus

of lung function in smokers slowed down to that in non-smokers when smoking was stopped.[49,50] For gastric ulcer it includes a randomized controlled trial in which the rate of healing was greater in patients advised to stop smoking (and greatest in those who accepted the advice) than in those not so advised.[51] For ischemic heart disease it includes the evidence that smoking increases the level of plasma fibrinogen[52] and serum apo-lipoprotein B[53] and decreases serum high-density lipoprotein and apolipoprotein A1,[54] all of which effects would increase the risk of the disease. For cancer of the bladder and myeloid leukemia it includes the identification in tobacco smoke of chemicals known to cause these diseases occupationally in humans (2-naphthylamine, benzene), while for cancer of the lung it includes the identification of benzo(a)pyrene which has been shown to form adducts in bronchial DNA that lead to mutations of the type that are sometimes found in lung cancer, particularly in the p53 gene.[55] For some other conditions, the conclusion about causality is

largely based on analogy with other diseases that have been studied more intensively.

Possibly harmful effects

Even these diseases may not constitute all the conditions produced by smoking, as there is some evidence of an increased risk of cataract,[46] impotence[56] and reduced production of sperm.[57] A few other major diseases or causes of death may also be partly due to smoking, though much, if not all, of the associated increase in risk is due to confounding with other etiological agents. These include cancer of the large bowel, cirrhosis of the liver, suicide and poisoning. Confounding with the consumption of alcohol and with personality probably explains most or all of the association with cirrhosis of the liver, suicide and poisoning, but how far the association with cancer of the large bowel can be explained similarly by confounding with alcohol and diet is uncertain.

Beneficial effects

Lastly, there are four diseases in men that occur less often than expected in smokers and may be alleviated or prevented by some of the chemicals in tobacco smoke: namely, Parkinson's disease, ulcerative colitis, aphthous ulcer and allergic alveolitis. Two are not fatal and the combined impact on mortality of their reduction in incidence as a result of smoking is less than 1% of that due to the increased incidence of the diseases caused by smoking that have been listed earlier.

Total effect on risk of death

The sum of all these effects is to double the risk of death in regular smokers after 30 years of age. Some small part of the increase is not directly due to smoking, as it includes the increase in a few causes of death due to confounding with personality, the consumption of alcohol and, to a small extent, a less healthy diet, which may account for about 5% of the excess mortality in cigarette smokers.

Confounding, however, can diminish the apparent effect of cigarette smoking as well as increase it, most notably confounding with the consumption of alcohol, as small or moderate amounts reduce the risk of vascular disease.[58] Precisely what effect this will have on the total risk for cigarette smokers is difficult to estimate and will vary from one population to another depending on the age distribution of the population, the background incidence of vascular disease, and the extent of alcohol use and abuse. In the UK in 1995, the proportion of all deaths over 35 years of age that was attributable to vascular disease in men was high (44%) and the total effect of confounding on the excess risk in middle aged and elderly cigarette smokers may have caused it to be underestimated rather than overestimated.

Benefit from stopping smoking

The harmful effects produced by smoking are, however, not inevitable for they can be reduced if smoking is stopped. Evidence to this effect was indeed part of the body of evidence that led to the conclusion that smoking was a cause of so many diseases. In recent years it has been demonstrated particularly clearly by the findings of two British studies. In one, the smoking habits of male doctors were recorded in 1951 and subsequently in 1957, 1961, 1972, 1978 and 1990 and comparisons could be made between the long-term survival of those who gave up at different ages and those who continued to smoke.[35] Those who stopped under 35 years of age (at a mean of 29 years) had a pattern of survival that did not differ significantly from that of lifelong non-smokers. For those who stopped later the survival was intermediate between that of non-smokers and that of continuing smokers: but even those who stopped at 65–74 years of age (mean 71 years) had age-specific mortality rates beyond 75 years that were appreciably lower than those who continued. The benefit of stopping in late middle or old age is, moreover, certainly underestimated in this analysis because some of those who stopped did so specifically because of illness.

In the other study, information was obtained about the smoking habits of nearly 1000 men and women with lung cancer and over 3000 controls in the years round 1990.[59] Many of the men had stopped smoking and it was estimated that, in the absence of other causes of death the cumulative risk of death from lung cancer by 75 years of age was 15.9% for continuing cigarette smokers and that it fell to 9.9, 6.0, 3.0 and 1.7%, respectively for those who stopped smoking round 60, 50, 40, and 30 years

of age. Very similar findings for the risk of lung cancer were also found in a large American study.[60]

Nicotine addiction

Unfortunately it is not always easy to stop smoking, as the nicotine in tobacco is an addictive drug and the addiction may be hard to break. For some smokers who have, perhaps, not been accustomed to inhale deeply, knowledge of the hazards of smoking and of its economic cost provides sufficient motivation to enable them to stop without great difficulty. For others, however, the withdrawal symptoms are severe and the craving for another cigarette may be overpowering. Addiction to this extent is not uncommon and needs to be treated like a disease by prescribing nicotine replacement therapy and providing psychological support while the therapy is gradually withdrawn. No therapy will work, however, unless the smoker is first mentally convinced of the need to stop.

Conclusion

Cigarette smoking is the single most important cause of death in cigarette smokers in developed countries, since it approximately doubles the risk after about 30 years of age and is consequently as important as all other causes combined. Apart from AIDS in some countries, it is likely to become the single most important cause of premature death in developing countries as well, if cigarette smoking is allowed to become prevalent for a long time. The disease that it produces most notably is cancer of the lung and this has already become the most common fatal cancer in the world. The worst effects can, however, be reduced by stopping smoking and, if it is stopped by or soon after 30 years of age, very little permanent harm is likely to have been done.

References

1. Tilley NW. The Bright Tobacco Industry, 1860–1929. Chapel Hill: University of North Carolina Press, 1948.
2. Sömmering ST. De morbis vasorum absorbentium corporis humani. Frankfurt: Varrentrapp & Wenner, 1795.

3. Bouisson EF. Du cancer buccal chez les fumeurs. Montpelier Med J 1859; 2: 539–99; 3: 19–41.

4. Virchow RL. Die Krankhaften Geschwülste. Berlin: A Hirschwald, 1863–7.

5. Anon. Cancer and smoking. BMJ 1890; 1: 748.

6. Beer GJ. Lehre von den Augenkrankheiten, vol II, Vienna, 1817. (Cited by Duke-Elder WSD. Textbook of Ophthalmology, vol 3, p.3009. London: Henry Kimpton).

7. Heaton JM, McCormick AJA, Freeman AG. Tobacco amblyopia. A clinical manifestation of vitamin B12 deficiency. Lancet 1958; 2: 286–90.

8. Erb W. Ueber dysbasia angiosclerotica ('intermittierendes Hinken'). Münchener med Woch 1904; 51: 905–8.

9. Buerger L. Thrombo-angiitis obliterans: a study of the vascular lesions leading to presenile spontaneous gangrene. Am J Med Sci 1908; 136: 567–80.

10. Hammer A. Ein fall von thrombotischen Verschlusse einer des Kranzarterien des Herzens. Wein Med Wochnschr 1878; 28: 97–102.

11. Herrick JB. Clinical features of sudden obstruction of the coronary arteries. JAMA 1912; 59: 2015–20.

12. Hoffman FL. Recent statistics of heart disease with special reference to its increasing incidence. JAMA 1920; 74: 1364–71.

13. English JP, Willius FA, Berkson J. Tobacco and coronary disease. JAMA 1940; 115: 1327–9.

14. Doll R. Major epidemics of the 20th century: from coronary thrombosis to AIDS. J Roy Stat Soc Series A 1987; 150: 373–95.

15. Rottmann H. Über primäre lungencarcinoma. Inaugural dissertation. Universität Würzburg, 1898.

16. Adler I. Primary Malignant Growths of the Lung and Bronchi. London: Longmans Green & Co., 1912.

17. Tylecote FE. Cancer of the lung. Lancet 1927; 2: 256–7.

18. Lickint F. Ätiologie und Prophylaxe des Lungenkrebes. 2. Statistische Voraussetzungen zur Klärung des Tabakrauchätiologie des Lungenkrebses. Leipzig: Theodor Steinkopff, 1953: 76–102.

19. Hoffman FL. Cancer and smoking habits. Ann Surg 1931; 93: 50–67.

20. Arkin A, Wagner DH. Primary carcinoma of the lung. JAMA 1936; 106: 587–91.

21. Ochsner A, De Bakey M. Carcinoma of the lung. Arch Surg 1941; 42: 209–58.

22. Roffo AH. Durch Tabak bein Kaninchen entwick-ettes Carcinom. Z Krebsforsch 1931; 33: 321–32.

23. Roffo AH. Der Tabak als Krebserzeugende Agens. Deutsche Med Wochnschr 1937; 63: 1267–71.

24. Cooper EA, Lamb FWM, Sanders E, Hirst EL. The role of tobacco-smoking in the production of cancer. J Hyg Lond 1932; 32: 293–300.

25. Müller FH. Tabakmissbrauch und lungencarcinoma. Z Krebsforsch 1939; 49: 57–85.

26. Schairer E, Schöniger E. Lungenkrebs und tabakverbrauch. Z Krebsforsch 1943; 54: 261–9.

27. Wassink WF. 'Onstaansvoorwarden voor Longkanker'. Ned Tijdschr Geneesk 1948; 92: 3732–47.

28. Doll R, Hill AB. Smoking and carcinoma of the lung. Preliminary report. BMJ 1950; 2: 739–48.

29. Wynder EL, Graham EA. Tobacco smoking as a possible etiologic factor in bronchogenic carcinoma. JAMA 1950; 143: 329–36.

30. Chen ZM, Xu Z, Collins R, Li W-X, Peto R. Early health effects of the emerging tobacco epidemic in China: a 16-year prospective study. JAMA 1997; 278: 1500–4.

31. Akiba S, Hirayama T. Cigarette smoking and cancer mortality: risk in Japanese men and women – results from reanalyses of the six-prefecture cohort study data. Environ Health Perspect 1990; 87: 19–26.

32. Lund E, Zeiner-Henriksen T. Smoking as a risk factor for cancer among 260 000 Norwegian males and females (Norw.). Tidsskv Nor Laegeforen 1981; 101: 1937–40.

33. Cederlöf R, Friber G, Hrubec Z, Lorich U. The relationship of smoking and some social variables to mortality and cancer morbidity. The Department of Environmental Hygiene. The Kasolinski Institute, Stockholm, 1971.

34. Best EWR, Josie GH, Walker CB. A Canadian study of mortality in relation to smoking habits. A preliminary report. Can J Public Health 1961; 52: 99–106.

35. Doll R, Peto R, Wheatley K, Gray R, Sutherland I. Mortality in relation to smoking: 40 years' observations on male British doctors. BMJ 1994; 309: 901–11.

36. Thun MJ, Day-lalley CA, Calle EE, Flanders WD, Heath CA. Excess mortality among cigarette smokers: changes in a 20-year interval. Am J Public Health 1995; 85: 1223–30.

37. Office of population censuses and surveys. 1993 Mortality Statistics, Cause. Series DH2 no. 20. London: HMSO, 1995.

38. Doll R. Cancers weakly associated with smoking. Br Med Bull 1996; 52: 39–49.

39. International Agency for Research on Cancer. IARC Monographs on the Evaluation of Cancer Risk of Chemicals to Humans. 2004.

40. International Agency for Research on Cancer. IARC Monographs on the Evaluation of Cancer Risk of Chemicals to Human Tobacco Smoking. International Agency for Research on Cancer, Lyon. 1986; 38.

41. Logan RFA. Smoking and inflammatory bowel disease. In: Wald N, Baron J (eds). Smoking and Hormone-related Disorders. Oxford: Oxford University Press, 1990: 122–34.

42. Law M. Smoking and osteoporosis. In: Wald N, Baron J (eds). Smoking and Hormone-related Disorders. Oxford: Oxford University Press, 1990: 83–92.

43. Eggar P, Duggleby S, Hobbs R, Fall C, Cowper C. Cigarette smoking and bone mineral density in the elderly. J Epidemiol Commun Health 1996; 50: 43–50.

44. Haber J. Smoking is a major risk factor for periodontitis. Curr Opin Periodontol 1994; 12–18.

45. Freeman AG. Optic neuropathy and chronic cyanide intoxication: a review. J Roy Soc Med 1988; 81: 103–6.

46. Christen WG, Glynn RJ, Manson JE, Ajani UA, Buring JE. A prospective study of cigarette smoking and risk of age-related macular degeneration in men. JAMA 1996; 276: 1147–51.

47. Seddon JM, Willett WS, Speizer FE, Hankinson SE. A prospective study of cigarette smoking and age-related vascular degeneration. JAMA 1996; 276: 1141–6.

48. Vingerling JR, Hofman A, Grobee DE, De Jong PTVM. Age-related macular degeneration and smoking. Arch Ophthalmol 1996; 114: 1193–6.

49. Hughes EF, Brennan BG. Does cigarette smoking impair natural and assisted fecundity? Fertil Steril 1996; 66: 679–89.

50. Fletcher CM, Peto R. The natural history of chronic airflow obstruction. BMJ 1977; 1: 1645–8.

51. Doll R, Jones FA, Pygott F. Effect of smoking on production and maintenance of gastric and duodenal ulcer. Lancet 1958; 1: 657.

52. Meade JW, Imeson J, Stirling Y. Effects of changes in smoking and other characteristics on clotting factors and the risk of ischaemic heart disease. Lancet 1987; ii: 986–8.

53. Parish S, Collins R, Peto R et al. For the International Studies of Infarct Survival (ISIS) Collaborators. Cigarette smoking, tar yields, and non-fatal myocardial infarction: 14 000 cases and 32 000 controls in the United Kingdom. BMJ 1995; 311: 471–7.

54. Craig WY, Palomaki GE, Maddow JE. Cigarette smoking and serum lipid and lipoprotein concentrations: an analysis of published data. BMJ 1989; 298: 784–8.

55. Denisenko MF, Pao A, Tang M, Pfeifer GP. Preferential formation of benzo(a)pyrene adducts at lung cancer mutational hot spots in P53. Science 1996; 274: 430–2.

56. Manino DM, Klevers M, Flanders DW. Cigarette smoking: an independent risk factor for impotence? Am J Epidemiol 1994; 140: 1003–8.

57. Nagler HM. Smoking and urology: male fertility and sexuality dysfunctions. In: London WM, Whelan EM, Case AG (eds). Cigarettes: What the Warning Label Doesn't Tell You. New York: American Council on Science and Health, 1996; 96–100.

58. Doll R. The benefit of alcohol in moderation. Drug Alcohol Rev 1998; 17: 353–63.

59. Peto R, Darby S, Deo H et al. Smoking, smoking cessation and lung cancer in the UK since 1950: combination of national statistics with two case-control studies. BMJ 2000; 321: 323–9.

60. Halpern MJ, Gillespie BW, Warner KE. Patterns of absolute risk of lung cancer mortality in former smokers. J Natl Cancer Inst 1993; 85: 457–64.

Further reading

Hill AB. Principles of Medical Statistics, 8th edn. London: The Lancet 1966: 305–13.

Peto R, Lopez AD, Boreham J, Heath C, Thun M. Mortality from Tobacco in Developed Countries, 1950–2000. Oxford: Oxford University Press, 1994.

Segi M, Fukushima L, Fujisako S, et al. An epidemiological study on cancer in Japan. Gann 1957; 48 (Suppl): 1–63.

Simpson WJ. A preliminary report on cigarette smoking and the incidence of prematurity. Am J Obstet Gynecol 1957; 73: 808–15.

Study Group on Smoking and Health. Joint report of study group on smoking and health. Science 1957; 125: 1129–33.

Sugiura K. Experimental production of carcinoma in mice with cigarette smoke tar. Gann 1956; 47: 243–4.

Surgeon General. Smoking and Health. Report of the Advisory Committee to the Surgeon General of the Public Health Service. US Department of Health,

Education and Welfare. Washington, DC: Public Health Services, US Government Printing Office, 1964.

Van Duuren BL. Identification of some polynuclear aromatic hydrocarbons in cigarette smoke condensate. J Natl Cancer Inst 1958; 21: 1–16.

World Health Organization. Epidemiology of cancer of the lung. Report of a study group. WHO Tech Rep Ser 192. Geneva: World Health Organization, 1960.

Wynder EL, Graham EA, Croninger AB. Experimental production of carcinoma with cigarette tar. Part I. Cancer Res 1953; 13: 855–64.

CHAPTER 38

Men as risk takers

Rod Griffiths

Men suffer more mortality, women suffer more morbidity. It is therefore no surprise that there have been many campaigns to improve women's health and to provide services aimed at women despite the fact that men die several years before women.

Men die more often from things that appear self-inflicted, at least to some degree. They die from accidents and the diseases caused by lifestyle factors like smoking and excessive alcohol consumption. It leads to the conclusion that men take risks and that their approach to risk is somehow part of the problem.

Taking risks is not easy to quantify; when risks go wrong the result is obvious but gambles that pay off can also look like skill. Nassim Nicholas Taleb in *Fooled by Randomness*[1] goes to great lengths to show that it is a big mistake to confuse luck with skill. If you get lucky and think you were skillful then you may take a bigger risk next time. Eventually your luck will run out and the resulting failure will be bigger as a result. On the other hand if you mistake skill for luck, then you are less likely to gamble bigger and also more likely to get it right next time – a much safer option. Taleb uses examples from the stock market but the same lessons apply to climbing mountains or driving fast cars.

Many people are poor at measuring risk or assessing probability. Public health professionals are taught statistics but often the media make simple mistakes. In an interview on the BBC's radio 4 'Today' program (the BBC's flagship current affairs program in the UK), a cleric said several times that randomized trials of prayer had produced a positive result 50% of the time; so there must be something in it, he said. He clearly had no understanding of probability but he was not challenged by the interviewers. Ideally there should have been a meta-analysis taking account of methods and sample sizes but saying that there 'must be something in' something that works half the time is like saying, 'I get a coin toss right 50% of the time so I must be a fortune teller'. Given that level of ignorance about probability in the media, it is no surprise that we are all poor at judging risk. But why should men be any different from women?

Bronsen and Howard, in a study typical of many, reviewed sex differences in risk-taking behavior in their students.[2] While it could be argued that taking a sample of psychology students is hardly random, their findings accord with many others. They found that there were many areas where males were bigger risk takers than females, but it was not all one way. Women were more likely to go white water rafting, to be hypnotized (is that risky?), and to skip classes, whereas men were more likely to drive while drunk, drive well over the speed limit, ride a motorcycle, get into a car with a stranger, and get onto the roof of a moving car (you have to admire the originality of some of the questions). The sexes were about equal in riding roller coasters, quitting jobs without another job to go to, shoplifting, and bungee jumping. Men were also more likely to take illegal drugs and to have unprotected sex.

Large institutions, such as insurance companies, build this sort of knowledge into their risk analysis and their premiums. Men pay more for car insurance because they cost the insurance companies more.

In a much bigger study Dohmen and colleagues,[3] in 2005, extracted data from the German socio-economic panel (SOEP) study, which is a large, wide-ranging and representative longitudinal study of private households in Germany. It provides information on all household members, including the old and new German States, foreigners, and recent immigrants to Germany. The Panel was started in 1984. In 2006, there were nearly 11 000 households, and more than 20 000 persons sampled. Some of the many topics include household composition, occupational biographies, employment, earnings, and health and satisfaction indicators; in 2004 the survey included some questions about risk. The survey found that willingness to take risks is negatively related to age and being female, and positively related to height and parental education. Women were less willing to take risks than men, at all ages; increasing age was associated with decreasing willingness to take risks; taller people were more willing to take risks. The education of parents is more complex and has a different impact depending on the nature of the risk studied, but in general the better educated the mother the more likely that the child would be a risk taker, with the father's education showing a weaker effect; however, in the case of financial risks the father's education has more effect.

In this study, the researchers used the SOEP and then followed up with an experiment in which participants were given hypothetical money to invest in various scenarios. Those who claimed in interviews to be willing to take risks also showed a high degree of willingness to take risks in the experiment, in which a relatively large sum of money was at stake. Various statistics collected from other organizations and linked to the sample also seemed to confirm the results: thus, the number of traffic offenses almost paralleled the readiness to take risks in the age group concerned – in other words, the younger the driver, the more carelessly he or she drove. In general the study bore out the idea, prominent in most economic analyses, that risk taking is a general characteristic that plays in a similar way across all sorts of risk. Closer analysis in this study showed that there were more complex responses underneath that general effect so that some people might approach a health risk, for example, in a different way from a sporting risk or a financial risk. When the analysis focused on health, for instance, they found that: 'Willingness to take risks in general has a strong positive impact on the propensity to smoke, but willingness to take risks in the domain of health has an even greater impact.'[3]

Even when these individual types of risk are analyzed independently, the same pattern of males taking more risks than females, the young taking more risks than the old, the tall taking more risks than the short, and better parental education increasing risk taking, tended to hold.

Is it genetic or cultural?

It is not easy to answer the question of whether these differences are genetic or cultural, particularly since the answer may be a bit of both. That doesn't stop fashions in science and the media leaping to conclusions. In the recent past there has been a gene for everything. Eventually the human genome project came to the conclusion that there were a lot fewer genes than originally expected, so a gene for every trait seems less likely; genes may well work together, play off each other, or be triggered by environmental factors to do different things in different circumstances.

It is easy to see why people might think that some of the differences in risk-taking behavior between males and females is genetic. I recently walked my 4-year-old grand-daughter home from school with two 4-year-old male friends of hers. The boys felt compelled to rush ahead and hide behind every available obstacle, to turn down every possible side road. 'Boys will be boys', one might say, but how long does it take for them to learn from other boys what boys do?

The relationship between age and risk taking could be genetic, if different genes turn on at different times; it could be a learned response; it could be a cohort effect because people at different ages have been through different circumstances; or it could just be that older people don't have the energy.

Taller people taking more risks could push the thinking towards the genetic side. However, the detail is more complex: people who were tall as teenagers but who ended up at average height took more risks than those who didn't have an early growth spurt – that feels more like a learned response. The impact of parental education could be placed on either side of the fence – it feels like a social or cultural influence but of course intelligence is inherited to some extent.

The media seem to have a passion for chasing genes. Roger Lancaster, who writes brilliantly on the subject, says, 'In 1996, *The New York Times* inaugurated the silly season of a decade characterized by an unwarranted faith in the power of science to answer questions about the meaning of human existence (and marked in particular by a mania for genetic explanations of the same).'[4] Indeed, in 1996 the paper had reported with a front page headline 'Variant gene tied to a love of new thrills'.[5] Thus was born the 'thrill-seeking gene', a term that circulated widely in print and broadcast news stories, joined heady debates, and quickly entered into vernacular English. Similar excessive enthusiasm surrounded the discovery of a so-called gay gene, but the failure to replicate the initial findings gets less publicity.[6–12] It is understandable that the media would want to be at the front of reporting new discoveries and perhaps understandable why the refutations and failures to replicate findings don't get reported on the front page, but the media also misconstrue the science. Amy Harmon wrote a series in *The New York Times* in the first half of 2006.[13,14] In 'That wild streak? Maybe it runs in the family', she says, 'The recent discoveries include genes that seem to influence whether an individual is fat, has a gift for dance or will be addicted to cigarettes.'[13] The fat gene paper that she refers to describes a gene found in 10% of the population; it may be a contributor, but given that a much greater percentage of the population than that are overweight it can't be the only cause, particularly since the percentages have changed in less than a generation. The 'smoking gene' that she refers to actually controls the rate of metabolism of nicotine – if you have it you could smoke less for the same effect, but

it doesn't make you smoke. To call it a smoking gene is a wild interpretation – perhaps there's a gene for wild interpretations that makes people become journalists.

Why are we so keen to attribute traits that we don't like to our genes? Do we think it absolves us from responsibility in some way? Why does no-one ask the questions: 'What did the smoking gene do before tobacco was discovered? What did the bungee jumping gene do before elastic?' Even if risk taking in general was driven to some extent by genetics and was a characteristic that we were born with, we still have some choice over what risks we take and about any actions we might take to make the activity safer. Even if there was a motorcycling gene it seems unlikely that there would be a motorcycling-without-crash-helmets gene and a motorcycling-with-crash-helmets gene.

The hunt for genes, which still seems insatiable in some parts of the media, throws up some fascinating side stories. Amy Harmon in the same series of articles in *The New York Times* quotes Tony Frudakis, the research director at DNAPrint, who said that the 3-year-old company had coined the term 'American Indian princess syndrome' to describe the insistent pursuit of Indian roots among many newly minted genetic genealogists.[14] If the tests fail to turn up any, Frudakis added, 'this type of customer is frequently quite angry'. DNAPrint calls the ethnic ancestry tests 'recreational genomics' to distinguish them from the more serious medical and forensic applications of genetics. Some of the anger is driven by the fact that there are special funds and scholarships available to certain ethnic groups. It might come as no surprise to find that money is behind some of the enthusiasm for genes but similar vehemence is often attached to belief that particular behavior is related to genetics. How often have you heard someone say, 'I can't help it, it's my genes'?

What should we do about it?

If men are more likely to die young as a result of risk-taking behavior then it is unlikely that market forces will cure the problem. If the very men who ought to demand more safety are themselves dead then the solution has to come from analysis of the statistics and development of effective strategies by society as a whole.

It does not matter whether maleness and risk taking is socially determined or a survival advantage from our evolutionary past; whatever the cause, we can make dangerous activities safer. Perhaps the most extreme example is in Formula 1 racing over the 55 years of its existence. It is now very unusual for a driver to be injured despite there being some massive crashes. It is reasonable to assume that the champions share similar skills and propensity for taking risks, so changes in racing-related fatalities among champions are most likely to have been determined by making the business safer rather than by changes in the behavior of the drivers. Of the 31 people who have been world champions since 1950, four died in motor racing accidents, three of them in the first 20 years of Formula 1 and only one in the next 35 years. These numbers are too small for formal statistical analysis but anyone who doesn't think that Formula 1 cars are now safer than they used to be should see the details of Robert Kubica's crash in 2007: he hit a concrete wall at over 140 miles per hour.[15] A few minutes on the website Youtube allows comparison with the crashes that killed Jochen Rindt in 1970 and Wolfgang Von Trips in 1961 – the damage done to the cars is similar, the difference is that Kubica left hospital the next day. During the 1980s the underlying attitudes in Formula 1 changed from laughing in the face of danger to engineering every element of the business to deliver as much excitement as possible with the maximum elimination of risk. In countless other areas there have been similar changes at the detailed level; in almost every aspect of society there are regulations and regulatory bodies that have specific remits to deliver a safer and more predictable world. Outside formal regulation, the concept of due diligence lays a responsibility on almost anyone to be as safe as might reasonably be expected in almost any activity. Change is possible.

Making dangerous activities safe is easier than creating safe lifestyles as a whole, but the past few years have also shown that apparently entrenched habits like smoking can be changed by social pressures. Effective leadership, particularly in the Republic of Ireland, showed how the social environment and attitudes to smoking can be changed.

Over the past century many formerly accepted behaviors have been altered – the emancipation of women and the universal education of children on the scale that has taken place would have been outside the average imagination a hundred years ago – but most of these changes have not been aimed at male behaviors associated with premature mortality.

Much of the analysis that might underpin change has been done, what are missing are the strategies and determination to make a difference. There is no point in men dying 4 or 5 years before women, but society has just not got around to doing anything about it. Some change in the future will happen as a side effect of reducing smoking, but we need to go further. It is fascinating to speculate as to why there has been no political will to do something about male mortality at either end of the age spectrum. It appears that society does not mind if old men die before their wives, nor does it mind if young men die. In middle life it seems quite clear that there is an expectation that men will work and that society expects this and rewards it. At the same time there seems to be some confusion as to what young men are for; there is little interest in their development, they are more likely to fail at school than girls and more likely to take up crime, to take drugs, or to kill themselves through suicide or accidents. At the other end of life we have become used to there being more women alive, and grandmothers appear to have clearer roles than grandfathers.

There needs to be a new debate, a new social contract. If society expects men to continue to use their youth to test themselves, we need to find ways to do it more safely and to create a culture that can deal with failure as part of learning and development. It's not the adventure that kills, it's when it goes wrong, and that is true whether it's driving a car or trying to form relationships. We need to create safe ways to fail and to celebrate the learning that comes from it.

In later life the situation is also complex and makes no sense, and it is in everyone's interest to change it. Men who are widowed tend to get more resources from the health and care systems because there is an unspoken view that men are less able to look after themselves. Widows, age for age, get less help than widowers. We live in a society where it is common for young men to marry girls younger than themselves, and the end result is thus an even longer period of widowhood and relative neglect for their wives. Widows often depend on a pension that is reduced when the husband dies. In the past few years there has been considerable discussion of aging and it's economic consequences but little discussion of the differential mortality between the sexes. Failing to keep men healthy and to deal with early male mortality is condemning many women to end their lives alone and poor. This is a system that is failing everyone.

References

1. Taleb NN. Fooled by Randomness: The Hidden Role of Chance in Life and in the Markets. London: Penguin, 2007.
2. Bronsen ME, Howard E. Gender Differences and their Influence on Thrill Seeking and Risk Taking. St Joseph, Missouri: Missouri Western State University, 2008 [http://clearinghouse.missouriwestern.edu/manuscripts/365.asp].
3. Dohmen T, Falk A, Huffman D, et al. Individual Risk Attitudes: New Evidence from a Large, Representative, Experimentally-Validated Survey. Discussion Paper No. 1730. Bonn: Forschungsinstitut zur Zukunft der Arbeit (Institute for the Study of Labor), 2005. [http://ftp.iza.org/dp1730.pdf].
4. Lancaster RN. Sex and Race in the Long Shadow of the Human Genome Project. New York: Social Science Research Council, 2006 [http://raceandgenomics.ssrc.org/Lancaster/].
5. Angier N. Variant gene tied to a love of new thrills. The New York Times, 2 January 1996.
6. Rice G, Anderson C, Risch N, Ebers G. Male homosexuality: absence of linkage to micro-satellite markers at Xq28. Science 1999; 284; 665–7.
7. Bailey JM, Dunne MP, Martin NG. Genetic and environmental influences in sexual orientation and its correlates in an Australian twin sample. J Pers Soc Psychol 2000; 78: 524–36.
8. Byne W, Tobet S, Mattiace LA et al. The interstitial nuclei of the human anterior hypothalamus: an investigation of variation with sex, sexual orientation, and HIV status. Horm Behav 2001; 40: 86–2.
9. Lancaster R. The Trouble with Nature: Sex in Science and Popular Culture. Berkeley, California: University of California Press, 2003: 268–71.
10. Marshall E., NIH's 'gay gene' study questioned. Science 1995; 268: 1841.
11. Finn R. Biological determination of sexuality heating up as a research field. The Scientist 1996; 10: 13–16.
12. Kaiser J. No misconduct in 'gay gene' study. Science 1997; 275: 1251.
13. Harmon A. Seeking ancestry in DNA ties uncovered by tests. The New York Times, 12 April 2006.
14. Harmon A. That wild streak? Maybe it runs in the family. The New York Times, 15 June 2006.
15. Stringent safety measures save Kubica. Automative FIA Sport, 2 July 2007 [http://www.fia.com/automotive/issue10/sport/article1.html].

CHAPTER 39

Keeping fit: avoiding and diagnosing chronic soft-tissue injuries

David Sutherland Muckle

Introduction

Keeping fit should be easy, but it isn't! Sedentary lifestyles, regular use of transportation, good food and drink, plus the increasing demands of a stressful life, have placed fitness on the back-burner of many people's lives. Sport is important for the obvious reasons – it maintains cardiovascular health, strengthens bones and muscles, uses up excess calories, promotes a feeling of wellbeing and relaxation, fosters discipline, and releases tensions and aggression in a controlled manner. There is no better way to bond with one's peers and form close relationships. However, sport need not be unduly vigorous to be effective, and it can be carried out at any age – a good, brisk walk with a rambling club over 10–20 km is easily achieved into the 70s or even 80s.

But one must be fit to train – as well as train to be fit. Simply to burst forth, in an uncontrolled release of enthusiasm to get fit, will result in injury. To see men wobbling at a walking pace in an effort to jog on hard surfaces sends shivers down the most hardened sports doctor's spine, as well as sending unnatural forces up the spine of the jogger.

First of all, lose weight! Walking briskly and running can magnify the body's weight by four to six times through the lower limb joints. Do not embark on long-distance running or raquet or contact sports without a period of diet and lighter exercise. This can be swimming (when the body is relatively weightless) and walking (increasing the pace and distance with time). Of course dietary intake should be controlled. Most people can lose 0.5–1 kg each week – regimens that say otherwise are not usually speaking the truth.

Over 3–4 weeks of increasing light exercise, the muscle fibers will begin to increase in size (hypertrophy), and this includes the heart muscle. More blood is ejected with each beat and so the pulse falls for a given cardiac output. Even moderate athletes have a lower resting pulse and blood pressure than others. Joints and soft tissues become more flexible. Now the chosen sport can be commenced – with the right equipment and on the right surface. For example, fancy running shoes look good in the shop but may irritate the Achilles tendon or predispose to ankle sprains or metatarsal fractures.

Humans are forest creatures. They were born to run on relatively soft, grassy surfaces, in and out of shade, in a moderately moist environment. Instead we now have concrete and synthetic surfaces. So the forces generated by exercise (and a falling man has enough energy to fracture any bone he wishes) judders up the soft tissues (ligaments, muscles, tendons and fascia), through lower limb joints, and up the spine.

Without an adequate warming up period of 15 minutes (and a similar warming down period at the end) the tissues are unprepared for any exertion. So, in time, frozen shoulder, tennis elbow, golfer's elbow, groin strain, adductor tendinitis, hamstring tears, shin splints and Achilles tendinitis can occur, amongst others (Fig. 39.1).

In such cases we look to the soft tissues for pathology – micro-tears, scarring, hematoma formation, and calcification; but often no obvious defect is found. Still the sportsman struggles on – with an array of therapies, including corticosteroid injections, ultrasonics, and massage. Surgical intervention may even be needed. However, it must be recalled that in any soft tissue injury there may be a spontaneous resolution in time, even without any form of intervention.

In some patients, when the chronic discomfort of a soft tissue injury becomes refractory to treatment, one may have to look to the spine for the root of the problem. Several years ago, I was struck by the frequency of tennis elbow in a certain age group which mirrored the onset of cervical disc degeneration and prolapse. The use of magnetic resonance imaging (MRI) scanning often indicated degeneration and prolapse of one or more discs in the cervical spine in cases of refractory tennis elbow (lateral epicondylitis). In such cases, neck therapy proved beneficial. Not all chronic injuries are a reflection of spinal problems, but one must keep such disorders in mind, especially in troublesome cases.

Frozen shoulder

Classically a frozen shoulder limits abduction to below 70°, and tenderness is found over the anterior capsule with a subacromial bursitis. The bursa may respond to corticosteroid injections and physiotherapy. Sometimes the small tendon of supraspinatus becomes frayed, torn, or even converted into soft calcified tissue (like toothpaste). Gymnasium enthusiasts who exceed their comfortable weight or repetition program can suffer suprapinatus pain and weakness, when the arm cannot be comfortably lifted from the side. Ultrasonic or MRI scanning will give an accurate diagnosis, and surgery usually leads to an excellent cure.

In older men the outer joint of the clavicle (with the acromial process of the scapula) becomes irregular or even spiky. Such shoulder pathology is found in golf and tennis players, for example. It can be treated by the trimming of the encroaching bone using an arthroscopic method.

In some cases of frozen shoulder (pericapsulitis), arthroscopic studies have often shown a band of inflamed synovium across the anterior aspect of the capsule (in the distribution of the C5–C6 nerve) beneath the subscapularis muscle. Scanning may show pathology in the cervical spine at this level, indicating a combined spinal and peripheral problem. The restriction of shoulder abduction occurs because there is thickening, pain and tightness of the anterior capsule, for abduction of the shoulder beyond 90° requires external rotation of the arm. Therapy to restore full external rotation is mandatory, and sometimes release of the anterior capsule by an arthroscopic technique is required.

Raquet players may also detach part of the glenoid labrum as well as damaging the subscapularis muscle at the front of the shoulder. Scanning and surgery are sometimes needed.

Tennis elbow and golfer's elbow

Tennis and golfer's elbow conditions are a problem in tennis, squash, golf, throwing sports, and rowing. The muscle–tendon junction generally tears, owing to repetitive action, although both conditions can reflect pathology at C5–C6 through the recurrent branch of the radial nerve from a double crush (neck/peripheral compression) situation. The ulnar nerve can become scarred from minor bleeds and need freeing from this scar tissue in its groove behind the elbow, while a small branch of the ulnar nerve as it passes behind the medial humeral epicondyle can be implicated in golfer's elbow. Therapy should be directed to the neck, if involved, as well as the limb.

Groin strain

In almost 40 years of treating sportspeople, I have found that two conditions occur more frequently than previously; these are groin strain and stress fractures of the lumbar spine. Could they be related in any way? Stretching or tearing of the lower abdominal muscles around the inguinal rings in footballers and rugby players can lead to a fatty hernia or even a small bowel hernia. The mechanism

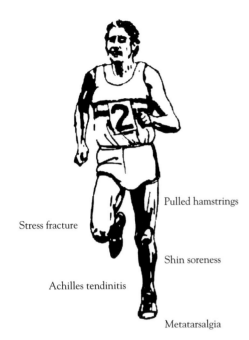

Figure 39.1. *Repetitive trauma of long distance running.*

cited is the repeated internal and external rotation of the lower limb. However, this explanation ignores the simple fact that such rotation is at the hip alone and all muscles that rotate arise from the pelvic wall below the inguinal rings, apart from the psoas major, which originates from the lumbar vertebrae.

The mechanism of kicking in rugby and football demands extension of the back and hip, with the psoas major muscle pulled taut to flex the lower limb powerfully and, as a secondary feature, to produce internal rotation of the limb (Fig. 39.2). The short external rotators must counterbalance this internal rotation and keep the foot pointing forwards. Thus the psoas tendon, external rotators, and back are all at risk. Weight-lifting (which most sportsmen seem to find mandatory) and an excessively strenuous training schedule can, by their repetitive nature, cause back and lower abdominal muscle overloading, the latter leading to weakness around the inguinal rings.

The simple repair of all groin strains by suturing the weakened inguinal area is effective in over 90% of patients. However, there is a small percentage of

cases in which the lumbar spine is involved. One can identify and treat L3–L4 or L4–L5 discs as the cause of the groin pain. This level of disc therapy seems to 'fly in the face' of the anatomy books, which state that the groin area is only supplied by L1 and L2 nerves (i.e. over the inguinal ring and inner upper thigh). However, the obturator nerve (anterior division) arises from L3–L4, and when compressed by a disc bulge, can produce pain in the groin and also over the adductor longus tendon, where it forms a plexus of nerves with the femoral nerve.

Hamstring injuries

Football is ballet with a ball. As the lower limb reaches towards a right angle with the trunk to collect a waist-high ball the hamstrings are pulled taut at the ischial tuberosity. Anyone dealing with chronic back problems notes that the patient cannot carry out a straight-leg-raising test (often beyond 50°) or touch the toes.

With lower lumbar problems, the hamstrings tighten both reflexly and through a lack of active stretching as a result of pain. Thus, when the footballer is asked to trap or collect a high ball or produce a sudden sprint, the tight hamstring muscle fibers tear – usually at the tendon–muscle interface. The lateral hamstring (biceps femoris) has the common peroneal (lateral popliteal) almost adherent to its lower third, and pain can be severe. One common cause of hamstring problems in footballers is a stress lesion affecting either L5–S1 or L4–L5, sometimes with a forward slipping of one vertebral body on another. With a forward slip, the disc between the vertebrae may be disrupted, which adds to the nerve root irritation, at L5, S1 and S2. Lumbar discs can on their own, of course, produce nerve irritation and muscle spasm. The back needs investigation by isotope or MRI scanning in all cases of recurrent hamstring injury.

Shin soreness

Micro-fractures in the tibia or scarring of the leg muscles cause shin pains; any faulty running

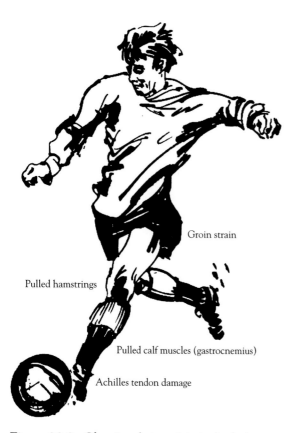

Groin strain

Pulled hamstrings

Pulled calf muscles (gastrocnemius)

Achilles tendon damage

Figure 39.2. *Chronic soft tissue injuries in the lower limb.*

hamstring pulls) to irritation of the lumbo-sacral nerve roots.

Achilles tendonitis

The Achilles tendon can tighten as a result of repetitive strains (especially running on hard surfaces) as a result of inadequate footwear, thus producing abnormal pronation–supination of the foot. Tendon degeneration may cause micro-tears, which sometimes coalesce to a sudden rupture. Surgery is often used when conservative measures fail. However, an area of the calf is supplied by lumbosacral nerves, and disc or facet joint changes at this level can result in Achilles tightness (a mild spasticity) and tearing. As for example with tennis elbow, the prevalence of Achilles tearing mirrors the onset of disc problems, usually in persons in their late 30s. Once again, it may be wise to investigate the lower lumbar spine.

Conclusion

This brief chapter is to promote fitness in the overweight and unfit. It is not intended to catalog so many complaints that participants will be deterred from sport. It is meant to inform and warn of the risks, which are low when exercise is sensibly approached. There are usually fitness coaches in most clubs and gymnasiums who are willing to advise on warming up and warming down, stretching exercises, diet, and nutrition. Many doctors take an active interest in sport and in sports medicine. An early consultation is best, before any injury has had the chance to become chronic. Finally, it is also a chapter to stimulate and aid in the reappraisal of chronic soft tissue injuries in sport, especially the associated spinal problem, which can easily be overlooked.

technique may be corrected by podiatry measures, including the use of inserts in the footwear, and by avoiding hard surfaces. Physiotherapy is beneficial, but sometimes surgical release of the thickened fascia that binds the tibial muscle is needed. Isotope bone scanning identifies the micro-fractures; cessation from exercise for 2–4 months allows the bone to heal. Gastrocnemius strain can be linked (like

CHAPTER 40

Men's body image

Donald R McCreary

Introduction

Over the past few decades, there has been a plethora of research studying women's body image. However, during the same time period, researchers focused very little energy studying men's body image. Several relatively robust and consistent factors combined to create this knowledge gap. First, researchers had shown that, compared with women, men were much less concerned or dissatisfied with their bodies.[1] Second, men tended not to be as concerned as women with their degree of body fat and, even though they were more likely than women to be overweight,[2] they were less likely to be dieting to lose weight. Third, men were much less likely than women to experience clinical eating disorders such as anorexia nervosa and bulimia nervosa, men representing approximately 5–15% of anorexics and 0.4–20% of bulimics.[3] These types of sex differences led many researchers and clinicians to assume that men are relatively happy with their bodies and do not have significant body image concerns.[1]

However, what this generation of researchers failed to address was that the social standard of attractiveness for men's bodies is qualitatively different from the social standard for women's bodies. That is, while the female standard is focused on a thin ideal, the male standard is focused on a muscular ideal: what Mishkind et al. described as the muscular mesomorphic shape.[4] In other words, Western society does not want its men to be small and thin, it wants them to be big and muscular.

Supporting evidence for society's focus on the muscular standard of bodily attractiveness for men comes in many forms. Media portrayals often provide an indication of the body stereotypes associated with men in the greater culture. Several studies have shown the media's increasing emphasis on men's muscularity over the past 25 years. For example, researchers have shown that some of the most popular action figures among North American boys (GI Joe, Batman, Superman) changed substantially over the years.[5,6] Between 1964 and 1996, the GI Joe action figure alone became so muscular that even competitive body builders could not hope to achieve the equivalent degree of muscularity (33-inch waist, 62-inch chest, 32-inch arms). This hyper-muscularization is not limited to action figures, for researchers have shown that portrayals of men in other forms of media also have become more muscular.[7,8]

A second area of research that shows society's emphasis on the muscular male physique comes from men's and women's expectations of what is the most attractive body type for men, as well as what type of body heterosexual men think women want in a man. Men and women commonly rate a muscular mesomorphic physique as the most desirable body shape for men,[9] and women rate men with a broad chest, wide shoulders, and narrow waist (i.e., the classic V-shape) as more attractive than men whose chest and shoulders do not form such a V-shape.[10] In addition, men tend to think that women want a man who is more muscular than he really is.[11,12]

Other evidence of the importance of the muscular ideal comes from the social pressure exerted on boys by parents and peers to be muscular.[13] There is growing evidence that parents (especially fathers) can strongly influence boys' motivation to develop a more muscular body. In fact, some studies have shown that parents exert more of an influence than the media with regard to boys' desires to become more muscular.[14] But peers, especially same-sex peers, appear to have the strongest influence on boy's body image.[14] Peers use social pressure, teasing, and popularity concerns to shape the muscular ideal in boys and male adolescents.[13,15,16]

The impact that the muscular ideal has on men's health and wellbeing is explored throughout the rest of this chapter. Four specific topics are focused upon: body dissatisfaction, the drive for muscularity, muscle dysmorphia, and supplement use. The chapter concludes with a discussion of clinical implications.

Body dissatisfaction

Typical studies of body dissatisfaction have focused on men's and women's perceptions of their body weight or adiposity. While there are several different ways in which this has been assessed, the most common procedures have involved using categorical or Likert-scale self-reports and silhouette ratings. Researchers using categorical or Likert-scale self-report methods typically ask participants to rate their current weight status (e.g. along a continuum – from thin to very overweight – or categorically – such as overweight, normal weight, underweight). Alternatively, the researchers may categorize participants' weight themselves, based on anthropomorphic measurements [e.g. body mass index (BMI)]. In addition to categorizing their weight, researchers also ask participants questions about how satisfied they are with their weight, their body, or their life. In some instances the researchers assess general or specific aspects of participants' mental health (e.g. self-esteem, depression). The presence of differences between weight status groups on these types of outcome ratings is an indication that body dissatisfaction is present in some groups to a greater extent than in other groups. Silhouette rating studies use a different approach. When using this method,

men and women are presented with a set of nine same-sex silhouettes that range from very thin to very overweight. The participants are typically asked to indicate the silhouette that corresponds most closely to their perceptions of their *current body size*; participants are then asked to repeat the process by indicating the silhouette that is closest to their *ideal body size*. The difference between the current and ideal ratings is used as an indication of body dissatisfaction.

Two convergent themes about men's body dissatisfaction have emerged from these different lines of research. The first finding is that men, like women, appear to experience body image misperceptions. However, whereas women tend to think they are heavier or bigger than they really are, men tend to think they are lighter or smaller than they actually are.[17] For example, researchers using adiposity-based silhouettes have shown that more than half of men want an ideal body that is bigger than their perceptions of their current body.[9] Similarly, studies comparing men's perceived weight status to their BMI-based weight status (overweight, underweight, normal weight, using international guidelines) have shown that, among men 20–64 years of age, 30–50% of objectively overweight men think they are normal weight.[17] Another study replicated these findings, but also showed that 25% of normal-weight men in their 20s believed they were underweight.[18] The fact that men think they are small and light may be a factor behind the results from research showing that between 20% and 68% of men and boys are on diets to gain weight.[19]

The second theme to emerge from research on men's body dissatisfaction is that being thin is the most undesirable body size for men. This has been demonstrated in studies that show that:

- men who perceive themselves to be underweight are more dissatisfied with their weight than men who think they are overweight;[19,20]
- underweight men see themselves as less attractive and less healthy than overweight men;[18]
- underweight men are more at risk than normal or overweight men for depression, suicide ideation, and suicide attempts.[21]

Thus, men tend to see themselves as smaller and lighter than they really are, and this misperception is associated with adverse psychological outcomes. However, when men look at themselves in the mirror and see someone smaller than they would like, are they picturing an ideal physique that is bigger because it has more body fat or because it has more muscle? Furthermore, when men say they are dieting to gain weight, are they attempting to add physical bulk in the form of body fat or are they increasing their caloric intake (or the use of specific types of food) to support a weight-training regimen? Does it matter to men whether they add bulk in the form of body fat or muscle, or is it just better to be big no matter what form that bulk takes? These are important issues to consider and are addressed next.

Drive for muscularity

Given that the social standard of bodily attractiveness for men is based on the muscular ideal, to what extent does the research on men's body dissatisfaction reflect a desire to be more muscular rather than fatter? Researchers have just begun to examine this question in a focused manner,[22] with initial research suggesting that men equate dieting and being thin with women and femininity, and being muscular with men and masculinity.[23,24]

One of the most commonly used approaches to ask men about their desire to become more muscular has been the use of pencil-and-paper questionnaires. The Drive for Muscularity Scale[25] is the most commonly used and most thoroughly validated measure to date.[26] The Drive for Muscularity Scale is a 15-item questionnaire that asks respondents to describe their attitudes about their muscularity and the behaviors they engage in to become more muscular. Other measures include the Swansea Muscularity Attitudes Questionnaire[27] and the Drive for Muscularity Attitudes Questionnaire.[28]

Findings from the use of these questionnaires have shown that those with a higher drive for muscularity also tend to report higher levels of depression symptomatology, social physique anxiety, neuroticism, narcissism, and perfectionism, as well as poorer self-esteem. People with a high drive for muscularity also appear to be highly focused on their bodies, reporting higher levels of fitness and

appearance orientation and a greater tendency to be regular weight-trainers, and they are more likely to be dieting to gain weight to support their weight-training regime.[19,26] The drive for muscularity also has been linked to men's perceptions of their masculinity. Men with higher scores on the Drive for Muscularity Scale report having more traditional sex roles, including an unhealthy focus on the self to the exclusion of others, an emphasis on status, toughness, and anti-femininity, and a heightened need to win at all costs.[26]

Other researchers have adapted the adiposity-based silhouettes for use in assessing men's desire to be muscular. Initially, this involved creating a series of figures that ranged from not at all muscular to very muscular.[29] An example of this type of silhouette-based measure can be found in Fig. 40.1.[30] When these types of silhouettes were used, men reported an ideal figure that was significantly more muscular than their perceptions of their current degree of muscularity.[29] However, there are two problems with using these types of silhouettes. First, they confound body fat with muscularity (i.e. muscle is found under a layer of body fat). For muscle to be shown at its best, the percentage of body fat must be low. However, this is not always the case: men with high levels of body fat also may be very muscular, but it would be less evident because it would be hidden to a greater degree. The second limitation is that different researchers have created their own sets of silhouette figures and these can vary substantially in terms of the degree of muscularity ascribed to each figure. This means that the findings reported by researcher A may not be generalizable to the findings reported by researcher B because the two sets of silhouette figures were not equivalent in their degree of muscularity.

The Somatomorphic Matrix (SM) addresses these two limitations.[31] The SM is a 10×10 matrix of figures of men whose anthropometric characteristics vary along two dimensions: body fat (x-axis) and muscularity (y-axis). Each of the figures has a known body fat percentage and fat-free mass index (i.e. an index of the amount of lean muscle mass). Participants use the matrix to identify the figure that most closely approximates their perceptions of their body as it currently is. They then identify the body that most closely represents their ideal.

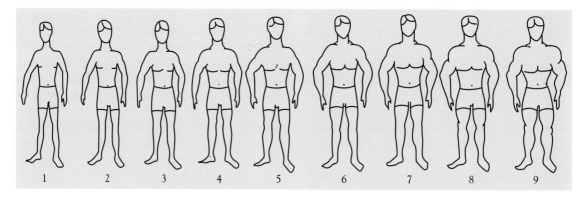

Figure 40.1. *An example of a set of muscle-based figure silhouettes used to assess muscularity dissatisfaction and the drive for muscularity in men. Adapted from reference 30.*

Using the SM, it can be determined whether the desire to be more muscular that was found in previous studies actually represents a desire to increase muscle mass rather than physical bulk (which could be a combination of the two), as well as whether there is a corresponding desire to have less body fat so that the muscle can be shown off to its best advantage.

Findings from studies using the SM have shown that men typically see their ideal body as being an average of 8–13 kg more muscular than their current one, with either no, or just a slight, reduction in body fat.[12,32] Furthermore, men believe that women want them to have approximately 14 kg more muscle than they currently have on their bodies.[12] The more muscular men want to be, the more symptoms of depression they report, the lower their self-esteem, and the greater likelihood they are using performance-enhancing substances such as creatine, ephedrine, and adrenal steroids.[32]

In sum, it appears as though men have internalized the muscular ideal society places on men's bodies. Those who have internalized the social standard more completely have a higher drive for muscularity, and those with a higher drive for muscularity report more adverse psychological outcomes. But is there such a thing as having too strong a drive for muscularity? As Olivardia[33] notes, 'Although there is nothing wrong with a healthy pursuit of muscularity and being fit, there exists a clinical phenomenon at the severe end of this continuum that is anything but healthy.' The phenomenon

being referred to here is muscle dysmorphia, a subset of body dysmorphia, which is a clinical obsession with being muscular. However, there is another related problem that may come from taking the muscular ideal too far: utilizing dangerous and untested performance-enhancing supplements, such as anabolic androgenic steroids (AASs). Both of these issues are discussed next.

Body dysmorphic disorder and muscle dysmorphia

Body dysmorphic disorder (BDD) is a psychological disorder defined by three general criteria. First, the person has a preoccupation with an imagined defect in his or her physical appearance. Second, the preoccupation leads to a clinically significant amount of distress that may result in an impairment in one's social activities, occupational pursuits, or other important aspects of day-to-day living. And third, the preoccupation should not be a symptom of another psychological disorder (e.g. anorexia nervosa or bulimia nervosa). Researchers studying BDD have shown both sex similarities and differences in the prevalence and characteristics of this disorder.[34] The prevalence of BDD appears to be the same in men and women, and the two sexes appear to experience BDD in relatively similar ways, with two exceptions: women appear to have an earlier onset of the disorder, and men's symptoms seem to be more severe and they appear to have a poorer level of functioning. But it is when one focuses on the imagined physical deficit that the sex difference becomes most apparent: men tend to focus on the size of their genitals, their degree of muscularity, and thinning hair, whereas women focus mostly on a wide variety of weight-related issues.[34]

The tendency for men to be obsessively preoccupied with their muscularity has been termed muscle dysmorphia.[35] Newly recognized and not yet part of the Diagnostic and Statistical Manual (DSM) of Mental Disorders, muscle dysmorphia is considered to be a form of BDD. Those with muscle dysmorphia tend to be mostly men who have a high drive for muscularity[36] and engage in persistent activities designed to increase their muscle mass (e.g. weight-training, high-protein diets, use of supplements, use of AASs), even though they already are excessively muscular. Their perceived lack of muscularity causes them a great degree of distress and they organize their daily activities around maximizing the time they can devote to becoming more muscular. As a result, they tend to isolate themselves from their larger social network because they are embarrassed to show their bodies in public.[33,35,37]

The diagnostic criteria for muscle dysmorphia are similar to the criteria for body dysmorphic disorder. Olivardia[38] outlines them as follows:

1. The person has a preoccupation with the idea that his or her body is not sufficiently lean and muscular.
2. The preoccupation causes clinically significant distress or impairment in social, occupational, or other important areas of functioning as demonstrated by at least two of the following four criteria:

    a. The individual frequently gives up important social, occupational, or recreational activities because of a compulsive need to maintain his or her workout and diet schedule.

    b. The individual avoids situations in which his or her body is exposed to others, or endures such situations only with marked distress or intense anxiety.

    c. The preoccupation about the inadequacy of body size or musculature causes clinically

significant distress or impairment in social, occupational, or other important areas of functioning.

    d. The individual continues to work out, diet, or use performance-enhancing substances despite knowledge of adverse physical or psychological consequences.

3. The primary focus of the preoccupation and behaviors is on being too small or inadequately muscular, and not on being fat, as in anorexia nervosa, or on other aspects of the appearance, as in other forms of BDD (p. 255).

As this is a relatively new phenomenon, there are currently no conclusive data on the population prevalence of muscle dysmorphia, its comorbidities, or assessment options and treatment effectiveness. What is known about muscle dysmorphia is that it is found mostly in men. Current estimates suggest there are several hundred thousand men in the USA alone who could meet the full diagnostic criteria, with thousands more who could meet the subclinical threshold.[33] The disorder may reach clinical significance in the late teens or early 20s, but there are younger teenage boys manifesting symptoms of the disorder.[37] In addition, the presence of muscle dysmorphia has been associated with current or prior diagnoses of mood disorders, a past or current eating disorder, and current AAS use.[36,37,39]

With regard to assessment options, it appears that two self-report measures might be useful pre-screening tools: the Muscle Appearance Satisfaction Scale[40] and the Muscle Dysmorphia Inventory.[41] Although the utility of the Drive for Muscularity Scale in this context still needs to be determined,[33] using the other two scales as initial screening tools allows for broad sampling of large groups of men by those with only minimal training. When measures such as these identify those with a potential diagnosis of muscle dysmorphia, a structured clinical interview would then be conducted by a trained interviewer.[33] If a muscle dysmorphia diagnosis follows, treatment options include psychoeducational interventions addressing topics such as the health implications of excessive exercise, AAS use, and balanced diets, as well as body image ideals and the various sociocultural factors that influence our perceptions of them. Another treatment option that has proven effective is cognitive behavioral therapy.[33]

Finally, there is only a limited understanding of the etiology of muscle dysmorphia at the present time. Biopsychosocial models describing the factors that are believed to contribute to the development of muscle dysmorphia are only now being developed.[33,42] Various models suggest that muscle dysmorphia and obsessive–compulsive disorders share a similar biological or genetic predisposition.[33] In addition, lack of desired body mass may prove to be a trigger for the onset of the disorder.[42] Psychological variables that are associated with muscle dysmorphia include high levels of the drive for muscularity and poor self-esteem. Also, perfectionism and negative affect have been implicated in the development of muscle dysmorphia.[42] Various cultural factors are also thought to influence the development of this disorder, specifically media portrayals of men's physiques, and peer and parental socializing influences.[42] It should be noted that, while there is evidence to support the correlations between some of these variables and the drive for muscularity, the evidence linking them to muscle dysmorphia (especially as causal factors) is limited at best. Similarly, being actively involved in weight-training does not appear to predispose a person to muscle dysmorphia. A recent study, for example, showed that regular weight-trainers can be classified into one of five groups, and the muscle dysmorphia group represented only 18% of the sample. The remaining 82% were psychologically healthy.[39] Thus, until researchers delineate the disorder and its antecedents and consequences more completely, models such as these should be considered guides only.

Anabolic-androgenic steroid use

For a body to develop muscularity, it relies on testosterone. However, there are biological limitations to the degree of hypertrophy that men can attain, so some men ingest or inject one of many synthetic derivatives of testosterone, the AASs. AASs accelerate the body's natural ability to masculinize and build muscle tissue, often allowing men to develop a degree of muscularity that they would not be able to

attain naturally. However, AASs have a wide range of physical and psychological side effects. Adverse physical effects include testicular atrophy, kidney and liver damage (especially for oral AASs), infertility, reduced immune system functioning, coronary artery disease, musculoskeletal problems, acne, various tumors and cysts, and increased risk for HIV and AIDS (via contaminated needles). The most common psychological side effects are negative affect and general irritability, as well as an increased tendency toward uncontrollable aggression (often referred to colloquially as 'roid rage').[43] In most Western countries, AASs are available legally only through a physician, and most men who use AASs buy them illicitly.

The use of AASs varies widely. Much of the research emanates from the USA and focuses on abuse in adolescents and athletes, though the assumption is that many adolescents use AASs to enhance their athletic performance.[44] However, there is also growing evidence to suggest that more and more non-athletes are using AASs in order to achieve a hyper-muscular physique, and that non-athletic users might actually outnumber athletes who use AASs.[45,46]

Those who use AASs often fail to understand the risks. For example, in a study of British weight-trainers, many believed that AASs were only harmful if used excessively.[47] The irony was that most of these respondents were stacking[43] AASs in dangerous quantities (with some taking as many as 15 doses in a single day).[47] AAS users in this study also were more likely than non-users to believe that many people who weight-train take AASs (i.e. they experience what health risk researchers call pluralistic ignorance). Lastly, AAS users are not deterred by the side effects. At least one study suggests that the more side effects a person experiences, the more satisfied they are with the drugs.[48]

Given the risks associated with taking AASs, the fact that men go to great lengths to find and use them suggests that muscularity might be an obsession with this group of men. For AAS users, becoming muscular is the ultimate goal and they will ignore the risks in order to achieve that outcome. It has been suggested that AAS use in men might be a proxy for BDD or muscle dysmorphia. Furthermore, comparing the prevalence of AAS use in men with the prevalence of anorexia and bulimia in women might provide an indication of sex similarities in body image disturbance. Although the rates of all three are thought to be underestimated, it has been suggested that in men the prevalence of AAS use is greater than the rate in women of anorexia, and equal to the rate in women of bulimia.[49]

There are few studies evaluating the treatment options for those who abuse AASs, though problems with withdrawal symptoms often are mentioned.[43] More emphasis has been put into studying the effectiveness of psychoeducational interventions targeted at preventing AAS use in high-risk populations and, especially, youth.[43] These studies show that organized psychoeducational interventions are somewhat effective at reducing AAS over the short- and long-term.[43]

Conclusions and clinical implications

This overview of the current scientific literature of men's body image reveals several key points. First, the social standard of bodily attractiveness for men is the muscular ideal, which differs from the thin ideal for women. Second, men tend to underestimate their weight, whereas women tend to overestimate theirs (e.g. a large number of overweight men actually think they are normal weight). Third, thinking one is small and light is associated with several adverse outcomes for men, including depression and suicide risk. Fourth, men who diet are more likely to be dieting to gain weight than dieting to lose weight. Fifth, men's desire to be big reflects a desire to be muscular, especially larger pectorals, biceps, wrists, shoulders, or forearms, and flatter abdominal muscles.[25] Sixth, men with a higher drive for muscularity tend to have poorer levels of psychological functioning (e.g. higher depression, lower self-esteem). Seventh, an obsession with one's muscularity (i.e. muscle dysmorphia) is a particular outcome that appears to be gaining in prevalence. And lastly, AAS use is associated with the desire to be muscular and represents a further physical health risk to those who have internalized the social standard of male bodily attractiveness to an unrealistic degree.

These findings have several implications for clinicians. The first implication has to do with treating overweight men. Overweight men are less likely than overweight women to believe they need to lose weight, and therefore are less likely to be dieting to lose weight. Given that men associate dieting with women and femininity,[23] getting men to diet may be difficult. The second implication is that, given the societal emphasis on muscular men, clinicians may underestimate men's risk for developing eating disorders (e.g. anorexia or bulimia). Third, clinicians need to educate themselves about muscle dysmorphia, including its symptoms, causes, and treatment options. Lastly, clinicians need to develop a more thorough understanding of the prevalence and treatment options for those abusing AASs.

References

1. Feingold A, Mazzella R. Gender differences in body image are increasing. Psychol Sci 1998; 9: 190–5.
2. Must A, Spadano J, Coakly EH et al. The disease burden associated with overweight and obesity. JAMA 1999; 282: 1523–9.
3. Olivardia R, Pope HG, Mangweth B et al. Eating disorders in college men. Am J Psychiatry 1995; 152: 1279–85.
4. Mishkind ME, Rodin J, Silberstein LR et al. The embodiment of masculinity: cultural, psychological, and behavioral dimensions. Am Behav Sci 1986; 29: 545–62.
5. Pope HG, Olivardia R, Gruber A et al. Evolving ideals of male body image as seen through action toys. Int J Eating Disord 1999; 26: 65–72.
6. Baghurst T, Hollander DB, Nardella B et al. Change in sociocultural ideal male physique: an examination of past and present action figures. Body Image 2006; 3: 87–91.
7. Harrison K, Bond BJ. Gaming magazines and the drive for muscularity in preadolescent boys: a longitudinal examination. Body Image 2007; 4: 269–77.
8. Leit RA, Pope HG, Gray JJ. Cultural expectations of muscularity in men: The evolution of Playgirl centerfolds. Int J Eating Disord 2001; 29: 90–3.
9. Jacobi L, Cash TF. In pursuit of the perfect appearance: Discrepancies among self-ideal perceptions of multiple physical attributes. J Appl Social Psychol 1994; 24: 379–96.

10. Swami V, Tovée MJ. Male physical attractiveness in Britain and Malaysia: A cross-cultural study. Body Image 2005; 2: 383–93.

11. Lavine H, Sweeney D, Wagner SH. Depicting women as sex objects in television advertising: Effects on body dissatisfaction. Person Social Psychol Bull 1999; 25: 1049–58.

12. Pope HG, Gruber AJ, Mangweth B et al. Body image perception among men in three countries. Am J Psychiatry 2000; 157: 1297–301.

13. Gray JJ, Ginsberg RL. Muscle dissatisfaction: an overview of psychological and cultural research and theory. In: Thompson JK, Cafri G, eds. The Muscular Ideal: Psychological, Social, and Medical Perspectives. Washington, DC: American Psychological Association, 2007: 15–39.

14. McCabe MP, Ricciardelli LA. Sociocultural influences on body image and body changes among adolescent boys and girls. J Social Psychol 2003; 143: 5–26.

15. Jones DC, Crawford JK. Adolescent boys and body image: weight and muscularity concerns as dual pathways to body dissatisfaction. J Youth Adolesc 2005; 34: 629–36.

16. Jones DC. Body image among adolescent girls and boys: a longitudinal study. Dev Psychol 2004; 40: 823–35.

17. McCreary DR. Gender and age differences in the relationship between body mass index and perceived weight: exploring the paradox. Int J Mens Health 2002; 1: 31–42.

18. McCreary DR, Sadava SW. Gender differences in relationships among perceived attractiveness, life satisfaction, and health in adults as a function of Body Mass Index and perceived weight. Psychol Men Muscul 2001; 2: 108–16.

19. McCreary DR, Sasse DK. Gender differences in high school students' dieting behavior and their correlates. Int J Mens Health 2002; 1: 195–213.

20. Page R, Allen O. Adolescent perceptions of body weight and weight satisfaction. Percept Mot Skills 1995; 81: 81–2.

21. Carpenter KM, Hasin DS, Allison DB et al. Relationships between obesity and DSM-IV major depressive disorder, suicide ideation, and suicide attempts: results from a general population study. Am J Pub Health 2000; 90: 251–7.

22. Thompson JK, Cafri G. The Muscular Ideal: Psychological, Social and Medical Perspectives. Washington, DC: American Psychological Association, 2007.

23. Grogan S, Richards H. Body image: focus groups with boys and men. Psychol Men Muscul 2002; 4: 219–32.

24. McCreary DR, Saucier DM, Courtenay WH. The drive for muscularity and masculinity: Testing the associations among gender role traits, behaviors, attitudes, and conflict. Psychol Men Muscul 2005; 6: 83–94.

25. McCreary DR, Sasse DK. Exploring the drive for muscularity in adolescent boys and girls. J Am Coll Health 2000; 48: 297–304.

26. McCreary DR. The Drive for Muscularity Scale: description, psychometrics, and research findings. In: Thompson JK, Cafri G, eds. The Muscular Ideal: Psychological, Social, and Medical Perspectives. Washington, DC: American Psychological Association, 2007: 87–106.

27. Edwards S, Launder C. Investigating muscularity concerns in male body image: Development of the Swansea muscularity attitudes questionnaire. Int J Eating Disord 2000; 28: 120–4.

28. Morrison TG, Morrison MA, Hopkins C et al. Muscle mania: development of a new scale examining the drive for muscularity in Canadian males. Psychol Men Muscul 2004; 5: 30–9.

29. Lynch SM, Zellner DA. Figure preferences in two generations of men: the use of figure drawings illustrating differences in muscle mass. Sex Roles 1999; 40: 833–43.

30. Peters MA, Phelps L. Body image dissatisfaction and distortion, steroid use, and sex differences in college age body builders. Psychol Schools 2001; 38: 283–9.

31. Gruber AJ, Pope HG, Borowiecki J et al. The development of the somatomorphic matrix: A biaxial instrument for measuring body image in men and women. In: Olds TS, Dollman J, Norton KI, eds. Kinanthropometry VI. Sydney: International Society for the Advancement of Kinanthropometry, 1999: 217–31.

32. Olivardia R, Pope HG, Borowiecki JJ et al. Biceps and body image: The relationship between muscularity and self-esteem, depression, and eating disorder symptoms. Psychol Men Muscul 2004; 5: 112–20.

33. Olivardia R. Muscle dysmorphia: Characteristics, assessment and treatment. In: Thompson JK, Cafri G, eds. The Muscular Ideal: Psychological, Social, and Medical Perspectives. Washington, DC: American Psychological Association 2007: 123–40.

34. Phillips KA, Menard W, Fay C. Gender similarities and differences in 200 individuals with body dysmorphic disorder. Compr Psychiatry 2006; 47: 77–87.

35. Pope HG, Gruber AJ, Choi P et al. Muscle dysmorphia: an underrecognized form of body dysmorphic disorder. Psychosomatics 1997; 38: 548–57.

36. Maida DM, Armstrong SL. The classification of muscle dysmorphia. Int J Mens Health 2005; 4: 73–91.

37. Olivardia R, Pope HG, Hudson JI. Muscle dysmorphia in male weightlifters: a case-control study. Am J Psychiatry 2000; 157: 1291–6.

38. Olivardia R. Mirror, mirror on the wall, who's the largest of them all? The features and phenomenology of muscle dysmorphia. Harv Rev Psychiatry 2001; 9: 254–9.

39. Hildebrandt T, Schlundt DG, Langenbucher J et al. Presence of muscle dysmorphia symptomology among male weightlifters. Comprehensive Psychiatry 2006; 47: 127–35.

40. Mayville SB, Williamson DA, White MA et al. Development of the muscle appearance satisfaction scale: A self-report measure for the assessment of muscle dysmorphia symptoms. Assessment 2002; 9: 351–60.

41. Rhea DJ, Lantz CD, Cornelius AE. Development of the muscle dysmorphia inventory (MDI). J Sports Med Phys Fitness 2004; 44: 428–35.

42. Grieve FG. a conceptual model of factors contributing to the development of muscle dysmorphia. Eating Disord 2007; 15: 63–80.

43. National Institute on Drug Abuse. Anabolic Steroid Abuse (NIH Publication Number 06-3721). Washington, DC: National Institute of Health, 2006.

44. Goldberg L, Elliot DL. The prevention of anabolic steroid use among adolescents. In: Thompson JK, Cafri G, eds. The Muscular Ideal: Psychological, Social, and Medical Perspectives. Washington, DC: American Psychological Association, 2007: 161–80.

45. Korkia P, Stimson GV. Indications of prevalence, practice, and effects of anabolic steroid use in Great Britain. Int J Sports Med 1997; 18: 557–62.

46. Perry HM, Wright D, Littlepage BN. Dying to be big: a review of anabolic steroid use. Br J Sports Med 1992; 26: 259–61.

47. Wright S, Grogan S, Hunter G. Motivation for anabolic steroid use among bodybuilders. J Health Psychol 2000; 5: 566–71.

48. Hildebrandt T, Langenbucher J, Carr S et al. Predicting intentions for long-term anabolic-androgenic steroid use among males: a covariance structure model. Psychol Addict Behav 2006; 20: 234–40.

49. Spitzer B L, Henderson KA, Zivian MT. Gender differences in population versus media body sizes: a comparison over four decades. Sex Roles 1999; 40: 545–65.

SECTION **8**

Miscellaneous topics

CHAPTER 41

Men and help seeking

Alan White, Ian Banks

Introduction

Gender has long been accepted as an important dimension of health inequalities, and more recent research and policy development have begun to focus on men's disadvantage in health as well as women's.[1,2] From an international perspective, analysis of morbidity and mortality data[3,4] show that countries differ with respect to overall life expectancies and the principal causes of death, but a common feature is that men's rate of premature death is still higher than women's across the majority of disease states and that there are also significant differences between men depending on cultural and socioeconomic circumstances.

In 2001, a scoping study on men's health[5] was conducted and found four key areas as being central to the discussion on factors influencing men and their health:

- Access to health services
- Lack of awareness of their health needs
- Inability to express their emotions
- Lack of social networks.

The majority of the respondents in this study saw men's reluctance to access health services as the principal issue facing men. Excellent healthcare services can be provided, but unless the man walks through the door then they will not have any impact. A prime example of this relates to the delay some men have in seeking medical assistance when faced with acute chest pain – millions of dollars are spent on the development of thrombolytic drugs, but they are effective only if administered within a short time period after myocardial infarction. Well man clinics have been tried in many different forms, but the majority have found very little uptake, unless by those men in the middle and upper social classes whose overall health is already improving, the groups that need the service the most being the least likely to attend.

This delay in seeking help has repercussions on men's health in terms of the degree of morbidity when they do present and the risk of avoidable premature death. It also has financial implications for caring for the chronically sick, with its health and social care components, as opposed to eliciting a cure, and for the inappropriate use of accident and emergency services if the general practitioner (GP) is avoided.

Nevertheless, though there is a lot we know about consultations with health professionals, there is also much we are still uncertain of; principally there is still a dearth of epidemiological analysis of actual healthcare usage broken down by sex to allow exploration of when and why men and women use the health services.

Data on men and help seeking

The number of consultations for a typical practice in England was estimated as 29 446 in 2006, which equates to an estimated annual volume of consultations in England of 289.8 million.[6] Though we know the average number of visits by age and even by socioeconomic circumstances, we do not know for certain why patients had the consultation in the first place or what the outcomes were.

We also know that GP partners held an average of 87 surgery consultations per week, equivalent to an average of 11.7 minutes per consultation (an increase from 8.4 minutes in 1992–1993). In addition they had an average of 17 telephone consultations that lasted on average 7.1 minutes each. Unfortunately the length of consultations is estimated by dividing the average length of surgeries by the average number of patients seen and so it is not possible to break the consultation duration down by sex.[7]

When we look for quantitative studies that have explored men's experience of using health services there are few to consider. There is little dispute that men do not have as many GP consultations in their early adulthood as women (Fig. 41.1). However, it is not clear what the reasons are for these visits or whether they indicate delay in seeking help and therefore have an overall effect on treatment options and patient outcomes.

A large-scale study undertaken in Denmark[8] that was based on a total of 35.8 million contacts with GPs and 1.2 million hospitalizations in 2005 showed a male pattern of lower contact rates with the GP but higher hospitalization and mortality rates (Fig. 41.2). This is compatible with a scenario in which men react later to severe symptoms than women so that they are more likely to be hospitalized for or die from the causative condition.

The latest publicly available detailed data on GP consultations come from the *Morbidity Statistics from General Practice Fourth National Study 1991–1992*.[9] Examination of these data does seem to suggest that men are presenting later in their illness. A higher proportion of men than women seem to present within the 'serious' category of severity for the majority of health conditions (Fig. 41.3), and this trend seems to go across the age span (Fig. 41.4). A particular concern with men is in the early adult years when various studies have shown they are at particular risk of developing and prematurely dying from a range of health conditions.[3,4] When the data for the age range 25–44 are considered it can be seen that for all disorders except conditions relating to endocrine, nutritional, metabolic, and immune problems, men were more likely to present within the 'serious' category of severity (Fig. 41.5).

It is also worth noting from the *Living in Britain: General Household Survey 2002*,[10] that when respondents were asked about inpatient stay in the previous 12 months, nearly twice as many men as women in the 65–74 age group reported hospitalization (Fig. 41.6), which would also tend to support the findings of the Danish study by Juel and Christensen.[8]

White[11] undertook an analysis of the data presented in a US health report.[12] The data suggest that over the entire lifespan there is little difference between men and women with regard to the

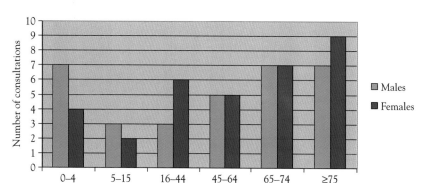

Figure 41.1. *Average number of general practice consultations per person per year by sex and age, England and Wales, 2002.*[10]

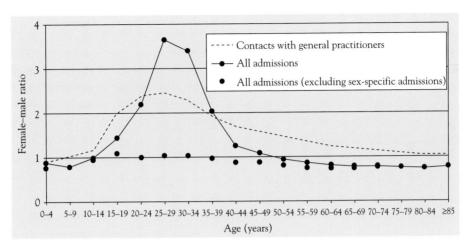

Figure 41.2. *Female–male ratio of contacts with general practitioners and hospital admissions in Denmark, 2005.[8] By permission of Oxford University Press.*

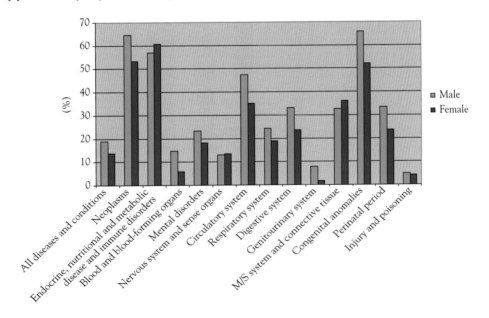

Figure 41.3. *Proportion of male to female consultations with a medical practitioner (rates per 10 000 person-years at risk) by 'serious' category of severity by sex. Calculated from McCormick et al.[9]*

distribution of ambulatory visits by primary diagnosis, but when the data are broken down by age the pattern changes. Though the assumption is that the higher usage of the healthcare system by women in the 18–44 year age group can be attributed to their peak years of reproductive health, it is also notable that women also have a higher consumption of

prescription medications generally, and when the specific data on prescription trends were explored, women were found to have a higher rate of prescription utilization for every category of medication surveyed.

Examination of prescription trends in the 45–64-year age group again revealed a higher utilization

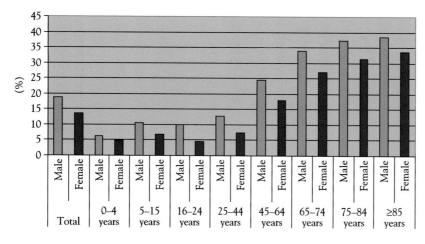

Figure 41.4. *Proportion of male to female consultations (rates per 10 000 person-years at risk) with medical practitioner, by 'serious' category of severity, by sex and age. Calculated from McCormick et al.[9]*

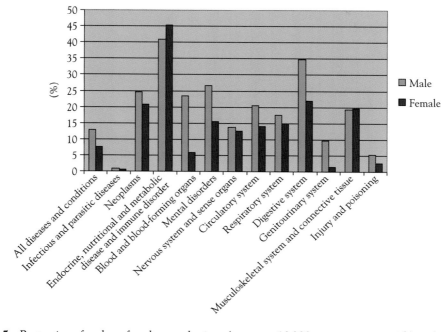

Figure 41.5. *Proportion of male to female consultations (rates per 10 000 person-years at risk) with medical practitioner, by 'serious' category of severity, by sex, in those aged 25–44 years. Calculated from McCormick et al.[9]*

rate for women than that for men for the majority of medication classifications, with the exceptions to this trend including anti-hyperlipidemic agents, angiotensin converting enzyme (ACE) inhibitors, and non-narcotic analgesics.

The analysis also suggested that women are more likely to receive preventive healthcare services from primary care specialists than age-matched male controls above the age of 15 years. It also revealed that a larger percentage of men have admitted to having no regular and definable access to healthcare (21.8% of men compared with 11.6% of women). It also showed that 21.8% of women compared with 18.2% of men visited the emergency department one or more times over the course of 2003 and that 8.4% of women compared with 5.6% of men had two or more visits over the same time period, which seems to cast doubt on the myth that men tend to use the emergency department instead of their family doctor.

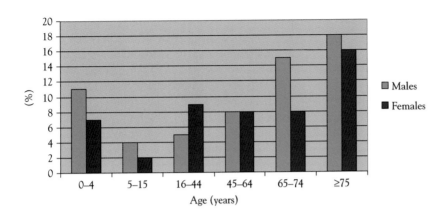

Figure 41.6. *Inpatient stays in the 12 months before interview, by sex and age, England and Wales, 2002.*[10]

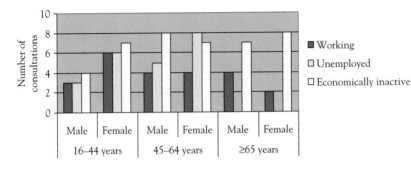

Figure 41.7. *Average number of consultations per person per year, by sex, age, and economic activity status, England and Wales.*[10]

Impact of socioeconomic status

The data on usage of health services by socioeconomic status show that men who are unemployed and in manual work tend to have higher rates of attendance at health centers as shown by prescription rates. The 'Living in Britain' study[10] demonstrates that a higher proportion of males living in households whose household reference person was in the routine and manual group consulted a doctor in the 2 weeks prior to interview than of males in intermediate group households and managerial and professional group households (Fig. 41.7).

Economically inactive men were over twice as likely to consult a doctor in the 2 weeks before interview as those who were working. The differences were evident in all age groups. It also showed that men who were economically inactive had an average of 6.5 consultations per year, whereas those who were working had an average of 3.5. Among people who had consulted a GP in the 2 weeks before interview, those living in households where

the household reference person was in the routine and manual group were more likely to receive a prescription than those in managerial and professional households.

Men and help seeking

There are conflicting messages from the literature and from research that has looked specifically at men's help-seeking behavior. Review of one study[13] showed no concrete evidence that men were less willing to report health-related symptoms or to seek healthcare and that there was no difference in the degree of suffering that men in comparison with women experienced prior to seeking help. Wyke et al.[14] using the same dataset found that though women reported more symptoms than men there was no difference in the likelihood of women reporting them. Similarly Adamson et al.[15] found no difference between men and women in the likelihood of their seeking health advice, the differences being based on socioeconomic and ethnic background.

Nevertheless across a broad band of health issues men are reported to delay in seeking help from the conventional services. This includes men with HIV and AIDS,[16,17] men with cancer,[18,19] men with emotional problems,[20,21] and men with chest pain.[22,23] There are also specific groups of men who are reluctant users of the health services, such as homeless men[24,25] and young men.[26–28] (See also the comprehensive review of the literature by Addis and Mahalik.[29])

The relationship between masculinity and reluctance to seek help has been at the center of a number of recent studies. White, when studying the impact of chest pain on men, found that there was a significant delay between the onset of the first signs of a problem and gaining assistance.[22,30] This persisted for some even when the pain was unendurable, with many different excuses made for the pain. In most cases the man's spouse was the person the man turned to to help validate his decision to seek assistance. The problem seemed to be focused around uncertainty over the meaning of the pain, worry over being seen to be a 'fraud' through calling for help when it was not necessary, and a reluctance to lose control over one's own health (i.e. the man had to accept that he couldn't manage the problem himself and that he would need help).

In a development from this study, Galdas compared the experiences of Caucasian men with those of men of South Asian descent.[23] He found that for the majority there was a feeling that they should 'act like a man', but this differed between the Caucasian men and the South Asian men. For the Caucasian men the dominant, or hegemonic, representation of masculinity that seemed to be the greatest influence was the belief that chest pain alone was a symptom unworthy of concern, and there was a perceived need to display a high tolerance for pain and a fear of being seen by others to be acting 'soft' if medical help was sought. By contrast, for the South Asian men, chest pain was a symptom worthy of concern, coupled with a willingness to discuss their symptoms with others and to seek help from their GP.

A study that looked at this issue from a different perspective was undertaken by O'Brien et al., whose research was focused onto different groups of men and how they saw the relationship between society's expectations of them as men and how they managed their health.[31] What emerged from the research was that they all recognized the pressure to conform to the hegemonic form of masculinity and that they should be reluctant to seek help, but help seeking was more quickly embraced when it was perceived as a means to preserve or restore another, more valued, enactment of masculinity – for instance, among men in the fire service who were very concerned about their health because it was seen as a necessity to be fit and well for the good of the team and their role, or in cases in which sexual function was impaired.

The problem of men accepting that they needed help was also explored by Richardson, who found the way men perceived their health needs changed depending on the nature of their illness, with it being easier to accept that help was required with 'normal' physical problems than with embarrassing conditions, such as erectile dysfunction (which seems at odds considering the findings noted above), depression, or health problems more associated with women (e.g. osteoporosis and breast cancer).[32] There were other factors that were associated with increased help seeking, which included: increased feeling of responsibility following such life events as becoming a father; experience of ill-health in others or previous experiences of personal delay and its implications; faith in their medical practitioners; having a partner who instigated help-seeking behavior; increasing age coupled with a growing sense of vulnerability; and when services were convenient. The men in Richardson's study also reported significant difficulties in relation to accessing the health centers, with concern over opening times, the female-orientated waiting rooms, the time disparity between their appointment time and actually getting to see the doctor, and the feeling of incomplete or rushed consultations; moreover, almost half the respondents felt that they were left with unanswered questions. There were also significant issues around the challenge that seeking help made on their sense of self-worth and masculinity.

Robertson's interview-based study of men's health practices found a tendency for the health center to be a 'feminised space'; one familiar to women in relation to health screening and checks but only for use by men when actually 'ill'.[33] There was a tension men felt in relation to 'healthy lifestyle' and health-seeking behavior. On one hand, as 'real men' they were expected not to show care or concern about health and well-being, but, on the other hand, as good citizens, there is a moral obligation to show care and concern, to live well and seek appropriate help. Robertson termed this the 'don't care/should care' dichotomy that men face. Consequently, any use of health services had to be legitimized for the men in some way; 'health' could not be done for its own sake. Examples of what could legitimate engaging with health services included:

- Observing ill health in close friends or relatives
- Having a family history of particular health problems
- Having a level of injury or symptoms or impairment that meant that seeking help was justified – not to do so would be irrational
- Being encouraged to seek help by significant others (usually the spouse or a female family member).

What these studies seem to be implying is that though it is blatantly wrong to judge all men the same, it is possible to discern components of their health behavior that have been influenced by socialization processes that affect a significant proportion of men. A consequence of the social expectations men have experienced from birth is that they have affected how men seek help, and this can have negative consequences on health outcomes.

Lessons learnt from community-based initiatives

There has been an increase over the past 5 years in community-based services that have recognized this difficulty and have set about specifically targeting men. These services have been based on the premise that if men find accessing traditional health center-based services problematic then it is better to go to where the men are and offer them a more male-focused service than to have men miss out altogether

on preventative healthcare. Three of these initiatives have been the subject of substantial research projects. Different models of delivery have been trialled; two recent ones include those seen in the Bradford and Airedale Health of Men Initiative and the Preston Men's Health Project.

Bradford and Airedale Health of Men Initiative

The Bradford Health of Men team in West Yorkshire, UK were awarded a £1 million grant to develop services for men and boys, with matched funding from the local primary care trust. Their approach was to go into the community to offer male-focused services within schools, youth centers, places of worship, work environments, social settings such as community centers and pubs, and barber shops. The research study that followed this initiative focused on trying to understand why men used these new health initiatives and to explore how the team worked with the men to see what lessons could be learnt.[34]

The key findings from the study can be summarized.

- None of the 50 men interviewed gave the impression that they did not care about their health.
- Men will access health services for preventative care if it is made available to them in a form that they can easily access.
- Moving out from the health center brings primary care to many more people, but men will attend clinics if given a medical reason.
- Working with industry and community-based services is effective at opening new avenues for the delivery of primary care.
- The time it takes to set up services is longer than for women, owing to the need for credibility to be built up and for 'word-of-mouth' support to grow. Incentives are often necessary to get the men engaged.
- Health screening alone is only part of the effectiveness of the service; giving the men time to talk in confidence allows a much wider range of health issues to be identified.

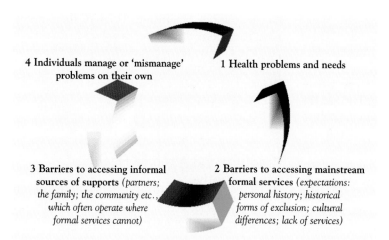

Figure 41.8. *The Preston Model of Service Need. Reprinted from reference 35, with permission from Elsevier.*

- Anonymity is as important as confidentiality for young men.
- Practitioners engaging with men in their settings need specific skills.
- Male-orientated resources need to be developed and tested.
- Having a team with a range of expertise enabled a broader range of activities to be supported.

The team also found that they could set up health checks within the health center when the men were invited through a letter giving an actual appointment time.

The Preston Men's Health Project

The Preston Men's Health Project[35] in Lancashire, UK ran from 2002 till 2006. It was funded by the Avenham Central Single Regeneration Budget and the Neighbourhood Renewal Fund and comprised outreach work by predominantly voluntary community partners with established groups of men. The eight initiatives included in the evaluation were: Homeless men and Nutrition, Young Men and Boys, Elderly Men, Gay and Bisexual men, African–Caribbean men, Asian men, Men with Disabilities, and a Nurse-led Outreach Project.

Many of the clients participating in these groups shared broadly similar life trajectories that impacted on their service needs in similar ways. The study found that their health needs and their difficulties in

seeking help can be explained through commonly experienced failures of informal support (from family or community) and formal support (institutional; medical; statutory), leading men to manage or mismanage their health in their own ways (Fig. 41.8).

From their work based on trying to understand men's health practices, it seems that services must do three things.

- Raise expectations – men are not going to use services if they don't think they are there for them to use.
- Repair informal networks – even when men are accessing services, following through on living with an illness or a particular problem requires a wide range of supports at a family and community level.
- Provide access to formal services – part of the solution is not simply designing men's health services, but practically working through how they are going to be accessed and sustained within the everyday routines of men's lives.

Conclusions

When the data relating to men's high rates of premature death are mapped against the studies, that have been done on men's usage of health services and help-seeking behavior it appears that there may be a relationship between the two; however, this relationship has not been fully tested and it is premature to make such claims. Nevertheless, it is worth recognizing that despite current advances, medical management is still much more effective if early diagnosis is made to maximize treatment options and to reduce the extent of morbidity and the risk of premature death.

To achieve the goal of early diagnosis there is a need to improve our outreach to men; in part this can be done by making current health centers more accessible, but there must be a recognition that we will not benefit from just making opening hours longer. The reality for many men is that they would still not access a GP if they did not feel unwell, and therefore there should be investment in finding ways of targeting men more effectively such that problems are identified before they become too advanced.

References

1. Acheson ED. Independent Inquiry into Inequalities in Health Report. London: Department of Health, 1998.
2. Mackenbach JP. Health Inequalities: Europe in Profile. Rotterdam: Erasmus MC, 2005. http://www.dh.gov.uk/assetRoot/04/12/15/84/04121584.pdf
3. White AK, Cash K. The State of Men's Health Across 17 European Countries. Brussels: The European Men's Health Forum, 2003.
4. White AK, Holmes M. Patterns of mortality across 44 countries among men and women aged 15–44. J Mens Health Gend 2006; 3: 139–41.
5. White AK. Scoping Study on Men's Health. London: Department of Health, 2001.
6. Hippisley-Cox J, Fenty J, Heaps M. Trends in Consultation Rates in General Practice 1995 to 2006: Analysis of the QRESEARCH Database. Final Report to the Information Centre and Department of Health. QResearch and The Information Centre for Health and Social Care, 2007.
7. 2006/07 UK General Practice Workload Survey. London: The Information Centre, Primary Care Statistics, 2007.
8. Juel K, Christensen K. Are men seeking help too late? Contacts to general practitioners and hospital admissions in Denmark 2005. J Public Health 2007.
9. McCormick A, Fleming D, Charlton J. Morbidity Statistics from General Practice Fourth National Study 1991–1992. London: HMSO, 1995.
10. Office for National Statistics. Living in Britain 2002: General Household Survey. London: Office for National Statistics, 2004.
11. White AK. Men and the problems of late diagnosis. In: Heidelbaugh JJ, ed. Clinical Men's Health: Evidence in Practice, 1st edn. Philadelphia: Elsevier, 2007; 31–43.
12. Health United States, 2005: With Chartbook on Trends in the Health of Americans. Hyattsville MD: National Center for Health Statistics, 2005.
13. Macintyre S, Ford G, Hunt K. Do women 'over-report' morbidity? Men's and women's responses to structured prompting on a standard question on long standing illness. Soc Sci Med 1999; 48: 89–98.
14. Wyke S, Hunt K, Ford G. Gender differences in consulting a general practitioner for common symptoms of minor illness. Soc Sci Med 1998; 46: 901–6.
15. Adamson J, Ben-Shlomo Y, Chaturvedi N, Donovan J. Ethnicity, socio-economic position and gender: do they affect reported health-care seeking behaviour? Soc Sci Med 2003; 57: 895–904.
16. Petchley RB, Farnsworth B, Williams J. 'The last resort would be to go to the GP.' Understanding the perceptions and use of general practitioner services among people with HIV/AIDS. Soc Sci Med 2000; 50: 233–45.
17. Randall M, Barroso J. Delayed pursuit of health care among HIV-positive gay men enrolled in a longitudinal research study. J Assoc Nurses AIDS Care 2002; 13: 23–31.
18. Evans REC, Brotherstone H, Miles A, Wardle J. Gender differences in early detection of cancer. J Mens Health Gend 2005; 2: 209–17.
19. Smith LK, Pope C, Botha JL. Patients' help-seeking experiences and delay in cancer presentation: a qualitative synthesis. Lancet 2005; 366: 825–31.
20. Green CA, Pope CR. Gender, psychosocial factors and the use of medical services: a longitudinal analysis. Soc Sci Med 1999; 48: 1363–72.
21. Möller-Leimkühler AM. Barriers to help seeking by men: a review of sociocultural and clinical literature with particular reference to depression. J Affect Disord 2002; 71: 1–9.
22. White AK, Johnson M. Men making sense of their chest pain – niggles, doubts and denials. J Clin Nurs 2000; 9: 534–41.

23. Galdas PM. The Influence of Masculinity on White and South Asian Men's Help-Seeking Behaviour for Chest Pain. Unpublished PhD Thesis. Leeds, UK: University of Leeds, 2006.

24. Brush BL, Powers EM. Health and service utilization patterns among homeless men in transition: exploring the need for on-site, shelter based nursing care. Scholarly Inquiry Nurs Pract 2001; 15: 143–54.

25. Shiner M. Adding insult to injury: homeless and health service use. Sociol Health Illn 1995; 17: 525–49.

26. Davies J, McCrae BP, Frant J. Identifying male college students' perceived health needs, barriers to seeking help, and recommendations to help men adopt healthier lifestyles. J Am Coll Health 2000; 48: 259–67.

27. Richardson CA, Rabiee F. A question of access: an exploration of the factors that influence the health of young males aged 15–19 living in Corby and their use of health care services. Health Educ J 2001; 60: 3–16.

28. Lloyd T, Forrest S. Boy's and young men's health: literature and practice review. An Interim Report. London: Health Development Agency, 2001.

29. Addis M, Mahalik JR. Men, masculinity, and the contexts of help seeking. Am Psychol 2003; 58: 5–14.

30. White AK. 'I feel a fraud': men and their experiences of acute admission following chest pain. Nurs Crit Care 1999; 4: 67–73.

31. O'Brien RK, Hunt K, Hart G. 'It's caveman stuff, but that is to a certain extent how guys still operate': men's accounts of masculinity and help seeking. Soc Sci Med 2005; 61: 503–16.

32. Richardson N. Men's Health Practices and the Construction of Masculinities. Unpublished PhD thesis. Bristol, UK: University of the West of England, 2007.

33. Robertson S. Understanding Men and Health: Masculinities, Identity and Well-being. Buckingham, UK: Open University Press, 2007.

34. White A, Cash K, Conrad D, Branney P. The Bradford and Airedale Health of Men Initiative: a study of its effectiveness in engaging with men. Leeds: Leeds Metropolitan University, 2008.

35. Kierans C, Robertson S, Mair MD. Formal health services in informal settings: findings from the Preston Men's Health Project. J Mens Health Gend 2007; 4: 440–7.

CHAPTER 42

Men's health in primary care: an emerging paradigm of sexual function and cardiometabolic risk

Martin M Miner, Richard Sadovsky

Introduction

Gender-based medicine – specifically recognizing the differences in the health of men and women – drew much attention in the 1990s. The US National Institutes of Health (NIH) Office of Research on Women's Health was established in 1990, and in 1994 the US Food and Drug Administration (FDA) created an Office of Women's Health, resulting in a dramatic increase in the quantity and quality of research devoted to examining numerous aspects of women's health such that today women's health research is clearly mainstream.[1]

While decades of research have yielded many important findings about health and disease in men, this knowledge has not resulted in the benefits expected. Men are still less likely than women to seek medical care and are nearly half as likely as women to pursue preventive health visits or undergo screening tests.[2] Recent data indicate that 68.6% of men aged 20 years and older are overweight,[3] and life expectancy of men in the USA continues to trail that of women by 5.3 years in 2003.[4]

Men's health as a concept and discipline is in a prehistoric state compared with women's health. Most clinicians and the public consider men's health to be a field concerned only with the prostate and sexual function. Men's health has recently become a hot topic in these specific areas with large amounts of money being spent on remedies for prostate health, improved urinary flow, and enhanced erections and a smaller amount directed to overall improved health.[5]

Men do not use or react to health services in the same way as women.[6] Men are less likely to go to healthcare providers for preventative healthcare visits.[7] Men are also less likely to follow medical regimens, and are less likely to achieve control with long-term therapeutic treatments.[8,9] The Commonwealth Fund did a mass survey and found that 'an alarming proportion of American men have only limited contact with physicians and the health care system generally. Many men fail to get routine check-ups, preventive care, or health counseling and they often ignore symptoms or delay seeking medical attention when sick or in pain.'[10] This report concludes by noting the need for increased efforts to address the special needs of men as well as attitudes toward healthcare. Men are more likely to be motivated to visit the doctor for conditions that specifically affect men most, such as baldness, sports injuries, or erectile dysfunction (ED). The presentation of a man to the clinician's office with a sexual health complaint can present an opportunity for a more complete evaluation, most notably with the complaint of erectile dysfunction. In a landmark article published in December, 2005, Thompson et al. confirmed what had been long believed: that ED is a sentinel marker and risk factor for future cardiovascular events.[11] After adjustment, incident ED occurring in the 4300 men without ED at study entry enrolled in the prostate cancer prevention trial (PCPT) was associated with a hazard ratio of 1.25 for subsequent cardiovascular events during the 9-year study follow-up (1994–2003). For men with either incident or prevalent ED, the hazard ratio was 1.45. Thus, men with ED are at risk for developing cardiac events over the next 10 years, with ED as strong a risk factor as current smoking or premature family history of cardiac disease. Never before has the association of ED or a male sexual dysfunction been so strongly linked as a harbinger of cardiovascular clinical events in men.

Historically, the office visit for a man complaining of sexual dysfunction focused solely upon ED, and this was the narrow definition of men's health. Over the past few years epidemiologic studies and novel data have mandated that the clinician redirect this office visit to include both a broader definition of sexual function and dysfunction: premature ejaculation, libido, and hypogonadism. Given the value of Thompson's study,[11] a cardiovascular assessment and an even broader cardiometabolic risk assessment should be performed in light of the data suggesting that ED may be a sentinel sign of cardiovascular disease. This chapter provides the rationale for this global assessment paradigm in primary care and other men's health topics, including sexual issues, but it does not include other pertinent topics of men's health, such as affective and mood disorders, domestic and partner violence, and other sex-specific issues. Disparities that exist between socioeconomic stratification of men regarding prevalence and access to care are beyond the scope of this chapter.

The office visit as a portal to men's health: male sexual evaluation

Erectile dysfunction

Definition

For years, the terms 'impotence' and 'erectile dysfunction' were used interchangeably to denote the inability of a man to achieve or maintain erection sufficient to permit satisfactory sexual intercourse.[12] Social scientists objected to the impotence label, because of its pejorative implications and lack of precision.[13] An NIH Consensus Development Conference[14] advocated that 'erectile dysfunction' be used in place of the term 'impotence'. ED or impotence was now defined as 'the inability of the male to achieve an erect penis as part of the overall multifaceted process of male sexual function'. This definition de-emphasizes intercourse as the *sine qua non* of sexual life and gives equal importance to other aspects of male sexual behavior.

Epidemiology

It is estimated that at least 10–20 million males in the USA suffer from ED.[15,16] Laumann et al.[16] have shown that the prevalence of male sexual dysfunction approaches 31% in a population survey of approximately 1400 men aged 18–59. Hypogonadism (in 5% of men surveyed), erectile dysfunction (in 5%), and premature ejaculation (in 21%) were the three most common male sexual dysfunctions noted.

The Massachusetts Male Aging Study,[15] a large epidemiologic study, asked men between the ages of 40 and 70 years to categorize their erectile function as either completely impotent, moderately impotent, minimally impotent, or not impotent. Fifty-two percent of the sample reported some degree of ED. This study demonstrated that ED is an age-dependent disorder: between the ages of 40 and 70 years the probability of complete impotence tripled from 5.1% to 15%, the probability of moderate impotence doubled from 17% to 34%, and the probability of minimal impotence remained constant at 17%. By age of 70, only 32% portrayed themselves as free of ED. Finally, cigarette smoking increased the probability of total ED in men with treated heart disease, hypertension, or untreated arthritis. It similarly increased the probability for men on cardiac, antihypertensive, or vasodilator medications.

After the data were adjusted for age, men treated for diabetes (28%), heart disease (39%), and hypertension (15%) had significantly higher probabilities for ED (28%, 39%, and 15% respectively) than the sample as a whole (9.6%). Men with untreated ulcer (18%), arthritis (15%) and allergy (12%) were also significantly more likely to develop ED (18%, 15%, and 12%, respectively). Although ED was not associated with total serum cholesterol, the probability of dysfunction varied inversely with high-density lipoprotein cholesterol.

Certain classes of medication were related to increased probability for total ED. The percentage of men with complete ED taking hypoglycemic agents, antihypertensives, vasodilators and cardiac drugs (26%, 14%, 36%, and 28%, respectively) was significantly higher than the sample as a whole (9.6%).

More recent data added greater depth to the national estimates of ED in the USA. The National Health and Nutrition Examination Survey (NHANES), conducted by the National Center for Health Statistics, collected data by household interview supplemented by medical examination. The sample size for the entire survey for the 2-year period was 11 039, with a response rate of 71.1% for men aged 20 years and older. Data include medical histories in which specific queries are made regarding sexual function. In men aged 20 years and older, ED affected almost one in five respondents. Hispanic men were more likely to report ED [odds ratio (OR), 1.89], after controlling for other factors.

The prevalence of ED increased dramatically with advanced age; 77.5% of men 75 years and older were affected. In addition, there were several modifiable risk factors that were independently associated with ED, including diabetes mellitus (OR, 2.69), obesity (OR, 1.60), current smoking (OR, 1.74), and hypertension (OR, 1.56).[17]

Relationship between erectile dysfunction and cardiovascular disease

Data specific to ED and related diseases have emerged recently (Fig. 42.1) and serve to support the relationship between ED and cardiovascular disease. Seftel et al.[18] quantified the prevalence of diagnosed hypertension, hyperlipidemia, diabetes mellitus, and depression in male health plan members in the USA with ED, using a nationally representative managed care claims database that covered 51 health plans with 28 million lives for 1995–2002. Based on 272 325 identified patients with ED, population and age-specific prevalence rates were

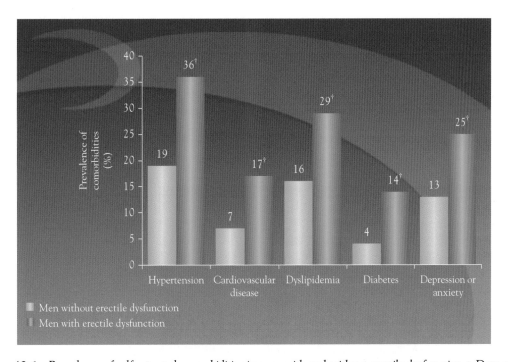

Figure 42.1. *Prevalence of self-reported comorbidities in men with and without erectile dysfunction.* Data relate to 27 839 men aged 25–70 years.[†] p < 0.0001 vs men without erectile dysfunction. Adapted with permission from Rosen et al.[106]

calculated for the same period. Crude population prevalence rates in this study population were 41.6% for hypertension, 42.4% for hyperlipidemia, 20.2% for diabetes mellitus, 11.1% for depression, 23.9% for hypertension and hyperlipidemia, 12.8% for hypertension and diabetes mellitus, and 11.5% for hyperlipidemia and depression.[18] The crude age-specific prevalence rates varied across age groups significantly for hypertension (4.5–68.4%), hyperlipidemia (3.9–52.3%), and diabetes mellitus (2.8–28.7%), and significantly less for depression (5.8–15.0%). Region-adjusted population prevalence rates were 41.2% for hypertension, 41.8% for hyperlipidemia, 19.7% for diabetes mellitus, and 11.9% for depression. These data suggested and confirmed that hypertension, hyperlipidemia, diabetes mellitus, and depression were prevalent in patients with ED.[18] This evidence supported the proposition that ED shares common risk factors with these four concurrent conditions, supporting the view that ED could be viewed as a potential observable marker for these concurrent cardiovascular disease (CVD) risk conditions.

Important epidemiologic data have suggested that ED may be an early marker for actual CVD. Min et al.[19] studied 221 men referred for stress myocardial perfusion single-photon emission computed tomography (MPS), which is commonly used to diagnose and stratify CVD. They found that 55% of the patients had ED, and that these men exhibited more severe coronary heart disease (MPS summed stress score >8) (43% vs 17%; $p = 0.001$) and left ventricular dysfunction (left ventricular ejection fraction <50%) (24% vs 11%; $p = 0.01$) than those without ED. These data suggested that ED was associated as an independent predictor of more severe coronary artery disease and high-risk MPS findings.

Further data support the ED–CVD paradigm. A sample of nearly 4000 Canadian men, aged 40–88 years, seen by primary care clinicians reported ED with the use of the International Index of Erectile Function (IIEF).[20] The presence of CVD or diabetes mellitus increased the probability of ED, and among those men without CVD or DM, the calculated 10-year Framingham coronary risk and fasting glucose level increase were independently associated with ED (Fig. 42.2). ED was also independently associated with undiagnosed hypergylcemia (OR, 1.46), impaired fasting glucose (OR, 1.26), and the metabolic syndrome (OR, 1.45).

The prospective analysis discussed in the introduction by Thompson et al.[11] of the nearly 9500 men randomly assigned to the placebo arm of the PCPT revealed that men with ED are at significantly greater risk ($p < 0.001$) of having a cardiovascular event – angina, myocardial infarction, or stroke – than those without ED. Furthermore, the findings indicate that the relationship between incident ED (the first report of ED of any grade) and CVD is comparable to that associated with current smoking, family history of myocardial infarction, or hyperlipidemia (Table 42.1) Subsequent to the analysis by Thompson et al.[11] and lending further support to the idea of ED as a precursor of CVD,

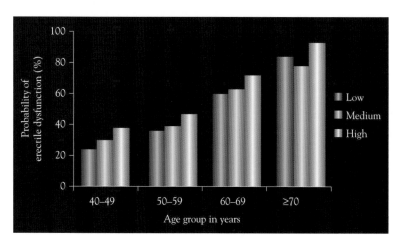

Figure 42.2. *Probability of erectile dysfunction increases with higher coronary risk. From Grover et al.[20]*

Table 42.1. *Erectile dysfunction (ED) as a harbinger of cardiovascular (CV) events*

End-points	Adjusted* hazard ratio for ED (95% CI)	P value
Angina	1.72 (1.26–2.33)	0.001
Myocardial infarction	1.50 (1.20–1.87)	<0.001
Stroke	1.79 (1.15–2.80)	0.01
First CV event	1.45 (1.25–1.69)	<0.001

Data relate to 8063 men ≥55 years of age evaluated every 3 months for ED and CVD between 1994 and 2003. *Adjusted for covariates: age, body mass index, systolic blood pressure, diabetic blood pressure, total cholestrol, high-density lipoprotein cholesterol, history of diabetes, close relative with a history of myocardial infarction, current use of antihypertensives, physical activity, and self-reported global health status. ED, erectile dysfunction; CV, cardiovascular. Data from Thompson et al.[11]

Montorsi et al.[21] investigated 285 patients with coronary artery disease. A key finding is that nearly all patients who developed symptoms of coronary artery disease symptom experienced ED first, on average 3 years beforehand.

The studies noted above suggest that a presentation of ED should trigger an assessment of cardiovascular risk factors, and if appropriate, vigorous intervention. The Second Princeton Consensus Conference on sexual dysfunction and cardiac risk and a follow-up report recommend screening men with ED of uncertain etiology for vascular disease and abnormal metabolic parameters, including glucose, lipids and blood pressure. It stressed that men with ED and no cardiac disease should be considered at risk for CVD until proven otherwise.[22]

Psychosocial morbidity of erectile dysfunction

The impact of ED frequently extends beyond a man's physical function; it can have a psychological effect on the man and his partner, producing bother. Consequently, the emotional toll that ED can have on men and their partners should be considered in the diagnosis and management of ED. A global survey of 13 618 men from 29 countries found that 13–28% have ED[23] and a survey of 1481 men in the Netherlands found that, of those with ED, 67% were bothered by it, and 85% wanted help for their condition.[24] Left untreated, the emotional bother associated with ED can have a significant impact on important psychosocial factors, including self-esteem and confidence, and can damage personal relationships.[25–27] In their Consensus Development Panel on Impotence, the NIH recommended that studies continue to investigate the social and the psychological effects of ED in patients and their partners.[14] However, there are few data on the effect of ED and its treatment on bother associated with ED. This may be due in part to the absence of data from an instrument designed to assess the bother or distress that is specific to ED.

Summary and recommendations

ED is a common men's sexual health complaint, increases in prevalence with aging, is bothersome, and is a future marker for CVD. A verbal inquiry or a brief written five-item survey (sexual health inventory for men)[28] can be used to quantify the degree of ED, and thereby, the concomitant risk of CVD. ED is associated with hypertension, diabetes, depression, hyperlipidemia, smoking,[29,30] a sedentary lifestyle,[30] and obesity. Thus, the man presenting to the clinician complaining of ED should have these areas explored. In addition to defining and characterizing the specific sexual complaint (discussed below), a brief cardiovascular assessment of risk factors, including smoking, lifestyle, exercise, diet, blood pressure, lipids, weight, and distress, should all be part of the initial evaluation. A World Health Organization consensus panel has deliberated and agreed that these recommendations about associating ED with the need for a CVD evaluation are reasonable.[31]

Premature ejaculation

Premature ejaculation (PE) is a very timely topic: the epidemiology is under intense review, and two recent reviews have helped to synthesize the data that are presented in the narrative that follows.[32,33]

Definition

The definition of PE remains controversial. In the *Diagnostic and Statistical Manual of Mental Disorders Fourth Edition Text Revision* (DSM-IV-TR), which is issued by the American Psychiatric Association, it is defined as a 'persistent or recurrent ejaculation with minimal sexual stimulation before, on, or shortly after penetration and before the person wishes it'.[34] DSM-IV-TR further notes that 'the clinician must take into account factors that affect duration of the excitement phase, such as age, novelty of the sexual partner or situation, and recent frequency of sexual activity'. According to this definition PE can be diagnosed only when 'the disturbance causes marked distress or interpersonal difficulty'.

Historically, most clinicians have used 1–2 minutes as the cut-off for the diagnosis of PE. In a recent study, Patrick et al.[35] have attempted to offer time-related norms. In an attempt to define normal ejaculation time, a 4-week, multicenter, observational study of men aged 18 years or older and their female partners in monogamous relationships of ≥6 months' duration was conducted using intravaginal ejaculatory latency time (IELT), measured by a stopwatch held by the partner. IELT was recorded for each sexual intercourse experience. Median IELT was 1.8 minutes (range, 0–41 minutes) for men with PE and 7.3 minutes (range, 0–53 minutes) for non-PE subjects ($p < 0.0001$). More men with PE than non-PE subjects gave ratings of 'very poor' or 'poor' for control over ejaculation (72% vs 5%; $p < 0.0001$) and for satisfaction with sexual intercourse (31% vs 1%; $p < 0.0001$). More men with PE than non-PE subjects gave ratings of 'quite a bit' or 'extremely' for personal distress (64% vs 4%; $p < 0.0001$) and interpersonal difficulty (31% vs 1%; $p < 0.0001$). Subject and partner assessments showed similar patterns and correlated moderately (0.36–0.57). These data would seem to support a 1–2-minute

time frame, *ante portal* or using IELT, for PE. Of note, in the above study, there was considerable overlap in IELT between the men with and without PE, suggesting that IELT alone may not be a good discriminator between men with and without PE. IELT was a good discriminator for men who had IELTs of less than 1 minute. Many authorities feel that IELT alone is not sufficient to diagnose PE. Thus PE should be a multidimensional diagnosis including IELT, control, and distress.[36,37] Questionnaires for the diagnosis of PE and other ejaculatory disorders exist, but have not found their way into the mainstream of evaluation and treatment of PE or other ejaculatory disorders.[38–40]

Epidemiology

Results from the global study of sexual attitudes and behaviors found PE to be the most common sexual dysfunction in six of seven worldwide geographic regions studied.[41] Only in the Middle East was the prevalence of PE (12.4%) eclipsed by other sexual dysfunctions, including ED (14.1%) and lack of sexual interest (21.6%). The prevalence rates for the non-European West (27.4%), Central and South American (28.3%), East Asia (29.1%) and South-east Asia (30.5%) regions were roughly equivalent and in agreement with the data from the National Health and Social Life Survey.[16] Prevalence of PE in the Northern Europe (20.7%) and Southern Europe (21.5%) regions was slightly less. In 1999, Fugl-Meyer et al.[42] reported a prevalence of 4% (51 of 1281 subjects) in a large representative population study of Swedes aged 18–74 years. Remarkably low prevalence of other common forms of sexual dysfunction were also reported, with erectile difficulties reported by only 3% of men surveyed. These results suggest that Swedes have an unexplainably lower prevalence of PE and other sexual dysfunctions than can be found in the USA or other regions. Of course, this assumes that the study design allowed for an accurate representation of the entire Swedish population. Estimates of PE in the USA range around 31% of the male population aged 18–59 years afflicted with sexual dysfunction.[10]

Morbidity

According to the American Urological Association (AUA) guideline on the pharmacologic management of PE, treatment for PE should target improved patient and partner satisfaction.[43] One study found that healthy males and males with PE similarly reported their concern for their partner's satisfaction as high, and, as expected, males with PE were more concerned with ejaculatory control and the duration of intercourse than males without PE.[44] Owing to its psychological impact, PE can be destructive to a relationship, causing embarrassment, frustration, and perhaps the avoidance of sexual contact by the male and his partner. A patient-reported outcome-based study found that 28% of men with PE feared being left by their partner as a result of their PE.[45] Interestingly, the sexual partners of males with PE may feel that the disorder is purely psychological or that the male is being selfish or simply chooses not to extend his latency time, whereas partners of males with ED may be more willing to perceive it as a disease and to be more understanding. In an attempt to avoid the risk of embarrassment and partner-related stress, males with PE may avoid relationships altogether.[44,46,47]

Summary and recommendations

A new definition of PE has been proposed, in lieu of the 1–2-minute timeframe used historically. Many authorities rely on ejaculation time, patient control, and patient distress to define PE. Others incorporate questionnaires into the history. However, most clinicians still use a 1–2-minute ejaculation time, combined with some element of distress as the criterion for the diagnosis of PE. Treatment options currently available for PE include psychosocial, cognitive, and sex therapy approaches in addition to pharmacologic approaches of topical desensitizing techniques and off-label treatment with selective serotonin reuptake inhibitors or phosphodiesterase type 5 inhibitors, or both. Psychosocial techniques, including the stop–start technique[48] and the squeeze technique,[49] attempt to teach the male to recognize pre-ejaculatory signals and to control ejaculation. Cognitive therapy and sex therapy focus on decreasing stress and anxiety related to sex through improved communication between the male and his partner.[50–52] These approaches may not be practical for all males with PE, since they may be more effective for couples who are willing to approach the therapy together.

Hypogonadism (testosterone deficiency)

Definition

The US FDA has accepted a total testosterone (T) of 300 ng/dL as the lower limit of normal for serum T levels. Others have challenged this level, citing a variety of reasons why a level of 300 ng/dL is not a true reflection of hypogonadism. Reasons include a lack of age-specific norms, a lack of evidence that 300 ng/dL is a proper number, and a lack of symptoms reflecting what the T level represents. Clinicians have gravitated to the term 'late-onset hypogonadism' to suggest that an older group of men might be a more appropriate group upon whom we should focus with respect to T deficiency. An international consensus statement (published in three or four journals simultaneously) has been produced; it offers the following guidance:[53]

1. Definition of late-onset hypogonadism – a clinical *and* biochemical syndrome associated with advancing age and characterized by typical symptoms and a deficiency in serum T levels; it may result in significant detriment in the quality of life and adversely affect the function of multiple organ systems.

2. Late-onset hypogonadism is a syndrome characterized primarily by:

    a. the easily recognized features of diminished sexual desire (libido) and erectile quality and frequency, particularly nocturnal erections;

    b. changes in mood with concomitant decreases in intellectual activity, cognitive functions, spatial orientation ability, fatigue, depressed mood, and irritability;

    c. sleep disturbances;

    d. decrease in lean body mass with associated diminution in muscle volume and strength;

    e. increase in visceral fat;

    f. decrease in body hair and skin alterations; and

    g. decreased bone mineral density resulting in osteopenia, osteoporosis, and increased risk of bone fractures.

Epidemiology

A recent review of this topic sheds light on the epidemiology of hypogonadism.[54] In healthy, young eugonadal men, serum T levels range from 300 ng/dL to 1050 ng/dL, but levels decline with advancing age, particularly after 50 years.[55-57] Using a serum T level of 325 ng/dL, the Baltimore Longitudinal Study of Aging reported that approximately 12%, 20%, 30%, and 50% of men in their 50s, 60s, 70s, and 80s, respectively, are hypogonadal.

The hypogonadism in males study[58] estimated the prevalence of hypogonadism [total testosterone (TT) <300 ng/dL] in men aged >45 years visiting primary care practices in the USA. A blood sample was obtained between 8.00 a.m. and 12 noon and assayed for TT, free testosterone (FT), and bio-available testosterone (BAT). Common symptoms of hypogonadism, comorbid conditions, demographics, and reason for visit were recorded. Of 2162 patients, 836 were hypogonadal, with 80 receiving T replacement. The crude prevalence rate of hypogonadism was 38.7%. Similar trends were observed for FT and BAT.[58]

Longitudinal and cross-sectional studies have demonstrated annual T decrements of 0.5–2% with advancing age.[55-57,59,60] The rate of decline in serum T in men appears to be largely dependent on their age at study entry. In the Baltimore Longitudinal Aging Study, the average decline was 3.2 ng/dL per year among men age 53 years at entry. On the other hand, the New Mexico Aging Process Study of men aged 66–80 years at entry showed a decrease in serum T of 110 ng/dL every 10 years. Although serum T levels are generally measured in the morning when at peak, this circadian rhythm is often abolished in elderly men.[61]

The International Society of Andrology, International Society for the Aging Male, and European Association of Urology recommendations[53] note that in patients at risk for or suspected of hypogonadism in general and LOH in particular, a thorough physical and biochemical work-up is mandatory and, especially, the following biochemical investigations should be done. A serum sample for total T determination and sex hormone binding globulin (SHBG) should be obtained between 7.00 a.m and 11.00 a.m. The most widely accepted parameters to establish the presence of hypogonadism are the measurement of TT and FT calculated from measured TT and SHBG or measured by a reliable FT dialysis method.

There are no generally accepted lower limits of normal and it is unclear whether geographically different thresholds depend on ethnic differences or on the physicians' perception. There is, however, general agreement that TT levels above 12 nmol/L (346 ng/dL) or FT levels above 250 pmol/L (72 pg/mL) do not require replacement. Similarly, based on the data of younger men, there is consensus that serum TT levels below 8 nmol/L (231 ng/dL) or FT levels below 180 pmol/L (52 pg/mL) require replacement. Since symptoms of T deficiency become manifest between 12 nmol/L and 8 nmol/L, trials of treatment can be considered in those in whom alternative causes of these symptoms have been excluded. (Since there are variations in the reagents and normal ranges among laboratories, the cut-off values given for serum T and FT may have to be adjusted depending on the reference values given by each laboratory.) If testosterone levels are below or at the lower limit of the accepted normal adult male values, it is recommended that a second determination be performed, together with assessment of serum luteinizing hormone and prolactin.

A clear indication based on a clinical picture together with biochemical evidence of low serum T should exist prior to the initiation of T substitution.

The Endocrine Society has recently published its set of guidelines, entitled *Testosterone Therapy in Adult Men with Androgen Deficiency Syndromes: an Endocrine Society Clinical Practice Guideline*.[62] The Endocrine Society recommends making a diagnosis of androgen deficiency only in men with consistent symptoms and signs and unequivocally low serum T levels. These recommendations include the measurement of morning TT levels by a reliable assay as the initial diagnostic test. They suggest confirmation of the diagnosis by repeating the measurement of morning TT and in some patients by measurement of FT or BAT levels, using accurate assays. Overall, they recommend T therapy for symptomatic men with androgen deficiency who have low T levels, to induce and maintain secondary sex characteristics and to improve sexual function, sense of well-being, muscle mass and strength, and bone mineral density.

These recommendations prohibit starting T therapy in patients with breast or prostate cancer, a palpable prostate nodule or induration, or prostate-specific antigen (PSA) levels >3 ng/mL (without further urological evaluation), erythrocytosis (hematocrit >50%), hyperviscosity, untreated obstructive sleep apnea, severe lower urinary tract symptoms with International Prostate Symptom Score (IPSS) >19, or class III or IV heart failure. When T therapy is instituted, they suggest aiming at achieving T levels during treatment in the mid-normal range with any of the approved formulations, chosen on the basis of the patient's preference, consideration of pharmacokinetics, treatment burden, and cost. Men receiving T therapy should be monitored using a standardized plan.

In an insightful commentary on the Endocrine Society guidelines referenced above, Shames[63] of the US FDA states that, 'testosterone products are approved by the US. FDA as replacement therapy for men with classical androgen deficiency (i.e. men with very low serum T concentrations generally associated with specific medical disorders). This is referred to as classical hypogonadism. Many prescribers, however, advocate administration of T to older men with an array of signs and symptoms, many of which may be related to normal aging, and a 'low' serum T concentration based on normative values for young men. This condition is often referred to by its most popularly accepted name, andropause.'

In 2004, the Institute of Medicine (IOM) reviewed the current state of knowledge about T therapy in older men concluding, 'As the FDA-approved treatment for male hypogonadism, T therapy has been found to be effective in ameliorating a number of symptoms in markedly hypogonadal males. Researchers have carefully explored the benefits of T therapy particularly placebo-controlled randomized trials, in the population of middle-aged or older men who do not meet all the clinical diagnostic criteria for hypogonadism but who may have T levels in the low range for young adult males and show one or more symptoms that are common to both aging and hypogonadism.'[64] The IOM further concluded that 'assessments of risks and benefits have been limited and uncertainties remain about the value of this therapy in older men.'

Shames of the US FDA[63] concludes that 'we support the right of individual physicians to treat patients based on their own knowledge or advice from known experts in the field. However, patients should be able to choose therapies based on accurate and evidence-based medical information and consultation with well-informed healthcare providers. Clinical guidelines and patient guides should be based on solid clinical evidence and must convey this information clearly and accurately to physicians and patients.'

The IOM report also cited evidence for a possible association of low endogenous T levels with components of the metabolic syndrome,[64] which has been defined in various ways but generally includes insulin resistance, obesity, abnormal lipid profiles, and borderline or overt hypertension.[65] Recent studies have confirmed that hypogonadism predisposes men to these features.[65] In 2005, a systematic review concluded that evidence linking hypogonadism and metabolic syndrome is strong enough that the definition of metabolic syndrome in men may be expanded in the future to include hypogonadism as a diagnostic parameter.[65]

Among men with diabetes, the prevalence of hypogonadism has been reported to range from 20% to 64%.[66,67] A systematic review and meta-analysis of 43 prospective and cross-sectional studies concluded that men with type 2 diabetes had significantly lower concentrations of T than did men with normal fasting glucose.[68]

Recent clinical studies have confirmed that TT is inversely associated with body mass index, waist–hip ratio, and percentage of body fat and insulin resistance.[69–72] Insulin resistance among hypogonadal men may be an indirect effect of changes in body composition, inhibition of lipoprotein lipase, or decreased circulating free fatty acids.[73,74] A series of data analyses from the Kuopio Ischemic Heart Disease Risk Factor Study, conducted in Finland, reported that non-diabetic men were nearly four-fold more likely to develop metabolic syndrome if they were hypogonadal,[75] twice as likely to develop diabetes or metabolic syndrome within an 11-year period if they were in the lowest quartile for T levels,[76] and up to 2.9 times as likely to develop hypogonadism during the 11-year follow-up period if they had metabolic syndrome at baseline.[77] Therefore, it is highly evident that low T levels are positively correlated with the onset of metabolic syndrome and perhaps type 2 diabetes.

This correlation may have clinical and economic significance because of the high prevalences and substantial costs of diabetes and metabolic syndrome in the USA.[78–80]

Potential reversibility of the link between metabolic syndrome and hypogonadism was suggested by a recent observational study and a recent interventional study. In the observational study, new-onset hypogonadism was 5.7–7.4 times more common among men with metabolic syndrome at baseline and at final visit, and approximately three times more common among men who also had new-onset metabolic syndrome; however, no increased risk of hypogonadism was observed among men who had metabolic syndrome at baseline that had resolved by the final visit.[81] In the interventional study of 58 obese men with metabolic syndrome, the prevalence of hypogonadism (TT <317 ng/dL) was 48% at baseline, 9% after the men lost an average of 16.3 kg on a very low-calorie diet, and 21% when men regained approximately 2 kg on average during a 12-month weight-maintenance program.[82] Significant improvements in insulin sensitivity, fasting glucose, high-density lipoprotein (HDL) levels, and triglycerides were observed at the end of each treatment phase.[83]

Emerging evidence suggests that the opposite is true as well – namely, that T replacement therapy may ameliorate some of the elements of metabolic syndrome – but results of these studies have been mixed (Table 42.2) Several studies have reported that T replacement therapy in hypogonadal men decreased body weight, waist–hip ratio, and body fat, and improved glycemic control, insulin resistance, and the lipid profile.[82–87] However, some of these studies reported that one or more of the parameters of metabolic syndrome were not significantly improved by T replacement therapy. Additional long-term studies are needed to elucidate the role of T replacement therapy in improving body composition and clinical outcomes associated with the metabolic syndrome.

Summary and recommendations

Hypogonadism remains a controversial topic in terms of diagnosis, treatment, and the importance of physiologic comorbidites, as discussed above. The cautionary stance provided by the US FDA in the comments offered by Shames seems appropriate. Thus, it remains unclear as to the most appropriate T level that will allow for the definitive diagnosis of hypogonadism. It also seems reasonable that, irrespective of the T level that is chosen by the clinician for the diagnosis of hypogonadism, certain hypogonadism-associated symptoms should be sought out and detailed in the patient record. For those clinicians unfamiliar with these symptoms, the questionnaires (Table 42.3) should suffice. Caution must be the guide here, as we make slow steady progress in understanding T replacement issues. Prostate gland monitoring and PSA levels can be followed safely by the recommendations in Table 42.4. The overall recommendations noted in the two guidelines outlined above provide helpful guidance.

Cardiometabolic risk and erectile dysfunction: reversing the risk

While it has been long recognized that cardiovascular disease and ED were related by healthy endothelial function and vasuclar perfusion it is not surprising that ED and CVD have been linked through traditional cardiovascular risk markers, including cigarette smoking, hypertension, and dyslipidemia. However, there is now emerging the evolving concept of ED and its relationship to novel and broader cardiovacular markers tied to male waist circumference (WC) and obesity (Table 42.5), and its assoication with vascular disease in other prominent vascular beds, specifically the carotid and femoral arteries. Investigators from the Massacheuettes Male Aging Study found that ED was predictive of subsequent development of the metabolic syndrome (central obesity, insulin dysregulation, abnormal lipids, and borderline hypertension). The association was greatest with men whose initial body mass index was below 25 kg/m^2.[88]

This information provides some guidance about risk reduction opportunities. Esposito et al.[89] determined the effect of weight loss and increased physical activity on erectile and endothelial function in obese men. The 55 men randomly assigned to the intervention group received detailed advice about how to achieve a loss of 10% or more in their total

Table 42.2. *Testosterone and the reversibility of the metabolic syndrome:[107] studies published since the 2003 report from the Institute of Medicine[64]*

Study	Study design	Key findings
Fukui et al., 2003[72]	Cross-sectional study of 253 men with type 2 diabetes (mean ± SD age, 62.0 ± 9.9 years)	Correlations with total testosterone: ↓ patient age ↓ age of diabetes onset ↓ duration of type 2 diabetes ↑ total cholesterol ↓ intima media thickness ↔ cardiovascular disease ↔ cerebral infarction ↔ coronary artery disease
Corrales et al., 2004[67]	Cross-sectional study of 55 diabetic men aged >50 years, 8 aging controls, and 32 young controls	Correlations with total testosterone: ↔ fasting glucose ↔ fructosamine ↔ insulin ↔ C-peptide ↑ glycosylated hemoglobin Prevalence of hypogonadism 20–55% among diabetic men, depending on the criteria used
Pitteloud et al., 2005[69]	Cross-sectional study of 60 men; 27 with normal glucose tolerance, 12 with impaired glucose tolerance, and 21 with type 2 diabetes	Correlations with total testosterone: ↓ insulin resistance ↓ body mass index ↓ waist–hip ratio ↓ % body fat Hypogonadal men (total testosterone <9.7 nmol/L) were twice as insulin resistant 90% of hypogonadal men met the criteria for metabolic syndrome
Kalme et al., 2005[71]	Cross-sectional study of 335 men aged 70–89 years	Correlations with total testosterone: ↓ glucose ↓ insulin ↓ age ↓ body mass index ↓ triglycerides ↑ HDL cholesterol
Basaria et al., 2006[98]	Cross-sectional study of 52 men; 18 hypogonadal, androgen-deprived men with prostate cancer, 17 eugonadal men with prostate cancer, and 17 eugonadal healthy men	Correlations with total testosterone: ↓ glucose ↓ insulin ↓ insulin resistance ↓ leptin
Smith et al., 2006[70]	Single-arm treatment study of leuprolide depot and bicalutamide in 25 non-diabetic men with locally advanced or recurrent prostate cancer	Androgen blockade increased glycosylated hemoglobin, insulin level, insulin resistance, total cholesterol, HDL cholesterol, and triglycerides

HDL, high-density lipoprotein; ↑, positive correlation; ↓, negative correlation; ↔, no correlation
Used with Permission from Miner and Seftel.[107]

Table 42.3. *Questionnaires used to diagnose androgen deficiency in aging males*

Androgen Deficiency in Aging Males (ADAM) questionnaire[*96]	Massachusetts Male Aging Study (MMAS) questionnaire[†88]
1 Do you have a decrease in libido (sex drive)? 2 Do you have a lack of energy? 3 Do you have a decrease in strength and/or endurance? 4 Have you lost height? 5 Have you noticed a decreased 'enjoyment of life'? 6 Are you sad and/or grumpy? 7 Are your erections less strong? 8 Have you noted a recent deterioration in your ability to play sports? 9 Are you falling asleep after dinner? 10 Has there been a recent deterioration in your work performance?	Libido – 'How frequently do you feel sexual desire?' (1–8) Erectile dysfunction – 13-item composite (1–4) Depression – antidepressant use (yes/no) Lethargy – past week (1–4) Inability to concentrate – past week (1–4) Sleep disturbance – past week (1–4) Irritability – past week (1–4) Depressed mood – past week (1–4)

[*]A positive ADAM questionnaire was defined as a 'yes' answer to question 1, question 7, or any three other questions.
[†]A positive MMAS questionnaire was defined as three or more positive symptoms (1–2 for libido, 'yes' for antidepressant use, and 2–4 for all other items).

Table 42.4. *Recommendations for monitoring prostate health before and during testosterone replacement therapy[99–104]*

Before initiating therapy
 Normal digital rectal examination
 PSA <4.0 ng/mL
 Evaluate individual risk of prostate cancer

During therapy
 Measure PSA:
  at 3–6 months
  annually or semi-annually as long as treatment continues
 Perform digital rectal examination:
  annually or semi-annually as long as treatment continues
 Refer for urologic evaluation and possible prostate biopsy if:
  Prostate is abnormal on digital rectal examination
  or
  PSA >4 ng/mL
  or
  PSA increase >1 ng/mL after 3–4 months on testosterone treatment
  or
  PSA velocity >1.5 ng/mL/year or >0.75 ng/mL/year over 2 years
  or
  PSA velocity >0.4 ng/mL/year over an observation period of <3 years (with PSA after 6 months on testosterone therapy used as a reference point)

PSA, prostate-specific antigen.

body weight by reducing caloric intake and increasing their level of physical activity. Men in the control group (n = 55) were given usual information about healthy food choices and exercise. After 2 years, body mass index decreased more in the intervention group [from a mean (SD) of 36.9 (2.5) to 31.2 (2.1)] than in the control group [from 36.4 (2.3) to 35.7 (2.5)] ($p < 0.001$), as did serum concentrations of interleukin 6 ($p = 0.03$) and C-reactive protein ($p = 0.02$). The mean (SD) level of physical activity increased more in the intervention group [from 48 (10) to 195 (36) minutes per week; $p = 0.001$] than in the control group [from 51 (9) to 84 (28) minutes per week; $p = 0.001$]. The mean (SD) IIEF score improved in the intervention group [from 13.9 (4.0) to 17 (5); $p = 0.001$] but remained stable in the control group [from 13.5 (4.0) to 13.6 (4.1); $p = 0.89$]. In multivariate analyses, changes in body mass index ($p = 0.02$), physical activity ($p = 0.02$), and C-reactive protein ($p = 0.03$) were independently associated with changes in IIEF score. The authors concluded that lifestyle changes were associated with improvement in sexual function in about one-third of obese men with ED at baseline (Fig. 42.3).

If these clinical associations are valid, then one could argue that there should be mechanistic data supporting these concepts. Eaton et al.[90] evaluated the cross-sectional association between the degree of ED and levels of atherosclerotic biomarkers. Men with poor to very poor erectile function compared with men with good and very good erectile function had 2.9 the odds of having elevated factor VII levels ($p = 0.03$), 1.9 times the odds of having elevated vascular cell adhesion molecule ($p = 0.13$), 2.0 times the odds of having elevated intracellular adhesion molecule ($p = 0.06$), and 2.1 times the odds

Table 42.5. *Cardiometabolic risk factors*

Traditional risk factors	Emerging risk factors
■ Hypertension	■ Abnorminal obesity
■ Diabetes	■ Abnormal fasting
■ High LDL cholesterol	blood sugar
■ Cigarette smoking	■ Insulin resistance
■ Age	■ Slightly elevated
■ Male gender	triglycerides
■ Sedentary lifestyle	■ Moderate blood
■ Family history of	pressure elevation
Heart disease	■ Low HDL cholesterol
	■ Inflammation (hs CRP)
	■ Pro-thrombotic factors

LDL, low-density lipoprotein; HDL, high-density lipoprotein; hs CRP, highly sensitive C-reaction protein.

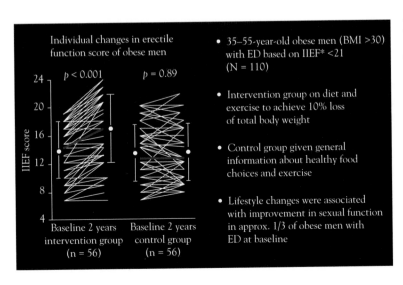

Figure 42.3. *Effect of weight loss on sexual function in obese men. ED, erectile dysfunction; IIEF, International Index of Erectile Function. Adapted from Esposito et al.*[89]

527

of having elevated total cholesterol–HDL ratio ($p=0.02$), comparing the top to bottom quintiles for each atherosclerotic biomarker after multivariate adjustment. Lipoprotein (a), homocysteine, interleukin-6, tumor necrosis factor receptor, C-reactive protein, and fibrinogen were not associated with the degree of erectile function after adjustment. The author concluded that selected biomarkers for endothelial function, thrombosis, and dyslipidemia but not inflammation were associated with the degree of ED in this cross-sectional analysis.

Recent clinical studies have investigated the prevalence of carotic and lower extremity arterial disease in men with vascular ED documented by penile ultrasound studies. Vicari et al.[91] found that penile artery insufficiency is associated with carotid or lower limb artery ultrasound abnomalities (atheroma or marked intima–media thickness) approximately 75% of the time. Another study found that the severity of ED based on penile Doppler ultrasound correlates with associated ultrasound abnormalities in the carotid artery, lower limb arteries, or both vascular beds. Men with ED and both carotid and lower limb abnormalities had the most severe penile artery disease based on ultrasound assessments of all vascular beds.[92] Both of these studies support the concept that many men with vascular ED should be regarded as having generalized vascular atherosclerosis. This is part of the emerging trend of utilizing ED as an early marker for increased global cardiometabolic risk.

Summary and recommendations

In additon to a work-up for cardiovascular risk, all men who present with ED should be assessed for the presence and severity of actual cardiovascular disease. High-risk patients with ED should undergo exercise or stress testing. In this context, high-risk patients are those with ED plus diabetes, a strong family history of CVD, three or more cardiovascular risk factors, angina, or a coronary heart disease risk equivalent.[93] Peripheral arterial disease, diabetes, and multiple risk factors with a 10-year coronary heart disease risk >20% constitute CHD risk equivalents.[94] Patients with ED and evidence of cerebrovascular disease (asymptomatic bruits or a history of transient ischemic events) should be assessed with carotid ultrasound. Symptoms of circulatory insufficiency that suggest peripheral vascular disease in men with ED should be evaluated using the ankle–brachial index. Obesity, while affecting one-third of US adults, clearly predisposes to cardiovascular risk factors, including insulin resistance, hypertension, and dyslipidemia. Body mass index has been used as the primary standard for outcomes in studies, but alternative measures including waist circumference and waist-to-hip ratio have demonstrated better correlations with CVD risk than body mass index.[95] Indicators of metabolic syndrome should be identified, highlighted to patients, and treated aggressively with risk reduction therapies, including exercise, diet, nutritional counseling, T replacement when indicated, and other pharmacotherapy.

Sexual medicine history and physical examination in primary care

It is vital to remember: if we do not ask, men will not tell. The office evaluation consists of a series of direct questions about the nature of the sexual dysfunction complaint. Questions should be direct yet inviting discussion (e.g. 'Do you have any concerns about your sexual functioning?') (Table 42.6). The interview should take place in a quiet room, in a non-judgmental fashion. These men are embarrassed and often need reassurance that this topic is acceptable to discuss. The questions should be asked in a gentle manner, avoiding any gestures or posturing that might be misconstrued.

In lieu of direct questions, many clinicians prefer to provide the patient with questionnaires that delve into the specific sexual complaint. Two examples are the Sexual Health Inventory for Men (SHIM) and the Androgen Deficiency in the Aging Male (ADAM) questionnaire.

The SHIM is a simple, five-question instrument that inquires about erectile function over the previous 6 months. It is an abridged and slightly modified version of the International Index of Erectile Function (IIEF).[28] This simpler version

Table 42.6. *Examples of the line of inquiry into male sexual dysfunction*

Characterize the sexual dysfunction

What type of sexual problem does the patient complain of?

Does he have erectile dysfunction?

If so, how long has he had the problem?

When was the last time he had intercourse?

When was the last time he had any sexual activity?

Does the erection problem bother him?

Does the erection problem bother his partner?

Did the problem arise suddenly (psychogenic) or has it arisen gradually?

Did the problem start when he started a new medication?

Does the problem occur with his partner only or does it also occur without his partner as well; for example with masturbation

Does the problem occur because he has no partner or an uninterested partner?

Does he have a partner outside of his main relationship?

Can he get an erection? If so, is it firm enough for penetration?

Can he maintain the erection for intercourse?

Does he have a problem with sexual desire?

How long has he lost sexual desire?

Has he lost sexual desire with all partners?

Has he lost desire under all circumstances?

Has he lost desire because he cannot get or maintain an erection?

Has he lost desire because his partner has lost desire?

Does the patient complain of other, associated symptoms, such as being tired, loss of stamina, loss of strength, loss of muscle mass, loss of muscle tone, recent weight gain, fatigue, sleep issues?

Is the patient depressed?

Does he have a problem with ejaculation?

What type of ejaculation problem does the patient complain of?

When did the problem start?

Is the problem bothersome to the patient?

Is the problem bothersome to the partner?

Does the problem occur under all circumstances?

allows the clinician to assess male ED with great security. It is scored as follows:

- Score 22–25 no ED
- Score 17–21 mild ED
- Score 12–16 mild-to-moderate ED
- Score 8–11 moderate ED
- Score 0–7 severe ED (in our experience consider psychogenic ED, or ED as seen after radical prostatectomy or pelvic surgery).

Table 42.7. *Physical examination for a man with sexual dysfunction*[105]

Height, weight, body mass index, waist size or waist-to-hip ratio

Blood pressure

Auscultation of heart and lungs

Pulses

Examination of abdomen (auscultation for bruits)

Examination of penis for plaques, lesions, urethral position

Examination of testis for size, lumps, masses, position

Examination of rectum for sphincter tone, prostate size, masses, lesions, bulbocavernosus reflex

Brief neurologic examination

Table 42.8. *Laboratory work-up for a man complaining of erectile dysfunction*

Fasting lipid panel

Fasting glucose

Total or free testosterone (morning collection preferred)

Prostate-specific antigen, mandatory if considering testosterone supplementation, otherwise may be optional

Optional laboratory tests:

Prolactin

Creatinine

Estradiol

Thyroid stimulating hormone

Luteinizing hormone

25-hydroxyvitamin D

Uninary microalbumin

Urine analysis

The SHIM gives a severity index and a common vocabulary, and it has supplanted vascular testing in many cases. However, it is not predictive of outcome.

The ADAM questionnaire, while not sensitive for hypogonadism, asks questions that are pertinent to the hypogonadal state.[96]

The physical examination for male sexual dysfunction evaluation in primary care is delineated in Table 42.7. This is a directed examination and is relatively straightforward. Table 42.8 describes the laboratory work that is suggested for male sexual dyfunctions as a whole, and that which is optional for the individual patient.

Summary

Men's health, now as an office evaluation in primary care, requires a thorough understanding of the implications of male sexual dysfunctions, hypogonadism and cardiometabolic risk stratification, and aggressive risk management. The paradigm of the men's

health office visit in primary care is the recognition and assessment of male sexual dysfunction, specifically ED, and its value as a signal of overall cardiometabolic health, including the emerging evidence linking low T levels and metabolic syndrome. A body of evidence from basic science and clinical research is rapidly emerging to make the compelling argument for endothelial cell dysfunction as a central etiologic factor in the development of CVD and other systemic vascular diseases (stroke, vascular claudication). Indeed, ED may now be thought of as a harbinger of cardiovascular clinical events in some men, with an association of risk for an incident cardiovascular event similar to that of current smoking or a family history of myocardial infarction.[11]

This awareness of ED as a barometer for vascular health and occult cardiovascular disease represents a unique opportunity for primary prevention of vascular disease in all men. However, for this to occur, both urologist and primary care doctor must work together to identify and treat modifiable risk factors. It is prudent for the urologist to note these risk factors in those men who present for sexual dysfunction, and ensure that they are evaluated fully by a knowledgeable primary care provider.

The optimal relationship between primary care doctor and urologist would involve a collaborative desire and communication to co-manage those issues vital to men's health: the enlarged prostate, prostate cancer detection and prevention, hormonal replacement therapy, post-prostatectomy penile rehabilitation, lower urinary tract symptoms, sexual dysfunctions of all types, and, finally, cardiovascular risk evaluation and reduction in men with ED. To paraphrase Richardson and Vinik: 'a flagging penis should raise the red flag of warning to evaluate the patient for arterial disease elsewhere.'[97] This collaborative or shared care model for male sexual dysfunction is being explored in Europe.

It is hoped that the data presented above will guide the clinician and allow for a successful evaluation and management of the patient in addition to the stratification of cardiovascular risk and the promotion of a healthy and satisfying lifestyle.

References

1. Fontanarosa PB, Cole HM. Improving men's health: evidence and opportunity. JAMA 2006; 296: 2373–5.
2. Agency for Healthcare Research and Quality. Rockville, MD: December 2005.
3. National Center for Health Statistics. Hyattsville, MD: December 2005.
4. Miniño AM, Heron M, Murphy SL, Kochanek KD. Deaths: final data for 2004. CDC National Center for Health Statistics [Available at: http://www.cdc.gov/nchs/products/pubs/pubd/hestats/finaldeaths04/finaldeaths04.htm].
5. Penson D, Kreiger JN. Men's health. Are we missing the big picture? J Gen Intern Med 2001; 16: 717–71.
6. O'Brien R, Hunt K, Hart G. 'It's caveman stuff, but that is to a certain extent how guys still operate': Men' accounts of masculinity and help seeking. Soc Sci Med 2005; 61: 503–16.
7. Courtenay WH. Constructions of masculinity and their influence on men's well being: a theory of gender and health. Soc Sci Med 2000; 50: 1385–401.
8. Rose I, Kim MT, Dennison CR et al. The contexts of adherence for African Americans with high blood pressure. J Adv Nurs 2000; 32: 587–94.
9. Plascencia A, Ostfield AM, Gruber SB. Effects of sex on differences in awareness, treatment, and control of blood pressure. Am J Prev Med 1988; 4: 315–26.
10. Sandman D, Simantov E, Anc. Out of touch: American men and the health care system. Commonwealth Fund, 2000 [Available at:www.cmwf.org].
11. Thompson IM, Tangen CM, Goodman PJ et al. Erectile dysfunction and subsequent cardiovascular disease. JAMA 2005; 294: 2996–3002.
12. Krane RJ, Goldstein I, Saenz de Tejada I. Impotence. N Engl J Med 1989; 321: 1648–59.
13. Rosen RC, Leiblum SR. Erectile disorders: an overview of historical trends and clinical perspectives. In: Rosen RC, Leiblum SR, eds. Erectile Disorders: Assessment and Treatment, New York: Guilford, 1992; 3–26.
14. NIH Consensus Conference. Impotence. NIH Consensus Development Panel on Impotence. JAMA 1993; 270: 83–90.
15. Feldman HA, Goldstein I, Hatzichristou DG et al. Impotence and its medical and psychosocial correlates: results of the Massachusetts Male Aging Study. J Urol 1994; 151: 54.
16. Laumann E, Paik A, Rosen RC. Sexual dysfunction in the United States: prevalence and predictors. JAMA 1999; 281: 537–44.
17. Saigal CS, Wessels H, Pace J et al. Predictors and prevalence of erectile dysfunction in a racially diverse population. Arch Intern Med 2006; 166: 207–12.
18. Seftel AD, Sun P, Swindle R. The prevalence of hypertension, hyperlipidemia, diabetes mellitus and depression in men with erectile dysfunction. J Urol 2004; 171: 2341–5.
19. Min JK, Williams KA, Okwuosa TM et al. Prediction of coronary heart disease by erectile dysfunction in men referred for nuclear stress testing. Arch Intern Med 2006; 166: 201–6.
20. Grover SA, Lowensteyn I, Kaouache M et al. The prevalence of erectile dysfunction in the primary care setting. Arch Intern Med 2006; 166: 213–19.
21. Montorsi P, Ravagnani PM, Galli S et al. Association between erectile dysfunction and coronary artery disease. Role of coronary clinical presentation and extent of coronary vessels involvement: the COBRA trial. Eur Heart J 2006; 27: 2632–9.

22. Kostis JB, Jackson G, Rosen R et al. Sexual dysfunction and cardiac risk (the Second Princeton Consensus Conference). Am J Cardiol 2005; 96: 313–21.

23. Laumann EO, Nicolosi A, Glasser DB et al. Sexual problems among women and men aged 40–80yr: prevalence and correlates identified in the global study of sexual attitudes and behaviors. Int J Impot Res 2005; 17: 39–57.

24. de Boer BJ, Bots ML, Lycklama a Nijeholt AA, Moors JPC, Verheij TJ. The prevalence of bother, acceptance, and need for help in men with erectile dysfunction. J Sex Med 2005; 2: 445–50.

25. Korenman SG. New insights into erectile dysfunction: a practical approach. Am J Med 1998; 105: 135–44.

26. Fugl-Meyer AR, Lodnert G, Branholm IB, Fugl-Meyer KS. On life satisfaction in male erectile dysfunction. Int J Impot Res 1997; 9: 141–8.

27. Rosen RC. Quality of life assessment in sexual dysfunction trials. Int J Impot Res 1998; 10: S21–3.

28. Rosen RC, Cappelleri JC, Smith MD, Lipsky J, Pena BM. Development and evaluation of an abridged, 5-item version of the International Index of Erectile Function (IIEF-5) as a diagnostic tool for erectile dysfunction. Int J Impot Res 1999; 11: 319–26.

29. Gades NM, Nehra A, Jacobson DJ et al. Association between smoking and erectile dysfunction: a population-based study. Am J Epidemiol 2005; 161: 346–51.

30. Bacon CG, Mittleman MA, Kawachi I et al. A prospective study of risk factors for erectile dysfunction. J Urol 2006; 176: 217–21.

31. Hatzichristou D, Rosen RC, Broderick G et al. A clinical evaluation and management strategy for sexual dysfunction in men and women. J Sex Med 2004; 1: 49–57.

32. Carson C, Gunn K. Premature ejaculation: definition and prevalence. Int J Impot Res 2006; 18: S5–13.

33. Segraves RT. Rapid ejaculation: a review of nosology, prevalence and treatment. Int J Impot Res 2006; 18: S24–32.

34. American Psychiatric Association. Diagnostic and Statistical Manual of Mental Disorders Fourth edition, Text Revision (DSM-IV-TR). Washington, DC: American Psychiatric Association, 2000.

35. Patrick DL, Althof SE, Pryor JL et al. Premature ejaculation: an observational study of men and their partners. J Sex Med 2005; 2: 358–67.

36. Waldinger M. Premature ejaculation: state of the art. Urol Clin North Am 2007; 34: 591–9.

37. Waldinger MD. The need for a revival of psychoanalytic investigations into premature ejaculation. J Mens Health Gender 2006; 3: 390–6.

38. Althof S, Rosen R, Symonds T et al. Development and validation of a new questionnaire to assess sexual satisfaction, control, and distress associated with premature ejaculation. J Sex Med 2006; 3: 465–75.

39. Symonds T, Perelman M, Althof S et al. Further evidence of the reliability and validity of the premature ejaculation diagnostic tool. Int J Impot Res 2007; 19: 512–25.

40. Rosen RC, Catania JA, Althof SE et al. Development and validation of four-item version of Male Sexual Health Questionnaire to assess ejaculatory dysfunction. Urol 2007; 69: 805–9.

41. Laumann EO, Nicolosi A, Glasser DB et al. Sexual problems among women and men aged 40–80 yr: prevalence and correlates identified in the global study of sexual attitudes and behaviors. Int J Impot Res 2005; 17: 39–57.

42. Fugl-Meyer AR, Sjogren K, Fugl-Meyer KS. Sexual disabilities, problems, and satisfaction in 18–74 year old Swedes. Scand J Sexol 1999; 3: 79–10.

43. Montague DK, Jarow J, Broderick G et al. AUA Guideline on the pharmacologic management of premature ejaculation. J Urol 2004; 172: 290–4.

44. Rowland D, Perelman M, Althof S et al. Self-reported premature ejaculation and aspects of sexual functioning and satisfaction. J Sex Med 2004; 1: 225–32.

45. Hartmann U, Schedlowski M, Kruger TH. Cognitive and partner-related factors in rapid ejaculation: differences between dysfunctional and functional men. World J Urol 2005; 23: 93–101.

46. Porst H, Montorsi F, Rosen RC et al. The Premature Ejaculation Prevalence and Attitudes (PEPA) survey: prevalence, comorbidities, and professional help-seeking. EUR Urol 2007; 51: 816–82.

47. Symonds T, Roblin D, Hart K, Althof S. How does premature ejaculation impact a man's life? J Sex Marital Ther 2003; 29: 361–70.

48. Semans J. Premature ejaculation: a new approach. South Med J 1956; 49: 353–8.

49. Masters W, Johnson V. Human Sexual Inadequacy. Boston, MA: Little, Brown, 1970.

50. Master VA, Turek PJ. Ejaculatory physiology and dysfunction. Urol Clin North Am 2001; 28: 363–75.

51. McCabe MP. Evaluation of a cognitive behavior therapy program for people with sexual dysfunction. J Sex Marital Ther 2001; 27: 259–71.

52. Hawton K, Catalan J. Prognostic factors in sex therapy. Behav Res Ther 1986; 24: 377–85.

53. Nieschlag E, Swerdloff R, Behre HM et al. Investigation, treatment, and monitoring of late-onset hypogonadism in males: ISA, ISSAM, and EAU recommendations. J. Androl 2006; 27: 135–7.

54. Seftel AD. Male hypogonadism. Part I: Epidemiology of hypogonadism. Int J Impot Res 2006; 18: 115–20.

55. Rhoden EL, Morgentaler A. Risks of testosterone-replacement therapy and recommendations for monitoring. N Engl J Med 2004; 350: 482–92.

56. Harman SM, Metter EJ, Tobin JD, Pearson J, Blackman MR. Longitudinal effects of aging on serum total and free testosterone levels in healthy men. Baltimore Longitudinal Study of Aging. J Clin Endocrinol Metab 2001; 86: 724–31.

57. Morley JE, Kaiser FE, Perry III HM et al. Longitudinal changes in testosterone, luteinizing hormone, and follicle-stimulating hormone in healthy older men. Metabolism 1997; 46: 410–13.

58. Mulligan T, Frick MF, Zuraw QC, Stemhagen A, McWhirter C. Prevalence of hypogonadism in males aged at least 45 years: the HIM study. Int J Clin Pract 2006; 60: 762–9.

59. Snyder PJ. Effects of age on testicular function and consequences of testosterone treatment. J Clin Endocrinol Metab 2001; 86: 2369–72.

60. Vermeulen A. Androgen replacement therapy in the aging male: a critical evaluation. J Clin Endocrinol Metab 2001; 86: 2380–90.

61. Bremner WJ, Vitiello MV, Prinz PN. Loss of circadian rhythmicity in blood testosterone levels with aging in normal men. J Clin Endocrinol Metab 1983; 56: 1278–81.

62. Bhasin S, Cunningham GR, Hayes F et al. Testosterone therapy in adult men with androgen deficiency syndromes: an Endocrine Society Clinical Practice Guideline. J Clin Endocrinol Metab 2006; 91: 1995–2010.

63. Shames D, Gassman A, Handelsman H. Commentary: guideline for male testosterone therapy: a regulatory perspective. J Clin Endocrinol Metab 2007; 92: 414–15.

64. Institute of Medicine Testosterone and Aging: Clinical Research Directions. Committee on Assessing the Need for Clinical Trials of Testosterone Replacement Therapy. Washington, DC: National Academics Press, 2003.

65. Makhsida N, Shah J, Yan G, Fisch H, Shabsigh R. Hypogonadism and metabolic syndrome: implications for testosterone therapy. J Urol 2005; 174: 827–34.

66. Dhindsa S, Prabhakar S, Sethi M et al. Frequent occurrence of hypogonadotropic hypogonadism in type 2 diabetes. J Clin Endocrinol Metab 2004; 89: 5462–8.

67. Corrales JJ, Burgo RM, Garca-Berrocal B et al. Partial androgen deficiency in aging type 2 diabetic men and its relationship to glycemic control. Metabolism 2004; 53: 666–72.

68. Ding EL, Song Y, Malik VS, Liu S. Sex differences of endogenous sex hormones and risk of type 2 diabetes: a systematic review and meta-analysis. JAMA 2006; 295: 1288–99.

69. Pitteloud N, Mootha VK, Dwyer AA et al. Relationship between testosterone levels, insulin sensitivity, and mitochondrial function in men. Diabetes Care 2005; 28: 1636–42.

70. Smith MR, Lee H, Nathan DM. Insulin sensitivity during combined androgen blockade for prostate cancer. J Clin Endocrinol Metab 2006; 91: 1305–8.

71. Kalme T, Seppala M, Qiao Q et al. Sex hormone-binding globulin and insulin-like growth factor-binding protein-1 as indicators of metabolic syndrome, cardiovascular risk, and mortality in elderly men. J Clin Endocrinol Metab 2005; 90: 1550–6.

72. Fukui M, Kitagawa Y, Nakamura N et al. Association between serum testosterone concentration and carotid atherosclerosis in men with type 2 diabetes. Diabetes Care 2003; 26: 1869–73.

73. Betancourt-Albrecht M, Cunningham GR. Hypogonadism and diabetes. Int J Impot Res 2003; 15(Suppl 4): S14–20.

74. Tsai EC, Matsumoto AM, Fujimoto WY, Boyko EJ. Association of bioavailable, free, and total testosterone with insulin resistance: influence of sex hormone-binding globulin and body fat. Diabetes Care 2004; 27: 861–8.

75. Laaksonen DE, Niskanen L, Punnonen K et al. Sex hormones, inflammation and the metabolic syndrome: a population-based study. Eur J Endocrinol 2003; 149: 601–8.

76. Laaksonen DE, Niskanen L, Punnonen K et al. Testosterone and sex hormone-binding globulin predict the metabolic syndrome and diabetes

in middle-aged men. Diabetes Care 2004; 27: 1036–41.

77. Laaksonen DE, Niskanen L, Punnonen K et al. The metabolic syndrome and smoking in relation to hypogonadism in middle-aged men: a prospective cohort study. J Clin Endocrinol Metab 2005; 90: 712–19.

78. Mokdad AH, Ford ES, Bowman BA et al. Prevalence of obesity, diabetes, and obesity-related health risk factors, 2001. JAMA 2003; 289: 76–9.

79. Sullivan PW, Morrato EH, Ghushchyan V, Wyatt HR, Hill JO. Obesity, inactivity, and the prevalence of diabetes and diabetes-related cardiovascular comorbidities in the U.S., 2000–2002. Diabetes Care 2005; 28: 1599–603.

80. Ford ES. Prevalence of the metabolic syndrome defined by the International Diabetes Federation among adults in the U.S. Diabetes Care 2005; 28: 2745–9.

81. Niskanen L, Laaksonen DE, Punnonen K et al. Changes in sex hormone-binding globulin and testosterone during weight loss and weight maintenance in abdominally obese men with the metabolic syndrome. Diabetes Obes Metab 2004; 6: 208–15.

82. Boyanov MA, Boneva Z, Christov VG. Testosterone supplementation in men with type 2 diabetes, visceral obesity and partial androgen deficiency. Aging Male 2003; 6: 1–7.

83. Steidle C, Schwartz S, Jacoby K et al. AA2500 testosterone gel normalizes androgen levels in aging males with improvements in body composition and sexual function. J Clin Endocrinol Metab 2003; 88: 2673–81.

84. Liu PY, Yee B, Wishart SM et al. The short-term effects of high-dose testosterone on sleep, breathing, and function in older men. J Clin Endocrinol Metab 2003; 88: 3605–13.

85. Malkin CJ, Pugh PJ, Jones RD et al. The effect of testosterone replacement on endogenous inflammatory cytokines and lipid profiles in hypogonadal men. J Clin Endocrinol Metab 2004; 89: 3313–18.

86. Kapoor D, Goodwin E, Channer KS, Jones TH. Testosterone replacement reduces insulin resistance in hypogonadal men with type 2 diabetes (abstract P1-394). Paper presented at: 87th Annual Meeting of the Endocrine Society, ENDO 2005, 4–7 June, 2005, San Diego, CA.

87. Pagotto U, Gambineri A, Pelusi C et al. Testosterone replacement therapy restores normal ghrelin in hypogonadal men. J Clin Endocrinol Metab 2003; 88: 4139–43.

88. Kupelian V, Shabsigh R, Araujo AB et al. Erectile dysfunction as a predictor of the metabolic syndrome in aging men: results from the Massachusetts Male Aging Study. J Urol 2006; 176: 201–6.

89. Esposito K, Giugliano F, Di Palo C et al. Effect of lifestyle changes on erectile dysfunction in obese men: a randomized controlled trial. JAMA 2004; 291: 2978–84.

90. Eaton CB, Liu YL, Mittleman MA et al. A retrospective study of the relationship between biomarkers of atherosclerosis and erectile dysfunction in 988 men. A retrospective study of the relationship between biomarkers of atherosclerosis and erectile dysfunction in 988 men. Int J Impot Res 2007; 19: 218–25.

91. Vicari E, Arcidiacono G, Di Pino L et al. Incidence of extragenital vascular disease in patients with erectile dysfunction of arterial origin. Int J Impot Res 2005; 17: 175–9.

92. Vicari E, Di Pino L, La Vignera S et al. Peak systolic velocity in patients with arterial erectile dysfunction and peripheral arterial disease. Int J Impot Res 2006; 18: 175–9.

93. Billups KL, Bank AJ, Padma-Nathan H, Katf SD, Williams RA. Erectile dysfunction as a harbinger for increased global cardiometabolic risk. Int J Impot Res. Advance online publication, January 2008.

94. Expert Panel on Detection, Evaluation, and Treatment of High Blood Cholesterol in Adults. Executive Summary of the third report of the National Cholesterol Education Program (NCEP) Expert Panel on Detection, Evaluation and Treatment of High Blood Cholesterol in Adults (Adult Treatment Panel III). JAMA 2001; 285: 2486–97.

95. Romero-Corral A, Montori VM, Somers VK et al. Association of bodyweight with total mortality and with cardiovascular events in coronary artery disease: a systematic review of cohort studies. Lancet 2006; 368: 666–78.

96. Morley JE, Charlton E, Patrick P et al. Validation of a screening questionnaire for androgen deficiency in aging males. Metabolism 2000; 49: 1239–42.

97. Richardson D, Vinik A. Etiology and treatment of erectile failure in diabetes mellitus. Curr Diab Rep 2002; 2: 501.

98. Basaria S, Muller DC, Carducci MA et al. Hyperglycemia and insulin resistance in men with

prostate carcinoma who receive androgen-deprivation therapy. Cancer 2006; 106: 581–6.

99. Morgentaler A, Rhoden EL. Prevalence of prostate cancer among hypogonadal men with prostate-specific antigen levels of 4.0 ng/mL or less. Urol 2006; 68: 1263–7.

100. Morales A. Monitoring androgen replacement therapy: testosterone and prostate safety. J Endocrinol Investig 2005; 28: 122–7.

101. Bhasin S, Singh AB, Mac RP et al. Managing the risks of prostate disease during testosterone replacement therapy in older men: recommendations for a standardized monitoring plan. J Androl 2003; 24: 299–311.

102. Thompson IM, Goodman PJ, Tangen CM et al. The influence of finasteride on the development of prostate cancer. N Engl J Med 2003; 349: 215–24.

103. Rhoden EL, Morgentaler A. Risks of testosterone-replacement therapy and recommendations for monitoring. N Engl J Med 2004; 350: 482–92.

104. Morgentaler A, Rhoden EL. Prevalence of prostate cancer among hypogonadal men with prostate-specific antigen levels of 4.0 ng/ml or less. Urol 2006; 68: 1223–67.

105. Miner M, Kuritzky L. Erectile dysfunction: a sentinel marker for cardiovascular disease in primary care. Cleve Clin J Med 2007; 74: S30–7.

106. Rosan RC, Fishor WA, Eardley I et al. The multinational Men's Attitude to Life Events and Sexuality (MALES) study: 1. Prevalence of erectile dysfunction and related health concerns in the general population. Curr Med Res Opin 2004; 20: 607–17.

107. Miner M, Seftel A. Testosterone and aging: what have we learned since the IOM report and what lies ahead. Int J Clin Pract 2007; 61: 622–32.

CHAPTER 43

The health of gay men

Justin Varney

Introduction

Approximately 6% of the population identify themselves as lesbian, gay, or bisexual according to the UK government,[1] this figure is comparable with the 7.9% of the UK population in the 2001 census who identified with a non-white ethnic minority group. In many countries, including the UK, gay men receive equal protection, in terms of employment and the provision of goods, services and facilities, against discrimination based on their sexual orientation and identity as do those from ethnic minorities and those living with disabilities. This protection includes the provision of healthcare and health services. Therefore it is important that healthcare professionals both understand concepts of sexual orientation, heterosexism, and homophobic discrimination, and develop knowledge of the physical and mental health issues that disproportionately affect gay men.

Sexual orientation, identity, and behavior

Sexual behavior can often be different from sexual identity and orientation. Many people at some point have a sexual fantasy or thought about another person of the same sex; however, this does not automatically mean that they would act out this fantasy or that the person instantly identifies as gay or lesbian.

The progression from sexual desire and attraction to behavior and then to defining an orientation and self-defined identity is not always linear and may change over time. A person who self-defines as celibate can still identify as heterosexual or straight despite having no active sexual behavior. When considering the gay aspects of a man it is worth recognizing the difference between sexual behavior of men who have sex with men and those who identify with the sexual orientation 'gay', which defines a sexual identity. Many men have some form of sexual activity with other men at some point during their lives, but not all of them identify as gay or bisexual. A man's sexual orientation and identity may change through his life or may remain the same. Alfred Kinsey's work[2] illustrated that human sexuality is a spectrum and that only a few men identify at either end of the spectrum, with the majority fluctuating throughout their lives and at some point having same-sex desires or actions.

This is often reflected in epidemiological studies in which men are categorized as 'men who have sex with men' or 'homosexually active men' in an attempt to capture data on all men engaging in same-sex sexual activity, including those who do not self-identify as gay or homosexual.

Sexual orientation and sexual identity are often used interchangeably. However, there are subtle but important differences between the two. 'Sexual orientation' describes the direction of a person's attraction and sexual desire towards people of a particular gender or sex; this is often categorized, using a binary model of gender and sex, into heterosexual (attracted to the opposite sex or gender), homosexual (attracted to the same sex or gender), or bisexual (attracted to both sexes or genders). 'Sexual identity' is slightly different and describes someone's personal identification with a sexual and social construct that reflects the sexual orientation (e.g. gay or lesbian). A person with a homosexual sexual orientation may actively engage in same-sex relationships but may not identify with a gay sexual identity and hence not respond to health services marketed to gay men.

A gay identity is, like most identities, culturally constructed, so what is considered 'gay' in one culture may not be in another, and similarly the language and 'tribal symbolism and totems' that may be markers of a gay identity in the UK may be very different in the Caribbean or in the USA. It is therefore essential that people are enabled and allowed to identify themselves rather than have practitioners assume an identity based on mannerisms, dress, or behavior. Asking about sexual orientation and identity is becoming more standard as part of routine demographic monitoring of staff (Box 43.1) and service users following the introduction of equality legislation in the UK, and there is readily available guidance on the correct language

---

Box 43.1. *Asking healthcare staff about sexual orientation*[54]

Monitoring can be conducted via:
- Anonymous staff satisfaction surveys
- Recruitment procedures
- All other policies, practices, and procedures where a person's sexual orientation might have had an impact on how he or she was treated, such as recruitment, appraisals, and training opportunities

When monitoring staff, organizations should ask whether staff are:
- Bisexual
- Gay man
- Gay woman or lesbian
- Heterosexual or straight
- Other
- Prefer not to say

---

and approach to be used. Also, many medical schools are now considering this as part of their core communication skills training.

Stigma and discrimination: barriers to health

In considering gay men's health it is important to recognize that gay men still face substantial stigma and discrimination in society. Legislation has progressed a long way since the Stonewall riots in 1969 and the first Gay Day in London in August 1970, and there is legal protection against discrimination in employment, education, and the provision of goods, services and facilities, including health services. However there remain over 1000 incidents of homophobic hate crime reported to the Metropolitan Police in London each year, and in both the UK and across the world gay men are murdered because of their sexual orientation, as happened to Matthew Sheppard[3] and David Morley.[4]

Discrimination against people based on perceptions about their sexual orientation and identity is often described as homophobia. Douglas Scott defined homophobia as 'an irrational fear and dislike of lesbian, gay and bisexual people, which can lead to hatred resulting in verbal and physical attacks and abuse'.[5]

Research has illustrated that whether actually experienced or not, gay men perceive that they will experience discrimination when accessing health services if their sexual orientation or identity is disclosed,[6] and that in order to enable disclosure gay men need to be given verbal or visual stimuli that acknowledge that the environment is safe and respectful of that disclosure. Often this decision about disclosure is complicated by the heterosexism of healthcare providers.

Tamsin Wilton defined heterosexism as 'the widespread social assumption that heterosexuality may be taken for granted as normal, natural and right'.[7] For example, when a person meets a palliative care team, the form they fill in may ask about the name of the person' husband or wife; this assumes a heterosexual married relationship rather than asking about the non-specific 'partner'. The use of heterosexual assumptions places a pressure on people to disclose their deviation from the assumed normality. This sets off a risk–benefit thought process, whereby the person assesses the risk of rejection and discrimination on disclosure leading to substandard or impaired support and care against the benefit of being able to be open about his or her relationship and family structure, which may be important in developing a suitable care plan and hence in the experience of the disease that is being managed.

Perception of discrimination is a major barrier to accessing services, and this can have implications in terms of health outcomes, leading to late presentation and hence the potential for worse prognosis because of more advanced pathology. Although there has been limited research on this amongst gay men, there is clear evidence of the impact of discrimination as a barrier amongst lesbians relating to uptake of screening services for breast cancer.[8] Discrimination as a barrier to health service will be a contributing factor to worse health outcomes for gay men across the board; however, there are some specific areas where sexual orientation and identity relate to health risk behavior and patterns of disease.

Health risk behavior

Health risk behavior is a term used to describe activities that lead to an increased likelihood of negative impacts on physical, mental, or social wellbeing. Risk behaviors include such things as smoking; eating high-fat, high-salt food; and not wearing a seat belt when driving.[9] There is now substantial evidence that rates of some health risk behaviors are significantly higher amongst gay men. Smoking rates are two or three times that of the general population,[10–12] and this picture of risk behavior is repeated for the use of recreational drugs[13] and alcohol.[14] There is little known about the eating patterns of gay men; however, there appears to be an increased prevalence of eating disorders amongst gay men.[15] There is also a growing body of research into the relationship gay men have with body image and cultural constructs of social body norms, which may contribute to eating disorders and steroid abuse.[16,17] There is substantial

research into sexual risk taking in the context of the HIV epidemic, and this is commented upon later in the chapter.

Significant effort has been put into understanding why people undertake health risk behaviors and the risk-versus-benefit deliberation, both conscious and unconscious, that leads to these negative impact actions. Although most of the research into risk motivation amongst gay men has focused on sexual risk behavior, the impact of these factors is likely to be common across risk behaviors. These factors include:

1. Perceptions and experiences of homophobia: such perceptions and experiences may lead to different communication and decision-making assessments, which is especially important in relation to accessing screening and health services. Experiences may also lead to an altered perception of longevity and poor self-esteem, which change a person's concept of risk versus benefit.

2. Limitations in safe social spaces (e.g. the feeling that the only 'gay space' is in a bar or pub): this may lead to normalization of alcohol and drug use in the context of a gay identity. When people start to explore their sexual identity, they will seek out spaces and other people who identify themselves as gay. The majority of such spaces are pubs and club venues; although in some areas there are alternatives such as lesbian, gay, bisexual, and/or transgender (LGBT) community centers. Coming into such a space has significant stressor factors and hence people may use drugs, cigarettes, or alcohol to help to manage that stress.[18]

3. Peer-group pressure and cultural media stereotype promotion of the risk behavior (e.g. the emphasis in the gay-targeted media that 'good' gay men have lots of sex, do drugs, and club every night): an informal survey of the gay media in the UK over a 1-month period in 2006 illustrated the predominance of muscled, waxed, tanned, white men on the cover of magazines and local press. This predominant image is paradoxical in the context of health risk because it portrays an object of physical health, yet research has illustrated that many gay men

attain this image through steroid[19] and recreational drug use[20] and significant health risk behavior. Furthermore, while gay men are up to 6% of the general population, it is suggested that 20% of men with anorexia identify as gay.[21] It is also worth noting that in some cases there has been direct marketing of products such as cigarettes to gay men.[22]

4. Impact of the AIDS epidemic and concepts of old age: the HIV epidemic had a disproportionate impact on the gay community and large numbers of gay men became infected and died young. However, since the mid 1990s improved treatment has led to increased life expectancy, which has translated HIV into a chronic terminal illness. The impact of the mass mortality in the 1980s may have contributed to an absence in the gay psyche of old age, which in turn means a disenfranchisement from the concept of investing in health in order to prepare for a healthy old age.

The concept of social marketing is predicated on the assumption that given the right triggers, through advertising and marketing approaches a person can be persuaded to move away from health risk behavior choices.[23] Although beyond the remit of this chapter, it is important to recognize that social marketing is based on a series of assumptions that stereotype the end-product consumer. This stereotyped consumer is usually assumed to be heterosexual; for example, an EU-wide social marketing campaign to reduce smoking used imagery of children and a fetus to stress the impact of smoking on fertility and parenthood. Although gay-identified men may have children, it remains relatively unusual that these are conceived through sexual intercourse unless during a previously heterosexual-identified period. Hence the imagery and language excluded gay men from the message being promoted at a population level. This, often unconscious, heterosexist approach has meant that many of the national-level social marketing campaigns have excluded gay men, which may in part explain the higher levels of health risk behaviors amongst this group.

The impact of higher levels of risk behaviors such as smoking and substance misuse is illustrated across the heterosexual population in chronic disease and premature mortality. Historically the gap in life expectancy between gay men and heterosexual men has been attributed to HIV and AIDS. However, advances in medication have mitigated this impact in the developed world. Therefore the impact of alcohol, drugs, and health risk behavior on this life expectancy gap will now become clearer, bringing home the realization of a hedonistic lifestyle.

Physical health

Relatively little is known about the non-sexual health aspects of gay men's physical health. This reflects the absence of sexual orientation monitoring in routine datasets[24] and the lack of funding for research into the health of gay men beyond the impact of HIV. The few published papers on the general health of gay men have illustrated higher self-reported ill health and indicators of chronic disease such as high blood pressure or high cholesterol.[25]

People's sexual orientation or identity is an important aspect of their physical healthcare. Perceptions of stigma and discrimination may act as a barrier to disclosure but without this information the physician may be unable to develop appropriate care plans and pathways and will innocently exclude significant partners and relationships from decision-making; this may be particularly important when planning support for old age[26] and end-of-life care.[27]

Cancer

Almost 4 million men across the world die every year from cancer. The most common cancers affecting men globally are of the lung, stomach, liver, colon and rectum, esophagus, and prostate.[28] All of these common cancers are affected by health risk behaviors that are more common among gay men, and hence one would expect a higher prevalence of these cancers among gay men. Despite this there is relatively little known about gay men and cancer.[29]

The one area of exception is anal cancer. Anal cancer is associated with human papilloma virus (HPV) infection, in a similar way to cervical cancer in women. In gay men who are HIV- and HPV-positive, there is a stark increase in the prevalence of anal cancer to an estimated 20 times higher rate than amongst heterosexual men.[30] Currently there is debate in many developed countries about the cost-effectiveness of anal pap cancer screening programs[31] at a national level for gay men; however, many practitioners have started to offer private anal cancer screening to gay men and in the future there may also be similar debates about the impact of HPV vaccination of men as a prevention intervention for anal cancer.

Two further cancers are associated with HIV infection. Kaposi's sarcoma is a rare vascular cancer thought to be linked to human herpes virus 8. The very visual purple skin lesions were a very public marker of the development of AIDS amongst many gay men, although the prevalence has reduced since the introduction of better HIV treatment. Lymphomas are between 50 and 100 times more common among people with HIV infection than among the general population, and since the improvement in HIV treatment there has been an increase in survival rates.[32]

HIV and AIDS

The HIV epidemic has been synonymous with the gay male identity across almost the entire developed world. The first reporting of the epidemic was amongst gay white men in the USA, and during the 1980s and 1990s almost entire age cohorts of gay men died from AIDS. Although much of the global epidemic is affecting heterosexuals, particularly in developing countries, men who have sex with men accounted for 44% of people living with HIV in the UK in 2006.[33]

The advent of highly active anti-retroviral treatment in the early 1990s has substantially changed the experience of living with HIV for gay men in developed countries. Whereas during the 1980s men infected with HIV expected to die within 5–10 years, the improvements in treatment and management of HIV have extended life expectancy with HIV to an almost normal lifespan, transforming HIV into a chronic terminal illness.

The culture of the gay community relating to HIV has evolved over the duration of the epidemic. In the 1980s vocal activist movements such as ACT UP used shock tactics and public demonstrations to move forward political action to fund prevention

and provide treatment for people living with HIV and AIDS. During the 1990s organizations such as the Terrance Higgins Trust transitioned from activism to become partners in the pan-government response to the epidemic, and across the world there was substantial investment in raising awareness and promoting a safer sex message.

In the new millennium there are new challenges to be faced. The shift to a 'chronic terminal disease' requires new ways of approaching prevention campaigns and the promotion of HIV testing, and a new paradigm for people living with HIV. Clinical care of people living with HIV has evolved from acute management of AIDS to the complexities of polypharmacy and comorbidities as these people develop coronary heart disease, cancer, and diabetes.

Sexual health

Although it is important to recognize that there is more to gay men than their sex lives, sexual health and wellbeing is an important aspect of any person's overall health. As with HIV, gay men are disproportionately represented in sexual health statistics, with higher rates of gonorrhea and syphilis. Often there are clustered outbreaks of sexually transmitted diseases associated with particular venues or cities. Since the mid-1990s there has been a year-on-year increase in the number of cases of gonorrhea amongst men who have sex with men, predominantly amongst those aged 25–44 years, and between 2005 and 2006 in the UK there was an increase of 10% in the total number of cases. Similarly the numbers infected with syphilis increased by two-thirds between 2001 and 2005.[33] Gay men are also disproportionately affected by genital warts and HPV infection compared with heterosexual men, and this has implications for anal cancer and the implementation of the developing HPV vaccines.

Although the stereotype of gay men as highly promiscuous is indeed a stereotype, there is a culture of sexual freedom within the gay community that is more visible than in the heterosexual community.[34] Most urban centers will have bath-houses, gymnasiums, or saunas where men can engage in sex with multiple partners, and some gay men will use 'cottages' (gay slang for public toilets) or go 'cruising' (hang out in public parks) for sex with strangers. It is important to recognize that, although some gay men engage in these sexual activities, not all do, and many of those who cottage or cruise identify themselves as heterosexual and, although often defined in epidemiological studies as men who have sex with men, they do not identify as gay men or use services targeted at this group.

Mental health

Mental health is a key aspect of any person's health and wellbeing. When considering the mental health of gay men it is useful to reflect on the impact of stigma and discrimination throughout life, which can be major factors leading to poor mental health. Bullying and abuse are a major factor affecting the mental and social wellbeing of gay men. Surveys have found that around 80% of gay men under 25 years of age experience verbal abuse, and up to 60% reported being physically attacked during their time at school.[35,36] One study found that 40% of those who had been bullied indicated that they had attempted suicide or self-harm on at least one occasion.[37] A national study in the UK into the mental health and wellbeing of gay men found that 68% of the gay men have been verbally harassed in the past 5 years, compared with 46% of heterosexual men. In the same study, 54% of the gay men had at some point self-harmed, compared with 41% of heterosexual men, illustrating that these experiences are not restricted to childhood.[38]

Although homosexuality is no longer being considered a mental illness, several studies have suggested that over a third of gay men experience negative or mixed reactions from mental health professionals when they are open about their sexuality,[39] and work looking at the attitudes of counselors found that up to a third had negative attitudes towards gay men.[40]

Social wellbeing

Social wellbeing is the third part of the World Health Organization's definition of health, there are many aspects of social wellbeing that relate to

people's engagement with social networks, their community, their employment, and their family.

In employment situations, discrimination can have significant negative effect on self-esteem and career progression. Gay men are significantly more likely to say they have been fired unfairly from their job because of discrimination.[41] The Department of Health commissioned a report into discrimination in the UK National Health Service, which found stark reports of experiences of discrimination in the workplace (Box 43.2).[42] In one survey of gay doctors in the UK 13% felt that being open about their sexual orientation had impaired their career progress.[43]

Experiences of social isolation and disenfranchisement can be compounded by other aspects of a man's identity, such as his age, disability, faith, or ethnicity. Often these issues are compounded by the lack of validation for these co-existent identities and an absence of safe and supportive spaces for their representation.

Younger gay men are often at increased risk of mental health problems and depression associated with experiences of bullying at school.[44] Research suggests that in comparison with heterosexual youth, gay men are seven times more likely to have attempted suicide.[45] Young gay men are also more likely to use illicit drugs than their heterosexual peers.[46]

Older gay men are often ignored since the concept of sexual behavior and identity associated with older people is socially challenging; however, aging for gay men presents serious issues and implications. Research suggests that compared with their heterosexual counterparts older gay men are two and a half times as likely to live alone, twice as likely to be single, and four and a half times as likely to have no children to call upon in times of need.[47] This absence of social support structures presents unique challenges for aging gay men, and this is compounded by perceptions and fear of stigma and discrimination from heath and social care staff.[48]

Very little is known about the health of gay men with disabilities. Research has suggested that gay men who have learning disabilities may experience a double 'coming out' process as disabled and as gay.[49] Coming out for a man with a disability can be more difficult because they may be reliant on family or social care for financial and physical support and so the implications of rejection may be more severe than for other gay men; in addition there is a general lack of validation for same-sex relationships for disabled men and a lack of acceptance in the non-disabled gay community.[50]

Similarly, little is know about the health of black and minority ethnic gay men or about gay men of faith. There is UK research that debunks the myth that all gay men are white and that in fact there is no evidence that sex between men is any more or less common among any ethnic group.[51] There has been some research done into the ethnicity of gay men affected by HIV, which suggests that in the UK African–Caribbean gay men are twice as likely to be living with diagnosed HIV infection than gay white men, whereas South Asian gay men were less likely to be doing so.[52] One study in London found that black and minority ethnic gay men were disproportionately affected by homophobic violence and abuse from strangers than their white counterparts.[53] It is also important to recognize that the language of gay identity may vary between BME communities and therefore when working with these communities it may be more useful to use the term men who have sex with men.

Summary

Gay men present an interesting opportunity to engage with a new and emerging cultural identity that debunks traditional models of masculinity and social constructs of gender. As with other minority identity groups there are limitations to the research and evidence base, particularly around the experiences and health of gay men with multiple aspects to their social and cultural identities.

What research exists suggests that gay men experience health inequalities that are similar to, and in some cases surpass, those experienced by other minority groups. Yet the understandable focus on the HIV epidemic has limited consideration of the wider physical, mental, and social health needs of this group.

Gay men often have huge personal resilience and competent life skills resulting from their experiences of discrimination and stigma, which provide consultations that are often challenging and enlightening. Working with gay men requires the same basic standards of dignity and respect that are the basis of healthcare professionalism and standards that any person should be entitled to.

References

1. Department of Trade and Industry, Women and Equalities Unit. Getting Equal: Proposals to Outlaw Sexual Orientation Discrimination in the Provision of Goods and Services. London: TSO, 2006.
2. Kinsey AC, Pomeroy WB, Martin CE. Sexual Behavior in the Human Male. Philadelphia: WB Saunders, 1948.
3. http://www.matthew shepard.org. Matthew Shepard Foundation.
4. http://david-morley.tabbyhost.co.uk. David Morley Tribute Website.
5. Douglas Scott S, Pringle A, Lumsdaine C. Sexual exclusion: homophobia and health inequalities: a review. London: UK Gay Men's Health Network, 2004.
6. Keogh P, Weatherburn P, Henderson L et al. Doctoring Gay Men: Exploring the Contribution of General Practice. London: Sigma Research, 2004.
7. Wilton T. Towards an understanding of the cultural roots of homophobia in order to provide a better midwifery service for lesbian clients. Midwifery 1999; 15: 154–64.
8. Fish J, Wilkinson S. Understanding lesbians' health-care behaviour: the case of breast self-examination. Soc Sci Med 2003; 56: 235–45.
9. Inequalities in Health: the Black report. Harmondsworth, UK: Pelican, 1992.

10. Stall RD, Greenwood GL, Acree M, Paul J, Coates TJ. Cigarette smoking among gay and bisexual men. Am J Public Health 1999; 89: 1875–8.

11. Gruskin EP, Greenwood GL, Matevia M, Pollack LM, Bye LM. Disparities in smoking between the lesbian, gay, and bisexual population and the general population in California. Am J Public Health 2001; 97: 1496–502.

12. Ryan H, Wortley PM, Easton A, Pederson L, Greenwood G. Smoking among lesbians, gays, and bisexuals: a review of the literature. Am J Prev Med 2001; 21: 142–9.

13. Hughes TL, Eliason M. Substance use and abuse in lesbian, gay, bisexual and transgender populations. J Prim Prev 2002; 22: 2.

14. Hughes TL, Eliason M. Substance use and abuse in lesbian, gay, bisexual and transgender populations. J Prim Prev 2002; 22: 263.

15. Feldman MB, Meyer IH. Eating disorders in diverse lesbian, gay, and bisexual populations. Int J Eat Disord 2007; 40: 218–26.

16. Levesque MJ, Vichesky DR. Raising the bar on the body beautiful: An analysis of the body image concerns of homosexual men. Body Image 2006; 3: 45–55.

17. Martins Y, Tiggemann M, Kirkbride A. Those speedos become them: the role of self-objectification in gay and heterosexual men's body image. Pers Soc Psychol Bull 2007; 33: 634–47.

18. Harris CE. Out in life; still up in smoke? J Gay Lesbian Med Assoc 1998; 2: 91–2.

19. Bolding G, Sherr L, Maguire M, Elford J. HIV risk behaviours among gay men who use anabolic steroids. Addict 1999; 94: 1829–35.

20. Steven P. Kurtz. Post-circuit blues: motivations and consequences of crystal meth use among gay men in Miami. AIDS Behav 2005; 9: 63–72.

21. Herzog D, Bradburn I, Newman K. Sexuality in males with eating disorders. In: Anderson AE, ed. Practical Comprehensive Treatment of Anorexia Nervosa and Bulimia. New York: Bruner Mazel, 1990: 40–53.

22. Goebel K. Lesbians and gays face tobacco targeting. Tob Control 1994; 3: 65–7.

23. Douglas Evans W. How social marketing works in health care. BMJ 2006; 332: 1207–10.

24. Sell RL, Becker JB. Sexual orientation data collection and progress toward healthy people 2010. Am J Public Health 2001; 91: 876–82.

25. Wang J, Häusermann M, Vounatsou P, Aggleton P, Weiss MG. Health status, behavior, and care utilization in the Geneva Gay Men's Health Survey. Prev Med 2007; 44: 70–5.

26. Hash K. Caregiving and post-caregiving experiences of midlife and older gay men and lesbians. J Gerontol Soc Work 2006; 47: 121–38.

27. Smolinski KM, Colon Y. Silent voices and invisible walls: exploring end of life care with lesbians and gay men. J Psychosoc Oncol 2006; 24: 51–64.

28. Cancer Factsheet 297. World Health Organization. July 2008 [available at: http://www.who.int/mediacentre/factsheets/fs297/en/index.html].

29. Blank TO. Gay men and prostate cancer: invisible diversity. J Clin Oncol 2005; 23: 2593–60.

30. Anderson JS, Vajdic C, Grulich AE. Is screening for anal cancer warranted in homosexual men? Sex Health 2006; 1: 137–40.

31. Goldie SJ, Kuntz KM, Weinstein MC, Freedberg KA, Palefsky JM. Cost-effectiveness of screening for anal squamous intraepithelial lesions and anal cancer in human immunodeficiency virus-negative homosexual and bisexual men. Am J Med 2000; 108: 634–41.

32. Chow KU, Mitrou PS, Geduldig K et al. Changing incidence and survival in patients with aids-related non-Hodgkin's lymphomas in the era of highly active antiretroviral therapy (HAART). Leuk Lymphoma 2001; 41: 105–16.

33. Health Protection Agency. A complex picture – HIV and other sexually transmitted infections in the United Kingdom. London: Health Protection Agency, 2006.

34. Elford J, Bolding G, Sherr L, Hart G. High-risk sexual behaviour among London gay men: no longer increasing. AIDS 2005; 19: 2171–4.

35. GALOP. Homophobic Violence Youth Survey. London: GALOP, 1997.

36. Rivers I. The bullying of sexual minorities at school. Educational Child Psychol 2001; 18: 32–46.

37. Rivers I. The long-term impact of peer victimisation in adolescence upon the well-being of lesbian, gay and bisexual adults. Paper presented at the Psychological Society of Ireland's Annual Conference, Dublin, Ireland, 13–15 November, 1997.

38. King M, McKeown E. Mental Health and Social Wellbeing of Gay Men, Lesbians and Bisexuals in England and Wales. A Summary of Findings. London: MIND, 2003.

39. McFarlane L. Diagnosis: homophobic – the experiences of lesbians, gay men and bisexuals in mental health services. London: PACE (The Project for Advice, Counselling and Education), 1998.

40. Rudolph J. Counsellors' attitudes towards homosexuality: a selective review of the literature. J Couns Dev 1988; 67: 165–68.

543

41.	Meyer IH. Prejudice, social stress and mental health in lesbian, gay and bisexual populations: conceptual issues and research evidence. Psychol Bull 129: 674–97.

42.	Hunt R, Cowan K, Chamberlin B. Being the gay one: experiences of Lesbian, Gay and Bisexual People Working in the Health and Social Care Sector. London: Stonewall, 2007.

43.	Hunt R, Cowan K. Harassment and sexual orientation in the health sector. London: Stonewall, 2006.

44.	Fergusson DM, Horwood LJ, Beautrais AL. Is sexual orientation related to mental health problems and suicidality in young people. Arch Gen Psychiatry 1999; 56: 876–80.

45.	Remafedi G, French S, Story M. The relationship between suicide risk and sexual orientation: results of a population-based study. Amer J Pub Health 1998; 88: 57–60.

46.	Ziyadeh NJ, Prokop LA, Fisher LB et al. Sexual orientation, gender and alcohol use in a cohort study of US adolescent girls and boys. Drug Alcohol Depend 2007; 86: 119–30.

47.	Knocker S. The Whole of Me: Meeting the Needs of Older Lesbians, Gay Men and Bisexuals Living in Care Homes and Extra Care Housing. London: Age Concern, 2006.

48.	Heaphy B, Yip A, Thompson D. Lesbian, Gay and Bisexual Lives over 50: A report on the project 'The Social and Policy Implications of Non-Heterosexual Ageing.' Nottingham: Trent University and York House Publication, 2003.

49.	Davidson-Paine C, Corbett J. A double coming out: gay men with learning disabilities. Br J Learn Disabil 1995; 23: 147–51.

50.	Abbott D, Howart J. Secret Loves, Hidden Lives: Exploring Issues for People with Learning Difficulties Who Are Gay, Lesbian or Bisexual. Bristol: Policy Press, 2005.

51.	Hickson F, Reid D, Weatherburn P et al. HIV risk, sexual risk and ethnicity among men in England who have sex with men. Sex Transm Infect 2004; 80: 443–50.

52.	Keogh P, Henderson L, Dodds C. Ethnic minority gay men: redefining community, restoring identity. Portsmouth: Sigma Research, 2004.

53.	GALOP. The Low Down: Black Lesbians, Gay Men and Bisexual People Talk About Their Experiences and Needs. London: Galop, 2001.

54.	Hunt R, Cowan K. Monitoring Sexual Orientation in the Health Sector. London: Stonewall, 2006.

CHAPTER 44

Men at work

Steven Boorman

Background

In the UK, projections of the size and composition of the workforce are regularly reviewed by the Office of National Statistics, for the interest of policy makers, business and those involved in socio-economic trends.[1] The size of the working population is expected to continue to grow until 2020, although the rate of increase will decline, peaking at around 32 million. As demographic trends tend towards an aging population and social and economic policy (avoiding discrimination or for pension and benefit reasons) seek to promote opportunities for the older worker, the average working age is becoming greater. The shift in population age is also increasing the dependency ratio (those above working age expressed as percentage of those working). More than three-quarters of adult men under the age of 65 years work (79% in 2004), compared with around two-thirds of women (67% in 2004), according to Equal Opportunities Commission data. Changes to the nature of work (decline in manufacturing, for example) and changes to legislative policy on discrimination and pensions issues underpin projected trends for future workforces to have greater equality of sex.

Many workplaces previously reserved to men, often because of the physical demands or other characteristics of the work, are changing to accommodate greater inclusivity. These changes, including adapting work to accommodate older workers, disabled workers and the promotion of sex equality, also widen access to the workplace to those less physically fit or agile. This is a trend that is also promoted by recognition of the high costs of retirement or workforce turnover. Unless an industry is actively seeking to reduce employee numbers, the costs of recruitment, retraining, lost opportunity, and lost experience and skills are substantial, and generally much greater than the costs of simple workplace changes required to widen accessibility to enable greater workforce diversity.

Is work healthy?

Work is important to good health, although until recently the evidence base for this has tended to focus on the more negative association between certain employments and ill health. Bernardino Ramazzini, often credited as the 'father' of occupational medicine after the publication of a carefully observed study of the link between different forms of work and disease, wrote in 1713, 'various and manifold is the harvest of diseases reaped by certain workers from crafts and trades they pursue'.[2]

Whilst even today some occupations are inherently hazardous, the perception of work as being a risky business is flawed – a thorough evidence-based review, commissioned by the Department for Work and Pensions,[3] sought to explore the difference between the negative health effects of long-term worklessness and the potential positive health benefits of being in work. Importantly, the reviewers confirm that work is good for health and wellbeing, concluding that the beneficial effects of work outweigh the adverse risks. There is also strong evidence that long-term worklessness caused by unemployment or sickness absence is harmful to health, with higher mortality, generally worse physical and mental ill health, and higher use of health services.

Many studies support the link between work and the necessary economic resources to participate fully in society. Aside from the psychosocial needs fulfilled by participating in work relationships, in many societies employment is regarded as 'normal' and central to concepts of social status, identity, and role.[4]

It is true that some occupations are associated with specific risks to health – many occupations have been long associated with known high morbidity or mortality, mining being an obvious example. Indeed, even in Egyptian times its hazards were sufficiently well recognized for this work to be reserved for criminals or slaves. Agricola in the 16th century described the risks to more highly skilled medieval artisans seeking silver in the Carpathian mountains and, importantly, the measures to improve mine design and ventilation to reduce these risks. However, a further 400 years were required before the true toxic workplace agent causing rampant 'consumption' (as the root cause for terrible mortality rates), was identified as uranium (for which mines are actively worked today).[5]

It was Percival Pott who first described clearly the link between a particular occupation and its impact on future men's health, when he recognized the link between scrotal cancer and exposure to soot for 'climbing boy' chimney sweeps.

Occupational medicine texts document the now well-described associations between a wide variety of occupations and exposure to physical, chemical, biological, and psychosocial hazards during work. Fortunately many such agents are now sufficiently well recognized that workplace exposures in developed countries are becoming rare and the conditions associated with them consigned to the history of textbooks. Despite this, occupation-related cancers (and other serious pathologies such as occupational lung diseases) may have long lead times between exposure to workplace risk and subsequent morbidity or mortality – in the UK during 2004, 1969

people died of mesothelioma,[7] a disease almost exclusively associated with workplace asbestos exposure common in industries such as ship building.

However, the majority of the working population in the UK, and a large proportion of working men, work in small businesses employing only a few workers with relatively low turnovers or profit margins. In such businesses, health and safety controls may be less rigorously adopted and enforcement activity is hard. Industrial workplaces of this nature often have predominantly male workforces, with a wide variety of physical and chemical hazards and variable standards of health and safety compliance.

Legislation, in the UK based on the Health and Safety at Work Act 1974, places onuses on employers to protect the health and safety of workers. Using a principle of simple risk assessment – identifying hazards and weighing the likelihood of harm arising – the law requires an employer to take steps to avoid work-related health risks. A simple hierarchy of control is recommended to help reduce the harm associated with risk exposure:

- elimination – where possible use of the hazardous agent should be completely avoided;
- substitution – if a less hazardous alternative exists it should be used in preference to the noxious agent;
- reduction – reducing the amount of exposure, either by reducing the quantity or reducing the amount of time that it is used for;
- containment – using engineering solutions to reduce contact between worker and hazard; and
- protection – as a last resort using personal protective equipment to avoid contact with hazard.

Employers have a responsibility to identify and provide safe systems of work, and workers are required to follow these.

It is difficult to estimate accurately the number of people working with chronic medical conditions (see Table 44.1). In a policy paper produced to support National Men's Health Week, the Men's Health Forum defined long-term health conditions as those that may be controlled but not at present cured. The most recent (2001) UK census

Table 44.1. *Estimates of numbers of people affected by common chronic medical conditions in the United Kingdom*

Condition	Est'd total no.	Information source
Anxiety and depression	4.3 million	National Statistics Online
Arthritis	9 million	Arthritis Care
Asthma (severe)	2.6 million	Asthma UK
Dementia	700 000	Alzheimer's Society
Diabetes types 1 and 2 (diagnosed)	2 million	Diabetes UK
Epilepsy	456 000	Epilepsy Action
Heart failure	740 000	National Statistics Online
HIV infection (diagnosed)	42 500	Terrence Higgins Trust
Inflammatory bowel disease	180 000	Nat. Assoc. for Colitis & Crohn's Disease
Multiple sclerosis	85 000	Multiple Sclerosis Society
Myalgic encephalomyelitis	250 000	ME Association
Parkinson's disease	120 000	Parkinson's Disease Society
Prostate cancer	150 000	Extrapolated for UK from Scottish data

Reproduced with permission from Men's Health Forum Policy Briefing Paper 2007: Men and Long Term Health Conditions

suggested that over 10 million people in the UK have a long-term illness, health problem, or disability that limits their work activity. The more recent 2004–2005 General Household Survey suggests that 15.9 million people have a long-term medical condition – although other sources estimate higher figures still (the Department of Health estimates that up to 60% of the population may have a chronic disease).[6]

Although good progress has been made in reducing workplace accidents (more than 10% reduction in past 10 years), there are still around 200 fatal injuries in the workplace each year (241 in 2006–2007, or 0.8 per 100 000 workers). These occur mainly to men – the majority within the construction industry, with agriculture, fishing and forestry being other high-risk occupations. Although fatalities and serious accidents are better reported, less serious injuries are subject to considerable under-reporting. Self-reporting from the Labour Force Survey would suggest that reportable injury rates of 1200 or so per 100 000 workers (in 2004–2005) should be expected, whilst employer reports made

under the reporting of Injuries, Diseases and Dangerous Occurrences Regulations (RIDDOR) are far fewer, at approximately 600 per 100 000 employees per year (146 076 in 2005–2006, equivalent to 562.4 per 100 000).[5,7]

Men, and particularly younger men, have lower perception of risk – and are more likely to accept risky working conditions or to adopt risk-taking behaviors; the consequence is greater likelihood of accident. Physically demanding manual work is more likely to result in accident than more sedentary employment, and when accidents do occur the consequence may be greater as a result of the greater physical forces involved. The greater numbers of men in such occupations therefore mean that fatal and serious workplace accidents more commonly involve men than women.

Revitalising health and safety

According to figures from the Health and Safety Executive, over 30 million working days are lost in the UK each year because of work-related ill health (24 million days) and workplace injury (6 million days).[7] Approximately 2 million people suffer from an illness that they believe is directly caused or made worse by the work that they undertake. Over half a million of these cases are new health problems arising within the previous 12 months.

Twenty-five years after the original Health and Safety at Work legislation the UK Deputy Prime Minister announced, in March 1999 the 'Revitalising Health and Safety' strategy,[8] with the aim of giving renewed priority to the issue of improved health and safety at work, with on emphasis on improving accidents and ill health caused by work, particularly among those working in smaller companies. The strategy statement set bold targets:

- To reduce working days lost from work-related injury and ill health by 30% by 2010
- To reduce the incidence rate of fatal and major injury accidents by 10% by 2010
- To reduce the incidence rate of cases of work-related ill health by 20% by 2010
- To achieve at least half of the improvements above by 2004.

From the data in previous paragraphs, the improvements to work-related ill health are on track to achieve the 10-year target, with continued improvement in 2005–2006. The number of days lost per worker has also improved and remains on track to achieve the stated target. Fatal and major injuries, despite improvement in 2005–2006, remain of concern and are currently behind target.

The bold targets were underpinned by a 10-point strategy and encouraged action plans to motivate employers to improve practices to reduce workplace risk. Small firms were targeted through a program of sector-specific guidance from the Health and Safety Executive and the development of grant schemes to support improvement, and occupational health coverage was highlighted as a key area for improvement – nearly 90% of UK workplaces do not have formal arrangements for occupational health cover, and access to appropriate occupational health support is inconsistent and poorer in smaller companies. Many large businesses benefit from well-organized multi-disciplinary occupational health teams – with specialist occupational physicians and occupational health nurses working alongside resources to support employee welfare, safety, or other specialist support functions. A small but increasing minority of UK businesses are also providing workplace-based treatment services, such as physiotherapy and cognitive behavioral therapy, and in some cases these have extended to specialist workplace-based rehabilitation facilities. Provision of such care can be effective for larger businesses funded by reductions in sickness absence, improved workplace morale (an engaged, motivated workforce is more productive), or reduced liabilities from claims due to work-related disability.

In 2006, collaboration between the UK Department of Health, the Department of Work and Pensions, and the Health and Safety Executive resulted in a collaborative strategy to improve the health of working-age people – 'Health, Work and Wellbeing – Caring for Our Future'.[9] Building on welfare reforms laid out in a white paper ('Choosing Health: Making Health Choices Easier', published in 2004), the strategy enables key stakeholders to work together to improve the health of the working-age population. The strategy resulted in the appointment of a National Director for Occupational Health – 'a czar role' similar to previous roles that have championed health improvement in specific health areas such as cancer or drug and alcohol issues. The core aims are to minimize the risks of employees becoming ill, and to improve their retention and rehabilitation if illness does occur.

A key challenge of this strategy is to improve working men's health. Working men, and particularly those in blue-collar, manual occupations, have relatively poorer access to healthcare services. Statistics from across Europe confirm generally higher mortality in men than in women for a range of common medical conditions, and reflect the fact that for many common medical issues men are more likely to ignore symptoms and present for medical care and advice later in the illness. Shift work, over-time, peer pressure, and attitudes to health behaviors are common reasons why men of working age access healthcare less frequently than women of a similar age.

Many sectors of the male working population also are less accessible to health-related messages carried in the electronic media or via magazines or other written health promotion material, and research in male working populations indicates that different styles of communication are required to promote health awareness for men from those used for women. Collaborative work done in the UK by the Men's Health Forum, a charity specializing in promoting health messages to men, has confirmed the need to develop health promotion materials in different formats and styles to encourage receptiveness from working men. A good example of this is the development of high-quality, well-researched health promotion manuals,[10] published in an identical style to popular workshop car maintenance manuals. Publishing materials in this way also enables distribution through channels more likely to be used by men (e.g. in car accessory and spares outlets). Subtle use of humor, pictorial material, and simple techniques such as attaching health messages to gadgets likely to be used by men can also improve uptake and awareness (e.g. delivering information in packaging with a pedometer).

Whereas women often attend primary care, either in a role as carers or for issues such as contraception, and may pick up health awareness materials from waiting rooms or from discussion with friends, this behavior is less common for men. Pilot studies among working men in the Midlands of England highlighted that delivering health messages and advice in local pubs was more likely to promote male understanding and stimulate acceptance than more traditional health-promotion campaigns delivered via general practice or secondary care.

Assessing fitness to work

Modern business practices highlight the importance of employee commitment and engagement to achieve high service and productivity standards. Programs to improve working conditions (which reduce risk of injury or disease caused by workplace hazards) are strong drivers of employee morale, as are programs aimed at promoting employee care. Large employers are adopting health promotion and other health-related proactive care programs

(e.g. provision of health screening via the workplace, employee assistance programs, or provision of healthcare insurance arrangements) as differentiators in a competitive employment market, believing that the provision of positive health-supporting measures enables the attraction and retention of better-quality workforces, as well as productivity benefits associated with reduced wastage from absence or ill-health retirement.

Ill health may reduce functional capacity to the extent that work cannot be undertaken. Even for very sedentary employment, issues such as coping with the journey to work or the nature of symptomatology may result in work becoming difficult or impossible to sustain. Often it is the primary carer who is involved in providing advice on fitness to work or who is required to certify patients as unfit to work for the purposes of eligibility for sick pay benefits. The primary carer is, however, not always well placed to make objective decisions in this difficult area – there may be limited time within an already full list of clinical appointments, limited access to information about the work requirements (and limited potential to modify or change them), limitations from the patient's perspective (often with misconceptions about the balance between positive benefits of remaining in work versus potential hazards of doing so), and limited access to occupational health support: these are all factors that may have an impact on the advice given.

For many medical conditions, remaining in work, or at least keeping the period of time required for diagnosis and intervention as short as possible, optimizes opportunities to maintain functional capacity and maintain employment. As a 'rule of thumb' the longer a person is away from the workplace, the lower the prospect of a successful and sustained return to work (with less than 50% achieving a return to work if sickness prevents work for more than 6 months). This was exemplified in data collated by the Clinical Standards Advisory Group on Back Pain,[11] as long ago as 1994, and it is true of other medical issues. Withdrawal from the workplace quickly results in loss of social stimuli, and working practices change and, as time goes by, it becomes harder and harder to overcome complex psychosocial barriers that make return to work increasingly difficult to achieve.

Inability to work is not a simple relationship between the work available and the medical condition – two people with similar work and similar pathology may differ enormously in their functional capacity, with biopsychosocial factors being used as the nomenclature to summarize the need to consider broadly the multiple drivers that influence attendance at work. Motivation and commitment, which are strongly related to job satisfaction, are prime influencers on individual desire to remain in work or not. Simple measures such as maintaining contact between worker and manager and flexibility in offering modified work arrangements are effective in enabling an early return to work following injury or illness. As referred to earlier in the chapter, men have generally less access to quality health information than women of similar social class or age. This can result in misconceptions about health and work, particularly for those in manual occupations. Clear and authoritative advice is helpful in encouraging return to work as part of a well-structured recovery program.

Large companies may provide such via in-house or out-sourced occupational health provision. Employers in the UK without such access can be assisted by the Employment Medical Advisory Service (available from the Health and Safety Executive), and increasingly advice may be available from National Health Services resources, within Hospital Trusts or Primary Care Trusts. Successful pilots have also been run to improve primary care access to advice on fitness for work, such as the work by Dr Cohen in Cardiff to provide general practitioners with interactive computer-based tools to provide training and assisted decision-making on return-to-work issues.

In assessing fitness for work, it is important to avoid generalizations and to consider each individual circumstance. Assuming an understanding of the work based on the job title is a common mistake – a postman, for example, may undertake very many different roles other than the traditional walking mail delivery, with very different physical and mental demands. Clear description of the work demands and potential alternatives can be crucial in advising on return to work. Understanding of likely barriers to return to work also requires an assessment of the contributory factors, such as social support,

travel requirements (e.g. cost and physical effort required to get to work in the first place) as well as other issues, such as the availability of retraining and individual motivation to return to work. Successful rehabilitation to work following chronic illness or significant injury requires a positive 'can-do' attitude, with willingness from all parties (patient, carer, and employer) to re-try when setbacks occur.

For most men the consequences of worklessness are much greater than the positive benefits gained from work, and successful medical management of clinical issues should encourage return to work or re-employment wherever feasible.

References

1. Madouros V. Labour Force Projections 2006 to 2020. Office of National Statistics, 2006 [Available at: http//www.statistics.gov.uk/CCI/article.asp?ID=1346].
2. Ramazzini B. Diseases of Workers. [Translated from Latin De Morbis articum by Bernardino Ramazzini 1713.] OH&S Press, 1993.
3. Wadell G, Burton AK. Is Work Good For Your Health and Well-Being? London: The Stationery Office, 2006.
4. Shah H, Marks N. A Well-being Manifesto For a Flourishing Society. London: New Economic Foundation, 2004.
5. Aw TC, Gardiner K, Harrington JM. Pocket Consultant Occupational Health. Oxford: Blackwell 2007.
6. Chronic Disease Management: a Compendium of Information. London: Department of Health, 2004.
7. HSE statistics: Key Figures for 2006/07 [Available at: www.hse.gov.uk/statistics].
8. Department of the Environment, Transport & The Regions Revitalising Health and Safety Strategy Statement, June 2000.
9. Health, Work and Wellbeing: Caring for our Future. London: Department for Work and Pensions, Department of Health, and the Health and Safety Executive, 2006.
10. Banks I. HGV man: reducing all large sizes; shapes and colours. Somerest, UK: Haynes and Co Ltd, 2005.
11. Report of a CSAG Committee on Back Pain. London, HMSO, 1994.

INDEX

Note: Page numbers in *italics* indicate figures and tables.